FITZPATRICK'S
COLOR ATLAS AND SYNOPSIS OF
CLINICAL DERMATOLOGY

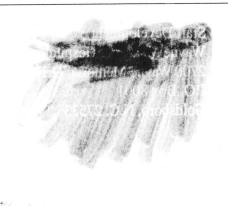

FITZPATRICK'S
COLOR ATLAS AND SYNOPSIS OF
CLINICAL DERMATOLOGY

EIGHTH EDITION

Klaus Wolff, MD, FRCP
Professor and Chairman Emeritus
Department of Dermatology
Medical University of Vienna
Chief Emeritus, Dermatology Service
General Hospital of Vienna
Vienna, Austria

Richard Allen Johnson, MDCM
Associate Professor of Dermatology
Massachusetts General Hospital
Harvard Medical School
Boston, Massachusetts

Arturo P. Saavedra, MD, PhD, MBA
Associate Professor of Dermatology
Massachusetts General Hospital
Vice Chair for Clinical Affairs
Harvard Medical School
Boston, Massachusetts

Ellen K. Roh, MD
Instructor in Dermatology
Massachusetts General Hospital
Boston, Massachusetts

Mc
Graw
Hill
Education

New York   Chicago   San Francisco   Athens   London   Madrid
Mexico City   Milan   New Delhi   Singapore   Sydney   Toronto

Fitzpatrick's Color Atlas and Synopsis of Clinical Dermatology, Eighth Edition

Copyright © 2017 by McGraw-Hill Education. All rights reserved. Printed in the United States of America. Except as permitted under the United States Copyright Act of 1976, no part of this publication may be reproduced or distributed in any form or by any means, or stored in a data base or retrieval system, without the prior written permission of the publisher.

Previous editions copyright © 2013, 2009, 2005, 2001, 1997, 1993, 1983 by The McGraw-Hill Companies, Inc.

1 2 3 4 5 6 7 8 9   LCR   22 21 20 19 18 17

ISBN 978-1-259-64219-7
MHID 1-259-64219-4

This book was set in Minion Pro by Aptara, Inc.
The editors were Karen G. Edmonson, Robert Pancotti, and Cindy Yoo.
The production supervisor was Richard Ruzycka.
Project management was provided by Indu Jawwad, Aptara, Inc.
The text designer was Alan Barnett; the cover designer was RANDOMATRIX.
LSC Communications was the printer and binder.

This book is printed on acid-free paper.

Library of Congress Cataloging-in-Publication Data

Names: Wolff, Klaus, 1935- author. | Johnson, Richard Allen, 1940- author. |
    Saavedra, Arturo P., author. | Roh, Ellen, author.
Title: Fitzpatrick's color atlas and synopsis of clinical dermatology / Klaus
    Wolff, Richard A. Johnson, Arturo P. Saavedra, Ellen Roh.
Other titles: Color atlas and synopsis of clinical dermatology
Description: Eighth edition. | New York: McGraw-Hill Education, [2017] |
    Includes index.
Identifiers: LCCN 2016030888 | ISBN 9781259642197 (pbk. : alk. paper) | ISBN
    1259642194 (pbk. : alk. paper)
Subjects: | MESH: Skin Diseases | Atlases
Classification: LCC RL81 | NLM WR 17 | DDC 616.5—dc23 LC record available at
    https://lccn.loc.gov/2016030888

International Edition ISBN 978-1-259-25122-1; MHID 1-259-25122-5.
Copyright © 2017. Exclusive rights by McGraw-Hill Education for manufacture and export. This book cannot be re-exported from the country to which it is consigned by McGraw-Hill Education. The International Edition is not available in North America.

McGraw-Hill Education books are available at special quantity discounts to use as premiums and sales promotions or for use in corporate training programs. To contact a representative, please visit the Contact Us pages at www.mhprofessional.com.

This eighth edition of
Fitzpatrick's Color Atlas and Synopsis of Clinical Dermatology
is dedicated to dermatology residents worldwide.

CONTENTS

SECTION 12

MELANOMA PRECURSORS AND PRIMARY CUTANEOUS MELANOMA   248

SECTION 13

PIGMENTARY DISORDERS   280

PART II   DERMATOLOGY AND INTERNAL MEDICINE   297

SECTION 14

THE SKIN IN IMMUNE, AUTOIMMUNE, AUTOINFLAMMATORY, AND RHEUMATIC DISORDERS   298

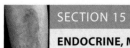

SECTION 15

ENDOCRINE, METABOLIC, AND NUTRITIONAL DISEASES   374

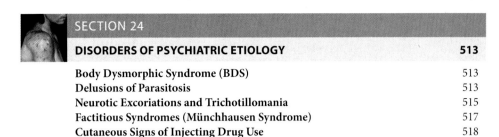

SECTION 24

DISORDERS OF PSYCHIATRIC ETIOLOGY 513

PART III   DISEASES CAUSED BY MICROBIAL AGENTS 521

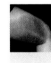

SECTION 25

BACTERIAL COLONIZATIONS AND INFECTIONS OF SKIN
AND SOFT TISSUES 522

SECTION 28

ARTHROPOD BITES, STINGS, AND CUTANEOUS INFESTATIONS   720

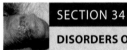

SECTION 34

DISORDERS OF THE GENITALIA, PERINEUM, AND ANUS   860

PREFACE

"Time is change; we measure its passage by how much things alter."
Nadine Gordimer

Thirty-four years ago in 1983, the first edition of this book appeared and has been expanded pari passu with the major developments that have occurred in dermatology over the past three and a half decades. Dermatology is now one of the most sought-after medical specialties because the burden of skin disease has become enormous and the many new innovative therapies available today attract large patient populations.

The *Color Atlas and Synopsis of Clinical Dermatology* has been used by thousands of primary care physicians, dermatology residents, dermatologists, internists, and other health care providers principally because it facilitates dermatologic diagnosis by providing color photographs of skin lesions and, juxtaposed, a succinct summary outline of skin disorders as well as the skin signs of systemic diseases.

The eighth edition has been extensively revised, rewritten, and expanded by new material. Around 30% of the old images have been replaced by new ones and additional images have been added. There is a complete update of etiology, pathogenesis, management, and therapy. There is also an online version. For this edition, videos containing clinical material relevant to the text are available at: mhprofessional.com/mediacenter.

ACKNOWLEDGMENT

Our secretary, Renate Kosma, worked hard to meet the demands of the authors. In the present McGraw-Hill team, we appreciated the counsel of Karen Edmonson, Senior Sponsoring Editor, and Robert Pancotti, Senior Project Development Editor.

Karen was the major force behind this edition. Her good nature, good judgment, loyalty to the authors, and, most of all, patience guided us to make an even better book.

HOW TO USE THIS BOOK

The *Color Atlas and Synopsis of Clinical Dermatology* is proposed as a "field guide" to the recognition of skin disorders and their management. The skin is a treasury of important lesions that can usually be recognized clinically. Gross morphology in the form of skin lesions remains the hard core of dermatologic diagnosis. Therefore, this text is accompanied by more than 900 color photographs illustrating skin diseases, skin manifestation of internal diseases, infections, tumors, and incidental skin findings in otherwise well individuals. We have endeavored to include information relevant to gender dermatology and a large number of images showing skin disease in different ethnic populations. This *Atlas* covers the entire field of clinical dermatology but does not include very rare syndromes or conditions. With respect to these, the reader is referred to another McGraw-Hill Publication: *Fitzpatrick's Dermatology in General Medicine*, 8th edition, 2012, edited by Lowell A. Goldsmith, Stephen I. Katz, Barbara A. Gilchrest, Amy S. Paller, David J. Leffell, and Klaus Wolff.

This text is intended for all physicians and other health care providers, including medical students, dermatology residents, internists, oncologists, and infectious disease specialists dealing with diseases with skin manifestations. For nondermatologists, it is advisable to start with "Approach to Dermatologic Diagnosis" and "Outline of Dermatologic Diagnosis" to familiarize themselves with the principles of dermatologic nomenclature and lines of thought.

The *Atlas* is organized into four parts, subdivided into 35 sections, and there are three short appendices. Each section has a color label that is reflected by the bar on the top of each page. This is to help the reader find his or her bearings rapidly when leafing through the book. Each disease is labeled with the respective ICD10 codes.

APPROACH TO DERMATOLOGIC DIAGNOSIS

There are two distinct clinical situations regarding the nature of skin changes:

I. The skin changes are *incidental* findings in *well* and *ill* individuals noted during the routine general physical examination:
   - "Bumps and blemishes": many asymptomatic lesions that are medically inconsequential may be present in well and ill persons, and may not be the reason for their visit to the physician; every general physician should be able to recognize these lesions to differentiate them from asymptomatic but important, e.g., malignant, lesions.
   - *Important skin lesions not* noted by the patient but that must not be overlooked by the physician: e.g., dysplastic nevi, melanoma, basal cell carcinoma, squamous cell carcinoma, café-au-lait macules in von Recklinghausen disease, and xanthomas.

II. The skin changes are the *chief complaint* of the patient:
   - "Minor" problems: e.g., localized itchy rash, "rash," rash in groin, nodules such as common moles and seborrheic keratoses.
   - "4-S": serious skin signs in sick patients.

SERIOUS SKIN SIGNS IN SICK PATIENTS

- **Generalized red rash with fever:**
  - Viral exanthems.
  - Rickettsial exanthems.
  - Drug eruptions.
  - Bacterial infections with toxin production.

- **Generalized red rash with blisters and prominent mouth lesions:**
  - Erythema multiforme (major).
  - Toxic epidermal necrolysis.
  - Pemphigus.

- Bullous pemphigoid.
- Drug eruptions.

- **Generalized red rash with pustules:**
  - Pustular psoriasis (von Zumbusch).
  - Drug eruptions.

- **Generalized rash with vesicles:**
  - Disseminated herpes simplex.
  - Generalized herpes zoster.
  - Varicella.
  - Drug eruptions.

- **Generalized red rash with scaling over whole body:**
  - Exfoliative erythroderma.

- **Generalized wheals and soft-tissue swelling:**
  - Urticaria and angioedema.

- **Generalized purpura:**
  - Thrombocytopenia.
  - Purpura fulminans.
  - Drug eruptions.

- **Generalized purpura that can be palpated:**
  - Vasculitis.
  - Bacterial endocarditis.

- **Multiple skin infarcts:**
  - Meningococcemia.
  - Gonococcemia.
  - Disseminated intravascular coagulopathy.

- **Localized skin infarcts:**
  - Calciphylaxis.
  - Atherosclerosis obliterans.
  - Atheroembolization.
  - Warfarin necrosis.
  - Antiphospholipid antibody syndrome.

- **Facial inflammatory edema with fever:**
  - Erysipelas.
  - Lupus erythematosus.
  - Dermatomyositis.

OUTLINE OF DERMATOLOGIC DIAGNOSIS

In contrast to other fields of clinical medicine, patients should be examined before a detailed history is taken because patients can see their lesions and thus often present with a history that is flawed with their own interpretation of the origin or causes of the skin eruption. Also, diagnostic accuracy is higher when objective examination is approached without preconceived ideas. However, a history should always be obtained but if taken during or after the visual and physical examination, it can be streamlined and more focused following the objective findings. Thus, recognizing, analyzing, and properly interpreting skin lesions are the sine qua non of dermatologic diagnosis.

PHYSICAL EXAMINATION

Appearance   Uncomfortable, "toxic," well.
Vital Signs   Pulse, respiration, temperature.
Skin: "Learning to Read"   The entire skin should be inspected and this should include mucous membranes, genital and anal regions, as well as hair and nails and peripheral lymph nodes. Reading the skin is like reading a text. The basic skin lesions are like the letters of the alphabet: their shape, color, margination, and other features combined will lead to words, and their localization and distribution to a sentence or paragraph. The prerequisite of dermatologic diagnosis is thus the recognition of (1) the type of skin lesion, (2) the color, (3) margination, (4) consistency, (5) shape, (6) arrangement, and (7) distribution of lesions.

Recognizing Letters: Types of Skin Lesions

- **Macule** (Latin: *macula*, "spot") A macule is a circumscribed area of change in skin color without elevation or depression. It is thus not palpable. Macules can be well defined and ill defined. Macules may be of any size or color (Fig. I-1). White, as in vitiligo; brown, as in café-au-lait spots; blue, as in Mongolian spots; or red, as in permanent vascular abnormalities such as port-wine stains or capillary dilatation due to inflammation (erythema). Pressure of a glass slide (*diascopy*) on the border of a red lesion detects the extravasation of red blood cells. If the redness remains under pressure from the slide, the lesion is purpuric, that is, results from extravasated red blood cells; if the redness disappears, the lesion is due to vascular dilatation. A rash consisting of macules is called a *macular exanthem*.

- **Papule** (Latin: *papula*, "pimple") A papule is a superficial, elevated, solid lesion, generally considered <0.5 cm in diameter. Most of it is elevated above, rather than deep within, the plane of the surrounding skin (Fig. I-2). A papule is palpable. It may be well defined or ill defined. In papules, the elevation is caused by metabolic or locally produced deposits, by localized cellular infiltrates, inflammatory or

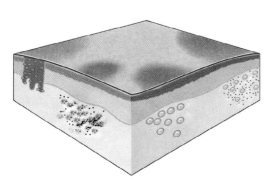
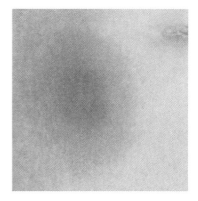

FIGURE I-1   Macule

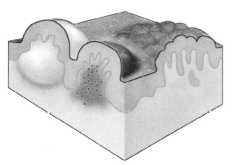
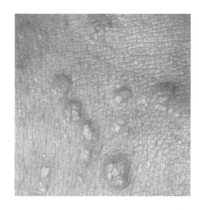

FIGURE I-2   Papule

noninflammatory, or by hyperplasia of local cellular elements. Superficial papules are sharply defined. Deeper dermal papules have indistinct borders. Papules may be dome-shaped, cone-shaped, or flat-topped (as in lichen planus) or consist of multiple, small, closely packed, projected elevations that are known as a *vegetation* (Fig. I-2). A rash consisting of papules is called a papular *exanthem*. Papular exanthems may be grouped ("lichenoid") or disseminated (dispersed). Confluence of papules leads to the development of larger, usually flat-topped, circumscribed, plateau-like elevations known as plaques (French: *plaque*, "plate"). See the following.

- **Plaque** A plaque is a plateau-like elevation above the skin surface that occupies a relatively large surface area in comparison with its height above the skin (Fig. I-3). It is usually well defined. Frequently, it is formed by a confluence of papules, as in psoriasis. *Lichenification* is a less well-defined large plaque where the skin appears thickened and the skin

markings are accentuated. Lichenification occurs in atopic dermatitis, eczematous dermatitis, psoriasis, lichen simplex chronicus, and mycosis fungoides. A *patch* is a barely elevated plaque—a lesion fitting between a macule and a plaque—as in parapsoriasis or Kaposi sarcoma.

- **Nodule** (Latin: *nodulus*, "small knot") A nodule is a palpable, solid, round, or ellipsoidal lesion that is larger than a papule (Fig. I-4) and may involve the epidermis, dermis, or subcutaneous tissue. The depth of involvement and the size differentiate a nodule from a papule. Nodules result from inflammatory infiltrates, neoplasms, or metabolic deposits in the dermis or subcutaneous tissue. Nodules may be well defined (superficial) or ill defined (deep); if localized in the subcutaneous tissue, they can often be better felt than seen. Nodules can be hard or soft upon palpation. They may be dome-shaped and smooth or may have a warty surface or crater-like central depression.

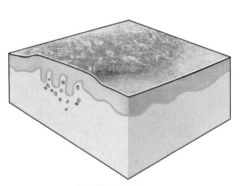

FIGURE I-3 Plaque

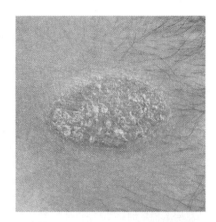

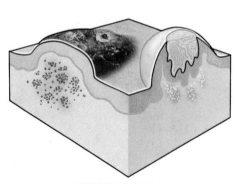

FIGURE I-4 Nodule

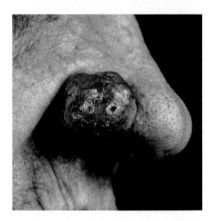

- **Wheal** A wheal is a rounded or flat-topped, pale red or white papule or plaque that is characteristically evanescent, disappearing within 24 to 48 h (Fig. I-5). It is due to edema in the papillary body of the dermis. If the edema is very pronounced, it will compress the dilated capillaries and the wheal will turn white (Fig. I-5). Wheals may be round, gyrate, or irregular with pseudopods—changing rapidly in size and shape due to shifting papillary edema. A rash consisting of wheals is called a *urticarial exanthema* or *urticaria*.

- **Vesicle-Bulla** (*Blister*) (Latin: *vesicula*, "little bladder"; *bulla*, "bubble") A vesicle (<0.5 cm) or a bulla (>0.5 cm) is a circumscribed, elevated, superficial cavity containing fluid (Fig. I-6). Vesicles are dome-shaped (as in contact dermatitis, dermatitis herpetiformis), umbilicated (as in herpes simplex), or flaccid (as in pemphigus). Often the roof of a vesicle/bulla is so thin that it is transparent, and the serum or blood in the cavity can be seen. Vesicles containing serum are yellowish; those containing blood from red to black. Vesicles and bullae arise from a cleavage at various levels of the superficial skin; the cleavage may be subcorneal or within the epidermis (i.e., intraepidermal vesication) or at the epidermal–dermal interface (i.e., subepidermal), as in Figure I-6. Since vesicles/bullae are always superficial they are always well defined. A rash consisting of vesicles is called a *vesicular exanthem*; a rash consisting of bullae a *bullous exanthem*.

- **Pustule** (Latin: *pustula*, "pustule") A pustule is a circumscribed superficial cavity of the skin that contains a purulent exudate (Fig. I-7), which may be white, yellow, greenish-yellow, or hemorrhagic. Pustules thus differ from vesicles in that they are not clear but have a turbid content. This process may arise in a hair follicle or independently. Pustules may vary in size and shape. Pustules are usually dome-shaped, but follicular pustules are conical and usually contain a hair in the center. The vesicular lesions of herpes simplex and varicella zoster virus infections may

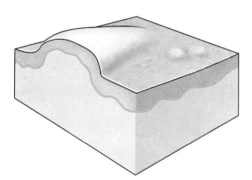

FIGURE I-5 **Wheal**

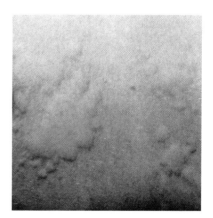

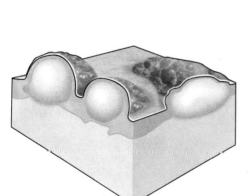

FIGURE I-6 **Vesicle**

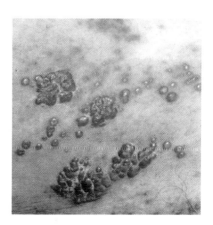

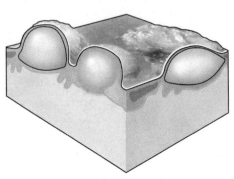

FIGURE I-7 Pustule

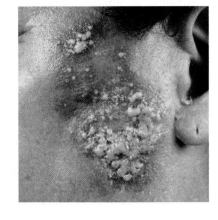

become pustular. A rash consisting of pustules is called a *pustular exanthem.*

- **Crusts** (Latin: *crusta*, "rind, bark, shell") Crusts develop when serum, blood, or purulent exudate dries on the skin surface (Fig. I-8). Crusts may be thin, delicate, and friable or thick and adherent. Crusts are yellow when formed from dried serum; green or yellow-green when formed from purulent exudate; or brown, dark red, or black when formed from blood. Superficial crusts occur as honey-colored, delicate, glistening particulates on the surface and are typically found in impetigo (Fig. I-8). When the exudate involves the entire epidermis, the crusts may be thick and adherent, and if it is accompanied by necrosis of the deeper tissues (e.g., the dermis), the condition is known as *ecthyma.*

- **Scales (squames)** (Latin: *squama*, "scale") Scales are flakes of stratum corneum (Fig. I-9). They may be large (like membranes, tiny [like dust], pityriasiform (Greek: *pityron*, "bran"),

adherent, or loose. A rash consisting of papules with scales is called a *papulosquamous exanthem.*

- **Erosion** An erosion is a defect only of the epidermis, not involving the dermis (Fig. I-10); in contrast to an ulcer, which always heals with scar formation (see the following), an erosion heals without a scar. An erosion is sharply defined, red, and oozes. There are superficial erosions, which are subcorneal or run through the epidermis, and deep erosions, the base of which is the papillary body (Fig. I-10). Except physical abrasions, erosions are always the result of intraepidermal or subepidermal cleavage and thus of vesicles or bullae.

- **Ulcer** (Latin: *ulcus*, "sore") An ulcer is a skin defect that extends into the dermis or deeper (Fig. I-11) into the subcutis and always occurs within pathologically altered tissue. An ulcer is therefore always a secondary phenomenon. The pathologically altered tissue that gives rise

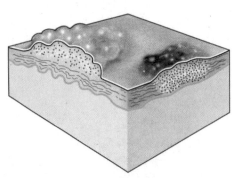

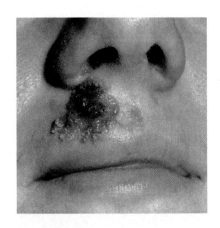

FIGURE I-8 Crust

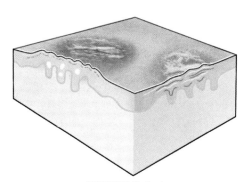

FIGURE I-9 Scale

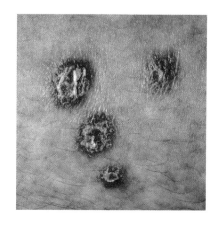

to an ulcer is usually seen at the border or the base of the ulcer and is helpful in determining its cause. Other features helpful in this respect are whether borders are elevated, undermined, hard, or soggy; location of the ulcer; discharge; and any associated topographic features, such as nodules, excoriations, varicosities, hair distribution, presence or absence of sweating, and arterial pulses. Ulcers always heal with scar formation.

• **Scar** A scar is the fibrous tissue replacement of the tissue defect by previous ulcer or a wound. Scars can be hypertrophic and

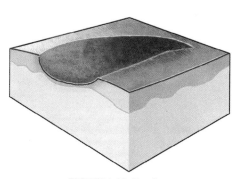

FIGURE I-10 Erosion

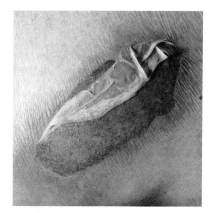

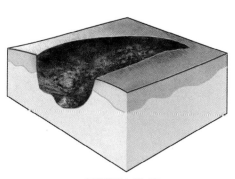

FIGURE I-11 Ulcer

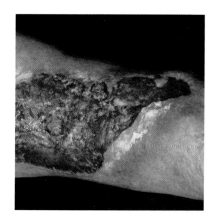

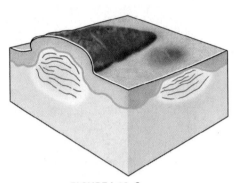

FIGURE I-12 Scar

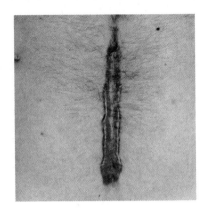

hard (Fig. I-12) or atrophic and soft with a thinning or loss of all tissue compartments of the skin (Fig. I-12).

- **Atrophy** This refers to a diminution of some or all layers of the skin (Fig. I-13). Epidermal atrophy is manifested by a thinning of the epidermis, which becomes transparent, revealing the papillary and subpapillary vessels; there

are loss of skin texture and cigarette paper-like wrinkling. In dermal atrophy, there is loss of connective tissue of the dermis and depression of the lesion (Fig. I-13).

- **Cyst** A cyst is a cavity containing liquid or solid or semisolid (Fig. I-14) materials and may be superficial or deep. Visually it appears like a spherical, most often dome-shaped papule or

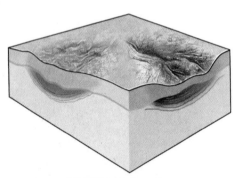

FIGURE I-13 Atrophy

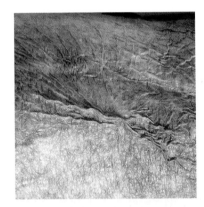

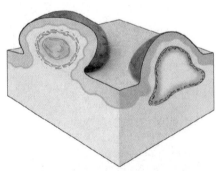

FIGURE I-14 Cyst

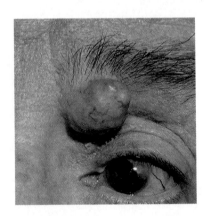

nodule, but upon palpation it is resilient. It is lined by an epithelium and often has a fibrous capsule; depending on its contents it may be skin colored, yellow, red, or blue. An epidermal cyst producing keratinaceous material and a pilar cyst that is lined by a multilayered epithelium are shown in Figure I-14.

Shaping Letters into Words: Further Characterization of Identified Lesions

- **Color** Pink, red, purple (purpuric lesions do not blanch with pressure with a glass slide [diascopy]), white, tan, brown, black, blue, gray, and yellow. The color can be uniform or variegated.

- **Margination** Well (can be traced with the tip of a pencil) and ill defined.

- **Shape** Round, oval, polygonal, polycyclic, annular (ring-shaped), iris, serpiginous (snakelike), umbilicated.

- **Palpation** Consider (1) *consistency* (soft, firm, hard, fluctuant, boardlike), (2) *deviation in temperature* (hot, cold), and (3) *mobility*. Note presence of *tenderness*, and estimate the *depth* of the lesion (i.e., dermal or subcutaneous).

Forming Sentences and Understanding the Text: Evaluation of Arrangement, Patterns, and Distribution

- **Number** Single or multiple lesions.

- **Arrangement** Multiple lesions may be (1) *grouped*: herpetiform, arciform, annular, reticulated (net-shaped), linear, serpiginous (snakelike) or (2) *disseminated*: scattered discrete lesions.

- **Confluence** Yes or no.

- **Distribution** Consider (1) *extent*: isolated (single lesions), localized, regional, generalized, universal, and (2) *pattern*: symmetric, exposed areas, sites of pressure, intertriginous area, follicular localization, random, following dermatomes or Blaschko lines.

Table I-1 provides an algorithm showing how to proceed.

HISTORY

Demographics   Age, race, sex, and occupation.

History

1. **Constitutional symptoms:**
   - "Acute illness" syndrome: headaches, chills, feverishness, and weakness.
   - "Chronic illness" syndrome: fatigue, weakness, anorexia, weight loss, and malaise.
2. **History of skin lesions. Seven key questions:**
   - When ¿ Onset
   - Where¿ Site of onset
   - Does it itch or hurt¿ Symptoms
   - How has it spread (pattern of spread)¿ Evolution
   - How have individual lesions changed¿ Evolution
   - Provocative factors¿ Heat, cold, sun, exercise, travel history, drug ingestion, pregnancy, season
   - Previous treatment(s)¿ Topical and systemic
3. **General history of present illness as indicated by clinical situation, with particular attention to constitutional and prodromal symptoms.**
4. **Past medical history:**
   - Operations
   - Illnesses (hospitalized¿)
   - Allergies, especially drug allergies
   - Medications (present and past)
   - Habits (smoking, alcohol intake, drug abuse)
   - Atopic history (asthma, hay fever, eczema)
5. **Family medical history (particularly of psoriasis, atopy, melanoma, xanthomas, tuberous sclerosis).**
6. **Social history, with particular reference to occupation, hobbies, exposures, travel, or injecting drug use.**
7. **Sexual history: history of risk factors of HIV: blood transfusions, IV drugs, sexually active, multiple partners, sexually transmitted disease?**

REVIEW OF SYMPTOMS

This should be done as indicated by the clinical situation, with particular attention to possible connections between signs and disease of other organ systems (e.g., rheumatic complaints, myalgias, arthralgias, Raynaud phenomenon, and sicca symptoms).

TABLE I-1 Algorithm for Evaluating Skin Lesions

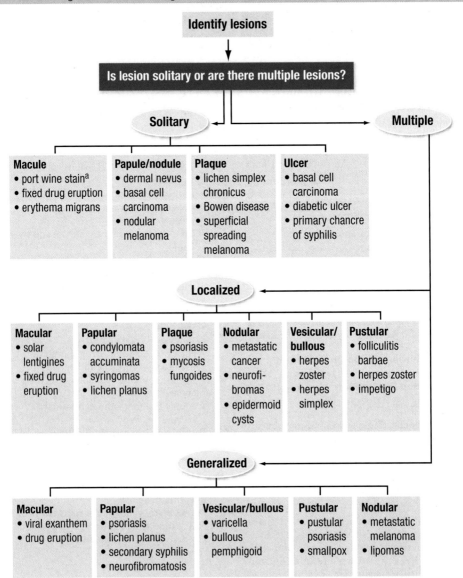

^aBulleted conditions are some examples.

SPECIAL CLINICAL AND LABORATORY AIDS TO DERMATOLOGIC DIAGNOSIS

SPECIAL TECHNIQUES USED IN CLINICAL EXAMINATION

Magnification with hand lens. To examine lesions for fine morphologic detail, it is necessary to use a magnifying glass (hand lens) ($7\times$) or a binocular microscope ($5\times$ to $40\times$). Magnification is especially helpful in the diagnosis of lupus erythematosus (follicular plugging), lichen planus (Wickham striae), basal cell carcinomas (translucence and telangiectasia), and melanoma (subtle changes in color, especially gray or blue); this is best visualized after application of a drop of mineral oil. Use of the dermatoscope is discussed below (see "Dermoscopy").

Oblique lighting of the skin lesion, done in a darkened room, is often required to detect slight degrees of elevation or depression, and it is useful in the visualization of the surface configuration of lesions and in estimating the extent of the eruption.

Subdued lighting in the examining room enhances the contrast between circumscribed hypopigmented or hyperpigmented lesions and normal skin.

Wood lamp (ultraviolet long-wave light, "black" light) is valuable in the diagnosis of certain skin and hair diseases and of porphyria. With the Wood lamp (365 nm), fluorescent pigments and subtle color differences of melanin pigmentation can be visualized. The Wood lamp also helps to estimate variation in the lightness of lesions in relation to the normal skin color in both dark-skinned and fair-skinned persons; e.g., the lesions seen in tuberous sclerosis and tinea versicolor are hypomelanotic and are not as white as the lesions seen in vitiligo, which are amelanotic. Circumscribed hypermelanosis, such as a freckle and melasma, is much more evident (darker) under the Wood lamp. By contrast, dermal melanin, as in a Mongolian sacral spot, does not become accentuated under the Wood lamp. Therefore, it is possible to localize the site of melanin by use of the Wood lamp. *However, this is more difficult or not possible in patients with brown or black skin.*

Wood lamp is particularly useful in the detection of the fluorescence of dermatophytosis in the hair shaft (green to yellow) and of erythrasma (coral red). A presumptive diagnosis of porphyria can be made if a pinkish-red fluorescence is demonstrated in urine examined with the Wood lamp; addition of dilute hydrochloric acid intensifies the fluorescence.

Diascopy consists of firmly pressing a microscopic slide or a glass spatula over a skin lesion. The examiner will find this procedure of special value in determining whether the red color of a macule or papule is due to capillary dilatation (erythema) or to extravasation of blood (purpura) that does not blanch. Diascopy is also useful for the detection of the glassy yellow-brown appearance of papules in sarcoidosis, tuberculosis of the skin, lymphoma, and granuloma annulare.

Dermoscopy (previously called *epiluminescence microscopy*). A hand lens with built-in lighting and a magnification of $10\times$ to $30\times$ is called a *dermatoscope* and permits the noninvasive inspection of deeper layers of the epidermis and beyond. This is particularly useful in the distinction of benign and malignant growth patterns in pigmented lesions. *Digital dermoscopy* is particularly useful in the monitoring of pigmented skin lesions because images are stored electronically and can be retrieved and examined at a later date to permit comparison quantitatively and qualitatively and to detect changes over time. Digital dermoscopy uses computer image analysis programs that provide (1) objective measurements of changes; (2) rapid storage, retrieval, and transmission of images to experts for further discussion (teledermatology); and (3) extraction of morphologic features for numerical analysis. Dermoscopy and digital dermoscopy require special training.

CLINICAL SIGNS

Darier sign is "positive" when a brown macular or a slightly papular lesion of urticarial pigmentosa (mastocytosis) becomes a palpable wheal after being vigorously rubbed with an instrument such as the blunt end of a pen. The wheal may not appear for 5 to 10 min.

Auspitz sign is "positive" when slight scratching or curetting of a scaly lesion reveals punctate bleeding points within the lesion. This suggests psoriasis, but it is not specific.

The *Nikolsky phenomenon* is positive when the epidermis is dislodged from the dermis by lateral, shearing pressure with a finger, resulting in an erosion. It is an important diagnostic sign in acantholytic disorders such as pemphigus or the staphylococcal scalded skin (SSS) syndrome or other blistering or epidermonecrotic disorders, such as toxic epidermal necrolysis.

CLINICAL TESTS

Patch testing is used to document and validate a diagnosis of allergic contact sensitization and identify the causative agent. Substances to be tested are applied to the skin in shallow cups (Finn chambers), affixed with a tape and left in place for 24 to 48 h. Contact hypersensitivity will show as a papular vesicular reaction that develops within 48 to 72 h when the test is read. It is a unique means of in vivo reproduction of disease in diminutive proportions, for sensitization affects all the skin and may therefore be elicited at any cutaneous site. The patch test is easier and safer than a "use test" with a questionable allergen, that for test purposes is applied in low concentrations in small areas of skin for short periods of time (see Section 2).

Photopatch testing is a combination of patch testing and UV irradiation of the test site and is used to document photo allergy (see Section 10).

Prick testing is used to determine type I allergies. A drop of a solution containing a minute concentration of the allergen is placed on the skin and the skin is pierced through this drop with a needle. Piercing should not go beyond the papillary body. A positive reaction will appear as a wheal within 20 min. The patient has to be under observation for possible anaphylaxis.

Acetowhitening facilitates detection of subclinical penile or vulvar warts. Gauze saturated with 5% acetic acid (or white vinegar) is wrapped around the glans penis or used on the cervix and anus. After 5 to 10 min, the penis or vulva is inspected with a 10× hand lens. Warts appear as small white papules.

LABORATORY TESTS

Microscopic Examination of Scales, Crusts, Serum, and Hair

Gram stains of smears and *cultures of exudates and of tissue minces* should be made in lesions suspected of being bacterial or yeast (*Candida albicans*) infections. Ulcers and nodules require a scalpel biopsy in which a wedge of tissue consisting of all three layers of skin is obtained; the biopsy specimen is divided into one-half for histopathology and one-half for culture. This is minced in a sterile mortar and then cultured for bacteria (including typical and atypical mycobacteria) and fungi.

Microscopic examination for mycelia should be made of the roofs of vesicles or of scales (the advancing borders are preferable) or of the hair in dermatophytoses. The tissue is cleared with 10 to 30% KOH and warmed gently. Hyphae and spores will light up by their birefringence (Fig. 26-25). Fungal cultures with Sabouraud medium should be made (see Section 26).

Microscopic examination of cells obtained from the base of vesicles (Tzanck preparation) may reveal the presence of acantholytic cells in the acantholytic diseases (e.g., pemphigus or SSS syndrome) or of giant epithelial cells and multinucleated giant cells (containing 10 to 12 nuclei) in herpes simplex, herpes zoster, and varicella. Material from the base of a vesicle obtained by *gentle* curettage with a scalpel is smeared on a glass slide, stained with either Giemsa or Wright stain or methylene blue, and examined to determine whether there are acantholytic or giant epithelial cells, which are diagnostic (Fig. 27-32). In addition, culture, immunofluorescence tests, or polymerase chain reaction for herpes have to be ordered.

Laboratory diagnosis of scabies. The diagnosis is established by identification of the mite, or ova or feces, in skin scrapings removed from the papules or burrows (see Section 28). Using a sterile scalpel blade on which a drop of sterile mineral oil has been placed, apply oil to the surface of the burrow or papule. Scrape the papule or burrow vigorously to remove the entire top of the papule; tiny flecks of blood will appear in the oil. Transfer the oil to a microscopic slide and examine for mites, ova, and feces. The mites are 0.2 to 0.4 mm in size and have four pairs of legs (see Fig. 28-16).

Biopsy of the Skin

Biopsy of the skin is one of the simplest, most rewarding diagnostic techniques because of the easy accessibility of the skin and the variety of techniques for study of the excised specimen (e.g., histopathology, immunopathology, polymerase chain reaction, and electron microscopy).

Selection of the site of the biopsy is based primarily on the stage of the eruption, and early lesions are usually more typical; this is especially important in vesiculobullous eruptions (e.g., pemphigus and herpes simplex), in which the lesion should be no more than 24 h old. However, older lesions (2 to 6 weeks) are often more characteristic in discoid lupus erythematosus.

A common technique for diagnostic biopsy is the use of a 3- to 4-mm punch, a small tubular knife much like a corkscrew, which by rotating movements between the thumb and index finger cuts through the epidermis, dermis, and subcutaneous tissue; the base is cut off with scissors. If immunofluorescence is indicated (e.g., as in bullous diseases or lupus erythematosus), a special medium for transport to the laboratory is required.

For nodules, however, a large wedge should be removed by excision including subcutaneous tissue. Furthermore, when indicated, lesions should be bisected, one-half for histology and the other half sent in a sterile container for bacterial and fungal cultures or in special fixatives or cell culture media, or frozen for immunopathologic examination.

Specimens for light microscopy should be fixed immediately in buffered neutral formalin. A brief but detailed summary of the clinical history and description of the lesions should accompany the specimen. Biopsy is indicated in *all* skin lesions that are suspected of being neoplasms, in all bullous disorders with immunofluorescence used simultaneously, and in all dermatologic disorders in which a specific diagnosis is not possible by clinical examination alone.

PART I

Disorders Presenting in the Skin and Mucous Membranes

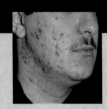

DISORDERS OF SEBACEOUS, ECCRINE AND APOCRINE GLANDS

ACNE VULGARIS (COMMON ACNE) AND CYSTIC ACNE ICD-10: L70.0

- An inflammation of pilosebaceous units, which is very common.
- Appears on the face, trunk, and rarely buttocks.
- Occurs most frequently in adolescents.
- Manifests as comedones, papulopustules, nodules, and cysts.
- Results in pitted, depressed, or hypertrophic scars.

EPIDEMIOLOGY

OCCURRENCE Very common, affecting approximately 85% of young people.

AGE OF ONSET Puberty; may appear for the first time around 25 years or older.

SEX More severe in males than in females.

RACE Lower incidence in Asians and Africans.

GENETIC ASPECTS Multifactorial genetic background and familial predisposition. Most individuals with cystic acne have a parent(s) with history of severe acne. Severe acne may be associated with XYY syndrome (rare).

PATHOGENESIS

Key factors are follicular keratinization, androgens, and *Propionibacterium acnes* (see Fig. 1-4).

Follicular plugging (comedone) prevents drainage of sebum; androgens (quantitatively and qualitatively normal in serum) stimulate sebaceous glands to produce more sebum. Bacterial (*p. acnes*) lipase converts lipids to fatty acids and produces proinflammatory mediators (IL-I, TNF-α), which lead to an inflammatory response. Distended follicle walls break; sebum, lipids, fatty acids, keratin, and bacteria enter the dermis, provoking an inflammatory and foreign-body response. Intense inflammation leads to scars.

CONTRIBUTORY FACTORS Acnegenic mineral oils, rarely dioxin, and others listed below.

Drugs. Lithium, hydantoin, isoniazid, glucocorticoids, oral contraceptives, iodides, bromides and androgens, and danazol.

Others. *Emotional stress* can cause exacerbations. *Occlusion* and *pressure* on the skin, such as leaning the face on the hands, is a *very important* and often unrecognized exacerbating factor (*acne mechanica*). Acne is not caused by any kind of food.

CLINICAL MANIFESTATION

DURATION OF LESIONS Weeks to months.

SEASON Often worse in fall and winter.

SYMPTOMS Pain in lesions (especially the nodulocystic type).

SKIN LESIONS *Comedones*—open (blackheads) or closed (whiteheads); *comedonal acne* (Fig. 1-1). *Papules* and *papulopustules*—i.e., a papule topped by a pustule; *papulopustular acne* (Fig. 1-2). *Nodules* or *cysts*—1 to 4 cm in diameter; *nodulocystic acne* (Fig. 1-3). Soft nodules result from repeated follicular ruptures and re-encapsulations with inflammation, abscess formation (cysts), and foreign-body reaction (Fig. 1-4). Round, isolated single nodules and cysts coalesce to linear mounds and sinus tracts (Figs. 1-3 and 1-5). *Sinuses*: draining epithelial-lined tracts, usually with nodular acne. *Scars*: atrophic depressed (often pitted) or hypertrophic (at times, keloidal). *Seborrhea* of the face and scalp are often present and sometimes severe.

Sites of Predilection. Face, neck, trunk, upper arms, and buttocks.

Special Forms

NEONATAL ACNE Occurs on the nose and cheeks in newborns or infants, and is related to glandular development; transient and self-healing.

ACNE EXCORIÉE Usually occurs in young women, and is associated with extensive excoriations and scarring resulting from emotional and psychological problems (obsessive compulsive disorder).

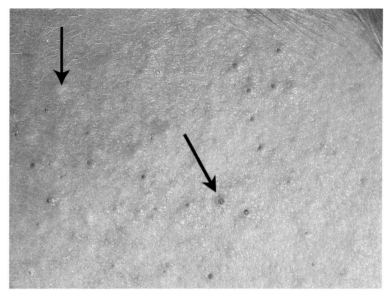

FIGURE 1-1 Acne vulgaris: comedones Comedones are keratin plugs that form within follicular ostia and are frequently associated with surrounding erythema and pustule formation. Comedones associated with small ostia are referred to as closed comedones or "white heads" (upper arrow); those associated with large ostia are referred to as open comedones or "black heads" (lower arrow). Comedones are best treated with topical retinoids.

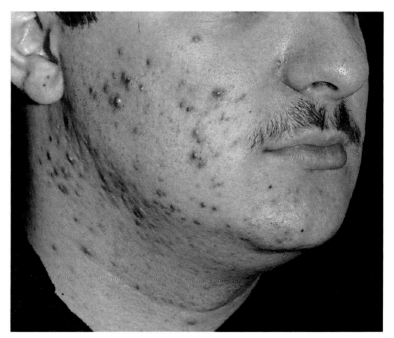

FIGURE 1-2 20-year-old male In this case of papulopustular acne, some inflammatory papules became nodular and thus represent early stages of nodulocystic acne.

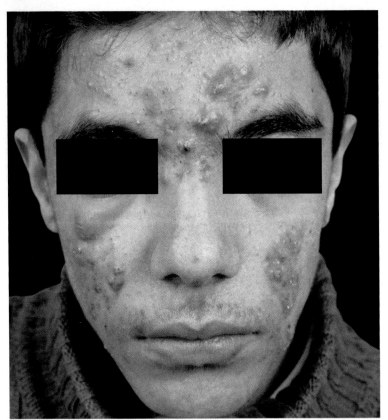

FIGURE 1-3 Nodulocystic acne A symmetric distribution in the face of a teenage boy. This image clearly shows that even nodulocystic acne starts with comedones—both open and closed comedones can be seen in his face—which then transform into papulopustular lesions that enlarge and coalesce, eventually leading to nodulocystic acne. It is not surprising that these lesions are very painful, and it is understandable that nodulocystic acne also severely impacts the social life of these adolescents.

ACNE MECHANICA Flares of acne occur on cheeks, chin, and forehead, because of leaning the face on the hands or forehead, and from the pressure of sports gear such as helmets.

ACNE CONGLOBATA Severe cystic acne (Figs. 1-5 and 1-6) occurs with more involvement of the trunk than the face, but also occurs on the buttocks. Coalescing nodules, cysts, abscesses, and ulceration. Spontaneous remission rare. Rarely seen in XYY genotype or polycystic ovary syndrome (PCOS).

ACNE FULMINANS Occurs primarily in teenage boys. *Acute onset*, severe cystic acne with suppuration and *ulceration*; malaise, fatigue, fever, generalized arthralgias, leukocytosis, and elevated ESR.

TROPICAL ACNE With severe folliculitis, inflammatory nodules, draining cysts on the trunk and buttocks, particularly in tropical climates; secondary infection with *Staphylococcus aureus*.

OCCUPATIONAL ACNE Caused by exposure to tar derivatives, cutting oils, chlorinated hydrocarbons (see "Chloracne" as follows). Not restricted to predilection sites, and can appear on other (covered) body sites, like arms, legs, or buttocks.

CHLORACNE Caused by exposure to chlorinated aromatic hydrocarbons in electrical conductors, insecticides, and herbicides. Sometimes very severe because of industrial accidents or intended poisoning (e.g., dioxin).

ACNE COSMETICA Caused by comedogenic cosmetics.

Pomade Acne. On the forehead, usually in Africans from applying pomade to hair.

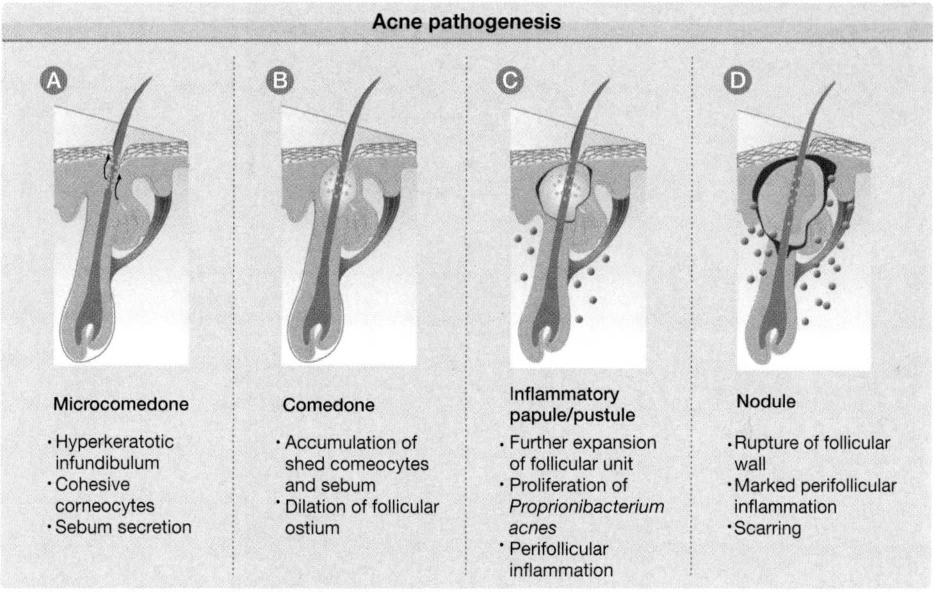

Acne pathogenesis

Microcomedone	Comedone	Inflammatory papule/pustule	Nodule
• Hyperkeratotic infundibulum • Cohesive corneocytes • Sebum secretion	• Accumulation of shed comeocytes and sebum • Dilation of follicular ostium	• Further expansion of follicular unit • Proliferation of *Proprionibacterium acnes* • Perifollicular inflammation	•Rupture of follicular wall •Marked perifollicular inflammation •Scarring

FIGURE 1-4 Acne pathogenesis (Reproduced with permission from Zaenglein AL, et al. Acne vulgaris and acneiform eruptions. In: Goldsmith LA, Katz SI, Gilchrest BA, et al, eds. *Fitzpatrick's Dermatology in General Medicine*. 8th ed. New York, NY: McGraw-Hill; 2012.)

SAPHO SYNDROME *S*ynovitis, *a*cne fulminans, *p*almoplantar pustulosis, *h*idradenitis suppurativa, *h*yperkeratosis, and *o*steitis; very rare.
PAPA SYNDROME Sterile *p*yogenic *a*rthritis, *p*yoderma gangrenosum *a*cne. An inherited autoinflammatory disorder; very rare.

Acne-Like Conditions Which Are Not Acne

STEROID ACNE No comedones. Following systemic or topical glucocorticoids. Monomorphous folliculitis—small erythematous papules and pustules on chest and back.
DRUG-INDUCED ACNE No comedones. Monomorphous acne-like eruption caused by phenytoin, lithium, isoniazid, high-dose vitamin B complex, epidermal growth factor inhibitors (see Section 23, ACDR-related to chemotherapy), and halogenated compounds.
ACNE AESTIVALIS No comedones. Papular eruption after sun exposure. Usually on forehead, shoulders, arms, neck, and chest.
GRAM-NEGATIVE FOLLICULITIS Multiple tiny yellow pustules on top of acne vulgaris in long-term antibiotic administration.

DIAGNOSIS AND DIFFERENTIAL DIAGNOSIS

Note: Comedones are required for diagnosis of any type of acne. Comedones are not a feature of acne-like conditions (see preceding), and

the following conditions: **Face**—*S. aureus* folliculitis, pseudofolliculitis barbae, rosacea, and perioral dermatitis. **Trunk**—*Malassezia* folliculitis, "hot-tub" pseudomonas folliculitis, *S. aureus* folliculitis, and acne-like conditions (see preceding).

LABORATORY EXAMINATION

No laboratory examinations required. In the overwhelming majority of acne patients, hormone levels are normal. If an endocrine disorder is suspected, determine free testosterone, follicle-stimulating hormone, luteinizing hormone, and DHEAS to exclude hyperandrogenism and PCOS. Recalcitrant acne can also be related to congenital adrenal hyperplasia (11β or 21β hydroxylase deficiency). If systemic isotretinoin treatment is planned, determine transaminase (ALT, AST), triglyceride, and cholesterol levels.

COURSE

Often clears spontaneously by the early twenties, but can persist to the fourth decade or older. Flares occur in the winter and with the onset of menses. The sequela of acne is scarring that may be avoided by treatment, *especially with oral isotretinoin early in the course of the disease* (see below).

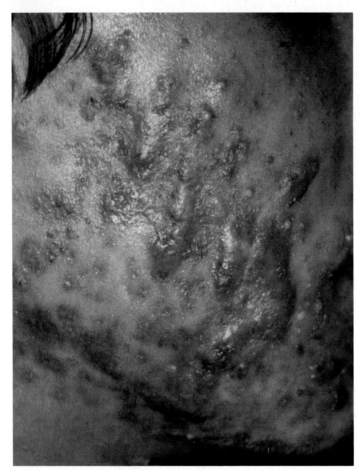

FIGURE 1-5 Acne conglobata In this severe nodulocystic acne, there are large confluent nodules and cysts forming linear mounds that correspond to interconnecting channels. There is pustulation, crusting, and scarring. Lesions are very painful.

MANAGEMENT

The goal of therapy is to remove any plugging of the pilar drainage, reduce sebum production, and treat bacterial colonization. The long-term goal is prevention of scarring.

Mild Acne

Use topical antibiotics (clindamycin and eryth-romycin) and benzoyl peroxide gels (2%, 5%, or 10%). Topical retinoids (retinoic acid, ada-palene, or tazarotene) require detailed instruc-tions regarding gradual increases in concentra-tion from 0.01% to 0.025% to 0.05% cream, gel, or liquid. Best combined with benzoyl peroxide–erythromycin gels.

Note: Acne surgery (extractions of comedo-nes) is helpful only when properly done and after pretreatment with topical retinoids.

MODERATE ACNE Add oral antibiotics to the above regimen. Minocycline is most effective, 50 to 100 mg/d, or doxycycline, 50 to 100 mg twice daily, tapered to 50 mg/d as acne lessens. Use of oral isotretinoin in moderate acne to prevent scarring has become much more com-mon and is very effective.

SEVERE ACNE In addition to topical treat-ment, systemic treatment with isotretinoin is indicated for cystic or conglobate acne, or any other acne refractory to treatment. This retinoid inhibits sebaceous gland function and keratinization, which is very effective. Oral

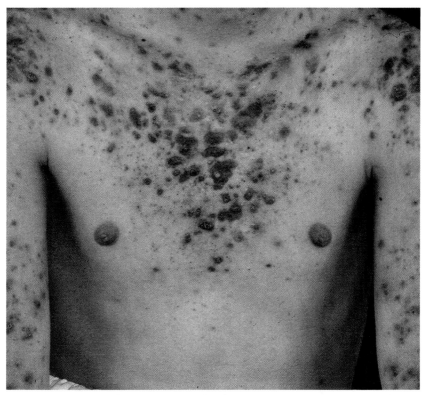

FIGURE 1-6 Acne conglobata on the trunk Inflammatory nodules and cysts have coalesced, forming abscesses that can lead to ulceration. There are many recent red scars following resolution of inflammatory lesions on the entire chest but also on the back.

isotretinoin leads to complete remission in almost all cases, lasting for months to years in the majority of patients.

Indications for Oral Isotretinoin. Moderate, recalcitrant, and nodular acne.

Contraindications. Isotretinoin is teratogenic and effective contraception is imperative. Concurrent tetracycline and isotretinoin may cause pseudotumor cerebri (benign intracranial swelling); therefore, the two medications should *never* be used together.

Warnings. Determine blood lipids, transaminases (ALT, AST) before therapy. Around 25% of patients can develop *increased plasma triglycerides*. Patients may develop mild-to-moderate elevation of transaminase levels, which normalize with reduction of the drug dosage. *Eyes: Night blindness* has been reported, and patients may have *decreased tolerance to contact lenses. Skin*: An eczema-like rash caused by drug-induced dryness can occur and responds dramatically to low potency (class III) topical glucocorticoids. Dry lips and cheilitis almost always occur and must be treated. Reversible thinning of hair may occur very rarely, as may paronychia. *Nose:* Dryness of nasal mucosa and nosebleeds occur rarely. *Other systems:* Rarely depression, headaches, arthritis, and muscular pain, but pancreatitis can occur. For additional rare possible complications, consult the package insert.

Dosage. Isotretinoin, 0.5 to 1 mg/kg given in divided doses with food. Most patients clear within 20 weeks with 1 mg/kg but 0.5 mg/kg is equally effective.

OTHER SYSTEMIC TREATMENTS FOR SEVERE ACNE
Adjunctive systemic glucocorticoids may be required in severe acne conglobata, acne fulminans, and SAPHO and PAPA syndromes. The TNF-α inhibitor infliximab and anakinra are investigational drugs in these severe forms and show promising effects. *Note:* For inflammatory cysts and nodules, intralesional triamcinolone is helpful (0.05 mL of a 3 to 5 mg/mL solution).

ROSACEA ICD-10: L71

- A common chronic inflammatory acneiform disorder of the facial pilosebaceous units.
- Coupled with an increased reactivity of capillaries leading to flushing and telangiectasia.
- May result in rubbery thickening of nose, cheeks, forehead, or chin caused by sebaceous hyperplasia, edema, and fibrosis.

EPIDEMIOLOGY

OCCURRENCE Common, affecting approximately 10% of fair-skinned people.
AGE OF ONSET From 30 to 50 years; peak incidence between 40 and 50 years.
SEX Females predominantly, but rhinophyma occurs mostly in males.
ETHNICITY Celtic persons (skin phototypes I and II) but also southern Mediterraneans; less frequent in pigmented persons (skin phototypes V and VI, i.e., brown and black).

STAGING (PLEWIG AND KLIGMAN CLASSIFICATION)

The rosacea diathesis: episodic erythema, "flushing and blushing."
Stage I: Persistent erythema with telangiectases.
Stage II: Persistent erythema, telangiectases, papules, and tiny pustules.
Stage III: Persistent deep erythema, dense telangiectases, papules, pustules, and nodules; rarely persistent "solid" edema on the central part of the face.

Note: Progression from one stage to another does not always occur. Rosacea may start with stage II or III and stages may overlap.

CLINICAL MANIFESTATION

History of episodic reddening of the face (flushing) in response to hot liquids, spicy foods, alcohol, or exposure to sun and heat. Acne may have preceded the onset of rosacea by years but rosacea usually arises de novo.
DURATION OF LESIONS Days, weeks, or months.
SKIN SYMPTOMS Concern about cosmetic facial appearance.
SKIN LESIONS Early. Stage I. Pathognomonic flushing—"red face" (Fig. 1-7). Stage II. Tiny papules and papulopustules (2 to 3 mm); pustules are often small (≤1 mm) and on the apex of the papule (Figs. 1-8 and 1-9). *No comedones.*
Late. Stage III. Red facies and dusky-red papules and nodules (Figs. 1-10 and 1-11). Scattered, discrete lesions. Telangiectases.

Marked sebaceous hyperplasia and lymphedema in chronic rosacea, causing disfigurement of the nose, forehead, eyelids, ears, and chin (Fig. 1-11). *Rhinophyma* (enlarged nose), *metophyma* (enlarged cushion-like swelling of the forehead), *blepharophyma* (swelling of the eyelids), *otophyma* (cauliflower-like swelling of the ear-lobes), and *gnathophyma* (swelling of the chin) result from marked sebaceous gland hyperplasia (Fig. 1-11) and fibrosis. Upon palpation: soft and rubber-like.
Distribution. Symmetric localization on the face (Fig. 1-10). Rarely neck, chest (V-shaped area), back, and scalp.
Associations. May be associated with seborrheic dermatitis.

Eye Involvement

"Red eyes" as a result of chronic blepharitis, conjunctivitis, and episcleritis. Rosacea keratitis, albeit rare, is a serious problem because corneal ulcers may develop.

LABORATORY EXAMINATIONS

BACTERIAL CULTURE Rule out *S. aureus* infection. Scrapings may reveal massive concurrent *Demodex folliculorum* infestation.
DERMATOPATHOLOGY Nonspecific perifollicular and pericapillary inflammation with occasional foci of "tuberculoid" granulomatous areas; dilated capillaries. *Later stages*: diffuse hypertrophy of the connective tissue, sebaceous gland hyperplasia, and epithelioid granuloma without caseation.

DIFFERENTIAL DIAGNOSIS

FACIAL PAPULES/PUSTULES Acne (in rosacea there are no comedones), periorificial dermatitis (see the following), *S. aureus* folliculitis, gram-negative folliculitis, and *D. folliculorum* infestation.
FACIAL FLUSHING/ERYTHEMA Seborrheic dermatitis, prolonged use of topical glucocorticoids, systemic lupus erythematosus; dermatomyositis.

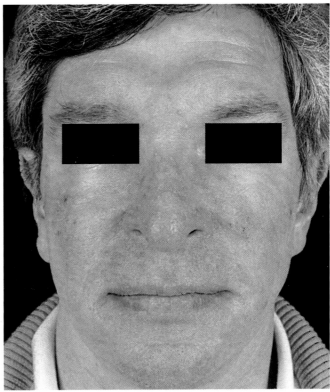

FIGURE 1-7 Erythematous rosacea (stage I) The early stages of rosa-cea often present by episodic erythema, "flushing and blushing," which is followed by persistent erythema caused by multiple tiny telangiectasias, resulting in a red face.

COURSE

PROLONGED Recurrences are common. After a few years, the disease may disappear sponta-neously but usually it is for lifetime. Men and very rarely women may develop rhinophyma, gnathophyma, etc.

MANAGEMENT

PREVENTION Marked reduction or elimination of alcohol and caffeine may be helpful in some patients.

Topical

Metronidazole gel or *cream*, 0.75% or 1%, once or twice daily. Ivermectin cream.
Topical antibiotics (e.g., erythromycin gel) is less effective.

SYSTEMIC Oral antibiotics are more effective than topical treatment.

Minocycline or doxycycline, 50 to 100 mg once or twice daily, first-line antibiotics; very effective. *Tetracycline*, 1 to 1.5 g/d in divided doses until clear; then gradually reduce to once-daily doses of 250 to 500 mg; oral met-ronidazole 500 mg bid, effective.

Maintenance Treatment. Minocycline or dox-ycycline 50 mg/d or 50 mg on alternate days.
ORAL ISOTRETINOIN For severe disease (especially stage III) not responding to antibiotics and topi-cal treatments. A low-dose regimen of 0.5 mg/kg body weight per day is effective in most patients, but occasionally 1 mg/kg may be required.
IVERMECTIN Single dose of 12 mg po in case of massive demodex infestation.
RHINOPHYMA AND TELANGIECTASIA Treated by surgery or laser surgery with excellent cosmetic results. The b-blocker carvedilol 6.5 mg PO reduces erythema and telangiectasia; topical brimonidin 0.5 % gel rapidly reduces erythema and teleangiectasia, but not in all cases.

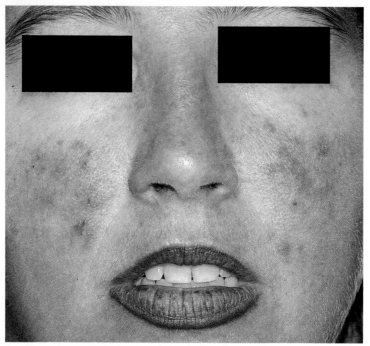

FIGURE 1-8 Rosacea Moderate rosacea in a 29-year-old female with persistent erythema, telangiectasia, red papules (stage II), and tiny pustules.

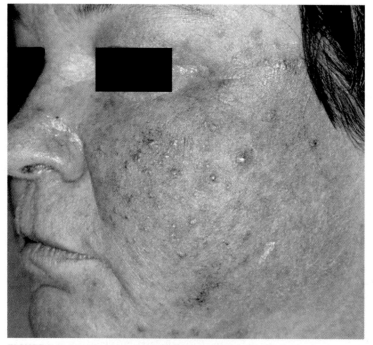

FIGURE 1-9 Rosacea (stages II–III) Telangiectasia, papules and pustules, and some swelling in a 50-year-old woman. There are no comedones.

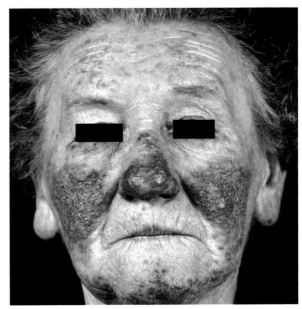

FIGURE 1-10 Papulopustular rosacea (stage III) In this 68-year-old female, rosacea involves almost the entire face, sparing only the upper and lower lip and temples. Papules and pustules have coalesced—again no comedones—and have already led to some swelling of the cheeks, which present "solid" edema.

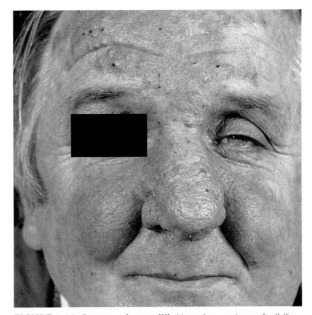

FIGURE 1-11 Rosacea (stage III) Here the persistent "solid" edema of the nose, forehead, and parts of the cheeks is the leading symptom. Papules, pustules, and crusted pustules are superimposed on this persistent edema. The enlarged nose feels rubbery and already represents rhinophyma. Note also blepharophyma of left upper eyelid.

PERIORIFICIAL DERMATITIS ICD-10: L71.0

- Discrete erythematous micropapules and microvesicles.
- Often confluent in the perioral and periorbital skin.
- Occurs mainly in young women but can occur in children and the old.

EPIDEMIOLOGY AND ETIOLOGY

AGE OF ONSET From 16 to 45 years, but can occur in children and the old.
SEX Females predominantly.
ETIOLOGY A variant of rosacea. May be markedly aggravated by potent topical (fluorinated) glucocorticoids.

CLINICAL MANIFESTATION

DURATION OF LESIONS Weeks to months. Skin symptoms perceived as cosmetic disfigurement; occasional itching or burning, feeling of tightness.
SKIN LESIONS 1- to 2-mm erythematous papulopustules on an erythematous background irregularly grouped (Fig. 1-12), symmetric. Lesions increase in number with central confluence and satellites (Fig. 1-13); confluent plaques may appear eczematous with tiny scales. There are no comedones.
Distribution. Initially perioral. Rim of sparing around the vermilion border of lips, nasolabial (Figs. 1-12 and 1-13); at times, in the periorbital area (Fig. 1-14). Uncommonly, only periorbital.

LABORATORY EXAMINATIONS

CULTURE Rule out *S. aureus* infection.

DIFFERENTIAL DIAGNOSIS

Allergic contact dermatitis, atopic dermatitis, seborrheic dermatitis, rosacea, acne vulgaris, and steroid acne.

COURSE

Appearance of lesions is usually subacute over weeks to months. At times, it is misdiagnosed as an eczematous or a seborrheic dermatitis and treated with a potent topical glucocorticoid preparation, aggravating perioral dermatitis, or inducing steroid acne.

MANAGEMENT

Topical

Avoid topical glucocorticoids; *metronidazole*, 0.75% gel two times daily or 1% once daily; *erythromycin*, 2% gel applied twice daily.

Systemic

Minocycline or *doxycycline*, 100 mg daily until clear, then 50 mg daily for another 2 months. (Caution: doxycycline is a photosensitizing drug.) Or *Tetracycline*, 500 mg twice daily until clear, then 500 mg daily for 1 month, followed by 250 mg daily for an additional month.

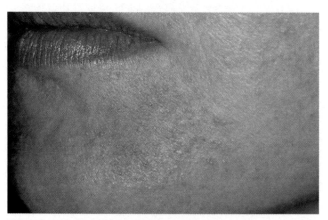

FIGURE 1-12 Perioral dermatitis Moderate involvement with early confluence of tiny papules and a few pustules in a perioral distribution in a young woman. Note typical sparing of the vermilion border (mucocutaneous junction).

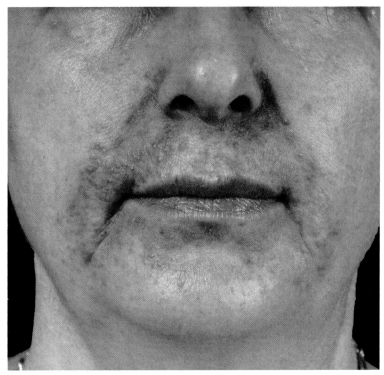

FIGURE 1-13 Perioral dermatitis Preferential location around the mouth and nasolabial folds and cheeks. This 38-year-old woman has been treated with fluorinated corticosteroids that led to a worsening of the condition.

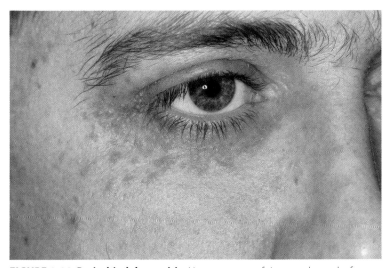

FIGURE 1-14 Periorbital dermatitis Note presence of tiny papules and a few pustules around the eye. This is a much less common site than lesions around the mouth.

MILIARIA ICD-10: L74

- A sweat retention disorder.
- Excessive sweating → maceration and blockage of eccrine ducts.
- Three types:
  - Crystallina (tiny, superficial clear vesicles), (Fig. 1-15),
  - Rubra (pruritic erythematous vesicles),
  - Profunda (white papules, caused by deeper ductal occlusion).
- Differential Diagnosis: Folliculitis, Grover's disease, or candidiasis.
- Therapy: Cool environment, topical corticosteroids, or calcineurin inhibitors.

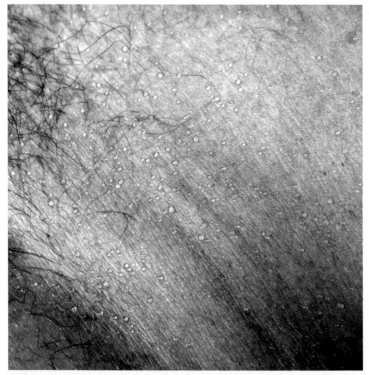

FIGURE 1-15 Miliaria crystallina Tiny, superficial, clear vesicles on the trunk after excessive sweating.

HYPERHIDROSIS ICD-10:R61

- Excessive production of eccrine sweat, with several types.
- Primary cortical hyperhidrosis. Usually palms, soles, axillae, occasionally face, symmetrical, or bilateral.
- Secondary cortical hyperhidrosis associated with palmoplantar keratodermas and epidermolysis bullosa.
- Secondary hypothalamic hyperhidrosis associated with systemic diseases, infections, and cancer.
- Secondary medullary hyperhidrosis (gustatory): facial sweating after ingestion of spicy foods. Frey's syndrome is gustatory sweating where disrupted nerves for sweat aberrantly connect with salivary nerves.
- Treatment: Topical antiperspirants containing aluminum salts. Injection of botulinum toxin type A where feasible. Tap water iontophoresis less effective.

CHROMHIDROSIS AND BROMHIDROSIS ICD-10:L75.1 and L75.0

- Colored sweat (green, black, yellow) in Chromhidrosis is caused by lipofuscin in apocrine glands, staining by clothing, or chromogenic bacteria or fungi (Fig. 1-16).
- The foul smelling sweat in bromhidrosis is caused by degradation of eccrine sweat by resident microflora (corynebacteria or micrococcus) or the degradation of apocrine sweat (usually triglycerides) also by skin flora.

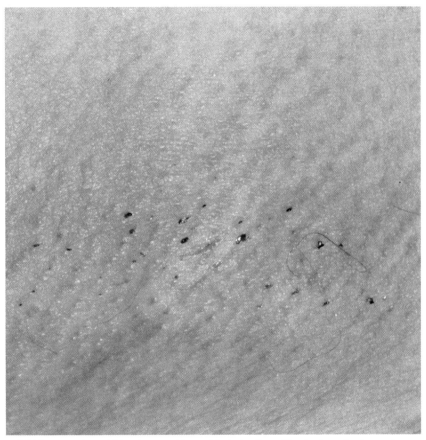

FIGURE 1-16 Chromhidrosis Note blue to black droplets of lipofuscin stained apocrine sweat in the glandular duct orifices. There is also a bluish sheen imparted to the entire axillary skin by lipofuscin in the glands deeper down in the tissue.

HIDRADENITIS SUPPURATIVA ICD-10: L73.2

- A chronic, suppurative, often cicatricial disease of apocrine gland-bearing skin.
- Involves the axillae, the inguinocrural, anogenital region, and rarely the scalp (called *dissecting perifolliculitis*).
- May be associated with severe nodulocystic acne or acne conglobata and pilonidal sinuses (also termed *follicular occlusion syndrome*).

Synonyms: Apocrinitis, hidradenitis axillaris, abscess of the apocrine sweat glands, acne inversa.

EPIDEMIOLOGY

AGE OF ONSET From puberty to climacteric.
SEX Affects more females than males; estimated to affect 4% of the female population. Males more often have anogenital whereas females experience axillary involvement.
RACE All races.
HEREDITY Mother–daughter transmission has been observed. Families give a history of nodulocystic acne and hidradenitis suppurativa occurring separately or together in blood relatives.

ETIOLOGY AND PATHOGENESIS

Etiology. Unknown. Predisposing factors: obesity, smoking, and genetic predisposition to acne.
PATHOGENESIS Keratinous plugging of the hair follicle → dilatation hair follicle and secondarily of the apocrine duct → inflammation → bacterial growth in dilated follicle and duct → rupture → extension of suppuration/tissue destruction → ulceration and fibrosis, sinus tract formation → scarring.

CLINICAL MANIFESTATION

Symptoms. Intermittent pain and marked point tenderness related to abscess.
SKIN LESIONS Open comedones, double comedones → *very tender*, red inflammatory nodules/abscesses (Fig. 1-17) → resolve or drain purulent/seropurulent material → moderately to exquisitely tender sinus tracts → fibrosis, "bridge" scars, hypertrophic and keloidal scars, contractures (Figs. 1-17, and 1-18). Rarely, lymphedema of the associated limb.
Distribution. Axillae, breasts, anogenital area, or groin. Often bilateral, but may extend over entire back, buttocks, perineum involving scrotum or vulva (Figs. 1-19 and 1-20), and scalp.

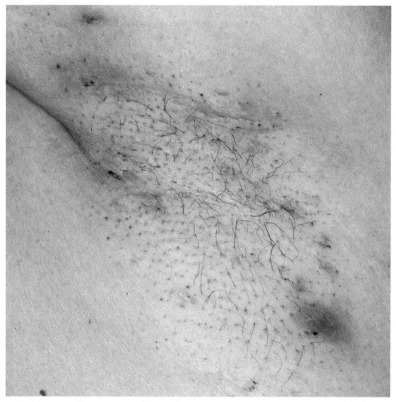

FIGURE 1-17 Hidradenitis suppurativa Many black comedones, some of which are paired, are a characteristic finding associated with deep, exquisitely painful abscesses and old scars in the axilla.

FIGURE 1-18 Hidradenitis suppurativa Multiple bulging and depressed scars, draining sinuses and larger ulcer in the axilla of a 24-year-old male.

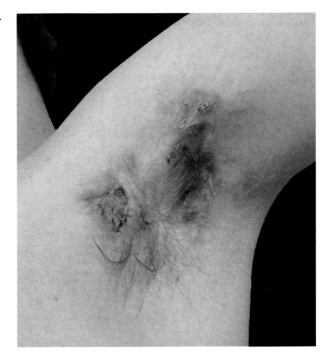

FIGURE 1-19 Hidradenitis suppurativa Severe scarring on the buttocks, inflammatory painful nodules with fistulas, and draining sinuses. When the patient sits down, pus will squirt from the sinus openings.

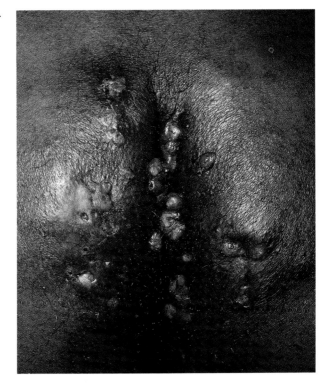

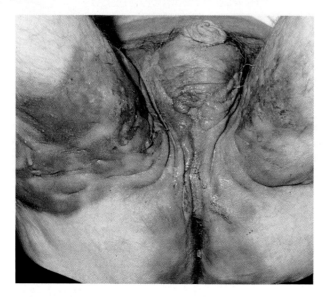

FIGURE 1-20 Hidradenitis suppurativa The entire perigenital and perianal skin as well as the buttocks and inner aspects of the thighs are involved in this 50-year-old male. There is considerable inflammation, and pressure releases purulent exudate from multiple sinuses. The patient had to wear a large diaper, because whenever he was seated, secretions would squirt from the sinuses.

Associated Findings. Cystic acne, pilonidal sinus. Often obesity.

LABORATORY EXAMINATIONS

BACTERIOLOGY Various pathogens may secondarily colonize or "infect" lesions. These include *S. aureus*, streptococci, *Escherichia coli*, *Proteus mirabilis*, and *Pseudomonas aeruginosa*.
DERMATOPATHOLOGY Keratin occlusion of hair follicle, ductal/tubular dilatation, inflammatory changes limited to follicular apparatus → destruction of apocrine/eccrine/pilosebaceous apparatus, fibrosis, or pseudoepitheliomatous hyperplasia in sinuses.

DIFFERENTIAL DIAGNOSIS

Painful papule, nodule, abscess in groin and axilla: furuncle, carbuncle, lymphadenitis, ruptured inclusion cyst, painful lymphadenopathy in lymphogranuloma venereum, or cat-scratch disease. *Also*: donovanosis, scrofuloderma, actinomycosis, sinus tracts, and fistulas associated with ulcerative colitis and regional enteritis.

COURSE AND PROGNOSIS

The severity varies considerably. Patients with mild involvement with recurrent, self-healing, tender red nodules often do not seek therapy. Usually a spontaneous remission with age (>35 years). Some course is relentlessly progressive, with marked morbidity related to chronic pain, draining sinuses, and scarring, with restricted mobility (Figs. 1-19 and 1-20). Rare complications: fistulas to urethra, bladder, and/or rectum; anemia; amyloidosis.

MANAGEMENT

Hidradenitis suppurativa is *not* simply an infection, and systemic antibiotics are only part of the treatment program. Combinations of (1) intralesional glucocorticoids, (2) surgery, (3) oral antibiotics, and (4) isotretinoin are used.

Medical Management

ACUTE PAINFUL *NODULE* AND ABSCESS Intralesional triamcinolone (3 to 5 mg/mL) into the wall followed by incision and drainage of abscess.
CHRONIC LOW-GRADE DISEASE Oral antibiotics: erythromycin (250 to 500 mg qid), tetracycline (250 to 500 mg qid), or minocycline (100 mg bid); or a combination of clindamycin, 300 mg bid, with rifampin (300 mg bid); resolution may take weeks or months.
PREDNISONE Concurrently, if pain and inflammation are severe: 70 mg daily for 2 to 3 days, tapered over 14 days.
ORAL ISOTRETINOIN Not useful in severe disease, but useful in early disease to prevent follicular plugging and when combined with surgical excision of individual lesions. TNF-α inhibitors (e.g., infliximab) show promising results in severe cases.

Surgical Management

- Incise and drain acute abscesses.
- Excise chronic recurrent, fibrotic nodules, or sinus tracts.
- With extensive, chronic disease, complete excision of axilla or involved anogenital area extending down to fascia, requires split skin grafting.

PSYCHOLOGICAL MANAGEMENT

Patients become very depressed because of pain, soiling of clothing by draining pus, odor, and the site of occurrence (anogenital area). Therefore, every effort should be made to deal with the disease, using every modality possible.

FOX FORDYCE DISEASE

- Rare, mostly in females, after puberty.
- Eruption consists of skin-colored or slightly erythematous papules localized to axillae and/or the genitofemoral region (Fig. 1-21).
- Very pruritic.
- Results from plugging of follicular infundibula → rupture → inflammation.
- Treatment: topical corticosteroids or calcineurin inhibitors, topical clindamycin, electrocoagulation, or liposuction/curettage.

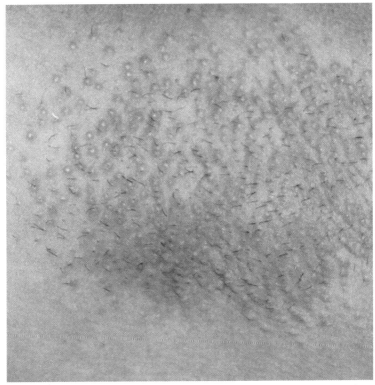

FIGURE 1-21 Fox Fordyce disease Skin colored follicular papules in the axilla which are very pruritic.

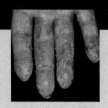

ECZEMA/DERMATITIS

The terms *eczema* and *dermatitis* are used interchangeably, denoting a polymorphic inflammatory reaction pattern involving the epidermis and dermis. There are many etiologies and a wide range of clinical findings. Acute eczema/dermatitis is characterized by pruritus, erythema, and vesiculation. Chronic eczema/dermatitis is characterized by pruritus, xerosis, lichenification, hyperkeratosis/scaling, and ± fissuring.

CONTACT DERMATITIS ICD-10: L25

Contact dermatitis is a generic term applied to acute or chronic inflammatory reactions to substances that come in contact with the skin. *Irritant contact dermatitis* (ICD) is caused by a chemical irritant. *Allergic contact dermatitis* (ACD) is caused by an antigen (allergen) that elicits a type IV (cell-mediated or delayed) hypersensitivity reaction.

ICD occurs after a single exposure to the offending agent that is toxic to the skin (e.g., croton oil) and in severe cases may lead to necrosis. It is dependent on concentration of the offending agent and occurs in everyone, depending on the penetrability and thickness of the stratum corneum. There is a threshold concentration for these substances above which they cause acute dermatitis and below which they do not. This sets ICD apart from ACD, which is dependent on sensitization and thus occurs only in sensitized individuals. Depending on the degree of sensitization, minute amounts of the offending agents may elicit a reaction. Since ICD is a toxic phenomenon, it is confined to the area of exposure and is therefore always sharply marginated and never spreads. ACD is an immunologic reaction that tends to involve the surrounding skin (spreading phenomenon) and may spread beyond affected sites.

IRRITANT CONTACT DERMATITIS (ICD) ICD-10: L24

- ICD is a localized disease confined to areas exposed to irritants.
- It is caused by exposure of the skin to chemical or other physical agents that are capable of irritating the skin.
- Severe irritants cause toxic reactions even after short exposure.
- Most cases are caused by chronic cumulative exposure to one or more irritants.
- The hands are the most commonly affected area.

TABLE 2-1 Most Common Irritant/Toxic Agents

- Soaps, detergents, waterless hand cleaners
- Acids and alkalis[a]: hydrofluoric acid, cement, chromic acid, phosphorus, ethylene oxide, phenol, metal salts
- Industrial solvents: coal tar solvents, petroleum, chlorinated hydrocarbons, alcohol solvents, ethylene glycol, ether, turpentine, ethyl ether, acetone, carbon dioxide, DMSO, dioxane, styrene
- Plants: Euphorbiaceae (spurges, crotons, poinsettias, manchineel tree), Ranunculaceae (buttercup), Cruciferae (black mustard), Urticaceae (nettles), Solanaceae (pepper, capsaicin), Opuntia (prickly pear)
- Others: fiberglass, wool, rough synthetic clothing, fire-retardant fabrics, "NCR" paper

[a]Lead to chemical burns and necrosis, if concentrated.

EPIDEMIOLOGY

ICD is the most common form of occupational skin disease, accounting for up to 80% of all occupational skin disorders. However, ICD need not be occupational and can occur in anyone being exposed to a substance irritant or toxic to the skin.

ETIOLOGY

ETIOLOGIC AGENTS (Table 2-1) Abrasives, cleaning agents, oxidizing agents; reducing agents, plants, and animal enzymes, secretions; desiccant powders, dust, and soils; excessive exposure to water.

PREDISPOSING FACTORS Atopy, fair skin, temperature (low), climate (low humidity), occlusion, and mechanical irritation.

OCCUPATIONAL EXPOSURE Individuals engaged in the following occupations/activities are at risk: medical, dental, or veterinary services; housekeeping, hairdressing, cleaning, floral arranging, agriculture, horticulture, forestry, food preparation and catering, printing, painting, metal work, mechanical engineering, car maintenance, construction, and fishing.

PATHOGENESIS

Irritants (both chemical and physical), if applied for sufficient time and in adequate concentration. The initial reaction is usually limited to the site of contact with the irritant.

Mechanisms involved in acute and chronic phases of ICD are different. Acute reactions result from direct cytotoxic damage to keratinocytes. Chronic ICD results from repeated exposures that cause damage to cell membranes, disrupting the skin barrier and leading to protein denaturation and then cellular toxicity.

ACUTE IRRITANT CONTACT DERMATITIS

CLINICAL MANIFESTATION

SYMPTOMS Subjective symptoms (burning, stinging, or smarting) can occur within seconds after exposure (immediate-type stinging), e.g., to acids, chloroform, and methanol. Delayed-type stinging occurs within 1 to 2 min, peaking at 5 to 10 min, fading by 30 min, and is caused by agents such as aluminum chloride, phenol, propylene glycol, and others. In delayed ICD, objective skin symptoms do not start until 8 to 24 h after exposure (e.g., anthralin, ethylene oxide, and benzalkonium chloride) and are accompanied by burning rather than itching.

SKIN FINDINGS Minutes after exposure or delayed up to ≥24 h. Lesions range from erythema to vesiculation (Figs. 2-1 and 2-2) and caustic burn with necrosis. Sharply demarcated erythema and superficial edema, corresponding to the application site of the toxic substance (Fig. 2-1). Lesions do not spread beyond the site of contact. In more severe reactions, vesicles and blisters (Figs. 2-1 and 2-2) → erosions and/or even frank necrosis, as with acids or alkaline solutions. No papules. Configuration is often bizarre or linear ("outside job" or dripping effect) (Fig. 2-1).

Distribution. Isolated, localized, or generalized, depending on contact with toxic agent.

Duration. Days, weeks, depending on tissue damage.

Constitutional Symptoms

Usually none, but in widespread acute ICD "acute illness" syndrome, fever may occur.

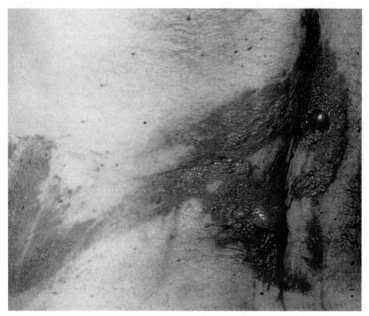

FIGURE 2-1 Acute irritant contact dermatitis following application of a cream containing nonylvanillamid and nicotinic acid butoxyethyl ester prescribed for lower back pain The "streaky pattern" indicates an outside job. The eruption is characterized by a massive erythema with vesiculation and blister formation, and is confined to the sites exposed to the toxic agent.

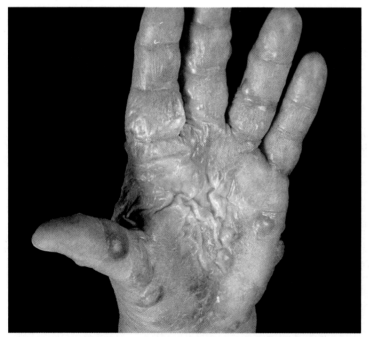

FIGURE 2-2 Acute irritant contact dermatitis on the hand resulting from an industrial solvent There is massive blistering on the palm.

CHRONIC IRRITANT CONTACT DERMATITIS

CUMULATIVE ICD Most common; develops slowly after repeated additive exposure to mild irritants (water, soap, detergents, etc.), usually on the hands. Repeated exposures to toxic or subtoxic concentrations of offending agents → disturbance of the barrier function that allows even subtoxic concentrations of the offending agent to penetrate into the skin and elicit a chronic inflammatory response. Injury (e.g., repeated rubbing of the skin), prolonged soaking in water, or chronic contact after repeated, cumulative physical trauma such as friction, pressure, and abrasions in individuals engaged in manual work (*traumatic ICD*).

CLINICAL MANIFESTATION

SYMPTOMS Stinging, smarting, burning, *and* itching; pain as fissures develop.
SKIN FINDINGS Dryness → chapping → erythema (Fig. 2-3) → hyperkeratosis and scaling → fissures and crusting (Fig. 2-4).

Sharp margination gives way to ill-defined borders, lichenification.
Distribution. Usually on the hands (Figs. 2-3 and 2-4). Usually starting at finger web spaces, spreading to the sides and dorsal surface of the hands, and then to the palms. In housewives, it often starts on the fingertips (*pulpitis*) (Fig. 2-3). Rarely seen in other locations exposed to irritants and/or trauma, e.g., in violinists on mandible or neck, or on exposed sites as in *airborne ICD* (see below).
Duration. Chronic or months to years.

Constitutional Symptoms

None, except when infection occurs. Chronic ICD (e.g., hand dermatitis; see below) can become a severe occupational and emotional problem.

LABORATORY EXAMINATION

HISTOPATHOLOGY In acute ICD, epidermal cell necrosis, neutrophils, vesiculation, and necrosis. In chronic ICD, acanthosis, hyperkeratosis, and lymphocytic infiltrate.
PATCH TESTS These are negative in ICD unless ACD is also present (see below).

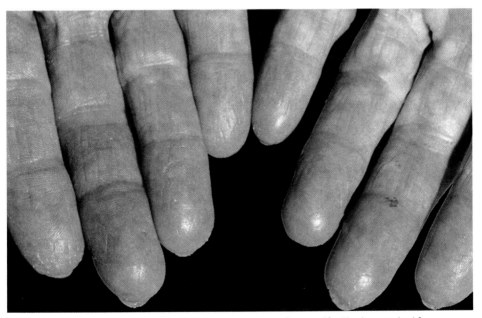

FIGURE 2-3 Early chronic irritant contact dermatitis in a housewife This has resulted from repeated exposure to soaps and detergents. Note glistening fingertips (pulpitis).

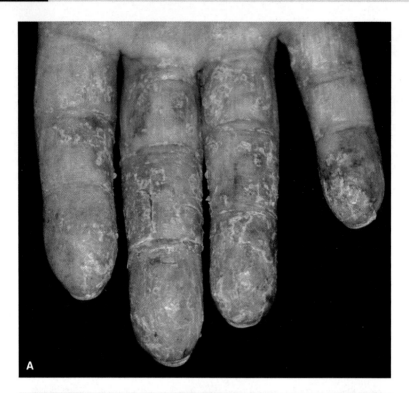

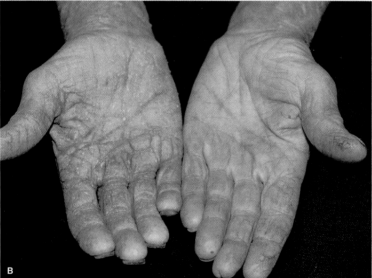

FIGURE 2-4 (A) Chronic irritant dermatitis with acute exacerbation in a housewife The patient used turpentine to clean her hands after painting. Erythema, fissuring, and scaling. Differential diagnosis is allergic contact dermatitis and palmar psoriasis. Patch tests to turpentine were negative. **(B) Irritant contact dermatitis in a construction worker who works with cement** Note the hyperkeratoses, scaling, and fissuring. There is also minimal pustulation. Note that right (dominant working) hand is more severely affected than the left hand.

SPECIAL FORMS OF ICD

Hand Dermatitis

Most cases of chronic ICD occur on the hands and are occupational. Often sensitization to allergens (such as nickel or chromate salts) occurs later, and then ACD is superimposed on ICD. A typical example is hand dermatitis in construction and cement workers. Cement is alkaline and corrosive, leading to chronic ICD (Fig. 2-4B); chromates in cement sensitize and lead to ACD (Allergic Contact Dermatitis, see below). In such cases, the eruption may spread beyond the hands and may even generalize.
AIRBORNE ICD Characteristically on the face, neck, anterior chest, and arms. Most frequent causes are irritating dust and volatile chemicals (ammonia, solvents, formaldehyde, epoxy resins, cement, fiberglass, or sawdust from toxic woods). This has to be distinguished from airborne *allergic* contact dermatitis (Airborne Allergic Contact Dermatitis, p. 32) and photoallergic contact dermatitis (Section 10).

Pustular and Acneiform ICD

ICD may target follicles and become pustular and papulopustular. Results from metals, mineral oils, greases, cutting fluids, and naphthalenes.

DIAGNOSIS AND DIFFERENTIAL DIAGNOSIS

Diagnosis is by history and clinical examination (lesions, pattern, and site). Most important differential diagnosis is ACD (Table 2-3). On the palms and soles, palmoplantar psoriasis; in exposed sites, photoallergic contact dermatitis.

COURSE AND PROGNOSIS

Healing usually occurs within 2 weeks of removal of noxious stimuli; in more chronic cases, 6 weeks or longer. In the setting of occupational ICD, only one-third of individuals have complete remission and two-thirds may require allocation to another job; atopic individuals have a worse prognosis. In cases of chronic subcritical levels of irritant, some workers develop tolerance or "hardening."

MANAGEMENT

Prevention

- Avoid irritant or caustic chemical(s) by wearing protective clothing (i.e., goggles, shields, and gloves).
- If contact does occur, wash with water or weak neutralizing solution.
- Barrier creams.
- In occupational ICD that persists in spite of adherence to the preceding measures, a change of job may be necessary.

TREATMENT

Acute. Identify and remove the etiologic agent. Apply wet dressings with Burow's solution, changed every 2 to 3 h. Larger vesicles may be drained. Topical class I–II glucocorticoid preparations. In severe cases, systemic glucocorticoids may be indicated. Prednisone: 2-week course, 60 mg initially, tapering by steps of 10 mg.
Subacute and Chronic. Remove etiologic/pathogenic agent. Potent topical glucocorticoids (betamethasone dipropionate or clobetasol propionate) and adequate lubrication. As healing occurs, continue with lubrication. The topical calcineurin inhibitors, pimecrolimus and tacrolimus, are usually not potent enough to sufficiently suppress the chronic inflammation on the hands.
 In chronic ICD of the hands, a "hardening effect" can be achieved in most cases with topical (soak or bath) PUVA therapy (page 60).
SYSTEMIC TREATMENT Alitretinoin (approved in Europe and Canada) 0.5 mg/kg body weight po for up to 6 months. Observe contraindications to systemic retinoids.

ALLERGIC CONTACT DERMATITIS (ACD) ICD-10: L24

- ACD is a systemic disease defined by hapten specific T-cell–mediated inflammation.
- One of the most frequent, vexing, and costly skin problems.
- An eczematous (papules, vesicles, or pruritic) dermatitis.
- Caused by re-exposure to a substance to which the individual has been sensitized.

EPIDEMIOLOGY

FREQUENT Accounts for 7% of occupationally related illnesses in the United States, but data suggest that the actual incidence rate is 10 to 50 times greater than reported in the U.S. Bureau of Labor Statistics data. Nonoccupational ACD is estimated to be three times greater than occupational ACD.

AGE OF ONSET All ages, but uncommon in young children and individuals older than 70 years.

OCCUPATION One of the most important causes of disability in industry.

PATHOGENESIS

ACD is a classic, delayed, cell-mediated hypersensitivity reaction. Exposure to a strong sensitizer results in sensitization in a week or so, while exposure to a weak allergen may take months to years for sensitization. Sensitized T cells circulate in the blood and home to the skin wherever the specific allergen is presented. Thus, *all* skin is hypersensitive to the contact allergen.

ALLERGENS

Contact allergens are diverse and range from metal salts to antibiotics and dyes to plant products. Thus, allergens are found in jewelry, personal care products, topical medications, plants, house remedies, and chemicals the individual may come in contact with. The most common allergens in the United States are listed in Table 2-2.

CLINICAL MANIFESTATION

The eruption starts in a sensitized individual 48 h or days after contact with the allergen; repeated exposures lead to a crescendo reaction, i.e., the eruption worsens. The site of the eruption is confined to the site of exposure.

SYMPTOMS Intense pruritus; in severe reactions, also stinging and pain.

CONSTITUTIONAL SYMPTOMS "Acute illness" syndrome, including fever, but only in severe ACD (e.g., poison ivy, see below).

Skin Lesions

Acute. Well-demarcated erythema and edema with superimposed closely spaced papules or nonumbilicated vesicles (Fig. 2-5); in severe reactions, bullae, confluent erosions exuding serum, and crusts. The same reaction can occur after several weeks at sites not exposed.

Subacute. Plaques of mild erythema showing small, dry scales, sometimes associated with small, red, pointed, or rounded erythematous firm papules and scales (Figs. 2-6 and 2-7).

TABLE 2-2 Top-Eleven Contact Allergens (North American Contact Dermatitis Group) and Other Common Contact Allergens[a]

Allergen	Principal Sources of Contact
Nickel sulfate	Metals in clothing, jewelry, catalyzing agents
Neomycin sulfate	Usually contained in creams, ointments
Balsam of Peru	Topical medications
Fragrance mix	Fragrances, cosmetics
Thimerosal	Antiseptics
Sodium gold thiosulfate	Medication
Formaldehyde	Disinfectant, curing agents, plastics
Quaternium-15	Disinfectant
Bacitracin	Ointments, powder
Cobalt chloride	Cement, galvanization, industrial oils, cooling agents, eyeshades
Methyldibromo glutaronitrile, phenoxyethanol	Preservatives, cosmetics

Others: Carba mix, Paraphenylenediamine, Thiuram, Parahydroxybenzoic acid ester, Propylene glycol, Procaine, benzocaine, Sulfonamides, Turpentine, Mercury salts, Chromates, Parabens, Cinnamic aldehyde, Pentadecylcatechols

[a]More than 3700 chemicals have been reported to cause allergic contact dermatitis.

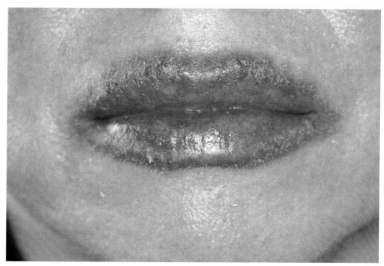

FIGURE 2-5 Acute allergic contact dermatitis on the lips caused by lip-stick The patient was hypersensitive to eosin. Note bright erythema, microvesiculation. At close inspection, a papular component can be discerned. At this stage, there is still sharp margination.

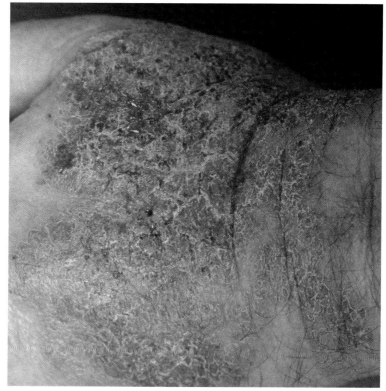

FIGURE 2-6 Allergic contact dermatitis of hands: chromates Confluent papules, vesicles, subacute erosions, and crusts on the dorsum of the left hand in a construction worker who was allergic to chromates.

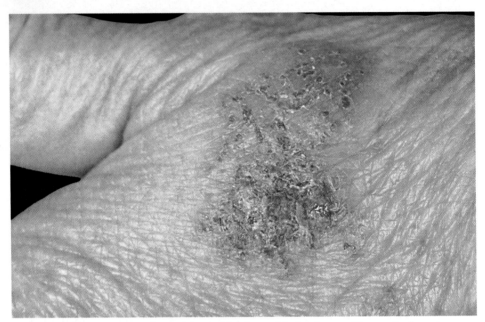

FIGURE 2-7 Allergic contact dermatitis resulting from nickel, subacute Note a mix of papular, vesicular, and crusted lesions and loss of sharp margination. The patient was a retired watchmaker who used a metal clasp on the dorsum of the left hand while repairing watches. He was known to be allergic to nickel.

Chronic. Plaques of lichenification (thickening of the epidermis with deepening of the skin lines in parallel or rhomboidal pattern), scaling with satellite, small, firm, rounded or flat-topped papules, excoriations, and pigmentation. **ARRANGEMENT** Initially, confined to the area of contact with the allergen [e.g., earlobe (earrings), dorsum of foot (shoes), wrist (watch or watchband), collar-like (necklace), and lips (lipstick)]. Often linear, with artificial patterns, an "outside job." Plant contact often results in linear lesions (e.g., *Rhus* dermatitis, see below). Initially confined to the site of contact, then later spreading beyond. **DISTRIBUTION Extent.** Isolated, localized to one region (e.g., shoe dermatitis) or generalized (e.g., plant dermatitis).

COURSE

EVOLUTION OF ACD The duration of ACD varies, resolving in around 1 to 2 weeks, but becomes worse as long as the allergen continues to come into contact with the skin.
Acute. Erythema → papules → vesicles → erosions → crusts → scaling.
Note: In the acute forms of contact dermatitis, papules occur only in ACD, not in ICD (see Table 2-3).

Chronic. Papules → scaling → lichenification → excoriations.
Note: ACD is always confined to the site of exposure to the allergen. Margination is originally sharp, but it spreads in the periphery beyond the actual site of exposure. In the case of strong sensitization, it spreads to other parts of the body and generalization can occur. The main differences between toxic irritant and ACD are summarized in Table 2-3.

LABORATORY EXAMINATIONS

DERMATOPATHOLOGY Acute. Prototype of spongiotic dermatitis, with intercellular edema (*spongiosis*), lymphocytes and eosinophils in the epidermis, and monocyte and histiocyte infiltration in the dermis.
Chronic. Also spongiosis plus acanthosis, elongation and broadening of papillae; hyperkeratosis; and a lymphocytic infiltrate.
PATCH TESTS In ACD, sensitization is present on every part of the skin. Therefore, application of the allergen to any area of normal skin provokes an eczematous reaction. A positive patch test shows erythema and papules, as well as possibly vesicles confined to the test site. Patch tests should be delayed until the dermatitis has subsided for at least 2 weeks and should be

TABLE 2-3 Differences Between Irritant and Allergic Contact Dermatitis[a]

		Irritant CD	Allergic CD
Symptoms	Acute	**Stinging, smarting → itching**	**Itching → pain**
	Chronic	Itching/pain	Itching/pain
Lesions	Acute	Erythema → vesicles → erosions → crusts → scaling	Erythema → **papules** →vesicles → erosions → crust → scaling
	Chronic	Papules, plaques, fissures, scaling, crusts	Papules, plaques, scaling, crusts
Margination and site	Acute	**Sharp, strictly confined to site of exposure**	Sharp, confined to site of exposure **but spreading in the periphery; usually tiny papules; may become generalized**
	Chronic	Ill defined	Ill defined, **spreads**
Evolution	Acute	**Rapid** (few hours after exposure)	**Not so rapid** (12 to 72 h after exposure)
	Chronic	Months to years of repeated exposure	Months or longer; exacerbation after every re-exposure
Causative agents		**Dependent on concentration of agent and state of skin barrier; occurs only above threshold level**	**Relatively independent of amount applied, usually very low concentrations, sufficient but depends on degree of sensitization**
Incidence		**May occur in practically everyone**	**Occurs only in the sensitized**

[a]Differences are printed in bold.

performed on a previously uninvolved site (see "Clinical Tests," Introduction).

DIAGNOSIS AND DIFFERENTIAL DIAGNOSIS

By history and clinical findings, including evaluation of site and distribution.

Histopathology may be helpful; verification of offending agent (allergen) by patch test. Exclude ICD (Table 2-3), atopic dermatitis (AD), seborrheic dermatitis (SD) (face), psoriasis (palms and soles), epidermal dermatophytosis (KOH), fixed drug eruption, and phytophotodermatitis.

SPECIAL FORMS OF ACD

ALLERGIC CONTACT DERMATITIS CAUSED BY PLANTS ICD-10:L23.7

■ Termed *allergic phytodermatitis* (APD).
■ Occurs in sensitized individuals after exposure to a wide variety of plant allergens.
■ Characterized by an acute, very pruritic, eczematous dermatitis, often in a linear arrangement.
■ In the United States, poison ivy/oak are by far the most common plants implicated.

Note: *Phytophotodermatitis* is a different entity. It is a photosensitivity reaction occurring in any individual with a photosensitizing plant-derived chemical on the skin and subsequent sun exposure (see Section 10).

EPIDEMIOLOGY AND ETIOLOGY

AGE OF ONSET All ages. Very young and very old are less likely to be sensitized. Sensitization is lifelong.

ETIOLOGY Pentadecylcatechols, present in the Anacardiaceae plant family, are the most common sensitizers in the United States. They cross-react with other phenolic compounds such as resorcinol, hexylresorcinol, and hydroxyquinones.

PLANTS Anacardiaceae Family. Poison ivy (*Toxicodendron radicans*), poison oak (*T. quercifolium, T. diversilobum*), and poison sumac (*T. vernix*). Plants related to poison ivy group: Brazilian pepper, cashew nut tree, ginkgo tree, Indian marker nut tree, lacquer tree, mango tree, and rengas tree.

GEOGRAPHY Poison ivy occurs throughout the United States (except in the extreme southwest) and southern Canada; poison oak is predominantly on the west coast. Poison sumac and poison dogwood occur in woody, swampy areas.

EXPOSURE Telephone and electrical workers working outdoors. Leaves, stems, seeds, flowers, berries, and roots contain milky sap that turns to a black resin upon exposure to air. Cashew oil, unroasted cashew nuts (heat destroys hapten); cashew oil in wood (Haitian voodoo dolls, swizzle sticks), resins, printer ink, and mango rind. Also occurs in the marking nut tree of India, the laundry marker (dhobi itch) and furniture lacquer from the Japanese lacquer tree.

SEASON APD usually occurs in the spring, summer, and fall. It can also occur year-round if exposed to stems or roots. In the United States southwest, it occurs year-round.

PATHOGENESIS

All *Toxicodendron* plants contain identical allergens. Oleoresins are present in milky sap in leaves, stems, seeds, flowers, berries, and roots, which are called *urushiol*. The haptens are the pentadecylcatechols (1,2-dihydroxybenzenes with a 15-carbon side chain in position three). Washing with soap and water removes oleoresins.

More than 70% of people can be sensitized. Dark-skinned individuals are less susceptible to APD. After first exposure (sensitization), dermatitis occurs 7 to 12 days later. In a previously sensitized person (maybe many decades before), dermatitis occurs in <12 h after reexposure.

Note: Blister fluid does not contain hapten and cannot spread the dermatitis.

CLINICAL MANIFESTATION

EXPOSURE Poison Ivy/oak Dermatitis. Direct plant exposure: plant brushes against exposed skin giving rise to linear lesions (Fig. 2-8);

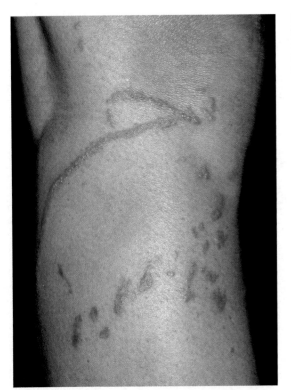

FIGURE 2-8 Allergic phytodermatitis of leg: poison ivy Linear vesicular lesions with erythema and edema on the calf at sites of direct contact to the skin 5 days after exposure to poison ivy leaves.

usually resin is not able to penetrate the thick stratum corneum of the palms/soles.

Food-Containing Urushiol. Lips exposed to unpeeled mango or unroasted cashew nuts. Mucous membranes uncommonly experience APD, but ingestion of urushiol can produce ACD of the anus and perineum.

SKIN SYMPTOMS Pruritus, mild to severe. Often sensed before any detectable skin changes. Pain in some cases.

CONSTITUTIONAL SYMPTOMS Sleep deprivation resulting from pruritus.

SKIN LESIONS Initially, well-demarcated patches of erythema, characteristic linear lesions (Fig. 2-8); → papules and edematous plaques; may be severe especially on the face and/or genitals, resembling cellulitis (Fig. 2-9) → microvesiculation → vesicles and/or bullae (Figs. 2-8 and 2-10) → erosions, crusts. Postinflammatory hyperpigmentation common in darker skinned individuals.

Distribution. Most commonly on exposed extremities, where contact with the plant occurs; blotting can transfer to any exposed site; the palms/soles are usually spared. However, lateral fingers can be involved.

Clothing-Protected Sites. Oleoresin can penetrate damp clothing onto covered skin; wearing clothing previously contaminated with resin can re-expose the skin.

Nonexposed Sites. "Id"-like reaction or some systemic absorption can be associated with disseminated urticarial, erythema multiforme-like, or scarlatiniform lesions away from sites of exposure in some individuals with well-established APD.

LABORATORY EXAMINATIONS

DERMATOPATHOLOGY See the previous discussion of ACD.

PATCH TESTS WITH PENTADECYLCATECHOLS *Contraindicated* as it can sensitize the individual to hapten.

DIAGNOSIS

By history and clinical findings only.

DIFFERENTIAL DIAGNOSIS

ACD to other allergens, phytophotodermatitis (see Section 10), soft-tissue infection (cellulitis, erysipelas), AD, inflammatory dermatophytosis, early herpes zoster, and fixed drug eruption.

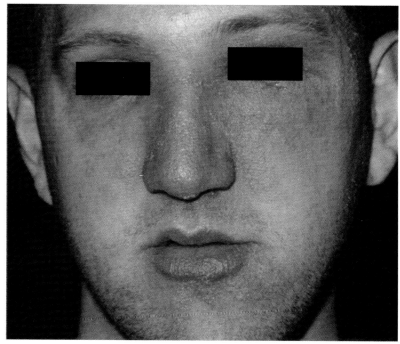

FIGURE 2-9 Allergic phytodermatitis of the face: poison ivy Extremely pruritic, erythema, edema, and microvesiculation in the periorbital and perioral area in a previously sensitized young man, occurring 3 days after exposure.

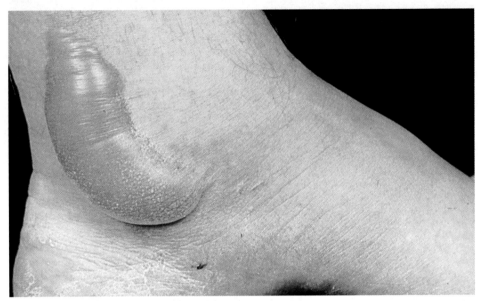

FIGURE 2-10 Acute allergic phytodermatitis, bullous This eruption occurred in a patient who had walked barefoot through a forest. It later spread as a papular eruption to the rest of the body. Similar lesions were present on the other foot and lower leg. Differential diagnosis included acute bullous contact dermatitis to caterpillars. Phytophotodermatitis was excluded because at the time of exposure, there was a heavily clouded sky and a papular eruption occurred later on. Caterpillar dermatitis was excluded because of the multiplicity of the lesions and because upon patch testing, the patient was positive to *Toxicodendron* haptens. Note, patch testing to urushiol is no longer done to avoid sensitization of patients.

OTHER SPECIAL FORMS OF ACD

SYSTEMIC ACD

- After systemic exposure to an allergen to which the individual had prior ACD.
- A delayed T-cell–mediated reaction.
- Examples: ACD to ethylenediamine → subsequent reaction to aminophylline (which contains ethylenediamine); poison ivy dermatitis → subsequent reaction to ingestion of cashew nuts; also antibiotics, sulfonamides, propylene glycol, metal ions, sorbic acid, and fragrances.

AIRBORNE ACD

- Contact with airborne allergens in exposed body sites, notably the face (Fig. 2-11) including the eyelids, "V" of the neck, arms, and legs.
- In contrast to airborne ICD, papular from the beginning, extremely itchy.
- Prolonged repetitive exposure leads to dry, lichenified ACD with erosions and crusting (Fig. 2-11).
- Caused by plant allergens, especially from compositae, natural resins, woods, and essential oils volatizing from aroma therapy.

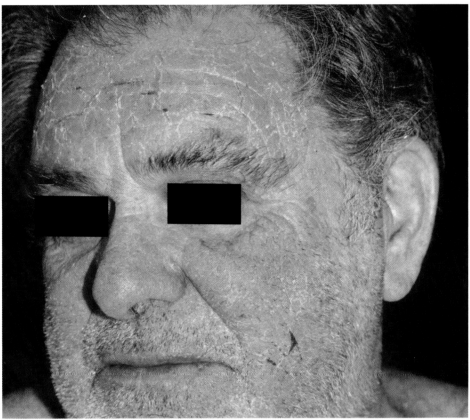

FIGURE 2-11 Airborne allergic contact dermatitis of the face Extremely itchy, confluent, papular, erosive, and crusted/scaly lesions with lichenification on the forehead, nose, and cheeks following exposure to pinewood dust.

MANAGEMENT OF ACD

TERMINATION OF EXPOSURE Identify and remove the etiologic agent.

TOPICAL THERAPY Topical glucocorticoid ointments/gels (classes I–III). Larger vesicles may be drained, but tops should not be removed. Wet dressings with cloths soaked in Burow's solution changed every 2 to 3 h. Airborne ACD may require systemic treatment.

Pimecrolimus and tacrolimus are effective in ACD but to a lesser degree than glucocorticoids.

SYSTEMIC THERAPY Glucocorticoids are indicated if severe and in airborne ACD. Prednisone beginning at 70 mg (adults), tapering by 5 to 10 mg/d over a 1- to 2-week period. In airborne ACD where complete avoidance of allergen may be impossible, immunosuppression with oral cyclosporine may become necessary.

ATOPIC DERMATITIS ICD-10: L20

- An acute, subacute, or chronic relapsing skin disorder.
- Very common in infancy. Prevalence peak of 15 to 20% in early childhood.
  - Characterized principally by dry skin and pruritus; consequent rubbing leads to increased inflammation and lichenification as well as to further itching and scratching: *itch–scratch cycle*.
- Diagnosis is based on clinical findings.
- Often associated with a personal or family history of AD, allergic rhinitis, and asthma; 35% of infants with AD develop asthma later in life.
- Associated with skin barrier dysfunction, IgE reactivity.
- Genetic basis influenced by environmental factors; alterations in immunologic responses in T cells, antigen processing, inflammatory cytokine release, allergen sensitivity, and infection.

Synonyms: IgE dermatitis, "eczema," atopic eczema.

EPIDEMIOLOGY

AGE OF ONSET First 2 months of life and by the first years in 60% of patients; 30% by age 5, and only 10% between age 6 and 20 years. Rarely AD has an adult onset.

GENDER Slightly more common in males than in females.

PREVALENCE Between 7% and 15% reported in population studies in Scandinavia and Germany.

GENETIC ASPECTS The inheritance pattern not yet ascertained. However, in one series, 60% of adults with AD had children with AD. The prevalence in children was higher (81%) when both parents had AD.

Skin Barrier Disruption. Decrease in barrier function resulting from impaired filaggrin production, reduced ceramide levels, and increased transepidermal water loss; dehydration of skin.

ELICITING FACTORS Inhalants. Specific aeroallergens, especially dust mites and pollens.

Microbial Agents. Exotoxins of *Staphylococcus aureus* acting as superantigens. Also, group A *streptococcus*, rarely fungus (*candida*).

Autoallergens. IgE antibodies directed at human proteins. Release of these autoallergens from damaged tissue could trigger IgE or T-cell responses, suggesting maintenance of allergic inflammation.

Foods. *Infants* and *children*, but not adults, have flares of AD with eggs, milk, peanuts, soybeans, fish, and wheat.

Other Exacerbating Factors

Season. In temperate climates, AD usually improves in summer and flares in winter.

Clothing. Pruritus flares *after* taking off clothing. Wool is an important trigger; wool clothing or blankets directly in contact with skin (also wool clothing of parents, fur of pets, and carpets).

Emotional Stress. Results from the disease or is itself an exacerbating factor in flares of the disease.

PATHOGENESIS

Complex interaction of skin barrier, genetic, environmental, pharmacologic, and immunologic factors. Type I (IgE-mediated) hypersensitivity reaction as a result of the release of vasoactive substances from mast cells and basophils sensitized by the interaction of the antigen with IgE (reaginic or skin-sensitizing antibody). High-affinity IgE receptors on Langerhans cells may mediate the eczema-like reaction. Acute AD is associated with a predominance of interleukin (IL) 4 and IL-13 expression, and chronic inflammation in AD with increased IL-5, granulocyte-macrophage colony-stimulating factor, IL-12, and interferon-γ. Thus, skin inflammation in AD shows a biphasic pattern of T-cell activation.

CLINICAL MANIFESTATION

SKIN SYMPTOMS Patients have dry skin. Pruritus is the sine qua non of AD—"eczema is the itch that rashes." The constant scratching leads to a vicious cycle of itch → scratch → rash → itch → scratch.

OTHER SYMPTOMS OF ATOPY Allergic rhinitis, obstruction of nasal passages, conjunctival and pharyngeal itching, and lacrimation; seasonal when associated with pollen.

SKIN LESIONS Acute. Poorly defined erythematous patches, papules, and plaques with or without scale. Edema with widespread involvement; skin appears "puffy" and edematous (Fig. 2-12). Erosions: moist, crusted. Linear or punctate, resulting from scratching. Secondarily infected sites: *S. aureus*. Oozing erosions (Fig. 2-12) and/or pustules (usually follicular). Skin is dry, cracked, and scaly (Figs. 2-12 and 2-13).

FIGURE 2-12 Atopic dermatitis: infantile Puffy face, confluent erythema, papules, microvesiculation, scaling, and crusting.

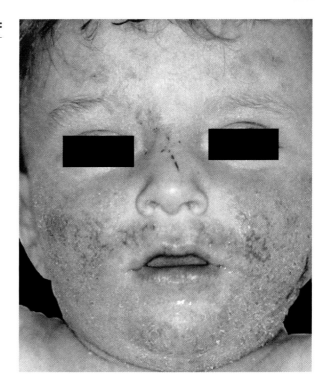

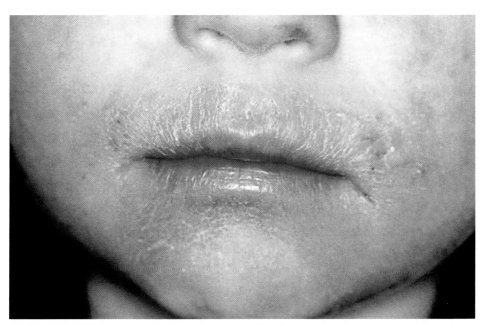

FIGURE 2-13 Childhood atopic dermatitis A typical localization of atopic dermatitis in children is the region around the mouth. In this child, there is lichenification and fissuring as well as crusting.

Chronic. Lichenification (thickening of the skin with accentuation of skin markings) (Figs. 2-14 and 2-15B); follicular lichenification (especially in brown and black persons) (Figs. 2-14B and 2-15B). Fissures: painful, especially in flexures (Fig. 2-14A), often on the palms, fingers, and soles. Alopecia: lateral one-third of the eyebrows as a result of rubbing. Periorbital pigmentation, also as a result of compulsive rubbing. Characteristic infraorbital fold below eyelids (Dennie–Morgan sign) (Adult Atopic Dermatitis, see Fig. 2-17).
Distribution. Predilection for the flexures, front and sides of the neck, eyelids, forehead, face, wrists, and dorsa of the feet and hands (Fig. 2-16). Generalized in severe disease (Figs. 2-15A and B).

Special Features Related to Age

Infantile AD. The lesions present as red skin, tiny vesicles on "puffy" surface. Scaling, exudation with wet crusts and cracks (fissures) (Figs. 2-12 to 2-13).
Childhood-Type AD. The lesions are papular, lichenified plaques, erosions, crusts, especially on the antecubital and popliteal fossae (Figs. 2-14A and B), the neck and face; may be generalized.
Adult-Type AD. There is a similar distribution, mostly flexural but also face and neck, with lichenification and excoriations being the most conspicuous symptoms (Figs. 2-15B and 2-17). May be generalized (Fig. 2-15B).

Special Features Related to Ethnicity

In African Americans and also in dark-brown skin, so-called follicular eczema is common, characterized by discrete follicular papules (Fig. 2-14B) involving hair follicles of the involved site.

Associated Findings

"WHITE" DERMATOGRAPHISM Stroking of involved skin will not lead to redness as in normal skin but to blanching; delayed blanch to cholinergic agents. *Ichthyosis vulgaris* and *keratosis pilaris* (see Section 4) occur in 10% of patients. *Vernal conjunctivitis* with papillary hypertrophy or cobblestoning of upper eyelid conjunctiva. Rare *atopic keratoconjunctivitis* is disabling and may result in corneal scarring. *Keratoconus* is rare. *Cataracts* occur in a very small percentage.

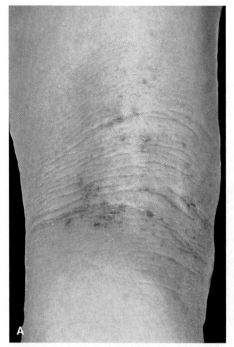
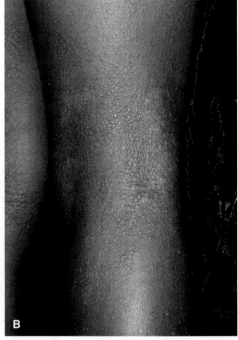

FIGURE 2-14 (A) Childhood atopic dermatitis One of the hallmarks of atopic dermatitis is lichenification in the flexural regions as shown in this picture. Note the thickening of the skin with exaggerated skin lines and erosions. **(B)** Atopic dermatitis in African-American child. Pruritic follicular papules on posterior leg. Follicular eczema pattern is more common in African and Asian children.

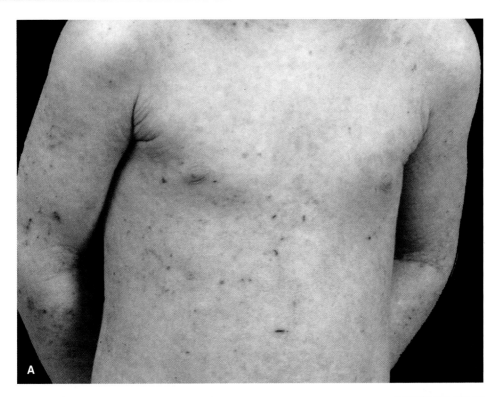

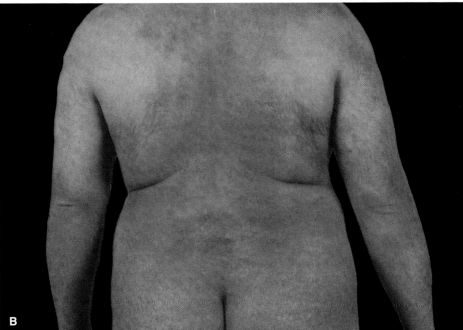

FIGURE 2-15 **(A) Childhood atopic dermatitis** This is a generalized eruption consisting of confluent, inflammatory papules that are erosive, excoriated, and crusted. **(B) Adult atopic dermatitis** Generalized eruption of follicular papules that are more heavily pigmented than normal skin in a 53-year-old woman of African extraction. There is extensive lichenification.

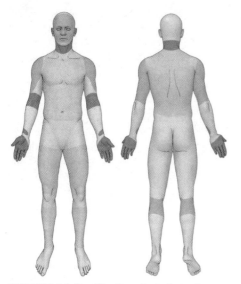

FIGURE 2-16   Predilection sites of atopic dermatitis.

DIAGNOSIS

History in infancy, clinical findings.

DIFFERENTIAL DIAGNOSIS

SD, ICD, ACD, psoriasis, nummular eczema, dermatophytosis, or early stages of mycosis fungoides. Rarely, acrodermatitis enteropathica, glucagonoma syndrome, histidinemia, phenyl-ketonuria; also, some immunologic disorders including Wiskott–Aldrich syndrome, X-linked agammaglobulinemia, hyper-IgE syndrome, and selective IgA deficiency; Langerhans cell histiocytosis, Letterer–Siwe type.

LABORATORY EXAMINATIONS

BACTERIAL CULTURE Colonization with *S. aureus* is very common in the nares and in the involved skin; almost 90% of patients with severe AD are secondarily colonized/infected. Look out for methicillin-resistant *S. aureus* (MRSA).

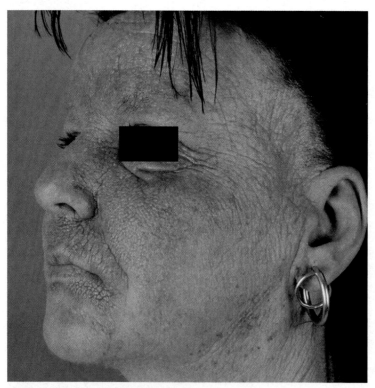

FIGURE 2-17   Adult atopic dermatitis Lichenification may also affect the face and neck as in this 32-year-old woman. Skin is exceedingly thickened and there is temporal alopecia and loss of lateral eyebrows caused by rubbing. Note typical infraorbital fold (Dennie Morgan sign).

VIRAL CULTURE Rule out herpes simplex virus (HSV) infection in crusted lesions (eczema herpeticum; see Section 27).
BLOOD STUDIES Increased IgE in serum, eosinophilia. HSV antigen detection for diagnosis of acute HSV infection.
DERMATOPATHOLOGY Various degrees of acanthosis with rare intraepidermal intercellular edema (spongiosis). The dermal infiltrate is composed of lymphocytes, monocytes, and mast cells with few or no eosinophils.

SPECIAL FORMS OF AD

Hand Dermatitis. Aggravated by wetting and washing with detergents, harsh soaps, and *disinfectants* leads to ICD in the atopic. Clinically indistinguishable from "normal" ICD (see page 20).
Exfoliative Dermatitis (see Section 8). Erythroderma in patients with extensive skin involvement. Generalized redness, scaling, weeping, crusting, lymphadenopathy, fever, and systemic toxicity.

COMPLICATIONS

Secondary infection with *S. aureus* and HSV (eczema herpeticum, see Section 27). Rarely keratoconjunctivitis and corneal ulcers caused by HSV.

COURSE AND PROGNOSIS

Untreated involved sites persist for months or years. Spontaneous, more or less complete remission during childhood occurs in >40% with occasional, recurrences during adolescence. In many patients, the disease persists for 15 to 20 years, but is less severe. Thirty to 50% of patients develop asthma and/or hay fever. *Adult-onset AD* exists and often runs a severe course. *S. aureus* infection leads to extensive erosions and crusting, and herpes simplex infection to eczema herpeticum, which may be life threatening (see Section 27).

MANAGEMENT

Education of the patient to avoid rubbing and scratching is most important. Use emollients.

An allergic workup is rarely helpful in uncovering an allergen. However, in patients who are hypersensitive to house dust mites, various pollens, and animal hair proteins, exposure to the appropriate allergen may cause flares. AD may exacerbate with emotional stress and sweating.

Patients should be warned of their special problems with herpes simplex and the superimposed staphylococcal infection.

Acute

1. Wet dressings and topical glucocorticoids; topical antibiotics (mupirocin ointment) when indicated.
2. Hydroxyzine, 10 to 100 mg four times daily for pruritus.
3. Oral antibiotics (dicloxacillin, erythromycin) to eliminate *S. aureus* and treat MRSA according to sensitivity as shown by culture.

Subacute and Chronic

1. Hydration (oilated baths or baths with oatmeal powder) followed by application of unscented emollients (e.g., hydrated petrolatum) is basic daily treatment to counteract xerosis; 12% ammonium lactate or 10% α-hydroxy acid lotion is very effective for xerosis. Soap showers are permissible for the body folds, but soap should seldom be used on the other parts of the skin surface.
2. Topical anti-inflammatory agents such as glucocorticoids, hydroxyquinoline preparations are the mainstays of treatment. Of these, glucocorticoids are the most effective. However, topical glucocorticoids may lead to skin atrophy if used for prolonged periods of time and if used excessively will lead to suppression of the pituitary–adrenal axis. Another problem is "glucocorticoid phobia." Patients or their parents are increasingly aware of glucocorticoid side effects and refuse their use, no matter how beneficial they may be.
3. The calcineurin inhibitors, tacrolimus and pimecrolimus, are gradually replacing glucocorticoids in most patients. They potently suppress itching and inflammation and do not lead to skin atrophy. They are usually not effective enough to suppress acute flares but work very well in minor flares and subacute AD.
4. Oral H_1-antihistamines are useful in reducing itching.
5. Systemic glucocorticoids should be avoided, except in rare instances of severe intractable disease in adults: prednisone, 60 to 80 mg daily for 2 days, then halving the dose each 2 days for the next 6 days. Patients with AD tend to become dependent on oral glucocorticoids. Often, small doses (5 to 10 mg) make the difference in control and can be reduced gradually to even 2.5 mg/d, as is often used for the control of asthma.

6. UVA–UVB phototherapy (combination of UVA plus UVB and increasing the radiation dose each treatment, with a frequency of two to three times weekly). Narrow band UV (311 nm) phototherapy and PUVA photo-chemotherapy are also effective.

7. In severe cases of adult AD and in normotensive healthy persons without renal disease, cyclosporine treatment (starting dose 5 mg/kg per day) is indicated when all other treatments fail, but should be monitored closely. Treatment is limited to 3 to 6 months because of potential side effects, including hypertension and reduced renal function. Blood pressure should be checked weekly and chemistry panels biweekly. Nifedipine can be used for moderate increases in blood pressure.

8. Patients should learn and use stress management techniques.

SUGGESTED ALGORITHM OF AD MANAGEMENT

- Baseline therapy of dryness with emollients.
- Suppression of mild-to-moderate AD by prolonged topical pimecrolimus or tacrolimus and continued emollients.
- Suppression of severe flares with topical glucocorticoids followed by pimecrolimus or tacrolimus and emollients.
- Oral and topical antibiotics to eliminate S. aureus.
- Hydroxyzine to suppress pruritus.

LICHEN SIMPLEX CHRONICUS (LSC) ICD-10: L28

- A special localized form of lichenification, occurring in circumscribed plaques.
- Occurs in individuals older than 20 years, is more frequent in women, and possibly more frequent in Asians.
- Results from repetitive rubbing and scratching.
- Skin symptoms consist of pruritus, often in paroxysms. The lichenified skin is like an erogenous zone as it becomes a pleasure (orgiastic) to scratch. The rubbing becomes automatic and reflexive, like an unconscious habit.
- Lichenification is a characteristic feature of AD, whether generalized or localized.
- A solid plaque of lichenification, arising from the confluence of small papules (Fig. 2-18). Skin is palpably thickened; skin markings (barely visible in normal skin) are accentuated and can be readily seen. Excoriations. Usually sharply defined. Isolated single lesion or several plaques. Nuchal area (female) (Fig. 2-18), scalp, ankles, lower legs, upper thighs, exterior forearms, vulva, pubis, anal area, scrotum, and groin. In African American and dark skin tones, lichenification may assume a special type of pattern consisting of multiple small (2 to 3 mm) closely set papules, a "follicular" pattern (as in Fig. 2-14B).
- LSC can last for decades unless the rubbing and scratching are stopped by treatment.
- Differential diagnosis includes a chronic pruritic plaque of psoriasis vulgaris, early stages of mycosis fungoides, ICD, ACD, and epidermal dermatophytosis.
- Management Difficult. Explain to the patient that rubbing and scratching must be stopped. Occlusive bandages can be used. Topical glucocorticoid preparations or tar preparations covered by occlusive dressings; if left for 24 h, glucocorticoids incorporated in adhesive plastic tape are also effective.
- Intralesional triamcinolone is often highly effective in smaller lesions (3 mg/mL; higher concentrations may cause atrophy). Oral hydroxyzine, 25 to 50 g at night, may be helpful.

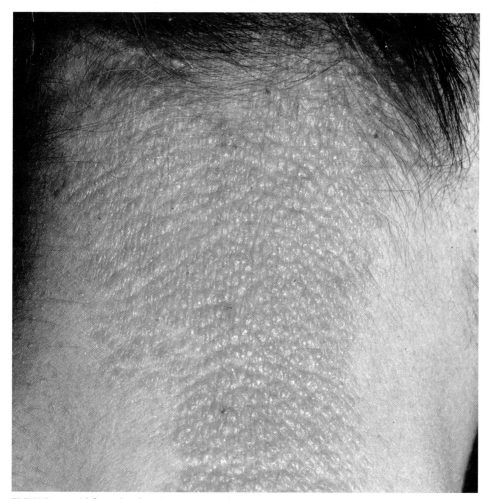

FIGURE 2-18 Lichen simplex chronicus Confluent, papular, follicular eczema, creating a plaque of lichen simplex chronicus of the posterior neck and occipital scalp. The condition had been present for many years as a result of chronic rubbing of the area.

PRURIGO NODULARIS (PN) ICD-10: L28.1

- Often associated with AD but can occur without AD.
- PN patients with AD are younger and have reactivity to environmental allergens; nonatopic PN patients are older and lack hypersensitivities to environmental allergens.
- PN usually occurs in younger or middle-aged females, who often exhibit signs of neurotic stigmatization.
- PN starts with piercing pruritus that leads to picking and scratching.
- Dome-shaped nodules—several millimeters to 2 cm—develop on sites in which persistent itching and scratching occur (Fig. 2-19). Nodules are often eroded, excoriated, and sometimes even ulcerated as patients dig into them with their nails.
- Usually multiple on the extremities.
- Lesions persist for months after the trauma has been discontinued.
- Treatment: intralesional triamcinolone, occlusive dressings with high-potency glucocorticoids. In severe cases, thalidomide 50 to 100 mg. Watch out for contraindications. Neurotonin 300 mg po tid is sometimes helpful.

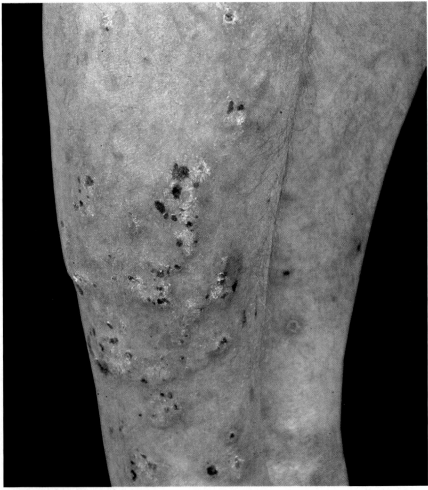

FIGURE 2-19 Prurigo nodularis Multiple, firm, excoriated nodules arising at sites of chronically picked or excoriated skin. Often occurring in patients with atopy but also without it. In this 56-year-old patient, the extreme pruritus necessitated multiple hospitalizations.

DYSHIDROTIC ECZEMATOUS DERMATITIS ICD-10: L30.1

- Dyshidrotic eczema is a special vesicular type of hand and foot dermatitis. Acute, chronic, or recurrent dermatosis of the fingers, palms, and soles.
- Sudden onset of many deep-seated pruritic, clear "tapioca-like" vesicles (Fig. 2-20).
- Large bullae can occur (pompholyx).
- Later scaling fissures and lichenification.
- Itching, when erosive painful.
- Secondary bacterial infection: pustules, cellulitis, lymphangitis, and painful lymphadenopathy.
- Recurrent attacks are the rule.
- Treatment: topical high-potency corticosteroids, intralesional triamcinolone 3 mg/mL for small areas; in severe cases, a short course of prednisone: starting with 70 mg and tapering by 10 or 5 mg over 7 or 14 days; systemic antibiotics for secondary infection and PUVA either oral or as "soaks" (page 60).

Synonyms: Pompholyx, vesicular palmar eczema.

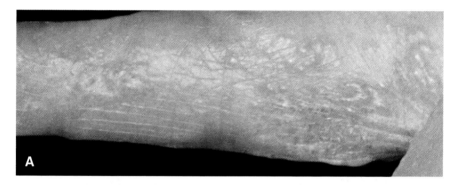

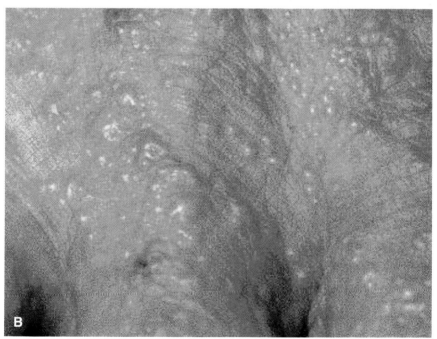

FIGURE 2-20 Dyshidrotic eczematous dermatitis Confluent tapioca-like vesicles on the lateral aspects of fingers (**A**) and finger webs and dorsa (**B**).

NUMMULAR ECZEMA ICD-10: L30.9

- Nummular eczema is a chronic, pruritic, inflammatory dermatitis occurring in the form of coin-shaped plaques composed of grouped small papules and vesicles on an erythematous base (Fig. 2-21).
- It is especially common on the extremities during winter months when xerosis is maximal; often seen in atopic individuals.
- *S. aureus* is often present but pathogenic significance has been not proven.
- Very pruritic. Course is chronic, lesions last from weeks to months.
- Management: Hydrate skin with moisturizer or moisturizing cream, topical glucocorticosteroids; PUVA or UVB-311 therapy can be very effective.

Synonyms: Discoid eczema, microbial eczema.

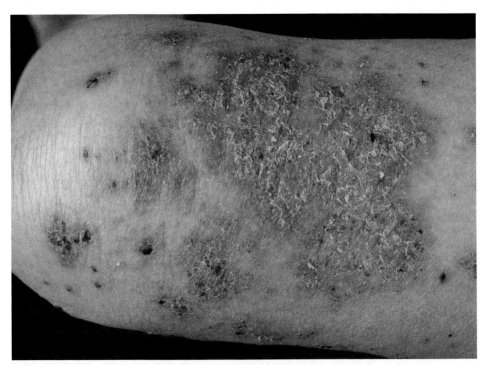

FIGURE 2-21 Nummular eczema Pruritic, round, nummular (coin-shaped) plaques with erythema, scales, and crusts that have coalesced on the upper arm.

AUTOSENSITIZATION DERMATITIS ICD-10: L30.9

- An often unrecognized generalized pruritic dermatitis directly related to a primary dermatitis elsewhere.
- For example, a patient with venous stasis dermatitis on the lower legs may develop pruritic, symmetric, scattered, erythematous, maculopapular, or papulovesicular lesions on the trunk, forearms, thighs, or legs.
- These persist and spread until the basic underlying primary dermatitis is controlled.
- Similarly, autosensitization may occur as an "id" reaction in inflammatory tinea pedis and manifests as a dyshidrosiform, vesicular eruption on the feet and hands (**Fig. 2-22**) and papulovesicular eczematoid lesions on the trunk.
- The phenomenon results from the release of cytokines in the primary dermatitis, as a result of sensitization. These cytokines circulate in the blood and heighten the sensitivity of the distant skin areas.
- The diagnosis of autosensitization dermatitis is often *post hoc*; i.e., the distant eruption disappears when the primary dermatitis is controlled.
- Oral glucocorticoids hasten the disappearance of the lesions.

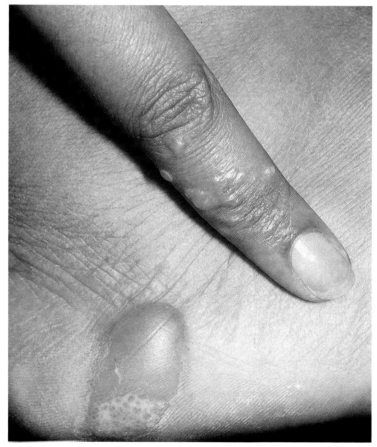

FIGURE 2-22 Autosensitization dermatitis ("id" reaction): dermatophytid Vesicles and bullae on the finger and the lateral foot of a 21-year-old female. Bullous (inflammatory) tinea pedis was present and was associated with dermatophytid reaction. Prednisone was given for 2 weeks; pruritus and vesiculation resolved.

SEBORRHEIC DERMATITIS ICD-10: L21.9

- A very common chronic dermatosis characterized by redness and scaling, which occurs in regions where the sebaceous glands are most active, such as the face and scalp, the presternal area, and in the body folds. Mild scalp SD causes flaking, i.e., dandruff.
- Hereditary diathesis, but *Malassezia furfur* may play a pathogenic role.
- Increased incidence in Parkinson disease and in immunosuppressed patients (HIV/AIDS).

Synonyms: "Cradle cap" (infants), pityriasis sicca (dandruff).

EPIDEMIOLOGY AND ETIOLOGY

AGE OF ONSET Infancy (within the first months), puberty, or most between often 20 and 50 years or older.
SEX More common in males.
INCIDENCE Two to five percent of the population.

PATHOGENESIS, PREDISPOSING, AND AGGRAVATING FACTORS

There is a hereditary diathesis, the so-called seborrheic state, with marked seborrheic and marginal blepharitis. May be associated with psoriasis as a "prepsoriasis state," and the mix of superficial scales on scalp and eyebrows and psoriasiform plaques on the trunk suggest the use of the term seborrhiasis. *M. furfur* may play a role as suggested by the response to ketoconazole and selenium sulfide. There is an increase in incidence in Parkinson disease and facial paralysis and in immunosuppressed patients (HIV/AIDS and cardiac transplants). SD-like lesions occur in nutritional deficiencies (zinc deficiency, niacin, and pyridoxine deficiency). Intractable SD should be a clue to the existence of HIV disease (see Section 27).

CLINICAL MANIFESTATION

DURATION OF LESIONS Gradual onset.
SEASONAL VARIATIONS Some patients are worse in winter in a dry, indoor environment. Sunlight exposure causes SD to flare in a few patients and promotes improvement of the condition in others.
SKIN SYMPTOMS Pruritus is variable, often increased by perspiration.
SKIN LESIONS Orange-red or gray-white skin, often with "greasy" or white dry scaling macules, papules of varying size (5 to 20 mm), or patches, rather sharply marginated (Fig. 2-23).

On the scalp, there is mostly marked scaling ("dandruff"), diffuse involvement of scalp. Scattered, discrete on the face. Nummular, polycyclic, and even annular on the trunk.
DISTRIBUTION AND MAJOR TYPES OF LESIONS (BASED ON LOCALIZATION AND AGE) Hairy Areas of Head. Scalp, eyebrows, eyelashes (blepharitis), beard (follicular orifices); cradle cap: erythema and yellow-orange scales and crusts on the scalp of infants.
Face. The flush ("butterfly") areas on forehead ("corona seborrhoica"), nasolabial folds, eyebrows, and glabella (Fig. 2-23). Ears: retroauricular, meatus, sticky crusts, and fissures.
Trunk. Simulating lesions of pityriasis rosea or pityriasis versicolor; yellowish-brown patches over the sternum common.
Body Folds. Axillae, groins, anogenital area, submammary areas, umbilicus, and diaper area in infants (Fig. 2-24)—presents as a diffuse, exudative, sharply marginated, brightly erythematous eruption; erosions and fissures common.
Genitalia. Often with yellow crusts and psoriasiform lesions.

DIAGNOSIS/DIFFERENTIAL DIAGNOSIS

Made on clinical criteria.
RED SCALY PLAQUES Common. Mild psoriasis vulgaris (sometimes may be indistinguishable), impetigo (rule out by smears for bacteria), dermatophytosis, pityriasis versicolor, intertriginous candidiasis (rule out dermatophytes and yeasts by KOH), subacute lupus erythematosus (rule out by biopsy), "seborrheic" papules in secondary syphilis (rule out *Treponema pallidum by dark field*); syphilis serology.
Rare. Langerhans cell histiocytosis (occurs in infants, often associated with purpura), acrodermatitis enteropathica, zinc deficiency, pemphigus foliaceus, glucagonoma syndrome.

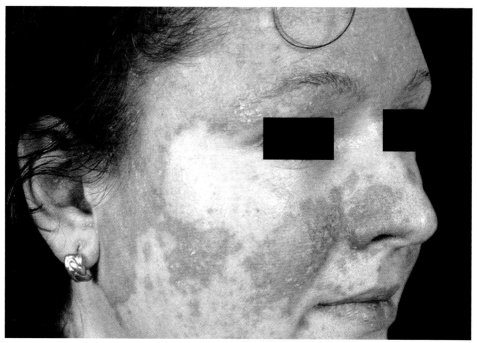

FIGURE 2-23 Seborrheic dermatitis of face: adult type Erythema and yellow-orange scaling of the forehead, cheeks, and nasolabial folds. Scalp and retroauricular areas were also involved.

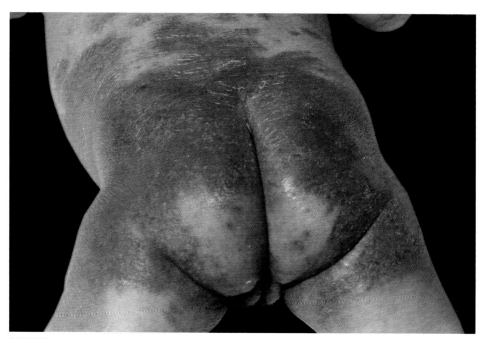

FIGURE 2-24 Seborrheic dermatitis: infantile type Erythema scales and crusting in the diaper region of an infant. This is difficult to distinguish in the diaper region from psoriasis and *Candida* has to be ruled out by KOH.

LABORATORY STUDIES

DERMATOPATHOLOGY Focal parakeratosis, with few neutrophils, moderate acanthosis, spongiosis (intercellular edema), and nonspecific inflammation of the dermis. Neutrophils at the tips of the dilated follicular openings, which appear as crusts/scales.

COURSE AND PROGNOSIS

The condition improves in the summer and flares in the fall. Recurrences and remissions, especially on the scalp, may be associated with alopecia in severe cases. Infantile and adolescent SD disappears with age. Seborrheic erythroderma may occur. *Seborrheic erythroderma with diarrhea and failure to thrive in infants (Leiner disease) is associated with a variety of immunodeficiency disorders including defective yeast opsonization, C3 deficiency, severe combined immunodeficiency, hypogammaglobulinemia, and hyperimmunoglobulinemia.*

MANAGEMENT

Requires initial therapy followed by chronic maintenance therapy.

Initial Topical Therapy

SCALP Adults. *Shampoos* containing selenium sulfide, zinc pyrithione, and/or tar. 2% ketoconazole shampoo is very effective; lather can be used on face and chest during shower. Low-potency *glucocorticoid* solution, lotion, or gels following a medicated shampoo (ketoconazole or tar) for more severe cases. Pimecrolimus, 1% cream, is very beneficial.

Infants. For cradle cap, removal of crusts with warm olive oil compresses, followed by baby shampoo, 2% ketoconazole shampoo, and application of 1 to 2.5% hydrocortisone cream, 2% ketoconazole cream, and 1% pimecrolimus cream.

FACE AND TRUNK *Ketoconazole shampoo*, 2%. Glucocorticoid cream and lotions. 2% ketoconazole cream, 1% pimecrolimus cream, and 0.03% or 0.1% tacrolimus ointment.

EYELIDS Gentle removal of the crusts in the morning with a cotton ball dipped in diluted baby shampoo. Sodium sulfacetamide in a suspension containing 0.2% prednisolone and 0.12% phenylephrine. Sodium sulfacetamide ointment alone is also effective, as is 2% ketoconazole cream, 1% pimecrolimus cream, or 0.03% tacrolimus ointment.

INTERTRIGINOUS AREAS *Ketoconazole, 2%.* If uncontrolled with these treatments, Castellani paint for dermatitis of the body folds is often very effective, but staining is a problem. Pimecrolimus cream, 1%; tacrolimus ointment, 0.03% or 0.1%.

Systemic Therapy

In severe cases, 13-*cis*-retinoic acid orally, 0.5 to 1 mg/kg, is highly effective. Contraception should be used in females of childbearing age. In milder cases, itraconazole 100 mg twice daily on two consecutive days, once a month, is effective.

Maintenance Therapy

Ketoconazole 2% shampoo, tar shampoos, and ketoconazole cream are effective. 1 to 2.5% hydrocortisone cream daily will work, but patients should be monitored for signs of atrophy; 1% pimecrolimus cream and 0.03% tacrolimus ointment are also safe and effective.

ASTEATOTIC DERMATITIS ICD-10: L30.9

- A common pruritic dermatitis that occurs especially in older persons, in temperate climates during the winter—related to the low humidity of heated houses.
- The sites of predilection are the legs (Fig. 2-25), arms, and hands but also the trunk.
- Dry, "cracked," superficially fissured skin with slight scaling.
- The incessant pruritus can lead to lichenification, which can even persist when the environmental conditions have been corrected.
- The disorder results from too frequent bathing in hot soapy baths or showers and/or in older persons living in rooms with a high environmental temperature and low relative humidity.
- Management: Avoiding overbathing with soap, especially tub baths, and increasing the ambient humidity to >50%, by using room humidifiers; also using tepid water baths containing bath oils for hydration, followed by immediate liberal application of emollient ointments, such as hydrated petrolatum. If skin is inflamed, use medium-potency glucocorticoid ointments, applied twice daily until the eczematous component has resolved.

Synonyms: Eczema *craquelé* (French *craquelé*, "marred with cracks," such as in old china and ceramic tile)

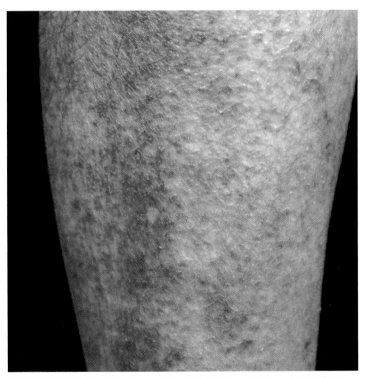

FIGURE 2-25 Asteatotic dermatitis In this 65-year-old man, lesions have coalesced to involve the entire skin of the lower leg.

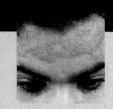

PSORIASIS, PSORIASIFORM, AND PITYRIASIFORM DERMATOSES

PSORIASIS

- Psoriasis affects 1.5 to 2% of the population in Western countries but has worldwide occurrence.
- A chronic disorder with polygenic predisposition and triggering environmental factors such as bacterial infection, trauma, or drugs.
- Several clinical expressions. Typical lesions are chronic, recurring, scaly papules, and plaques. Pustular eruptions and erythroderma occur.
- Clinical presentation varies among individuals, from those with only a few localized plaques to those with generalized skin involvement.
- Psoriatic erythroderma is psoriasis involving the entire skin.
- Psoriatic arthritis occurs in 10 to 25% of patients.

CLASSIFICATION

Psoriasis vulgaris
  Acute guttate
  Chronic stable plaque
  Palmoplantar
  Inverse

Psoriatic erythroderma
Pustular psoriasis
  Pustular psoriasis of von Zumbusch
  Palmoplantar pustulosis
  Acrodermatitis continua

PSORIASIS VULGARIS ICD-10: L40.0

EPIDEMIOLOGY

AGE OF ONSET All ages. *Early*: Peak incidence occurs at 22.5 years of age (in children, the mean age of onset is 8 years). *Late*: Presents around age 55. *Early onset* predicts a more severe and long-lasting disease, and there is usually a positive family history of psoriasis.
INCIDENCE Occurs in about 1.5 to 2% of the population in Western countries. In the United States, there are 3 to 5 million persons with psoriasis. Most have localized psoriasis, but in approximately 300,000 persons psoriasis is generalized.
SEX Equal incidence in males and females.
RACE Low incidence in West Africans, Japanese, and Inuits; very low incidence or absence in North and South American Indians.
HEREDITY Polygenic trait. When one parent has psoriasis, 8% of his or her offspring develop psoriasis; when both parents have psoriasis, 41% of their children develop psoriasis. HLA types most frequently associated with psoriasis

are HLA- B13, B37, -B57, and, most importantly, HLA-Cw6, which is a candidate for functional involvement.
TRIGGER FACTORS *Physical trauma* (rubbing and scratching) is a major factor in eliciting lesions. Acute streptococcal infection precipitates guttate psoriasis. *Stress* is a factor in flares of psoriasis and is said to be as high as 40% in adults and even higher in children. *Drugs*: Systemic glucocorticoids, oral lithium, antimalarial drugs, interferon, and β-adrenergic blockers can cause flares and cause a psoriasiform drug eruption. *Alcohol ingestion* is a putative trigger factor.

PATHOGENESIS

The most obvious abnormalities in psoriasis are (1) an alteration of the cell kinetics of keratinocytes with a shortening of the cell cycle resulting in 28 times the normal production of epidermal cells and (2) CD8+ T cells, which are the overwhelming T cell population in lesions. The epidermis and dermis react as an integrated system: the described changes in the germinative layer of the epidermis and inflammatory changes in the dermis, which trigger the epidermal changes. Psoriasis is a T cell–driven disease and the cytokine spectrum is that of a T_H1 response. Maintenance of psoriatic lesions is considered an ongoing autoreactive immune response driven by TNFα, IL-17 and IL-23.

CLINICAL MANIFESTATION

There are two major types:

1. *Eruptive, inflammatory type* with multiple small lesions and a greater tendency toward spontaneous resolution (Figs. 3-1 and 3-2); relatively rare (<2.0% of all psoriasis).
2. *Chronic stable (plaque) psoriasis* (Figs. 3-3 and 3-4). Majority of patients, with chronic indolent lesions present for months and years, changing only slowly.

SKIN SYMPTOMS Pruritus is reasonably common, especially in scalp and anogenital psoriasis.

Acute Guttate Type. Salmon-pink papules (guttate: Latin *gutta*, "drop"), 2.0 mm to 1.0 cm with or without scales (Figs. 3-1 and 3-2); scales may not be visible but become apparent upon scraping. Scales are lamellar, loose, and easily removed by scratching. Removal of scale results in the appearance of minute blood droplets (*Auspitz sign*). Scattered discrete lesions; generally on the trunk (Fig. 3-2); may resolve spontaneously or become recurrent and evolve into chronic, stable psoriasis.

Chronic Stable Type. Sharply marginated, dull-red plaques with loosely adherent, lamellar, silvery-white scales (Fig. 3-3). Plaques coalesce to form polycyclic, geographic lesions (Fig. 3-4) and may partially regress, resulting in annular, serpiginous, and arciform patterns. Lamellar scaling can easily be removed, but when the lesion is extremely chronic, it adheres tightly resembling an oyster shell (Fig. 3-3).

Distribution and Predilection Sites

Acute Guttate. Disseminated, generalized, mainly trunk.

Chronic Stable. Single lesion or lesions localized to one or more predilection sites: elbows,

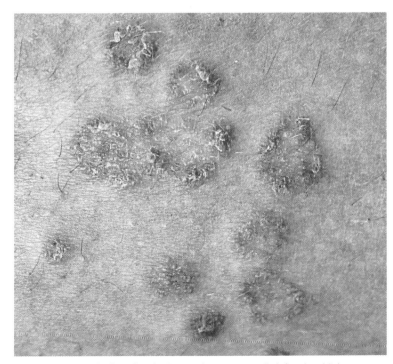

FIGURE 3-1 Psoriasis vulgaris Primary lesions are well-defined, reddish, or salmon-pink papules, droplike, with a loosely adherent silvery-white lamellar scale.

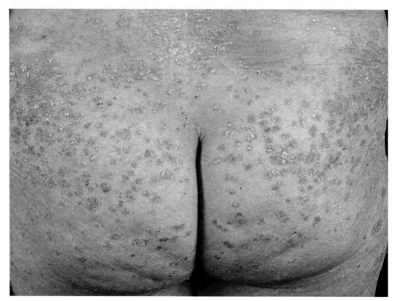

FIGURE 3-2 Psoriasis vulgaris: buttocks (guttate type) Small, discrete, erythematous, scaling, papules that tend to coalesce, appearing after a group A streptococcal pharyngitis. There was a family history of psoriasis.

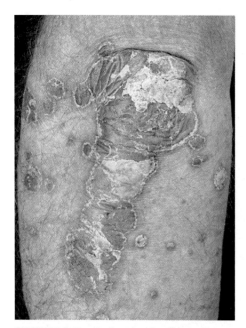

FIGURE 3-3 Psoriasis vulgaris: elbow Chronic stable plaque psoriasis on the elbow. In this location, scales can either accumulate to oyster shell-like hyperkeratosis, or are shed in large sheets revealing a beefy-red base. This plaque has arisen from the coalescence of smaller, papular lesions that can still be seen on the lower arm.

knees, sacral gluteal region, scalp, and palm/soles (Fig. 3-5). Sometimes only regional involvement (scalp), often generalized.
Pattern. Bilateral, often symmetric (predilection sites, Fig. 3-5); often spares exposed areas.
Psoriasis in Skin of Color. In people with darker skin tones, psoriasis lacks the bright red color. Lesions are brown to black but otherwise their morphology is the same as in lighter skin.

Special Sites

PALMS AND SOLES May be the only areas involved. There is massive silvery white or yellowish hyperkeratosis, which is not easily removed (Fig. 3-6B). The inflammatory plaque at the base is always sharply demarcated (Fig. 3-6A). There may be cracking, painful fissures and bleeding.
SCALP Plaques, sharply marginated, with thick adherent scales (Fig. 3-7). Often very pruritic. *Note:* Psoriasis of the scalp does not lead to hair loss. Scalp psoriasis may be part of generalized psoriasis or the only site involved.
FACE Uncommon but when involved, usually associated with a refractory type of psoriasis (Figs. 3-7 and 3-8).
CHRONIC PSORIASIS OF THE PERIANAL AND GENITAL REGIONS AND OF THE BODY FOLDS—INVERSE PSORIASIS Resulting from the warm and moist environment in these regions, plaques usually

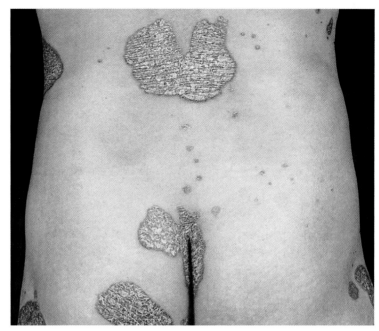

FIGURE 3-4 Psoriasis vulgaris: chronic stable type Multiple large scaling plaques on the trunk, buttock, and legs. Lesions are round or polycyclic and conflu-ent forming geographic patterns. Although this is the classical manifestation of chronic stable plaque psoriasis, the eruption is still ongoing, as evidenced by the small guttate lesions in the lumbar and lower back area. This patient was cleared by acitretin/PUVA combination treatment within 4 weeks.

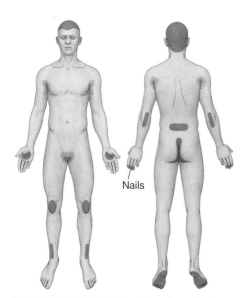

Nails

FIGURE 3-5 Predilection sites of psoriasis.

not scaly but macerated, often bright red and fissured (Fig. 3-9). Sharp demarcation permits distinction from intertrigo, candidiasis, and contact dermatitis.

NAILS Fingernails and toenails frequently (25%) involved, especially with concomitant arthri-tis (Fig. 3-10). Nail changes include pitting, subungual hyperkeratosis, onycholysis, and yellowish-brown spots under the nail plate—the *oil spot* (pathognomonic) (see Section 32, Disorders of the Nail Apparatus).

LABORATORY EXAMINATIONS

Dermatopathology

Marked overall thickening of the epidermis (acanthosis) and thinning of epidermis over elongated dermal papillae. Increased mitosis of keratinocytes, fibroblasts, and endothelial cells. Parakeratotic hyperkeratosis (nuclei retained in the stratum corneum). Inflammatory cells in

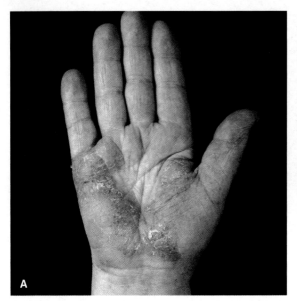
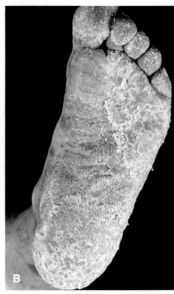

FIGURE 3-6 **(A) Psoriasis, palmar involvement** The palm shows adherent scales with fissures. The base is erythematous and there is a sharp margin on the wrist. **(B) Psoriasis vulgaris: soles** Erythematous plaques with thick, yellowish, lamellar scale and desquamation on sites of pressure arising on the plantar feet. Note sharp demarcation of the inflammatory lesion on the arch of the foot. Similar lesions were present on the palms.

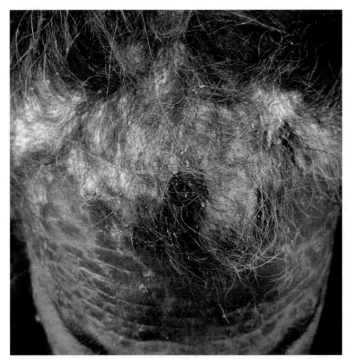

FIGURE 3-7 **Psoriasis of the scalp** There is massive compaction of horny material on the entire scalp. In some areas, the thick asbestos-like scales compact hairs but do not lead to alopecia. Note also that the forehead is involved.

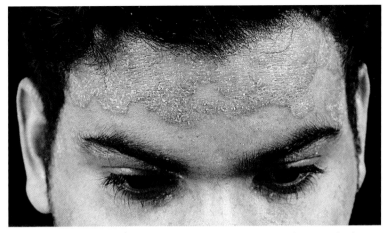

FIGURE 3-8 Psoriasis, facial involvement Classic psoriatic plaque on the forehead of a 21-year-old male who also had massive scalp involvement.

the dermis (lymphocytes and monocytes) and in the epidermis (lymphocytes and polymorphonuclear cells), forming microabscesses of Munro in the stratum corneum.

SERUM Increased antistreptolysin titer in acute guttate psoriasis with antecedent streptococcal infection. Sudden onset of psoriasis may be associated with HIV infection—do HIV serology. Serum uric acid is increased in 50% of patients, usually correlated with the extent of the disease; there is an increased risk of gouty arthritis.

CULTURE Throat culture for group A β-hemolytic streptococcus infection.

DIAGNOSIS AND DIFFERENTIAL DIAGNOSIS

Diagnosis is made on clinical grounds.

ACUTE GUTTATE PSORIASIS Any maculopapular drug eruption, secondary syphilis, pityriasis rosea.

SMALL SCALING PLAQUES *Seborrheic dermatitis*— may be indistinguishable from psoriasis.

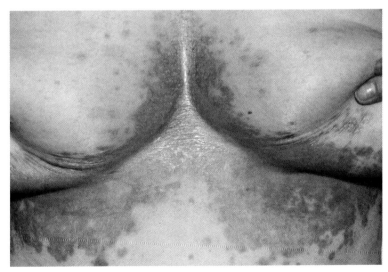

FIGURE 3-9 Psoriasis vulgaris: inverse pattern Because of the moist and warm environment in the submammary region, scales have been macerated and shed revealing a brightly erythematous and glistening base.

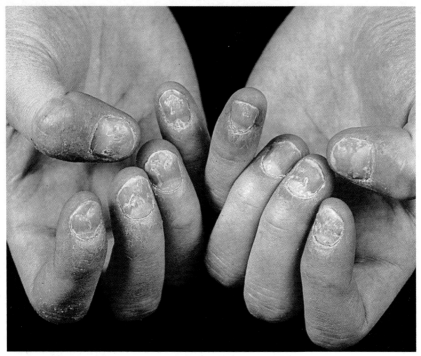

FIGURE 3-10 Psoriasis of the fingernails Pits have progressed to elkonyxis (holes in the nail plates), and there is transverse and longitudinal ridging. This patient also has paronychial psoriasis and psoriatic arthritis (for further images of nail involvement, see Section 32).

Lichen simplex chronicus. Psoriasiform drug eruptions—especially beta-blockers, gold, and methyldopa. *Tinea corporis*—KOH examination is mandatory, particularly in single lesions. *Mycosis fungoides*—scaling plaques can be an initial stage of mycosis fungoides. Biopsy.

LARGE GEOGRAPHIC PLAQUES Tinea corporis, mycosis fungoides.

SCALP PSORIASIS Seborrheic dermatitis, tinea capitis.

INVERSE PSORIASIS Tinea, candidiasis, intertrigo, extramammary Paget disease (Section 19). *Glucagonoma syndrome* (Section 19)—An important differential because this is a serious disease; the lesions look like inverse psoriasis. Langerhans cell histiocytosis (see Section 20), Hailey–Hailey disease (page 92).

NAILS Onychomycosis. KOH is mandatory.

COMORBIDITIES

Psoriasis is associated with increased morbidity and mortality from cardiovascular events. Metabolic syndrome is 3-fold more frequent in psoriatic patients, with hypertension and hyperlipidemia being the most common findings.

COURSE AND PROGNOSIS

Acute guttate psoriasis appears rapidly, a generalized "rash." Sometimes this type of psoriasis disappears spontaneously in a few weeks without any treatment. More often, it evolves into chronic plaque psoriasis. This is stable and may undergo remission after months or years, recur, then be a lifelong companion.

PUSTULAR PSORIASIS

- Characterized by pustules, not papules, arising on normal or inflamed, erythematous skin. Two types.

PALMOPLANTAR PUSTULOSIS ICD-10: L40.3

- Incidence low as compared with psoriasis vulgaris.
- A chronic relapsing eruption limited to palms and soles.
- Numerous sterile, yellow; deep-seated pustules (Fig. 3-11) that evolve into dusky-red crusts.
- Considered by some as localized pustular psoriasis (Barber-type) and by others a separate entity.

FIGURE 3-11 Palmar pustulosis Creamy-yellow pustules that are partially confluent on the palm of a 28-year-old female. Pustules are sterile and pruritic, and when they get larger, become painful. At the time of this eruption, there was no other evidence of psoriasis anywhere else on the body, but 2 years later the patient developed chronic stable plaque psoriasis on the trunk.

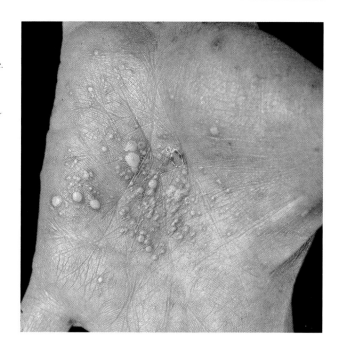

GENERALIZED ACUTE PUSTULAR PSORIASIS (VON ZUMBUSCH) ICD-10: L40.1

- A rare, life-threatening medical problem with abrupt onset.
- Burning, fiery-red erythema topped by pinpoint sterile yellow pustules in clusters spreading within hours over the entire body. Coalescing lesions form "lakes" of pus (Fig. 3-12). Easily wiped off.
- Waves of pustules follow each other.
- Fever, malaise, and leukocytosis.
- Symptoms: burning, painful; patient appears frightened.
- Onycholysis and shedding of nails; hair loss of the telogen defluvium type (Section 31), 2 to 3 months later; circinate desquamation of tongue.
- Pathogenesis unknown. Fever and leukocytosis result from release of cytokines and chemokines into circulation.
- Differential diagnosis: pustular drug eruption (see Section 23); generalized HSV infection (Section 27).
- May follow, evolve, or be followed by psoriasis vulgaris.
- Special types: *Impetigo herpetiformis*: generalized pustular psoriasis in pregnant woman with hypocalcemia. *Annular type*: in children with less constitutional symptoms (Fig. 3-13A). *Psoriasis cum pustulatione* (psoriasis vulgaris with pustulation: In maltreated psoriasis vulgaris. No constitutional symptoms. *Acrodermatitis continua of Hallopeau*: Chronic recurrent pustulation of nail folds, nail beds, and distal fingers leading to nail loss (Fig. 3-13B). Occurs alone or with generalized pustular psoriasis.

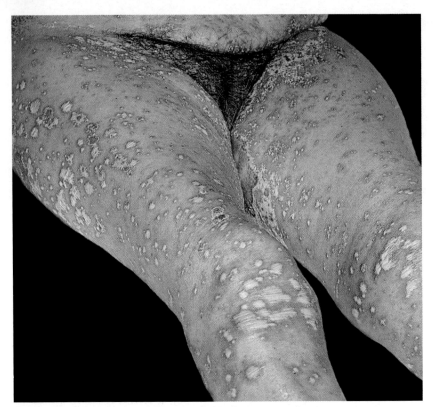

FIGURE 3-12 Generalized acute pustular psoriasis (von Zumbusch) This female patient was toxic and had fever and peripheral leukocytosis. The entire body was covered with showers of creamy-white coalescing pustules on a fiery-red base. Since these pustules are very superficial, they can be literally wiped off, which results in red, oozing erosions.

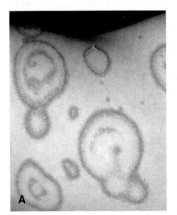

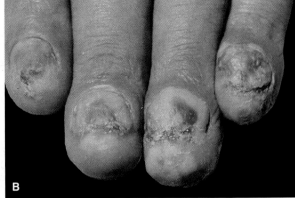

FIGURE 3-13 (A) Anular pustular psoriasis This rare condition occurs mainly in children and consists of expanding ring-like micropustular eruptions on a highly inflammatory base that is clear in the center and results in a collarette-like scaling at the margin. There is hardly any systemic toxicity. **(B) Acrodermatitis continua of Hallopeau** with acral pustule formation, subungual lakes of pus, and destruction of nail plates. This may lead to permanent loss of nails and scarring.

PSORIATIC ERYTHRODERMA ICD-10: L40

In this condition, psoriasis involves the entire skin. See Section 8.

PSORIATIC ARTHRITIS ICD-10: L40.5

- Seronegative. Psoriatic arthritis is included among the seronegative spondyloarthropathies, which include ankylosing spondylitis, enteropathic arthritis, and reactive arthritis.
- Asymmetric peripheral joint involvement of upper extremities and especially distal interphalangeal joints. Dactylitis—sausage fingers (Fig. 3-14).
- Axial form involves vertebral column, sacroiliitis.
- Enthesitis: inflammation of ligament insertion into bone.
  Mutilating with bone erosions, osteolysis, or ankylosis. Telescoping fingers. Functional impairment.
- Often associated with psoriasis of nails (Figs. 3-10 and 3-14).
- Associated with MHC class I antigens, whereas rheumatoid arthritis is associated with MHC class II antigens.
- Incidence is 5 to 8%. Rare before age 20.
- *May be present (in 10% of individuals) without any visible psoriasis; if so, search for a family history.*

MANAGEMENT OF PSORIASIS

Factors Influencing Selection of Treatment

1. Age: childhood, adolescence, young adulthood, middle age, >60 years.
2. Type of psoriasis: guttate, plaque, palmar and palmopustular, generalized pustular psoriasis, erythrodermic psoriasis.
3. Site and extent of involvement: *localized* to palms and soles, scalp, anogenital area, scattered plaques but <5% involvement; *generalized* and >30% involvement.
4. Previous treatment: ionizing radiation, systemic glucocorticoids, photochemotherapy (PUVA), cyclosporine (CS), and methotrexate (MTX).
5. Associated medical disorders (e.g., HIV disease).

Management of psoriasis is discussed in the context of types of psoriasis, sites, and extent of involvement. Psoriasis has to be managed by a dermatologist.

LOCALIZED PSORIASIS (Fig. 3-3)

- *Topical fluorinated glucocorticoid* covered with plastic wrap. Glucocorticoid-impregnated tape also useful. Beware of glucocosteroid side effects.
- *Hydrocolloid dressing,* left on for 24 to 48 h, is effective and prevents scratching.
- For small plaques (≤4 cm), *triamcinolone acetonide* aqueous suspension 3 mg/mL

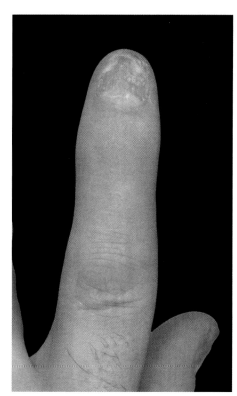

FIGURE 3-14 Psoriatic arthritis Dactylitis of index finger. Note sausage-like thickening over interphalangeal joints. There is psoriasis of the nail.

diluted with normal saline injected *intradermally* into lesions. Beware of hypopigmentation in skin of color.

- Topical *anthralin* is also effective but is an irritant.
- *Vitamin D analogues* (calcipotriene, ointment and cream) are good nonsteroidal antipsoriatic topical agents but less effective than corticosteroids; they are not associated with cutaneous atrophy; they can be combined with corticosteroids. Topical tacrolimus, 0.1%, is similarly effective.
- Topical pimecrolimus, 1%, is effective in inverse psoriasis and seborrheic dermatitis-like psoriasis of the face and ear canals.
- *Tazarotene* (a topical retinoid, 0.05 and 0.1% gel) has similar efficacy, best combined with class II topical glucocorticoids.
- All these topical treatments can be combined with 311-nm UVB phototherapy or PUVA.

SCALP Superficial scaling and lacking thick plaques: Tar or ketoconazole shampoos *followed by* betamethasone valerate, 1% lotion; if refractory, clobetasol propionate, 0.05% scalp application. In thick, adherent plaques (Fig. 3-7): scales have to be removed by 10% salicylic acid in mineral oil, covered with a plastic cap and left on overnight before embarking on topical therapy. If this is unsuccessful, consider systemic treatment (see below).

PALMS AND SOLES (Fig. 3-6) Occlusive dressings with class I topical *glucocorticoids*. If ineffective, *PUVA* either systemically or as *PUVA* soaks (immersion in 8-methoxypsoralen solution and subsequent UVA exposure). Retinoids (acitretin > isotretinoin), orally, removes the thick hyperkeratosis of the palms and soles. However, a combination with topical glucocorticoids or PUVA (re-PUVA) is much more efficacious. Systemic treatments should be considered.

PALMOPLANTAR PUSTULOSIS (Fig. 3-11) PUVA *soaks* and glucocorticosteroids are effective. Systemic treatment for recalcitrant cases.

Inverse Psoriasis (Fig. 3-9). *Topical glucocorticoids* (caution: these are atrophy-prone regions; steroids should be applied for only limited periods of time); switch to topical vitamin D derivatives such as tazarotene, topical tacrolimus, or pimecrolimus. If resistant or recurrent, consider systemic therapy.

NAILS (Fig. 3-10) Topical treatments of the fingernails are unsatisfactory. Systemic MTX and CS therapy are effective but take time and are thus prone to side effects.

GENERALIZED PSORIASIS

ACUTE, GUTTATE PSORIASIS (Fig. 3-2) Treat streptococcal infection with antibiotics. Narrowband (311 nm) UVB irradiation most effective.

GENERALIZED PLAQUE-TYPE PSORIASIS (Fig. 3-4) PUVA or systemic treatments that are given as either mono—or combined—or rotational therapy. Combination therapy denotes the combination of two or more modalities, while rotational therapy denotes switching the patient after clearing and a subsequent relapse to another different treatment.

NARROWBAND UVB PHOTOTHERAPY (311 nm) Effective only in thin plaques; effectiveness is increased by combination with topical glucocorticoids, vitamin D analogues, tazarotene, or topical tacrolimus/pimecrolimus.

ORAL PUVA Treatment consists of oral ingestion of 8-methoxypsoralen (8-MOP) (0.6 mg 8-MOP per kilogram body weight) or, in some European countries, 5-MOP (1.2 mg/kg body weight) and exposure to doses of UVA that are adjusted to the sensitivity of the patient. Most patients clear after 19 to 25 treatments, and the amount of UVA needed ranges from 100 to 245 J/cm^2. *Long-Term Side Effects* PUVA keratoses and squamous cell carcinomas in some patients who receive an excessive number of treatments.

ORAL RETINOIDS Acitretin and isotretinoin are effective in inducing desquamation but only moderately effective in clearing psoriatic plaques. Highly effective when combined with 311-nm UVB or PUVA (called re-PUVA). *The latter is in fact the most effective therapy to date for generalized plaque psoriasis.*

METHOTREXATE THERAPY Oral MTX is one of the most effective treatments but response is slow and long-term treatment is required. Hepatic toxicity may occur after cumulative doses in normal persons ($\geq$1.5 g). *The Triple-Dose (Weinstein) Regimen* Preferred by most over the single-dose MTX once weekly, 5 mg is given every 12 h for a total of three doses, i.e., 15 mg/week. Achieves an 80% improvement but total clearing only in some, and higher doses increase the risk of toxicity. When patients respond, the dose of MTX can be reduced by 2.5 mg periodically. Determine liver enzymes, complete blood count, and serum creatinine periodically. Be aware of the various drug interactions with MTX.

CYCLOSPORINE[1] CS treatment is highly effective at a dose of 3 to 5 mg/kg per day. If the patient responds, the dose is tapered to the lowest effective maintenance dose. Monitoring blood pressure and serum creatinine is mandatory because of the known nephrotoxicity of the drug. Watch out for drug interactions.

MONOCLONAL ANTIBODIES AND FUSION PROTEINS[1] (so-called biologicals). Some of these proteins, specifically targeted to pathogenically relevant receptors on T cells or to cytokines, have been approved and more are being developed. They should be employed only by specifically trained dermatologists who are familiar with the dosage schedules, drug interactions, and short- or long-term side effects.

Alefacept is a human lymphocyte function-associated antigen (LFA)-3-IgG1 fusion protein that prevents interaction of LFA-3 and CD2. Given intramuscularly once weekly leads to considerable improvement and there may be long periods of remissions, but some patients do not respond.

Tumor Necrosis Factor-Alpha (TNF-α) *antagonists* that are effective in psoriasis are infliximab, adalimumab, and etanercept. *Infliximab* is a chimeric monoclonal antibody to TNF-α. Administered intravenously at weeks 0, 2, and 6, it is highly effective in psoriasis and psoriatic arthritis. *Adalimumab* is a fully human recombinant monoclonal antibody that specifically targets TNF-α. It is administered subcutaneously every other week and is similarly effective as infliximab. *Etanercept* is a human recombinant, soluble TNF-α receptor that neutralizes TNF-α activity. Administered subcutaneously twice weekly and is less effective than infliximab and adalimumab but is highly effective in psoriatic arthritis.

Ustekinumab (Anti-Interleukin (IL) 12/Interleukin 23 p40) is a human IgG1κ monoclonal antibody that binds to the common p40 subunit of human IL-12 and IL-23, preventing its interaction with its receptor. Given every 4 months subcutaneously, it is highly effective.

Sekinumab is an anti-IL-17 recombinant fully human monocloncal antibody that neutralizes the proinflammatory cytokine IL-17A. It is

delivered subcutaneously at weeks 0, 1, 2, and 3 followed by monthly maintenance doses of 300 mg. It is rapidly effective, even more effective than Ustekinumab, and is approved by EMA for the treatment of plaque psoriasis in adults.

Apremilast is a "small molecule", phosphodiesterase-4 inhibitor which can be administered orally and leads to a reduction of proinflammatory cytokines (TNFα, IL-23, IL-17) and thus to a down regulation of the inflammatory process. Doses start with 10 mg PO daily, which is gradually increased to 300 mg bid. A PASI 75 response at 16 weeks is 33%, which means a significant improvement.

All these biologicals and others currently developed in clinical trials have side effects, and there are long-term safety concerns. Also, currently they are extremely expensive, which limits their use in clinical practice. For doses, see warnings and side effects.[1]

GENERALIZED PUSTULAR PSORIASIS (see Fig. 3-12)

Ill patients with generalized rash should be hospitalized and treated in the same manner as patients with extensive burns, toxic epidermal necrolysis, or exfoliative erythroderma—in a specialized unit. Isolation, fluid replacement, and repeated blood cultures are necessary. Rapid suppression and resolution of lesions is achieved by oral retinoids (acitretin, 50 mg/day). Supportive measures should include fluid intake, IV antibiotics to prevent septicemia, cardiac support, temperature control, topical lubricants, and antiseptic baths. Systemic glucocorticoids to be used only as a rescue intervention as rapid tachyphylaxis occurs. Oral PUVA is effective, but logistics of treatment are usually prohibitive in a toxic patient with fever.

ACRODERMATITIS CONTINUA HALLOPEAU

Oral retinoids as in von Zumbusch pustular psoriasis; MTX, once-a-week schedule, is the second-line choice (Figure 3-13B).

PSORIATIC ARTHRITIS

Should be recognized early in order to prevent bone destruction. MTX, once-a-week schedule as previously outlined; TNFα blockers and Ustekinumab are highly effective.

[1]For details and drug interaction, see S Richardson, J Gelfand. In: Goldsmith L, Gilchrest B, Katz S, Paller A, Leffel D, Wolff K. eds. *Fitzpatrick's Dermatology, in General Medicine* 8th ed. New York, NY. McGraw-Hill; 2013: pp 2814–2826.

PITYRIASIS RUBRA PILARIS (PRP) ICD-10: L44.4

- Rare, chronic, papulosquamous disorder often progressing to erythroderma.
- Six types exist.
- Follicular hyperkeratotic papules, reddish-orange progressing to generalized erythroderma. Sharply demarcated islands of unaffected (normal) skin.
- Waxy, diffuse, orange keratoderma of the palms and soles; the nails may be affected.
- Most effective therapy is MTX, systemic retinoids.

CLASSIFICATION[2]

Type 1: Classic Adult. Generalized, beginning on head and neck.

Type 2: Atypical Adult. Generalized, sparse hair.

Type 3: Classic Juvenile. Appears within the first 2 years of life, generalized.

Type 4: Circumscribed Juvenile. In prepubertal children, localized.

Type 5: Atypical Juvenile. Onset in first few years of life, familial, generalized.

Type 6: HIV-Associated. Generalized, associated with acne conglobata, hidradenitis suppurativa, and lichen spinulosus.

EPIDEMIOLOGY

Rare. Affects both sexes and occurs in all races.

ETIOLOGY AND PATHOGENESIS

Unknown.

CLINICAL MANIFESTATION

Both insidious and rapid onset occur.

SKIN LESIONS All types of PRP. An eruption of follicular hyperkeratotic papules of reddish-orange color usually spreading in a cephalo-caudal direction (Fig. 3-15). Confluence to a reddish-orange psoriasiform, scaling dermatitis with sharply demarcated islands of unaffected skin (Fig. 3-16). In darker skin tones, papules are brown.

Distribution. Types 1, 2, 3, 5, and 6: Generalized, classically beginning on the head and neck, then spreading caudally. Progression to erythroderma (except for types 2 and 4). In type 4, localized orange/red plaques (Fig. 3-17).

SCALP AND HAIR Scalp affected, as in psoriasis, often leading to asbestos-like accumulation of scale. Hair not affected except in type 2 where sparse scalp hair is observed.

MUCOUS MEMBRANES Spared.

PALMS AND SOLES (TYPE 1) Palm shows diffuse, waxy, yellowish/orange hyperkeratosis (Fig. 3-18).

NAILS Common but not diagnostic. Distal yellow-brown discoloration, nail plate thickening, subungual hyperkeratosis, and splinter hemorrhages. See Section 32.

ASSOCIATED CONDITIONS Ichthyosiform lesions on legs in type 2. Scleroderma-like appearance of hands and feet in type 5. Acne conglobata, hidradenitis suppurativa, and lichen spinulosus in type 6.

DIAGNOSIS AND DIFFERENTIAL DIAGNOSIS

The diagnosis is made on clinical grounds. The differential diagnosis includes psoriasis, follicular ichthyosis, erythrokeratodermia variabilis, and ichthyosiform erythrodermas.

LABORATORY EXAMINATIONS

HISTOPATHOLOGY Not diagnostic but suggestive: Hyperkeratosis, acanthosis with broad short rete ridges, alternating orthokeratosis, and parakeratosis. Keratinous plugs of follicular infundibula and perifollicular areas of parakeratosis. Prominent granular layer may distinguish PRP from psoriasis. Superficial perivascular lymphocytic infiltrate.

COURSE AND PROGNOSIS

A socially and psychologically disabling condition. Long duration; type 3 often resolves after 2 years; type 4 may clear. Type 5 has a very chronic course. Type 6 may respond to highly active antiretroviral therapy (HAART).

MANAGEMENT

Topical therapies consist of emollients, keratolytic agents, vitamin D_3 (calcipotriol),

[2]Griffiths WAD. *Clin Exp Dermatol.* 1980; 5:105 and Gonzáles-López A et al. *Br J Dermatol.* 1999; 140:931.

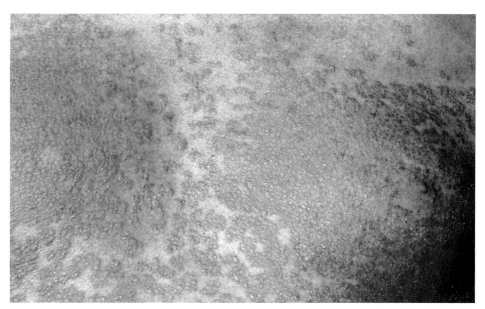

FIGURE 3-15 Pityriasis rubra pilaris (type 1, classic adult) Orange-red follicular papules beginning on the head and neck have coalesced on the chest of a 57-year-old male. There are sharply demarcated islands of unaffected normal skin.

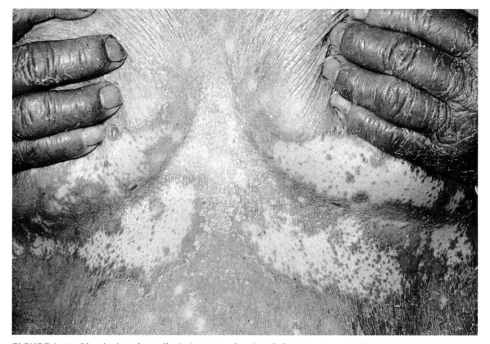

FIGURE 3-16 Pityriasis rubra pilaris (type 1, classic adult) Orange-reddish papules have coalesced to near erythroderma, sparing isolated islands of normal skin. Also note involvement of the hands in this 55-year-old woman.

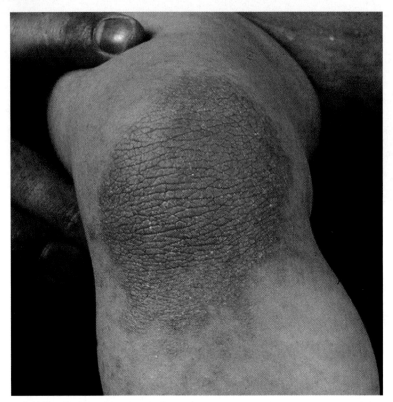

FIGURE 3-17 Pityriasis rubra pilaris (type 4) Localized orange plaque on the knee of an infant.

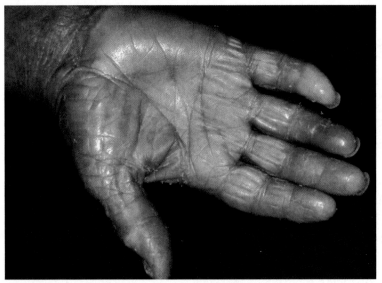

FIGURE 3-18 Pityriasis rubra pilaris on palms There is diffuse, waxy hyperkeratosis with an orange hue.

glucocorticoids, and vitamin A analogues (tazarotene). All are not very effective. Phototherapy (ultraviolet A phototherapy, narrowband ultraviolet B phototherapy, and photochemotherapy) is effective but only in some cases. Most effective treatment consists of systemic administration of MTX or retinoids (both as in psoriasis). In type 6: HAART. The anti-TNF agents, e.g., infliximab and etanercept are effective.

PITYRIASIS ROSEA ICD-10: L42

- An acute exanthematous eruption with a distinctive morphology and often with a characteristic self-limited course.
- Initially, a single (primary, or "herald") plaque lesion develops, usually on the trunk; 1 or 2 weeks later a generalized secondary eruption develops in a typical distribution pattern.
- The entire process remits spontaneously in 6 weeks.
- Reactivation of human herpesvirus-7 (HHV-7) and HHV-6 is the most probable cause.

EPIDEMIOLOGY AND ETIOLOGY

AGE OF ONSET Ten to 43 years, but can occur rarely in infants and old persons.
SEASON Spring and fall.
ETIOLOGY There is good evidence that pityriasis rosea is associated with reactivation of HHV-7 or HHV-6, two closely related β-herpes viruses.

CLINICAL MANIFESTATION

SKIN LESIONS Herald Patch. Occurs in 80% of patients, preceding exanthem. Oval, slightly raised plaque or patch 2 to 5 cm, salmon-red, fine collarette scale at periphery; may be multiple (Fig. 3-19A).
Exanthem. One to two weeks after herald patch. Fine scaling papules and patches with marginal collarette (Fig. 3-19B). Dull pink or tawny. Oval, scattered, with characteristic distribution following the lines of cleavage in a "Christmas tree" pattern (Fig. 3-20). Lesions usually confined to trunk and proximal aspects of the arms and legs. Rarely on face.
Atypical Pityriasis Rosea. Lesions may be present only on the face and neck. The primary plaque may be absent; may be the sole manifestation of the disease, or may be multiple. Most confusing are the examples of pityriasis rosea with vesicles or simulating erythema multiforme. This usually results from irritation and sweating, often as a consequence of inadequate treatment (*pityriasis rosea irritata*).

DIFFERENTIAL DIAGNOSIS

MULTIPLE SMALL SCALING PLAQUES *Drug eruptions* (e.g., captopril and barbiturates), *secondary syphilis* (obtain serology), *guttate psoriasis* (no marginal collarette), *small plaque parapsoriasis, erythema migrans* with secondary lesions, *erythema multiforme,* and *tinea corporis.*

LABORATORY EXAMINATION

DERMATOPATHOLOGY Patchy or diffuse parakeratosis, absence of granular layer, slight acanthosis, focal spongiosis, and microscopic vesicles. Occasional dyskeratotic cells with an eosinophilic homogeneous appearance. Edema of dermis and perivascular infiltrate of mononuclear cells.

COURSE

Spontaneous remission in 6 to 12 weeks or less. Recurrences are uncommon.

MANAGEMENT

SYMPTOMATIC Oral antihistamines and/or topical antipruritic lotions for relief of pruritus. Topical glucocorticoids. May be improved by UVB phototherapy or natural sunlight exposure if treatment is begun in the first week of eruption. A short course of systemic glucocorticoids is the best option.

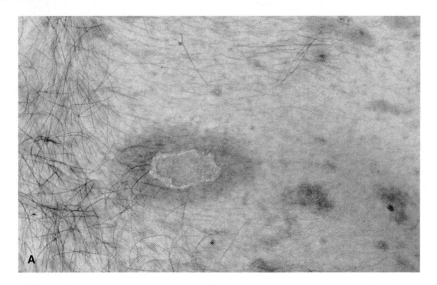

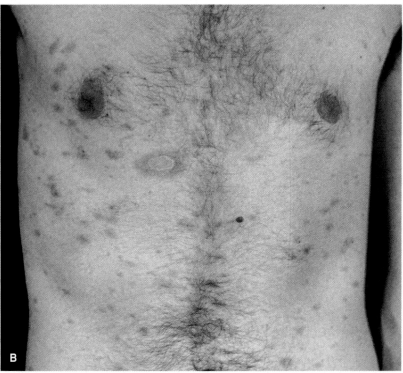

FIGURE 3-19   Pityriasis rosea   (A) Herald patch. An erythematous (salmon-red) plaque with a collarette scale on the trailing edge of the advancing border. Collarette means that scale is attached at periphery and loose toward the center of the lesion. **(B)** Overview of exanthem of pityriasis rosea with the herald patch shown in part **(A)**. There are papules and small plaques with oval configurations that follow the lines of cleavage. The fine scaling of the salmon-red papules cannot be seen at this magnification, whereas the herald patch's collarette is obvious.

FIGURE 3-20 Pityriasis rosea Distribution "Christmas tree" pattern on the back.

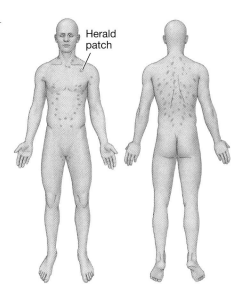

Herald patch

PARAPSORIASIS EN PLAQUES (PP)

- Rare eruptions with worldwide occurrence.
- Two types are recognized: small-plaque PP (SPP) and large-plaque PP (LPP).
- In SPP (ICD-10:L41.3), lesions are small (<5 cm), round to oval, or linear mostly on the trunk: "digitate dermatosis" (Fig. 3-21), slightly infiltrated, yellowish, or fawn-colored patches. Minimal scaling, asymptomatic, or mild pruritus.
- In LPP (ICD-10:L41.4), lesions are oval or irregularly shaped patches and >5 cm (Fig. 3-22). Minimal scaling, with and without atrophy. May be poikilodermatous.
- SPP does not progress to mycosis fungoides (MF). LPP, by contrast, exists on a continuum with patch-stage MF and can progress to overt MF.
- Treatment consists of topical glucocorticoids, phototherapy, narrowband 311-nm UV phototherapy, or PUVA.

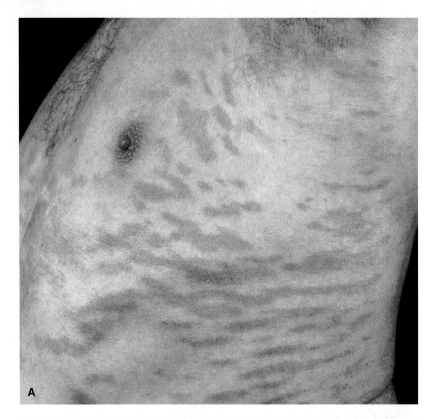

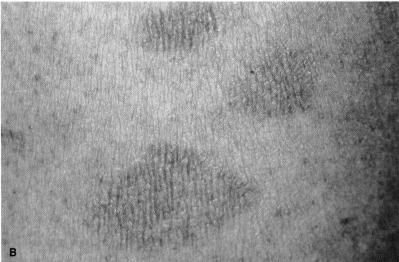

FIGURE 3-21 Digitate dermatosis (small-plaque parapsoriasis) (A) The lesions are asymptomatic, yellowish or fawn-colored, very thin, well defined, slightly scaly and superficially wrinkled patches. They are oval and follow the lines of cleavage of the skin, giving the appearance of a "hug" that left fingerprints on the trunk. The long axis of these lesions often reaches more than 5 cm. **(B)** Close up of smaller lesions showing wrinkling of surface.

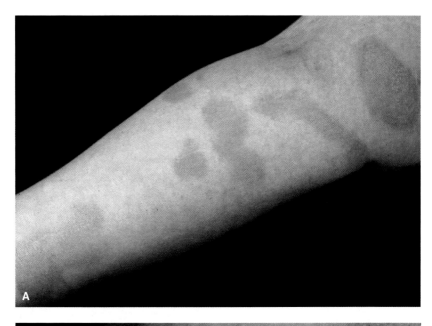

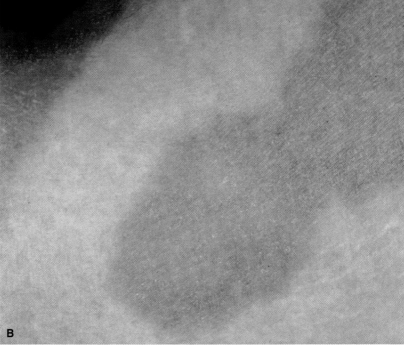

FIGURE 3-22   Large-plaque parapsoriasis (parapsoriasis en plaques) (A) The lesions are asymptomatic, well-defined, rounded, slightly scaly, thin plaques, or patches. The lesions can be larger than 10 cm and are light red-brown or salmon-pink. There may be atrophy in some areas. The lesions here are located on the extremities, but they are more commonly noted on the trunk. These lesions must be carefully followed, and repeated biopsies are necessary to detect mycosis fungoides. This entity may be considered as a prestage of mycosis fungoides but not all patients progress to MF. **(B)** Close up of lesions showing minimal scaling and wrinkled surface.

PITYRIASIS LICHENOIDES (ACUTE AND CHRONIC) (PL)   ICD-10: L41.0/L41.1

- PL is an eruption of unknown etiology, characterized clinically by successive crops of a wide range of morphologic lesions.
- Classified into an acute form, pityriasis lichenoides et varioliformis acuta (PLEVA), and a chronic form, pityriasis lichenoides chronica (PLC).
- However, most patients have lesions of PLEVA and PLC simultaneously.
- PLEVA is important because it can be mistaken for lymphomatoid papulosis (see Section 21).
- More common in males than females, adolescents, and young adults.
- Lesions tend to appear in crops over a period of weeks or months. Uncommonly, patients with an acute onset of the disorder may have symptoms of an acute infection with fever, malaise, and headache. Cutaneous lesions are usually asymptomatic but may be pruritic or sensitive to touch.
- **Lesions: PLEVA.** Randomly arranged, most commonly on trunk, proximal extremities but also generalized, including the palms and soles. Bright-red edematous papules (i.e., lichenoides), less commonly vesicles, which undergo central necrosis with hemorrhagic crusting (i.e., varioliformis, hence the designation *PLEVA*) (Fig. 3-23A and B). *PLC*. This is the chronic form, scaling papules of reddish-brown color, and a central mica-like scale (Fig. 3-23C). Postinflammatory hypo- or hyperpigmentation often presents after lesions resolve. PLEVA may heal with depressed or elevated scars.
- **Dermatopathology.** *Epidermis*: spongiosis, keratinocyte necrosis, vesiculation, ulceration; exocytosis or erythrocytes within epidermis. *Dermis*: Edema, chronic inflammatory cell infiltrate in wedge shape extending to deep reticular dermis.
- Clinical diagnosis is confirmed by skin biopsy. Differential diagnosis: varicella, guttate psoriasis, and lymphomatoid papulosis (which is clinically almost indistinguishable from PLEVA).
- New lesions appear in successive crops. PLC tends to resolve spontaneously after 6 to 12 months. In some cases, patients relapse after many months or years.
- Most patients do not require any therapeutic intervention. Oral erythromycin and tetracycline are effective in some cases. Ultraviolet radiation (whether natural sunlight or broadband UVB), 311-nm UVB, and PUVA are the treatments of choice if oral antibiotics fail after a 2-week trial.

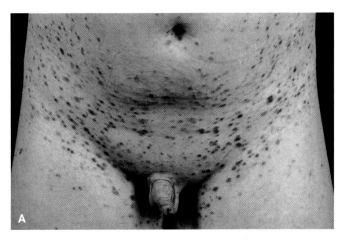

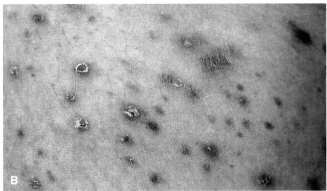

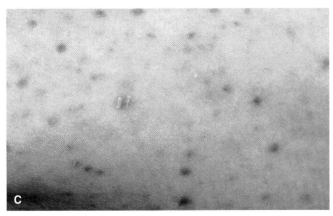

**FIGURE 3-23   Pityriasis lichenoides et varioliformis acuta
(PLEVA) (A)** Randomly distributed red papules of different size, some
of which show hemorrhagic crusting. In this 5-year-old child, the eruption appeared in crops over a period of 10 days. **(B) PLEVA** lesions in
a 38-year-old Indonesian man. Lesions are more hyperpigmented and
there is considerable scaling and crusting. **(C) Pityriasis lichenoides
chronica (PLC)** Discrete papules with fine mica-like scales that become
more visible after slight scraping. In contrast to PLEVA, there is no hemorrhagic crusting.

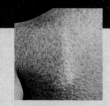

ICHTHYOSES

- A group of hereditary disorders characterized by an excess accumulation of cutaneous scale, varying from very mild and asymptomatic to life threatening.
- A relatively large number of types of hereditary ichthyoses exist; most are extremely rare and often part of multiorgan syndromes. The four most common and important types are discussed here along with a brief discussion of two syndromic ichthyoses and ichthyosis affecting the newborn.
- *Acquired* ichthyosis can be a manifestation of systemic disease, malignancy, drugs, endocrine disease, autoimmune disease, and HIV as well as other infections.
- Support groups such as Foundation for Ichthyosis and Related Skin Types (FIRST) exist.

CLASSIFICATION

Dominant ichthyosis vulgaris (DIV)
X-linked ichthyosis (XLI)
Lamellar ichthyosis (LI)
Epidermolytic hyperkeratosis (EH)

This simplified classification is presented here for clinical-diagnostic and didactical reasons.

A scientific classification based on molecular genetics is found in P. Fleckman and J. DiGiovanna: The Ichthyoses in Goldsmith, Katz, Gilchrest, Paller, Leffell, Wolff (eds.) Fitzpatrick's Dermatology in General Medicine, 8th edition, New York, McGraw-Hill, 2012, pp. 507–537.

DOMINANT ICHTHYOSIS VULGARIS (DIV) ICD-10: Q 80.0

- Characterized by usually mild generalized xerosis with scaling, most pronounced on lower legs; in severe cases large, tessellated scales.
- Hyperlinear palms and soles.
- Perifollicular hyperkeratosis (keratosis pilaris) usually on arms and legs.
- Frequently associated with atopy.

EPIDEMIOLOGY

AGE OF ONSET 3 to 12 months.
SEX Equal incidence in males and females. Autosomal dominant inheritance.
INCIDENCE Common (1 in 250).

PATHOGENESIS

Etiology unknown. There is reduced or absent filaggrin. Epidermis proliferates normally but keratin is retained with a resultant thickened stratum corneum.

CLINICAL MANIFESTATION

Very commonly associated with atopy. When hyperkeratosis is severe, many patients have a cosmetic concern.
SKIN LESIONS Xerosis (dry skin) with fine, powdery scaling but also larger, firmly adherent tacked-down scales in a fish-scale pattern (Figs. 4-1 and 4-2). Diffuse general involvement, accentuated on the shins, arms, and back, buttocks, and lateral thighs; axillae and the antecubital and popliteal fossae spared

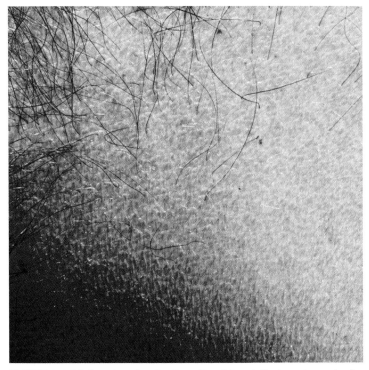

FIGURE 4-1 Ichthyosis vulgaris: chest Fine fish scalelike hyperkeratosis of the pectoral area. This is a mild form of ichthyosis vulgaris.

(Figs. 4-2 and 4-3). The face is usually spared but the cheeks and forehead may be involved. Keratosis pilaris is perifollicular hyperkeratosis with little, spiny hyperkeratotic follicular papules of normal skin color either grouped or disseminated, mostly on the extensor surfaces of the extremities (Fig. 4-4); in childhood, also on cheeks. The hands and feet usually spared, but palmoplantar markings are more accentuated (hyperlinear).

ASSOCIATED DISEASES More than 50% of individuals with DIV also have atopic dermatitis, rarely keratopathy.

LABORATORY EXAMINATION

DERMATOPATHOLOGY Compact hyperkeratosis; reduced or absent granular layer; small, poorly formed keratohyalin granules by electron microscopy, germinative layer flattened.

DIAGNOSIS

By clinical findings; absent or reduced keratohyalin granules in electron microscopy. Differential diagnosis includes all forms of xerosis and hyperkeratosis.

COURSE AND PROGNOSIS

Improvement in the summer, humid climates, and in adulthood. Keratosis pilaris occurring on the cheeks during childhood usually improves during adulthood.

MANAGEMENT

HYDRATION OF STRATUM CORNEUM Immersion in a bath followed by the application of petrolatum. Urea-containing creams bind water in the stratum corneum.

KERATOLYTIC AGENTS Propylene glycol–glycerin–lactic acid mixtures. Propylene glycol (44 to 60% in water); 6% salicylic acid in propylene glycol and alcohol, used under plastic occlusion (beware of hypersalicism). α-Hydroxy acids (lactic acid or glycolic acid) control scaling. Urea-containing creams and lotions (2 to 10%) are effective.

SYSTEMIC RETINOIDS Isotretinoin and acitretin are very effective, but careful monitoring for toxicity is required. Only severe cases may require intermittent therapy.

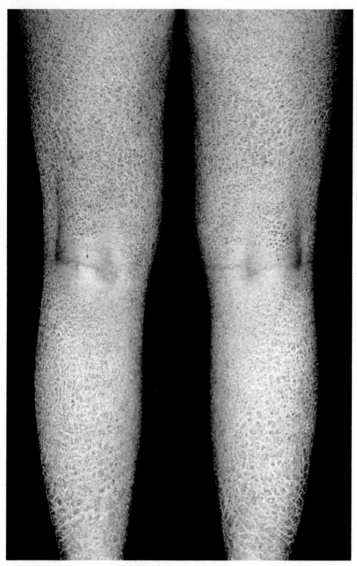

FIGURE 4-2 Ichthyosis vulgaris: legs Grayish tessellated (tilelike), firmly bound down scales. The similarity to fish skin or the skin of an amphibian is quite obvious. Note sparing of popliteal fossae. This is a more severe form of ichthyosis vulgaris.

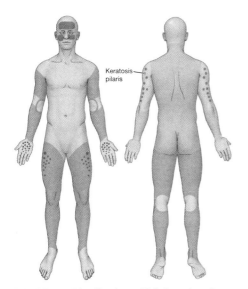

FIGURE 4-3 Distribution of ichthyosis vulgaris Dots indicate keratosis pilaris. Palms with increased skin markings (hyperlinearity).

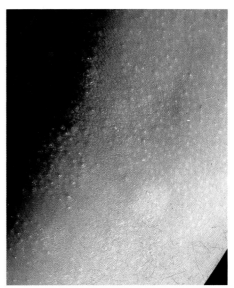

FIGURE 4-4 Ichthyosis vulgaris. Keratosis pilaris: arm Small, follicular, horny spines occur as a manifestation of mild ichthyosis vulgaris; arising mostly on the shoulders, upper arms, and thighs. Desquamation of the nonfollicular skin results in hypomelanotic (less pigmented) spots similar to pityriasis alba (compare with Fig. 13-18).

X-LINKED RECESSIVE ICHTHYOSIS (XLRI) ICD-10: Q 80.1

- Occurs in males, x-linked recessive; gene locus $X_p22.32$.
- Steroid sulfatase deficiency. Accumulation of cholesterol sulfate resulting in retention hyperkeratosis associated with normal epidermal proliferation.
- Incidence 1:2000 to 1:6000.
- Onset soon after birth.
- Prominent, dirty brown scales on the neck, extremities, trunk, and buttocks (Fig. 4-5).
- Involvement of flexural regions (Fig. 4-6).
- Absence of palm or sole involvement.
- Comma-shaped stromal corneal opacities (asymptomatic) in 50% of adult males. Present in some female carriers.
- Laboratory: Cholesterol sulfate level↑; increased mobility of β-lipoproteins in electrophoresis. Steroid sulfatase decreased or absent. Dermatopathology: Hyperkeratosis and granular layer present.
- Prenatal diagnosis: Amniocentesis, steroid sulfatase ↓ in chorionic villus samples.
- Course: No improvement with age. Worse in temperate climates and winter.
- Management: Hydration of stratum corneum and keratolytic agents as in ichthyosis vulgaris. Marked improvement with systemic retinoids (acitretin and isotretinoin), intermittent treatment with careful monitoring of toxicity.

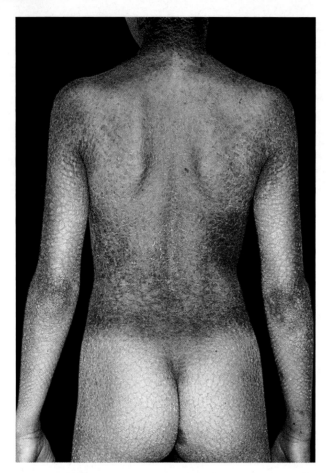

FIGURE 4-5 X-linked ichthyosis: trunk, buttocks, and arms Dark hyperkeratosis with tessellated scales gives a dirty appearance in this 12-year-old boy of African American ethnicity.

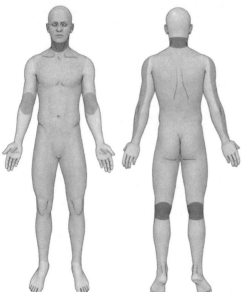

FIGURE 4-6 Distribution of X-linked ichthyosis.

LAMELLAR ICHTHYOSIS (LI) ICD-10: Q 80.2

- Onset at birth, usually as collodion baby (p. 80).
- Equally in both sexes; incidence ≤1:300,000.
- Autosomal recessive. Three types: (1) Mutation of gene encoding transglutaminase 1(TGM1); (2) Mutation of gene encoding an ABC lipid transporter; and (3) Mutation of gene encoding 2 lipoxygenases (ALOXIZB, ALOXE3).
- Soon after birth, collodion membrane shed with subsequent large, coarse, tessellated scales involving the entire body (Figs. 4-7 and 4-8). The scales are thick, brown, accumulated on lower extremities, flexural areas involved (Fig. 4-9).
- Hands, feet involvement varies; accentuation of palmar/plantar creases.
- Eyes: Extropium (Fig. 4-7) and eclabium.
- Scalp: Hairs bound down by scales; scarring alopecia.
- Mucous membranes; nails: Occasional dystrophy secondary to nail fold inflammation.
- Heat intolerance; obstruction of eccrine glands impairs sweating.
- Laboratory: Acanthosis; hyperkeratosis, granular layer present. Epidermal transglutaminase ↓ in transglutaminase-deficient subtype.
- Course: Persists throughout life, no improvement with age.
- Management: Newborn, see collodion baby, p. 80. Adults: Emollients, keratolytics, systemic retinoids as in DIV and XLI. Instruct about overheating.

FIGURE 4-7 Lamellar ichthyosis Parchment-like hyperkeratosis gives the impression of the skin being too tight on the face of this 6-year-old Arab boy. There is lamellar scaling hyperkeratosis, pronounced ectropium, and beginning alopecia.

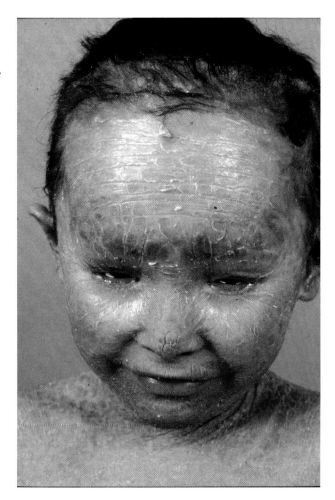

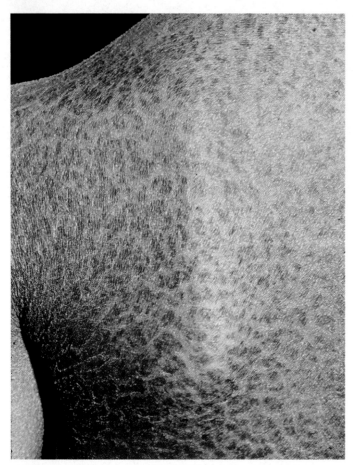

FIGURE 4-8 Lamellar ichthyosis Shoulder tesselated (tilelike) hyperkeratosis gives the appearance of reptilian scales on the shoulder and back. The entire body was involved, and there was ectropium.

FIGURE 4-9 Distribution of lamellar ichthyosis.

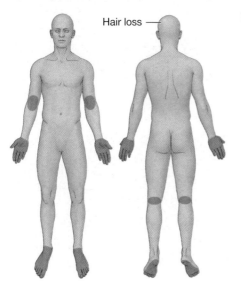

Hair loss

EPIDERMOLYTIC HYPERKERATOSIS (EH) ICD-10: Q 80.8

- Autosomal dominant. Mutation of genes that encode epidermal differentiation keratins, KRT1, and KRT10.
- Presents at or shortly after birth with erythroderma and blistering, generalized, or localized.
- With time becomes keratotic and verrucous (Fig. 4-10) but blisters continue (Fig. 4-10).
- Shedding of hyperkeratotic masses results in circumscribed areas of normal-appearing skin.
- Involvement of flexural areas and palmar and plantar skin (Fig. 4-11).
- Associated with unpleasant odor (like rancid butter).
- Secondary pyogenic infections.
- Dermatopathology: Giant coarse keratohyalin granules, vacuolization of granular layer → subcorneal blisters.
- Management: Topical α-hydroxy acids, systemic acitretin, or isotretinoin that initially lead to increased blister formation but later improve skin dramatically. Determine dose carefully, monitor side effects, and observe contraindications.

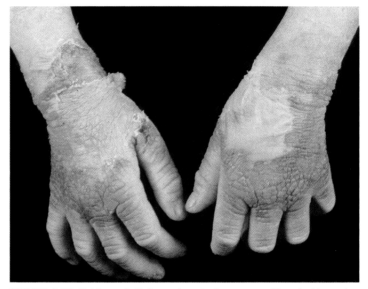

FIGURE 4-10 Epidermolytic hyperkeratosis: arms and hands Mountain rangelike hyperkeratosis of the dorsum of hands with blistering that results in erosions and shedding of large sheets of keratin.

FIGURE 4-11 Distribution of epidermolytic hyperkeratosis.

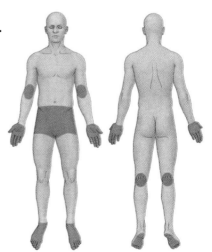

ICHTHYOSIS IN THE NEWBORN

COLLODION BABY ICD-10: Q 80.2

- Encasement of the entire baby in a transparent parchment-like membrane (Fig. 4-12A), which impairs respiration and sucking.
- Breaking and shedding of the collodion membrane initially leads to difficulties in thermoregulation and increased risk of infection.
- Skin is bright red and moist (Fig. 4-12A). After healing, skin appears normal for some time until signs of ichthyosis develop.
- Collodion baby may be the initial presentation of lamellar ichthyosis or some less common forms of ichthyosis not discussed here.
- Collodion baby also may be a condition that, after the collodion membrane is shed and the resultant erythema has cleared, will progress to normal skin for the rest of the child's life (Fig. 4-12B).
- Management: Keep the newborn in the incubator and monitor temperature, fluids, and nutrient replacement. Aggressive antibiotic therapy for skin and lung infection.

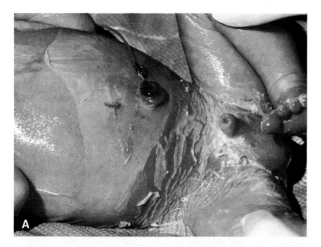

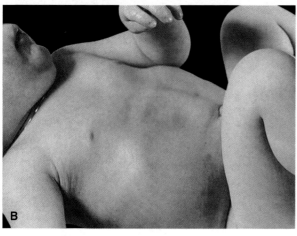

FIGURE 4-12 Ichthyosis in the newborn (A) "Collodion baby" shortly after birth with a parchment-like membrane covering the entire body. In some areas, the membrane has ruptured and is being shed leaving oozing, raw-looking skin. **(B)** At 8 months of age, the same infant is a beautiful baby with minimal residual scale and erythema.

HARLEQUIN FETUS ICD-10: Q 80.4

- Harlequin fetus is an extremely rare condition in which the child is born with very thick plates of stratum corneum separated by deep cracks and fissures (Fig. 4-13).
- Eclabium, ectropion, and absence of or rudimentary ears result in a grotesque appearance.
- These babies usually die shortly after birth, but there are reports of survival for weeks to several months.
- This condition is different from collodion baby and the other forms of ichthyosis, with an unusual fibrous protein within the epidermis.

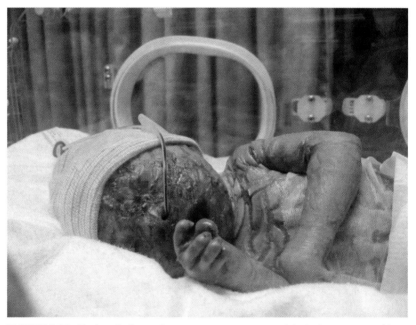

FIGURE 4-13   Harlequin fetus Stratum corneum consists of thick plates separated by deep cracks. (Reproduced with permission from Benjamin Solky, MD.)

SYNDROMIC ICHTHYOSES ICD-10: Q 80.9

- These are a number of rare syndromic ichthyoses where ichthyotic skin changes are associated with metabolic and/or functional and structural abnormalities.
- *For erythrokeratodermia variabilis (Fig. 4-14), keratitis–ichthyosis–deafness (KID) syndrome (Fig. 4-15), Child syndrome, and Netherton syndrome (Fig. 4-16), see P Fleckman, JJ DiGiovanna, in L Goldsmith et al: Fitzpatrick's Dermatology in General Medicine, 8th ed. New York, McGraw-Hill, pp. 507–538, 2012.*

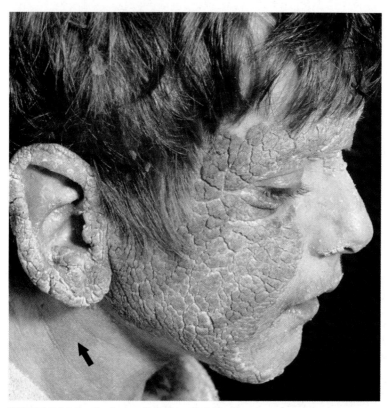

FIGURE 4-14 Erythrokeratodermia variabilis Note hyperkeratotic plaques on the face associated with migrating erythemas on the neck (arrow).

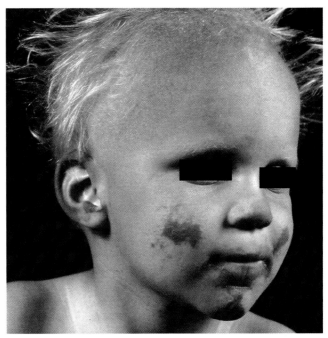

FIGURE 4-15 Keratitis-ichthyosis-deafness (KID) syndrome Hyper-keratosis on the cheeks, and the tip of the nose and ear and sparse hair are characteristic for this syndrome as are hyperkeratosis in the flexural folds, dorsa of hands. In addition, there is keratitis and loss of hearing.

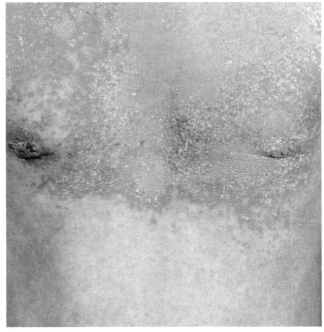

FIGURE 4-16 Netherton syndrome Ichthyosis linearis circumflexa consists of serpiginous psoriasiform erythemas with scaling and is asso-ciated with trichorrhexis nodosa (bamboo hairs).

ACQUIRED ICHTHYOSES ICD-10: L 85.0

- Occurs in adults.
- Associated with malignancies (Hodgkin disease but also non-Hodgkin lymphomas and other malignancies).
- Associated with AIDS.
- Associated with sarcoidosis.
- Associated with systemic lupus erythematosus, dermatomyositis, mixed connective tissue disease, and eosinophilic fasciitis.
- Associated with graft-versus-host disease.
- Associated with drugs (nicotinic acid, triparanol, butyrophenone, dixyrazine, and nafoxidine).
- Occurs in Kava drinkers: *Kava dermopathy*.

INHERITED KERATODERMAS OF PALMS AND SOLES ICD-10: Q 82.2

- Palmoplantar keratodermas (PPK) are a rare and diverse group of keratinization disorders.
- More than 20 different PKK exist that are either confined to palms and soles or concomitant with (related) lesions elsewhere on the body or are part of more complex syndromes.
- The genetic basis of most PPK involves mutations of keratin genes or genes encoding connexin or desmosomal proteins.
- Clinical classification distinguishes between diffuse (Fig. 4-17), punctate (Fig. 4-18), striate (Fig. 4-19), and focal PPK (callus-like circumscribed hyperkeratoses).
- Histopathologic distinction is made between epidermolytic and nonepidermolytic PPKs.
- Symptoms vary from inconvenience to functional disability. Plantar pain in focal PPK and hyperhidrosis may be debilitating.
- PPK do not improve with age, and often result in being an lifelong companion.
- Management: Physical debridement, topical keratolytic agents, systemic acitretin, or isotretinoin may be associated with increased sensitivity, difficulties with normal work and walking, particularly in the epidermolytic forms of PKK.

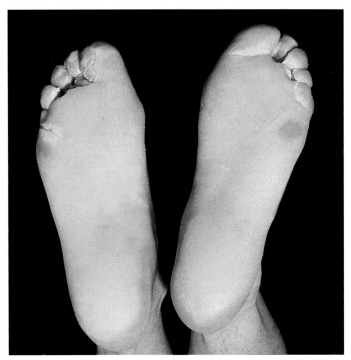

FIGURE 4-17 Plantar keratoderma, diffuse type Yellow waxy diffuse hyperkeratosis on both soles.

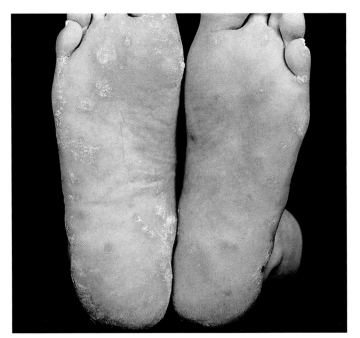

FIGURE 4-18 Punctate plantar keratoderma Multiple, discrete drop-like keratoses resembling plantar warts. Lesions had been present since late childhood and have become worse, particularly in the pressure areas.

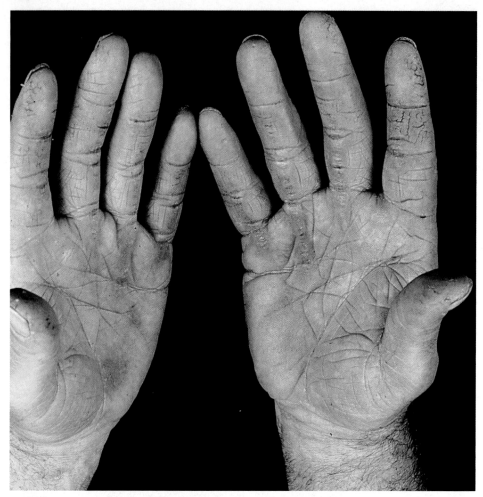

FIGURE 4-19 Striate palmar keratoderma There are linear verrucous hyperkeratoses extending from the palm onto the fingers. Manual work aggravates these lesions, which can become fissured and painful. In **focal palmar and plantar keratoderma**, there are large hyperkeratoses on pressure sites of soles and palms that can become quite painful.

MISCELLANEOUS EPIDERMAL DISORDERS

ACANTHOSIS NIGRICANS (AN) ICD-10: L 83

- Asymmetric velvety thickening and hyperpigmentation of the skin, seen chiefly on the neck, axilla, groins, and other body folds.
- May be hyperkeratotic and associated with skin tags.
- A cutaneous marker related to heredity, obesity, endocrine disorders (particularly diabetes), drug administration, and malignancy.
- Insidious onset; in malignancy, rapid.

CLASSIFICATION

Type 1: Hereditary Benign AN. No associated endocrine disorder.

Type 2: Benign AN. Endocrine disorders associated with insulin resistance: insulin-resistant type II diabetes mellitus, hyper-androgenic states, acromegaly/gigantism, Cushing disease, hypogonadal syndromes with insulin resistance, Addison disease, and hypothyroidism.

Type 3: Pseudo-AN. Associated with obesity; more common in patients with darker pigmentation. Common in metabolic syndrome. Obesity produces insulin resistance.

Type 4: Drug-Induced AN. Nicotinic acid in high dosage, stilbestrol in young males, gluco-corticoid therapy, diethylstilbestrol/oral contraceptive, and growth hormone therapy.

Type 5: Malignant AN. Paraneoplastic, usually adenocarcinoma of gastrointestinal or genito-urinary tract; less commonly, bronchial carcinoma and lymphoma.

EPIDEMIOLOGY

AGE OF ONSET Type 1: Occurs during childhood or puberty; other types dependent on associated conditions.

ETIOLOGY AND PATHOGENESIS

Dependent on associated disorder. In a subset of women with hyperandrogenism and insulin intolerance and AN, loss-of-function mutation in the insulin receptor or anti-insulin receptor antibodies can be found (types A and B).

It is postulated that excess growth factor stimulation in the skin leads to proliferation of keratinocytes and fibroblasts. In hyperinsu-linemia AN, excess insulin binding to insulin-like growth factor 1 receptor and fibroblast growth factor receptor has also been implicated. In malignancy-associated AN, trans-forming growth factor β released from tumor cells may stimulate keratinocyte proliferation via epidermal growth factor receptors.

CLINICAL MANIFESTATION

Insidious onset; in type 5 rapid. The first visible change is darkening of pigmentation.

SKIN LESIONS All types of AN: Darkening of pigmentation, skin appears dirty (Fig. 5-1). As skin thickens, it appears velvety; skin lines accentuated; surface becomes rugose, mammillated. Type 3: Velvety patch on inner, upper thigh at site of chafing; often has many skin tags in body folds and neck. Type 5: Hyperkeratosis and hyperpigmenta-tion more pronounced (Fig. 5-2A). Involve-ment of oral mucosa and vermilion border of lips (Fig. 5-2B). Hyperkeratosis of the palms/soles, with accentuation of papillary markings, "Tripe hands" (Fig. 5-2C).

DISTRIBUTION Most commonly, axil-lae (Fig. 5-1); neck (back, sides), groins (Fig. 5-2A), anogenitalie, antecubital fossae, knuckles, submammary, and umbilicus. In type 5, also periocular, peroral, mammilary, and the palms (tripe palms) (Fig. 5-2C).

MUCOUS MEMBRANES Oral mucosa: Velvety texture with delicate furrows. Type 5: Mucous membranes and mucocutaneous junctions

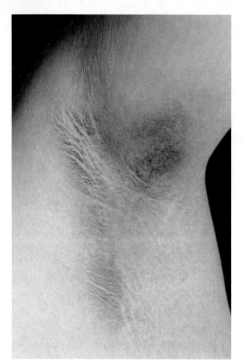

FIGURE 5-1 Acanthosis nigricans Velvety, dark-brown to gray thickening of the armpits with prominent skin folds and feathered edges in a 30-year-old obese woman from the Middle East. There were similar changes on the neck, the ante-cubital fossae, and on the knuckles.

commonly involved; warty papillomatous thickenings periorally (Fig. 5-2B).

General Examination

Examine for underlying endocrine disorders in overweight to morbidly obese persons; in type 5 wasting, search for malignancy.

DIAGNOSIS AND DIFFERENTIAL DIAGNOSIS

CLINICAL FINDINGS Dark thickened flexural skin: Confluent and reticulated papillomatosis (Gougerot–Carteaud syndrome), pityriasis versicolor, X-linked ichthyosis, retention hyperkeratosis, and nicotinic acid ingestion.

LABORATORY EXAMINATIONS

CHEMISTRY Rule out diabetes mellitus; meta-bolic syndrome.

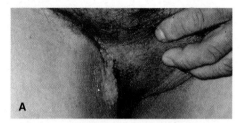

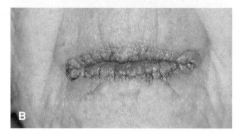

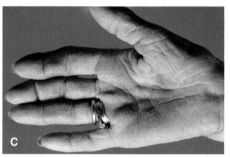

FIGURE 5-2 Acanthosis nigricans, type 5 (malignant) (A) Verrucous, papillomatous grayish-brown plaques in groins, medial aspects of the thigh, and scrotum. Similar lesions were found on neck and all other body folds. The patient had weight loss and wasting, and gastric adenocarcinoma was found. **(B)** Verrucous and papillomatous growths on the vermillion border of lips. Oral mucosa was velvety with deep fur-rows of the tongue. **(C)** Tripe palms. Palmar ridges show maximal accentuation resembling the mucosa of the stomach of a ruminant.

DERMATOPATHOLOGY Papillomatosis, hyperker-atosis; epidermis thrown into irregular folds, showing various degrees of acanthosis.

IMAGING AND ENDOSCOPY Rule out associated malignancy.

COURSE AND PROGNOSIS

Type 1: Accentuated at puberty but, at times, regresses when older. Type 2: Depends on underlying disturbance. Type 3: May regress after significant weight loss. Type 4: Resolves when causative drug is discontinued. Type 5: AN may precede other symptoms of malignancy by 5 years; removal of malignancy may be followed by regression of AN.

MANAGEMENT

Symptomatic. Treat associated disorder. Topical keratolytic and/or topical or systemic retinoids may improve AN but overall, they are not very effective.

DARIER DISEASE (DD) ICD-10: L 87

- A rare autosomal-dominant inherited disease with late onset.
- Multiple discrete scaling, crusted, and pruritic papules mainly in seborrheic and flexural areas.
- Malodorous and disfiguring, also involving nails and mucous membranes.
- Itching and/or painful.
- Histologically characterized by suprabasal acantholysis and dyskeratosis.
- Caused by loss-of-function mutation in the *ATP2A2* gene.
- *Synonym*: Darier–White disease, keratosis follicularis.

EPIDEMIOLOGY AND ETIOLOGY

Rare.

AGE OF ONSET Usually in the first or second decade; males and females are equally affected.

GENETICS Autosomal-dominant trait, new mutations common, penetrance >95%. Loss-of-function mutations in the *ATP2A2* gene encoding, sarco/endoplasmic reticulum calcium adenosine triphosphatase isoform 2 (SERCA 2), which impair intracellular Ca2+ signaling.

PRECIPITATING FACTORS Frequently worse in summer with heat and humidity; also exacerbated by UVB, mechanical trauma, and bacterial infections. Often associated with affective disorders and rarely with decreased intelligence.

CLINICAL MANIFESTATION

Usually insidious; abrupt onset occurs after precipitating factors; associated with severe pruritus and often pain.

SKIN LESIONS Multiple discrete scaling of crusted, pruritic papules (Fig. 5-3); when scaling crust is removed, a slitlike opening becomes visible (Fig. 5-4). Confluence to large plaques covered by hypertrophic warty masses that are foul smelling, particularly in intertriginous areas.

DISTRIBUTION Corresponding to the "seborrheic areas": chest (Fig. 5-3), back, ears, nasolabial folds, forehead (Fig. 5-4), and the scalp; axilla, neck, and the groin.

PALMS AND SOLES Multiple, flat, cobblestone-like papules.

APPENDAGES Hair not involved, but permanent alopecia may result from extensive scalp involvement and scarring. Nails thin, splitting distally, and showing characteristic V-shaped scalloping.

MUCOUS MEMBRANES White, centrally depressed papules on the mucosa of cheeks, hard and soft palate, and gums, "cobblestone" lesions.

DISEASE ASSOCIATION

Associated with *acrokeratosis verruciformis*, allelic with DD. Multiple, small flat-topped papules predominantly on the dorsa of the hands and feet.

LABORATORY EXAMINATION

DERMATOPATHOLOGY Dyskeratotic cells in the spinous layer (corps ronds) and stratum corneum (grains); suprabasal acantholysis and clefts (lacunae); and papillary overgrowth of the epidermis and hyperkeratosis.

DIAGNOSIS AND DIFFERENTIAL DIAGNOSIS

Diagnosis based on the history of familial involvement, clinical appearance, and histopathology. May be confused with seborrheic dermatitis, Grover disease, benign familial pemphigus (Hailey–Hailey disease), and pemphigus foliaceus. Acrokeratosis verruciformis: flat warts (verrucae planae juveniles).

COURSE AND PROGNOSIS

Persisting throughout life and not associated with cutaneous malignancies.

MANAGEMENT

Sunscreens, avoidance of friction and rubbing (turtle neck sweaters), antibiotic therapy (systemic and topical) to suppress bacterial infection, topical retinoids (tazarotene and adapalene), or, most effective, systemic retinoids (isotretinoin or acitretin).

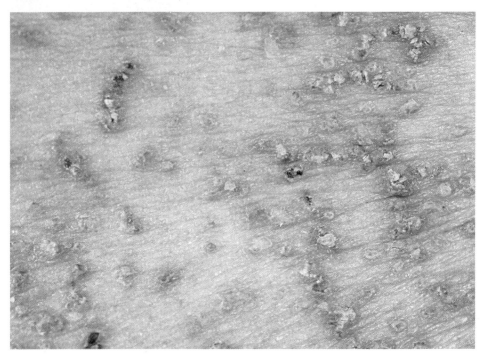

FIGURE 5-3 Darier disease: chest Primary lesions are reddish-brown, scaling, and crusted papules that feel warty when stroked. Where crusts have been removed, there are slitlike erosions that are later covered by hemorrhagic crusts.

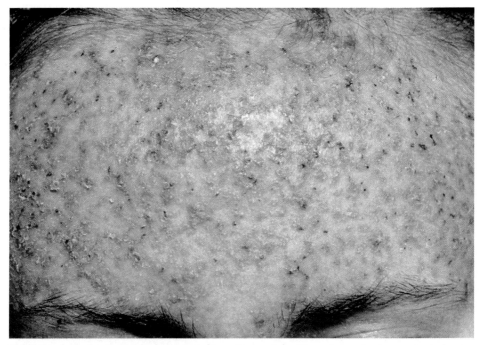

FIGURE 5-4 Darier disease: forehead Partly coalescing, hyperkeratotic papules that are eroded and crusted. The main concern of this young female was disfigurement.

GROVER DISEASE (GD) ICD-10: L 11.1

- A pruritic dermatosis located principally on the trunk, occurring as crops of discrete papular or papulovesicular lesions, sparse to numerous (Fig. 5-5). Similar to Darier's disease. Upon palpation smooth or warty.
- Occurs in adults (mean 50 years), males > females.
- Pruritus is the main symptom.
- Usually transient but a persistent form is recognized.
- Precipitating factors: heavy, sweat-inducing exercise, exposure to solar radiation, heat, and persistent fever, also in bedridden patients.
- Principal histopathologic feature: variable focal acantholysis and dyskeratosis.
- No evidence of genetic predisposition.
- Management: glucocorticosteroids under occlusion, UVB, or PUVA (photochemotherapy). Oral glucocorticosteroids, dapsone, and isotretinoin in refractory cases.
- Synonym: transient acantholytic dermatosis.

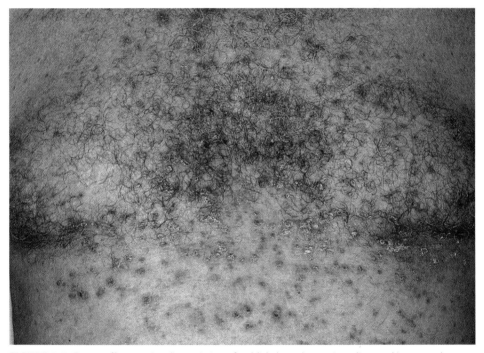

FIGURE 5-5 Grover disease A rash consisting of reddish, hyperkeratotic scaling, and/or crusted papules with a sandpaper feel upon palpation. Papules are discrete, scattered on the central trunk, and very pruritic.

HAILEY–HAILEY DISEASE (FAMILIAL BENIGN PEMPHIGUS) ICD-10: Q 82.8

- Hailey–Hailey disease, or familial benign pemphigus, is a rare genodermatosis with dominant inheritance that is classically described as a blistering disorder but actually presents as an erythematous, erosive, oozing condition with cracks and fissures localized to the nape of the neck, axillae (Fig. 5-6).
- Submammary regions, inguinal folds, and scrotum *are major sites of involvement*.
- Individual lesions consist of microscopically small flaccid vesicles on an erythematous background that soon turn into eroded plaques with the described, highly characteristic, fissured appearance (Fig. 5-6). Crusting, scaling, and hypertrophic vegetative lesions occur.
- The underlying pathologic process is acantholysis whereby the fragility of the epidermis results from a defect in the adhesion complex between desmosomal proteins and tonofilaments.
- The genetic abnormality lies in *ATP2CI*, which encodes an ATP-powered calcium pump.
- Onset is usually between the third and fourth decades.
- Crusting, scaling, and hypertrophic vegetative growths may occur.
- Histology explains the clinical appearance as epidermal cells lose their coherence with acantholysis throughout the epithelium, giving the appearance of a dilapidated brick wall.
- Colonization of the lesions, particularly by *Staphylococcus aureus and candida*, is a trigger for further acantholysis and maintenance of the pathologic process.
- Treatment rests on antimicrobial therapy, administered both topically and systemically; systemically, the tetracyclines seem to work better than most. Mupirocin topically. Topical glucocorticoids depress the anti-inflammatory response and accelerate healing. In severe cases, dermabrasion or carbon dioxide laser vaporization leads to healing with scars, which are resistant to recurrences. The condition becomes less troublesome with age.

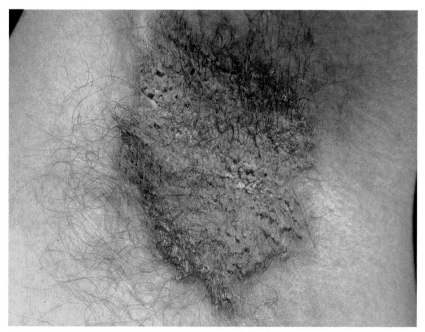

FIGURE 5-6 Hailey–Hailey disease This 46-year-old male had oozing lesions on both armpits, occasionally in the groins and nape of the neck for several years, which became worse during summer months. Father and sister have similar lesions. Lesions wax and wane, are painful, and show typical cracks and fissures within a partially erosive erythematous plaque.

DISSEMINATED SUPERFICIAL ACTINIC POROKERATOSIS (DSAP) ICD-10: Q 82.8

- DSAP is the most common form of the very rare porokeratoses.
- Uniformly small, annular flat papules range from 2 to 5 mm in diameter.
- Distributed symmetrically on the extremities and located predominantly in sun-exposed sites.
- Typically, it spares the palms, soles, and mucous membranes.
- Characteristic feature: well-demarcated hyperkeratotic border of individual lesions, usually <1 mm in height with a characteristic longitudinal furrow encircling the entire lesion (**Fig. 5-7**).
- As lesions progress, the central area becomes atrophic and anhidrotic.
- Symptoms: asymptomatic or mildly pruritic cosmetically disfiguring.
- Tends to be inherited as an autosomal-dominant disorder.
- Pathogenesis unknown.
- A benign condition, but rarely a precursor for in situ or invasive squamous cell carcinoma.
- Treatment: topical 5-fluorouracil, retinoids, and imiquimod.
- Patients should be monitored for SCC.

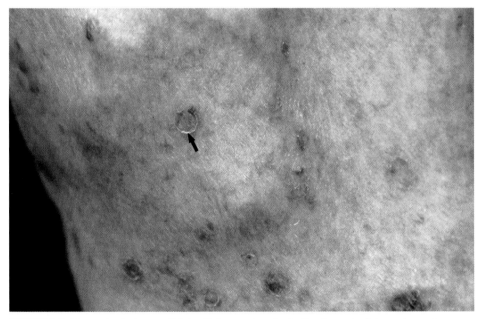

FIGURE 5-7 Disseminated superficial actinic porokeratosis Small annular flat papules up to 4 mm in diameter surrounded by a well-demarcated hyperkeratotic border (arrow) on the lower leg of a 55-year-old female. With a hand lens, the longitudinal furrow encircling the entire lesion can be seen.

OTHER POROKERATOSES ICD-10: 82.8

- Very rare, genetically heterogenous disorders which all have the porokeratotic ridge described for DSAP.
- These porokeratoses are porokeratosis of Mibelli, disseminated superficial porokeratosis (DSP), porokeratosis palmaris et plantaris disseminata, punctate porokeratosis, linear porokeratosis, and a syndromic form.

For details see G.M.O'Regan and A.D. Irvine, Dermatology in General Medicine, 8th edition. LA Goldsmith, SI Katz, BA Gilchrest, AS Paller, DJ Leffell, K Wolff eds. McGraw-Hill, NY, 2012, pp. 563–568.

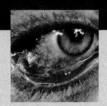

GENETIC AND ACQUIRED BULLOUS DISEASES

Bullous diseases are defined as conditions where cavities filled with fluid form in the superficial layers of the skin clinically manifesting as vesicles or blisters. Although vesicles and blisters can arise as secondary lesions in many conditions, in the bullous diseases they are the primary pathologic event. Genetic (hereditary) and acquired (mostly autoimmune) bullous diseases exist.

HEREDITARY EPIDERMOLYSIS BULLOSA (EB) ICD-10: Q 81

- A spectrum of rare genodermatoses in which a disturbed coherence of the epidermis and/or dermis leads to blister formation following trauma. Hence, the designation *mechanobullous dermatoses*.
- Disease manifestations range from very mild to severely mutilating and even lethal forms that differ in modes of inheritance, clinical manifestations, and associated findings.
- Classification based on the site of blister formation distinguishes three main groups: epidermolytic or EB simplex, junctional EB (JEB), and dermolytic or dystrophic EB (DEB).
- In each of these groups, there are several distinct types of EB based on clinical, genetic, histologic, and biochemical evaluation.

CLASSIFICATION

Based on the level of cleavage and blister formation, there are three main types:

- Epidermolytic. Cleavage occurs in keratinocytes: EB simplex (EBS).
- Junctional. Cleavage occurs in basal lamina: junctional EB (JEB).
- Dermolytic. Cleavage occurs in most superficial papillary dermis: dermolytic or dystrophic EB (DEB).

In each of these groups, there are several distinct types of EB based on clinical, genetic, histologic/electronmicroscopic, and biochemical evaluation (Table 6-1). Only the most important are discussed here.

EPIDEMIOLOGY

The overall incidence of hereditary EB is placed at 19.6 live births per 1 million births in the United States. Stratified by subtype, the incidences are 11 for EBS, 2 for JEB, and 5 for DEB. The estimated prevalence in the United States is 8.2 per million, but this figure represents only the most severe cases. It does not include the majority of very mild disease going unreported.

ETIOLOGY AND PATHOGENESIS

GENETIC DEFECTS Molecules involved are listed in Table 6-1 and localization in the tissue and sites of cleavage are shown in Figure 6-1.

CLINICAL PHENOTYPES

EB Simplex

A trauma-induced, intraepidermal blistering, based in most cases on mutations of the genes for keratins 5 and 14, resulting in a disturbance of the stability of the keratin filament network (Table 6-1). This causes cytolysis of basal keratinocytes and a cleft in the basal cell layer (Fig. 6-1). Different subgroups have considerable phenotypic variations (Table 6-1), and there are several distinct forms, most of which are dominantly inherited. The two most common are described in the following discussion. **Generalized EBS** (Table 6-1). The so-called Koebner variant is dominantly inherited, with onset at birth to early infancy. Generalized blistering following trauma with a predilection for traumatized body sites such as the feet, hands, elbows, and knees. Blisters tense or flaccid (Fig. 6-2) leading to erosions. Rapid healing and only minimal scarring at sites of repeated

TABLE 6-1 Classification of Epidermolysis Bullosa

Level of Separation	Disease	Defect
Simplex	Generalized/Koebner	KRT5/KRT14
Simplex	Herpetiformis/Dowling-Meara	KRT5/KRT14
Simplex	Localized/Weber-Cockayne	KRT5/KRT14
Simplex	Ogna	KRT5/KRT14/PLEC1
Simplex	Mottled pigmentation	KRT5/KRT14
Simplex	EB with muscular dystrophy	PLEC1
Simplex	Superficials	KRT5/KRT14
Simplex	Ectodermal dysplasia-skin fragility	PKP1
Junctional[a]	EB with pyloric atresia	ITGB4/ITGA6/PLEC1
Junctional	Herlitz	LAMB3/LAMA3/LAMG2
Junctional	Non-Herlitz (GABEB)	LAMB3/LAMA3/LAMG2/COL17A1
Junctional	Localized	COL17A1
Dystrophic	Generalized dominant	COL7A1
Dystrophic	Localized dominant	COL7A1
Dystrophic	Recessive	COL7A1
Dystrophic	Hallopeau-Siemens	COL7A1
Variable	Kindler syndrome	KIND1

[a]Alternatively classified as simplex.
COL7A1, collagen type VII, α_1; EB, epidermolysis bullosa; ITGB, integrin β; KRT, keratin; LAMA, laminin α; LAMB, laminin β; PKP, plakophilin; PLEC, plectin; GABEB, Generalized atrophic benign epidermolysis bullosa.

Source: Modified with permission from Marinkovich MP. Inherited epidermolysis bullosa. In: Goldsmith LA, Katz SI, Gilchrest BA, et al, eds. *Fitzpatrick's Dermatology in General Medicine*. 8th ed. New York, NY: McGraw-Hill; 2012, pp. 649–665.

FIGURE 6-1 Schematic of the components of dermal–epidermal basement membrane and levels of dermal–epidermal separation in hereditary and autoimmune bullous diseases with dermal–epidermal cleavage discussed in this Atlas EBS, epidermolysis bullosa simplex; BP, bullous pemphigoid; PG, pempihgoid gestationis; LAD, linear IgA disease; CP, cicatricial pemphigoid; EBA, epidermolysis bullosa acquisita; DEB, dermolytic epidermolysis bullosa. (Modified with permission from Marinkovich MP. Inherited epidermolysis bullosa. In: Goldsmith LA, Katz SI, Gilchrest BA, et al, eds. *Fitzpatrick's Dermatology in General Medicine*. 8th ed. New York, NY: McGraw-Hill; 2012, pp. 649–665.)

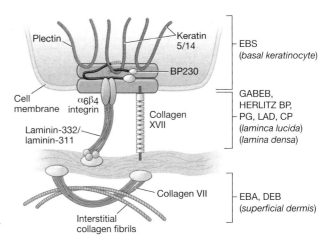

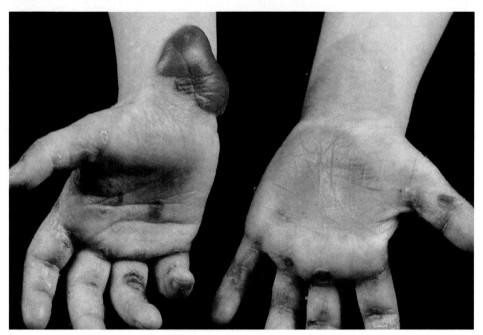

FIGURE 6-2 Generalized EBS (Koebner) This 4-year-old girl has had blistering since very early infancy with predilection for traumatized body sites such as the palms and soles and also the elbows and knees. Blistering also occurs in other areas such as the forearm, as shown here, and on the trunk. There is hardly any evidence of scarring.

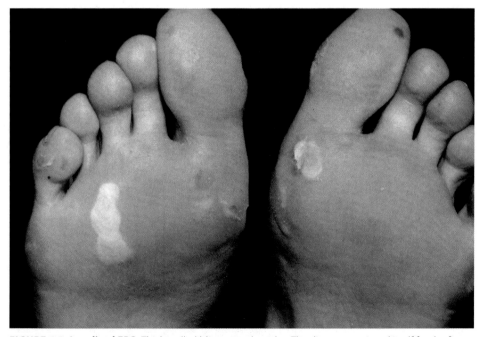

FIGURE 6-3 Localized EBS Thick-walled blisters on the soles. The disease presented itself for the first time during military training when this 19-year-old had to march over a long distance.

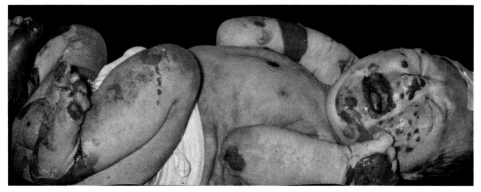

FIGURE 6-4 Junctional epidermolysis bullosa (Herlitz) There are large eroded, oozing, and bleeding areas that occurred intrapartum. When this newborn is lifted up, dislodgment of epidermis and erosions occur with manual handling.

blistering. Palmoplantar hyperkeratoses may be present. Nails, teeth, and oral mucosa are usually spared.

Localized EBS. Weber-Cockayne subtype (Table 6-1). The most common form of EBS. Onset in childhood or later. The disease may not present itself until adulthood, when thick-walled blisters on the feet and hands occur after excessive exercise, manual work, or military training (Fig. 6-3). Increased ambient temperature facilitates lesions. Hyperhidrosis of palms and soles; secondary infection of blisters.

Junctional EB

All forms of JEB share the pathologic feature of blister formation within the lamina lucida of the basement membrane (Fig. 6-1). Mutations are in the gene for collagen XVII and laminin (Table 6-1). Autosomal recessive, several clinical phenotypes (Table 6-1), three of which are described as follows.

Herlitz EB (JEB Gravis). Mortality rate is 40% during the first year of life. Generalized blistering at birth (Fig. 6-4) or distinctive and severe periorificial granulation, loss of nails, and involvement of most mucosal surfaces. The skin of these children may be completely denuded, representing oozing painful erosion. Associated findings include all symptoms resulting from generalized epithelial blistering with respiratory, gastrointestinal, and genitourinary organ systems involved.

Non-Herlitz EB JEB Mitis. These children may have moderate or severe JEB at birth but survive infancy and clinically improve with age. Periorificial nonhealing erosions during childhood.

Non-Herlitz EB Generalized Atrophic Benign Epidermolysis Bullosa (GABEB). Presents

at birth with generalized cutaneous blistering and erosions on the extremities, trunk, face, and scalp. Survival to adulthood is the rule, but blistering on traumatized areas continues (Fig. 6-5). Pronounced with increased ambient temperature, and there is atrophic healing of the lesions. Nail dystrophy, nonscarring or scarring alopecia, mild oral mucous membrane involvement, and enamel defects may occur. Mutations are in the genes for laminin and collagen XVII (Table 6-1).

Dystrophic Epidermolysis Bullosa (DEB)

DEB is a spectrum of dermolytic diseases where blistering occurs below the basal lamina (Fig. 6-1); healing is therefore usually accompanied by scarring and milia formation, hence, the name *dystrophic*. There are four principal subtypes, all caused by mutations in anchoring fibril VII collagen (Table 6-1), two of which are described as follows.

Dominant DEB. Cockayne-Touraine disease. Onset in infancy or early childhood with acral blistering and nail dystrophy; milia and scar formation, which may be hypertrophic or hyperplastic. Oral lesions are uncommon and the teeth are usually normal.

Recessive DEB (RDEB). Comprises a larger spectrum of clinical phenotypes. The localized, less severe form (RDEB mitis) occurs at birth, shows acral blistering, atrophic scarring, and little or no mucosal involvement. Generalized, severe RDEB, the Hallopeau-Siemens variant, is mutilating. There is generalized blistering at birth, then progression followed by repeated blistering at the same sites (Fig. 6-6) result in remarkable scarring and ulcerations, syndactyly with loss of nails (Fig. 6-7) and even

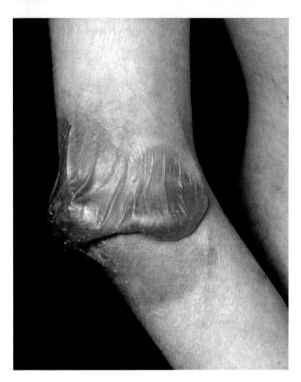

FIGURE 6-5 Generalized atrophic benign epidermolysis bullosa (GABEB) This 15-year-old boy has had cutaneous blistering since birth, with blisters and erosions arising on the elbows and knees and also on the trunk and arms following trauma. There is no scarring but some spotty atrophy will occur.

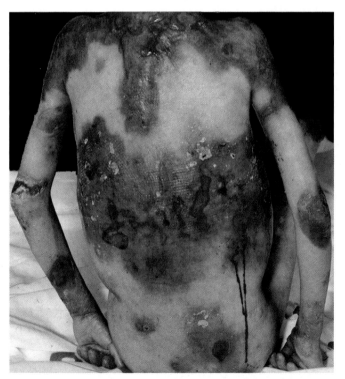

FIGURE 6-6 Generalized recessive dystrophic epidermolysis bullosa (RDEB) In this severe disease, blistering occurs often at the same sites, as in this 10-year-old girl. Blisters lead to erosions and these become ulcers that have a low tendency to heal. When healing occurs, it results in scarring. This girl also has enamel defects with caries, strictures of the esophagus, severe anemia, and considerable growth retardation. It is obvious that the large wounds are portal entries for systemic infection.

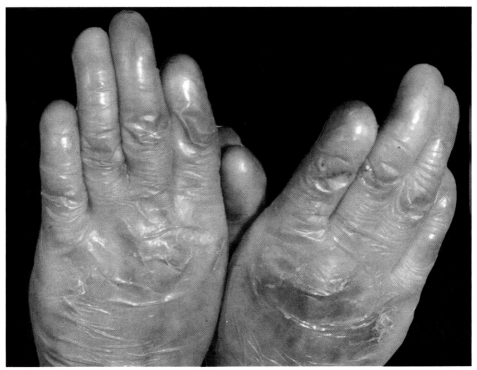

FIGURE 6-7 Generalized recessive dystrophic epidermolysis bullosa (RDEB) Loss of all finger-nails, syndactyly, and severe atrophic scarring on the dorsa of hands.

mitten-like deformities of the hands and feet, and flexion contractures. There are enamel defects with caries and parodontitis, strictures, and scarring in the oral mucous membrane and esophagus, urethral and anal stenosis, and ocular surface scarring; also malnutrition, growth retardation, and anemia. Squamous cell carcinoma in chronic recurrent erosions.

DIAGNOSIS

Based on clinical appearance and history. His-topathology determines the level of cleavage, which is further defined by electron micros-copy and/or immunohistochemical mapping. Western blot, Northern blot, restriction frag-ment length polymorphism analysis, and DNA sequences may then identify the mutated gene.

MANAGEMENT

There is as yet no causal therapy for EB, but gene therapy is being investigated.

Management is tailored to the severity and extent of skin involvement: supportive skin care, supportive care for other organ systems, and systemic therapies for complications. Wound management, nutritional support, and infection control are key.

In EBS, maintenance of a cool environ-ment and use of soft, well-ventilated shoes are important. Blistered skin is treated by saline compresses and topical antibiotics or, in the case of inflammation, with topical steroids. More severely affected JEB and DEB patients are treated like patients in a burn unit. Gentle bathing and cleansing are fol-lowed by protective emollients and nonad-herent dressings.

Although rare, EB and, in particular, JEB and DEB pose a major health and socioeconomic problem. Organizations such as the Dystrophic Epidermolysis Bullosa Research Association (DEBRA) offer assistance that includes patient education and support.

PEMPHIGUS ICD-10: L10

- A serious, acute or chronic, bullous autoimmune disease of skin and mucous membranes based on acantholysis.
- Two major types: Pemphigus vulgaris (PV) and pemphigus foliaceus (PF).
- PV: Flaccid blisters on skin and erosions on mucous membranes. PF: Scaly and crusted skin lesions.
- PV: Suprabasal acantholysis. PF: Subcorneal acantholysis.
- IgG autoantibodies to desmogleins, transmembrane desmosomal adhesion molecules.
- Serious and often fatal, unless treated with immunosuppressive agents.

CLASSIFICATION (see Table 6-2)

Epidemiology

PV: Rare, more common in the Jewish population and people of Mediterranean descent. In Jerusalem, the incidence is estimated at 16 per million, whereas in France and Germany, it is 1.3 per million.

PF: Also rare but endemic in rural areas in of Brazil (fogo selvagem), where the prevalence can be as high as 3.4%.

AGE OF ONSET Forty to 60 years; fogo selvagem also occurs in children and young adults.
SEX Equal incidence in males and in females, but predominance of females with PF are in Tunisia and Colombia.

ETIOLOGY AND PATHOGENESIS

An autoimmune disorder. Loss of cell-to-cell adhesion in the epidermis (*acantholysis*).

TABLE 6-2 Classification of Pemphigus

Pemphigus vulgaris
  Pemphigus vulgaris: localized and generalized
  Pemphigus vegetans: localized
  Drug induced

Pemphigus foliaceus
  Pemphigus foliaceus: generalized
  Pemphigus erythematosus: localized
  Fogo selvagem: endemic
  Drug induced

Paraneoplastic pemphigus (Paraneoplastic Autoimmune Multiorgan Syndrome, (PAMS): associated with malignancy

IgA pemphigus: subcorneal pustular dermatosis and intraepidermal neutrophilic IgA dermatitis[a]

[a]see F. Trautinger and H. Hönigsmann: Subcorneal pustular dermatosis (Sneddon-Wilkinson Disease) in LA. Goldsmith et al. Editors, *Fitzpatrick's Dermatology in General Medicine* 8th edition, New York, McGraw-Hill, 2012, pp. 383–385.

Occurs as a result of circulating antibodies of the IgG class, which bind to desmogleins, transmembrane glycoproteins in the desmosomes, members of the cadherin superfamily. Desmosomes hold epidermal cells (keratinocytes) together. In PV, desmoglein 3 (in some, also desmoglein 1). In PF, only desmoglein 1. Autoantibodies interfere with calcium-sensitive adhesion function and thus induce acantholysis.

CLINICAL MANIFESTATIONS

Pemphigus Vulgaris usually starts in the oral mucosa, but months may elapse before skin lesions occur. Less frequently, there may be a generalized, acute eruption of bullae from the beginning. No pruritus but burning and pain in erosions. Painful and tender mouth lesions may prevent adequate food intake. Epistaxis, hoarseness, and dysphagia. Weakness, malaise, and weight loss.

SKIN LESIONS Vesicles and bullae with serous content, flaccid (flabby) (Fig. 6-8), easily ruptured, and weeping (Fig. 6-9), arising on *normal* skin, randomly scattered, and discrete. Localized (e.g., to mouth or circumscribed skin area) or generalized with a random pattern. Extensive erosions bleed easily (Fig. 6-10), crusts particularly on scalp. Since blisters rupture so easily, only painful erosions in many patients.

Nikolsky Sign. Dislodging of normal-appearing epidermis by lateral finger pressure in the vicinity of lesions, which leads to an erosion. Pressure on bulla leads to lateral extension of the blister.

Sites of Predilection. Scalp, face, chest, axillae, groin, and umbilicus. In bedridden patients, there is extensive involvement of the back (Fig. 6-10).

MUCOUS MEMBRANES Bullae are rarely seen in erosions of the mouth (see Section 33) and nose, pharynx and larynx, or vagina.

OTHER TYPES (see Table 6-2)

Pemphigus Vegetans (PVeg). A PV variant. Usually confined to intertriginous regions, perioral area, neck, and scalp. Granulomatous vegetating purulent plaques that extend centrifugally. In

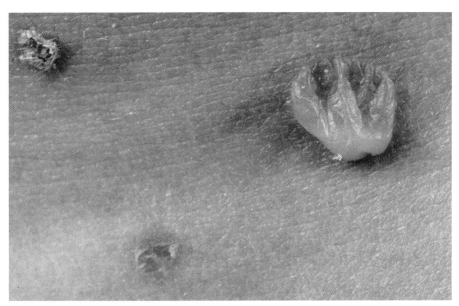

FIGURE 6-8 Pemphigus vulgaris This is the classic initial lesion: flaccid, easily ruptured bulla on normal-appearing skin. Ruptured vesicles lead to erosions that subsequently crust as seen in the two smaller lesions.

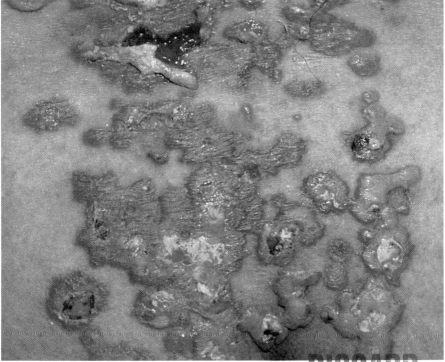

FIGURE 6-9 Pemphigus vulgaris Widespread confluent flaccid blisters on the lower back of a 40-year-old male who had a generalized eruption including scalp and mucous membranes. The eroded lesions are extremely painful.

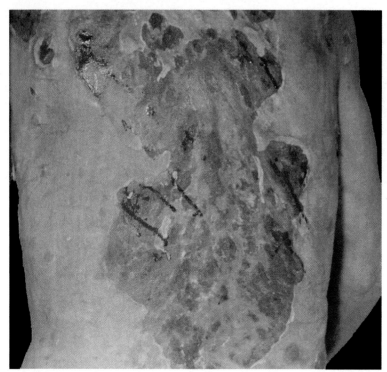

FIGURE 6-10 Pemphigus vulgaris Widespread confluent erosions that are very painful and bleed easily in a 53-year-old male. There are hardly any intact blisters because they are so fragile and break easily. The blood tracts go sideways because the patient had been lying on his right side before the photograph was taken.

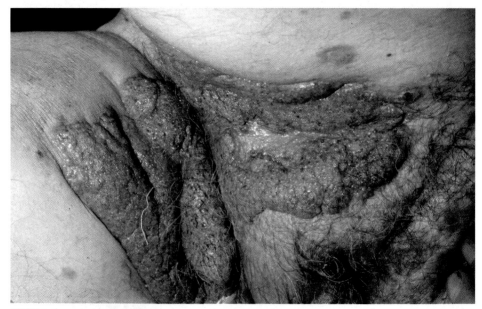

FIGURE 6-11 Pemphigus vegetans Papillomatous, cauliflower-like, oozing growths in the groin and pubis of a 50-year-old man.

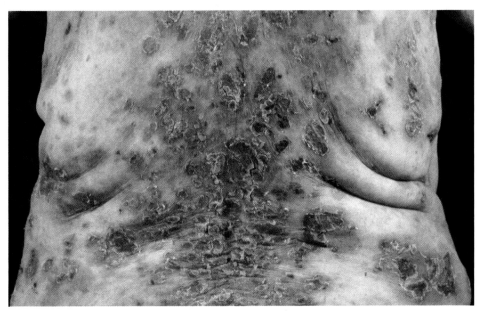

FIGURE 6-12 Pemphigus foliaceus The back of this patient is covered by scaly crusts and superficial erosions.

these patients, there is a granulomatous response to the autoimmune damage of PV (Fig. 6-11).
Drug-Induced PV. Clinically identical to sporadic PV. Several different drugs implicated, most significantly, captopril and D-penicillamine.
Pemphigus Foliaceus. PF has no mucosal lesions and starts with scaly, crusted lesions on an erythematous base, initially in seborrheic areas.
SKIN LESIONS Most commonly on the face, scalp, upper chest, and abdomen. Scaly, crusted erosions on an erythematous base (Fig. 6-12). In early or localized disease, sharply demarcated in seborrheic areas; they may stay localized or progress to generalized disease and exfoliative erythroderma. Initial lesion also a flaccid bulla, but this is rarely seen because of superficial location (see dermatopathology).
Brazilian Pemphigus (Fogo Selvagem). A distinctive form of PF endemic to south central Brazil. Clinically, histologically, and immunopathologically identical to PF. Patients improve when moved to urban areas but relapse after returning to endemic regions. Probably related to an arthropod-borne infectious agent, with clustering similar to that of the *black fly—simulium nigrimanum*. More than 1000 new cases per year are estimated to occur in the endemic regions.

Pemphigus Erythematosus (PE). *Synonym:* Senear-Usher syndrome. A localized variant of PF largely confined to seborrheic sites. Erythematous, crusted, and erosive lesions in the "butterfly" area of the face, forehead, and presternal and interscapular regions. May have antinuclear antibodies.
Drug-Induced PF. As in PV, associated with D-penicillamine and less frequently by captopril and other drugs. In most, but not all, instances, the eruption resolves after termination of therapy with the offending drug.
Neonatal Pemphigus. Very rare, transplacental transmission from diseased mother; spontaneous resolution.

PARANEOPLASTIC PEMPHIGUS (PARANEOPLASTIC AUTOIMMUNE MULTIORGAN SYNDROME)

This is a disease sui generis and is discussed in Section 19.

LABORATORY EXAMINATIONS

DERMATOPATHOLOGY PV: Light microscopy (select early small bulla or, if not present, margin of larger bulla or erosion). Separation of keratinocytes, suprabasally, leading to split

just *above* the basal cell layer and vesicles containing separated, rounded-up (acantholytic) keratinocytes. PF: Superficial form with acantholysis in the granular layer of the epidermis. **IMMUNOPATHOLOGY** Direct immunofluorescence (IF) staining reveals IgG and often C3 deposited in lesional and paralesional skin in *the intercellular substance of the epidermis*. In PE Ig and complement deposits also found at the dermal epidermal junction.
SERUM Autoantibodies (IgG) detected by indirect IF or ELISA. Titer usually correlates with activity of disease. In PV, autoantibodies against a 130-kDa glycoprotein, desmoglein 3, located in desmosomes of keratinocytes. In PF, autoantibodies to a 160-kDa intercellular (cell surface) antigen, desmoglein 1, in desmosomes of keratinocytes.

DIAGNOSIS AND DIFFERENTIAL DIAGNOSIS

Difficult problem if only mouth lesions are present. Aphthae, mucosal lichen planus, and erythema multiforme. Differential diagnosis includes all forms of acquired bullous diseases (see Table 6-3). Biopsy of the skin and mucous membrane, direct IF, and demonstration of circulating autoantibodies confirm a high index of suspicion.

COURSE

In most cases, the disease inexorably progresses to death unless treated aggressively with immunosuppressive agents. The mortality rate has been markedly reduced since treatment has become available. Currently, morbidity is mainly related to glucocorticoids and immunosuppressive therapies.

MANAGEMENT

Requires expertise and experience. Treatment to be performed by a dermatologist.
GLUCOCORTICOIDS 2 to 3 mg/kg body weight of prednisone until cessation of new blister formation and disappearance of the Nikolsky

sign. Then rapid reduction to about half the initial dose until the patient is almost clear, followed by very slow tapering of the dose to the minimal effective maintenance dose.
CONCOMITANT IMMUNOSUPPRESSIVE THERAPY Immunosuppressive agents are given concomitantly for their glucocorticoid-sparing effect:

Azathioprine. Determine thiopurine transferase. 2 to 3 mg/kg body weight until complete clearing, then tapered.
Methotrexate. Either orally or IM at doses of 25 to 35 mg/wk. Dose adjustments are made as with azathioprine.
Cyclophosphamide. 100 to 200 mg daily, with reduction to maintenance doses of 50 to 100 mg/d. Alternatively, cyclophosphamide "bolus" therapy with 1000 mg IV once a week or every 2 weeks in the initial phases, followed by 50 to 100 mg/d po as maintenance.
Mycophenolate mofetil. 1 g twice daily.
Plasmapheresis. In conjunction with glucocorticoids and immunosuppressive agents.
High-dose intravenous immunoglobulin (IVIG). 2 g/kg body weight every 3 to 4 weeks has glucocorticoid-sparing effects.
Rituximab. Monoclonal antibody to CD20 targets B cells, the precursors of (auto) antibody-producing plasma cells. For patients refractory to the treatments previously listed, intravenous therapy given once a week for 4 weeks shows dramatic effects in some and at least partial remission in other patients. Serious infections may be seen.

OTHER MEASURES Cleansing baths, wet dressings, topical and intralesional glucocorticoids, and antimicrobial therapy in documented bacterial infections. Correction of fluid and electrolyte imbalance.
MONITORING Clinical, for improvement of skin lesions and development of drug-related side effects. Laboratory monitoring of pemphigus antibody titers and for hematologic and metabolic indicators of glucocorticoid- and/or immunosuppressive-induced adverse effects.

TABLE 6-3 Differential Diagnosis of Important Acquired Bullous Diseases

Disease	Skin Lesions	Mucous Membranes	Distribution
PV	Flaccid bullae on normal skin, erosions	Almost always involved, erosions	Anywhere, localized or generalized
PVeg	Granulating plaques, occasionally vesicles at margin	As in PV	Intertriginous regions, scalp
PF	Crusted erosions, occasionally flaccid vesicles	Rarely involved	Exposed, seborrheic regions or generalized
Bullous pemphigoid	Tense bullae on normal and erythematous skin; urticarial plaques and papules	Mouth involved in 10–35%	Anywhere, localized or generalized
EBA	Tense bullae and erosions, noninflammatory or BP-, DH- or LAD-like presentation	May be severely involved (oral esophagus, vagina)	Traumatized regions or random
Dermatitis herpetiformis	Grouped papules, vesicles, urticarial plaques, crusted	None	Predilection sites: elbows, knees, gluteal, sacral, and scapular areas
Linear IgA dermatosis	Annular, grouped papules, vesicles, and bullae	Oral erosions and ulcers, conjunctival erosions and scarring	Anywhere

Disease	Histopathology	Immunopathology/Skin	Serum
PV	Suprabasal acantholysis	IgG intercellular pattern	IgG AB to intercellular substance of epidermis (IIF) ELISA: AB to desmoglein 3 >>> desmoglein 1
PF	Acantholysis in granular layer	IgG, intracellular pattern	IgG AB to intercellular substance of epidermis (IIF) ELISA: AB to desmoglein 1 only
PVeg	Acantholysis ± intraepidermal neutrophilic abscesses, epidermal hyperplasia	As in PV	As in PV
Bullous pemphigoid	Subepidermal blister	IgG and C3 linear at BMZ	IgG AB to BMZ (IIF); directed to BPAG1 and BPAG2
EBA	Subepidermal blister	Linear IgG at BMZ	IgG AB to BMZ (IIF) directed to type VII collagen (ELISA, Western blot)
Dermatitis herpetiformis	Papillary microabscesses, subepidermal vesicle	Granular IgA in tips of papillae	Antiendomysial antibodies
Linear IgA dermatosis	Subepidermal blister with neutrophils	Linear IgA at BMZ	Low titers of IgA AB against BMZ

AB, antibody; BMZ, basement membrane zone; BP, bullous pemphigoid; DH, dermatitis herpetiformis; EB, epidermolysis bullosa acquisita; ELISA, enzyme-linked immunosorbent assay; IIF, indirect immunofluorescence; LAD, linear IgA dermatosis; PF, pemphigus foliaceus; PV, pemphigus vulgaris; PVeg, pemphigus vegetans.

BULLOUS PEMPHIGOID (BP) ICD-10: L12.0

- A bullous autoimmune disease usually in elderly patients.
- Pruritic papular and/or urticarial lesions with large tense bullae.
- Subepidermal blisters with eosinophils.
- C3 and IgG at epidermal basement membrane, antibasement membrane IgG autoantibodies in serum.
- Autoantigens are keratinocyte hemidesmosome proteins.
- Therapy includes topical and systemic glucocorticoids and other immunosuppressives.

EPIDEMIOLOGY

AGE OF ONSET Sixty to 80 years.
SEX Equal incidence in males and in females. No known racial predilection.
INCIDENCE The most common bullous autoimmune disease. Seven per million in Germany and France. Far more common in authors' experience in very old people.

ETIOLOGY AND PATHOGENESIS

Interaction of autoantibody with BP antigen [BPAG1 (BP230) and BPAG2 (type XVII collagen)] in hemidesmosomes of basal keratinocytes (Fig. 6-1) is followed by complement and mast cell activation, attraction of neutrophils and eosinophils, and release of multiple bioactive molecules from inflammatory cells.

CLINICAL MANIFESTATION

Often starts with a prodromal eruption (urticarial, papular lesions) and evolves in weeks to months to bullae that may appear suddenly as a generalized eruption. Initially moderate or severe pruritus; later, tenderness of eroded lesions. No constitutional symptoms, except in widespread, severe disease.

SKIN LESIONS Erythematous, papular, or urticarial-type lesions (Fig. 6-13) may precede bullae formation by months. Bullae: small (Fig. 6-13) or large (Fig. 6-14) tense, firm-topped, oval or round; arise in normal, erythematous, or urticarial skin and contain serous (Fig. 6-14) or hemorrhagic fluid. Localized or generalized, usually scattered but also grouped in arciform and serpiginous patterns. Bullae rupture less easily than in pemphigus,

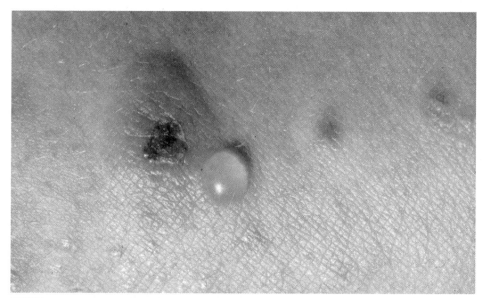

FIGURE 6-13 Bullous pemphigoid Early lesions in a 75-year-old female. Note urticarial plaques and a small, tense blister with a clear serous content.

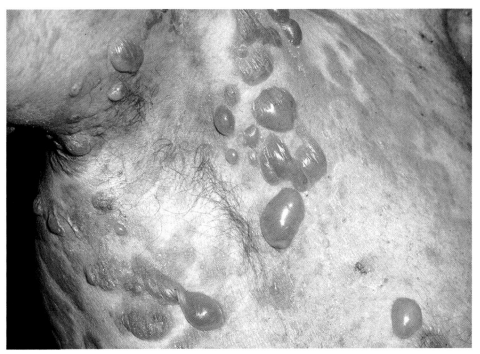

FIGURE 6-14 Bullous pemphigoid This 77-year-old male has a generalized eruption with confluent urticarial plaques and multiple tense blisters. The condition is severely pruritic.

but sometimes large, bright red, oozing, and bleeding erosions occur. Usually bullae collapse and transform into crusts.

Sites of Predilection. Axillae; medial aspects of thighs, groins, and abdomen; flexor aspects of forearms; lower legs (often first manifestation); generalized.

MUCOUS MEMBRANES Practically only in the mouth (10 to 35%); less severe and painful, and less easily ruptured than in pemphigus (see Section 33).

LABORATORY EXAMINATIONS

DERMATOPATHOLOGY Light Microscopy. Neutrophils in "Indian-file" alignment at dermal–epidermal junction; neutrophils, eosinophils, and lymphocytes in papillary dermis; *subepidermal* bulla.

Electron Microscopy. Junctional cleavage, i.e., split occurs in lamina lucida of basement membrane (see Fig. 6-1).

IMMUNOPATHOLOGY Linear IgG deposits along the basement membrane zone. Also C3, which may occur in the absence of IgG.

SERUM Circulating antibasement membrane IgG antibodies detected by IIF in 70% of patients. Titers do not correlate with the course of disease. Autoantibodies recognize two types of antigens. BPAG1 is a 230-kDa glycoprotein that has high homology with desmoplakin I and is part of hemidesmosomes. BPAG2 is a transmembranous 180-kDa polypeptide (type XVII collagen) (see Fig. 6-1).

HEMATOLOGY Eosinophilia (not always).

DIAGNOSIS AND DIFFERENTIAL DIAGNOSIS

Clinical appearance, histopathology, and immunology permit a differentiation from other bullous diseases (see Table 6-3).

MANAGEMENT

Systemic prednisone with starting doses of 50 to 100 mg/d continued until clear, either alone or combined with azathioprine, 150 mg daily, for remission induction and 50 to 100 mg for maintenance; in refractory cases, IVIG; plasmapheresis. Rituximab i.v. effective in some cases, whereas in others it helps sparing corticosteroids. In milder cases, sulfones (dapsone), 100 to 150 mg/d. Low-dose methotrexate 2.5

to 10 mg weekly PO is effective and safe in the elderly. In very mild cases and for local recurrences, topical glucocorticoid or topical tacrolimus therapy may be beneficial. Tetracycline ± nicotinamide has been reported to be effective in some cases.

COURSE AND PROGNOSIS

Patients often go into a permanent remission after therapy and do not require further therapy; local recurrences can sometimes be controlled with topical glucocorticoids. Some cases go into spontaneous remission without therapy.

CICATRICIAL PEMPHIGOID ICD-10: L12.1

- A rare disease, largely of the elderly.
- Ocular involvement may initially manifest as unilateral or bilateral conjunctivitis with burning, dryness, and foreign-body sensation.
- Blisters that rupture easily and erosions resulting from epithelial fragility in the conjunctivae, mouth, oropharynx, and, more rarely, the nasopharyngeal, esophageal, genital, and anal mucosae.
- Chronic involvement results in scarring, symblepharon (**Fig. 6-15**), and, in severe disease, fusion of the bulbar and palpebral conjunctiva. Entropion and trichiasis result in corneal irritation, superficial punctate keratinopathy, corneal neovascularization, ulceration, and blindness.
- Scarring also in the larynx; stricture formation in the esophagus, dysphagia, or dynophagia.
- Blisters on the skin in roughly 30% of patients.
- *Brunsting-Perry pemphigoid* describes a subset of patients whose skin lesions recur at the same sites, mainly on the head and neck and scalp, which can also lead to scarring.
- Antigens to which autoantibodies may be directed include BPAG1, BPAG2, integrin subunits β_4 and α_6, type VII collagen, and laminin 332 (see **Fig. 6-1**).
- *Management*: Mild involvement—topical corticosteroids, calcineurin inhibitors (tacrolimus, pimecrolimus). Moderate and severe involvement: dapsone in combination with prednisone. Some patients require more aggressive immunosuppressive treatment with cyclophosphamide or azathioprine, in combination with glucocorticoids, also high-dose IVIGs, or rituximab. Surgical intervention for scarring and supportive measures.
- *Synonym*: Mucous membrane pemphigoid.

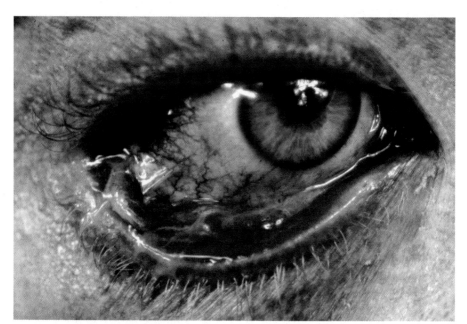

FIGURE 6-15 Cicatricial pemphigoid This condition in a 78-year-old female started with bilateral conjunctival pain and foreign body sensation as the first symptoms. The conjunctiva then became erosive with scarring and fibrous tracts between eyelids and the eye.

PEMPHIGOID GESTATIONIS (PG) ICD-10: L12.8

- A rare pruritic and polymorphic inflammatory bullous dermatosis of pregnancy and the postpartum period.
- Estimated incidence from 1 in 1700 to 1 in 10,000 deliveries.
- Extremely pruritic eruption mainly on the abdomen but also on other areas, with sparing of the mucous membranes. Lesions vary from erythematous, edematous papules, and urticarial plaques (Fig. 6-16) to vesicles and tense bullae (Fig. 6-16 inset).
- Usually begins from the fourth to the seventh month of pregnancy, but can also occur in the first trimester and in the immediate postpartum period. May recur in subsequent pregnancies; if it does, it is likely to begin earlier.
- PG can be exacerbated by the use of estrogen and progesterone-containing medications.
- Histopathologically, it is a subepidermal blistering condition with linear deposition of C3 along the basement membrane zone with concomitant IgG deposition in roughly 30% of patients.
- Serum contains IgG antibasal membrane antibodies, but these are detected in only 20% of patients by IIF. ELISA and immunoblotting assays detect autoantibodies in >70%, directed to BP180 (type XVII collagen) in hemidesmosomes (see Fig. 6-1). They are avid complement-fixing IgG1 antibodies that bind to the amniotic epithelial basement membrane.
- Some 5% of babies born to mothers with PG have urticarial, vesicular, or bullous lesions, which resolve spontaneously during the first weeks. There is a slight increase in premature and small-for-gestational-age births. Some reports revealed significant fetal death and premature deliveries, whereas others have suggested no increase in fetal mortality.
- *Management*: Prednisone, 20 to 40 mg/d, but sometimes higher doses are required; during the postpartum period, taper gradually.

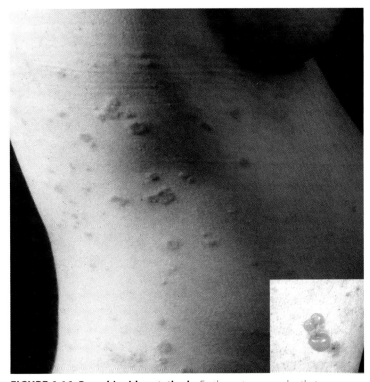

FIGURE 6-16 Pemphigoid gestationis Erythematous papules that were highly pruritic and had appeared on the trunk and abdomen of this 33-year-old pregnant female (third trimester). At this time, there were no blisters and diagnosis was established by biopsy and immunopathology. Inset: Urticarial lesions and vesicles in another patient who had similar eruptions in previous pregnancies.

DERMATITIS HERPETIFORMIS (DH) ICD-10: L13.0

- A chronic, recurrent, intensely pruritic eruption occurring symmetrically on the extremities and the trunk.
- Consists of tiny vesicles, papules, and urticarial plaques that are arranged in groups.
- Associated with gluten-sensitive enteropathy (GSE).
- Characterized histologically by papillary collection of neutrophils.
- Granular IgA deposits in paralesional or normal skin are diagnostic.
- Responds to sulfa drugs and, to a lesser extent, a gluten-free diet.

EPIDEMIOLOGY

Prevalence in Caucasians varies from 10 to 39 per 100,000 persons.
AGE OF ONSET Most common at 30 to 40 years; may occur in children.
SEX Male:female ratio is 2:1.

ETIOLOGY AND PATHOGENESIS

The GSE probably relates to IgA deposits in the skin. Patients have antibodies to transglutaminases (Tgs) that may be the major autoantigens. Epidermal Tg autoantibody probably binds to Tg in the gut and circulates either alone or as immune complexes and deposits in the skin. IgA activates complement via the alternative pathway, with subsequent chemotaxis

of neutrophils releasing their enzymes and producing tissue injury.

CLINICAL MANIFESTATION

Pruritus, intense, episodic; burning or stinging of the skin; rarely, pruritus may be absent. Symptoms often precede the appearance of skin lesions by 8 to 12 h. Ingestion of iodides and overload of gluten are exacerbating factors.
SYSTEMS REVIEW Laboratory evidence of small-bowel malabsorption is detected in 10 to 20% of patients. GSE occurs in nearly all patients and is demonstrated by small-bowel biopsy. There are usually no systemic symptoms.
SKIN LESIONS Erythematous papules or wheal-like plaques (Fig. 6-17); tiny firm-topped vesicles, sometimes hemorrhagic (Fig. 6-18);

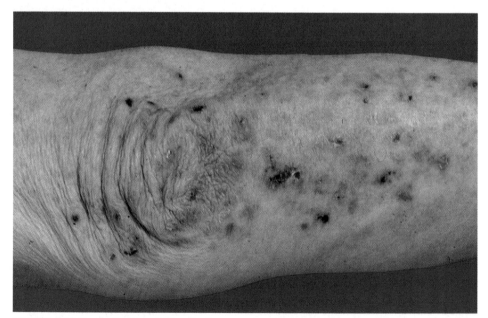

FIGURE 6-17 Dermatitis herpetiformis These are the classic early lesions. Papules, urticarial plaques and excoriated small grouped vesicles, and crusts on the elbow of a 23-year-old male.

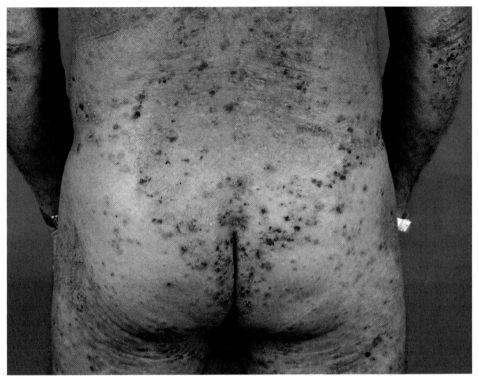

FIGURE 6-18 Dermatitis herpetiformis A 56-year-old male patient with a generalized highly pruritic eruption. The diagnosis can be made upon first sight by the distribution of the lesions. Most heavily involved are the sacral and gluteal areas (note butterfly-like distribution) and (not seen in this picture) the knees and elbows; the scapular areas. Upon close inspection, there are grouped papules, small vesicles, crusts, and erosions on an erythematous base as well as postinflammatory hypo- and hyper-pigmentation.

occasionally bullae. Lesions are arranged in groups (hence the name *herpertiformis*). Scratching results in excoriations, crusts (Fig. 6-18). Postinflammatory hyper- and hypo-pigmentation at sites of healed lesions. **Sites of Predilection.** Typical and almost diagnostic: Extensor areas—elbows (Fig. 6-18), knees. Strikingly symmetrical. Buttocks, scapular, and sacral areas (Figs. 6-18 and 6-19). Here, often in a "butterfly" fashion. Scalp, face, and hairline.

LABORATORY EXAMINATIONS

IMMUNOGENETICS Association with HLA-B8, HLA-DR, and HLA-DQ.

DERMATOPATHOLOGY Biopsy is best from early erythematous papule. Microabscesses (polymorphonuclear cells and eosinophils) at the tips of the dermal papillae. Dermal infiltration of neutrophils and eosinophils. *Subepidermal vesicle.*

IMMUNOFLUORESCENCE Of *perilesional* skin, best on the buttocks. Granular IgA deposits in

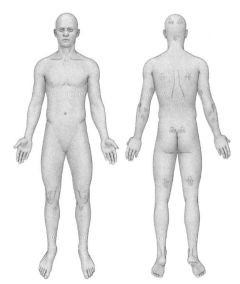

FIGURE 6-19 Dermatitis herpetiformis
Pattern of distribution.

tips of papillae. Diagnostic. Also found are C3 and C5 and alternative complement pathway components.

CIRCULATING AUTOANTIBODIES Antireticulin antibodies of the IgA and IgG types, thyroid antimicrosomal antibodies, and antinuclear antibodies can be present. Putative immune complexes in 20 to 40% of patients. IgA antibodies binding to the intermyofibril substance of smooth muscles (*antiendomysial antibodies*) are present in most patients and have specificity for Tgs.

OTHER STUDIES Steatorrhea (20 to 30%) and abnormal D-xylose absorption (10 to 73%). Anemia secondary to iron or folate deficiency. *Endoscopy of small bowel*: blunting and flattening of the villi (80 to 90%) in the small bowel as in celiac disease. Lesions are focal; verification is by small-bowel biopsy.

DIAGNOSIS AND DIFFERENTIAL DIAGNOSIS

Grouped papulovesicles at predilection sites accompanied by severe pruritus are highly suggestive. Biopsy usually diagnostic, but IgA deposits in perilesional skin detected by IF are the best confirming evidence. Differential diagnosis is to allergic contact dermatitis, atopic dermatitis, scabies, neurotic excoriations, papular urticaria, and bullous autoimmune disease (see Table 6-3).

COURSE

Prolonged, for many years, with a third of patients eventually having a spontaneous remission.

MANAGEMENT

SYSTEMIC THERAPY Dapsone. 100 to 150 mg daily, with gradual reduction to as low as 50 mg twice a week. Dramatic response, often within hours. Obtain a glucose-6-phosphate dehydrogenase level before starting sulfones; obtain methemoglobin levels in the initial 2 weeks and follow blood counts carefully.

Sulfapyridine. 1 to 1.5 g/d, with plenty of fluids, if dapsone contraindicated or not tolerated. Monitor for casts in urine and kidney function.

DIET A gluten-free diet *may* suppress the disease or allow reduction in the dosage of dapsone or sulfapyridine, but response is very slow.

LINEAR IGA DERMATOSIS (LAD) ICD-10: L13.819, L13.820

- A rare, immune-mediated, subepidermal blistering skin disease defined by the presence of homogeneous linear deposits of IgA at the cutaneous basement membrane zone (Fig. 6-1).
- No association with GSE.
- LAD most often occurs after puberty. However, it is identical with *chronic bullous disease of childhood* (CBDC), which is a rare blistering disease that occurs predominantly in children <5 years.
- Clinically similar to DH, but there is more blistering. Patients present with annular or grouped papules, vesicles, and bullae, distributed symmetrically on trunk and extremities (Figs. 6-20 and 6-21). Very pruritic but less severe than DH.
- Mucosal involvement ranges from asymptomatic oral erosions and ulceration to severe oral disease alone, or severe generalized cutaneous involvement and oral disease similar to that in cicatricial pemphigoid.
- Circulating autoantibodies against various epidermal basement membrane antigens.
- LAD has been associated with drugs: vancomycin, lithium, phenytoin, sulfamethoxazole/trimethoprim, furosemide, captopril, diclofenac, and others.
- There is a small risk of lymphoid malignancies, and associated ulcerative colitis has been reported.
- *Management:* Patients respond to dapsone or sulfapyridine but in addition, most may require low-dose prednisone. *Patients do not respond to a gluten-free diet.*

FIGURE 6-20 Linear IgA dermatosis
There are multiple grouped, confluent vesicles, bullae, and crusts on an urticarial and erythematous base. There were similar lesions on the trunk and the upper extremities.

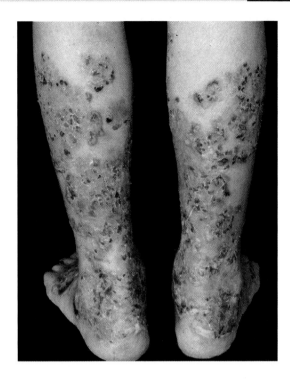

FIGURE 6-21 Linear IgA dermatosis (chronic, bullous disease of childhood) Extensive blistering on the upper extremities and trunk in a 7-year-old child. Note: Blisters are both tense and flaccid. They are grouped and there is no notable inflammation.

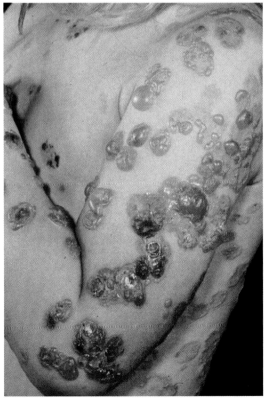

EPIDERMOLYSIS BULLOSA ACQUISITA (EBA) ICD-10: L12.3

- A chronic subepidermal bullous disease associated with autoimmunity to the type VII collagen within the anchoring fibrils in the basement membrane zone (see Fig. 6-1).
- Four types: The *classic mechanobullous presentation* is a noninflammatory, blistering eruption with acral distribution that heals with scarring and milia formation. It is a mechanobullous disease marked by skin fragility. Scars in traumatized regions such as the dorsa of the hands, knuckles, elbows, knees, sacral area, and toes. Resembling porphyria cutanea tarda (see Section 10) or hereditary epidermolysis bullosa.
- *Bullous pemphigoid–like presentation:* Widespread inflammatory vesiculobullous eruption associated with erythematous or urticarial skin lesions involving the trunk, skin folds, and in addition the extremities (Fig. 6-22).
- *Cicatricial pemphigoid–like presentation* has prominent mucosal involvement—erosions and scarring in the mouth, esophagus, conjunctiva, anus, and vagina.
- The *linear IgA bullous dermatosis–like presentation* shows vesicles arranged in an annular fashion, reminiscent of linear IgA bullous dermatosis, DH, or CBDC.
- Histopathology: Subepidermal blisters.
- Immunopathology: linear IgG (plus IgA, gM, factor B, and properdin) at the dermal–epidermal junction.
- Antibodies in sera bind to a 290-kDa band in Western blots containing type VII collagen. ELISA specific for antibodies to type VII collagen.
- Treatment: Difficult. In the mechanobullous form, patients are refractory to high doses of systemic glucocorticoids, azathioprine, methotrexate, and cyclophosphamide, which are somewhat helpful in the inflammatory BP-like form of the disease. Some EBA patients improve on dapsone and high doses of colchicine. Supportive therapy.

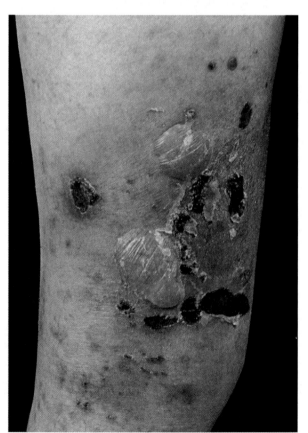

FIGURE 6-22 Epidermolysis bullosa acquisita This is the bullous pemphigoid-like presentation with tense bullae, erosions, and crusts on an erythematous base. There is also postinflammatory pigmentation resulting from previous blistering.

NEUTROPHIL-MEDIATED DISEASES

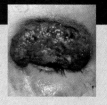

PYODERMA GANGRENOSUM (PG) ICD-10: L88

- PG is an idiopathic, either acute or chronic, severely debilitating skin disease.
- It is characterized by neutrophilic infiltration, destruction of tissue, and ulceration.
- It occurs most commonly in association with a systemic disease, especially arthritis, inflammatory bowel disease, hematologic dyscrasias, and malignancy, but may also occur alone.
- Characterized by the presence of painful, irregular, boggy, blue-red ulcers with undermined borders and purulent necrotic bases.
- There is no laboratory test that establishes the diagnosis.
- The mainstays of treatment are immune-suppressive or -modulating agents.
- Relapses occur in most patients and there is significant morbidity.

EPIDEMIOLOGY

Rare, prevalence unknown. All age groups affected with a peak between 40 and 60 years. Slight preponderance of females.

ETIOLOGY AND PATHOGENESIS

Unknown. Although called pyoderma, it does not have a microbial etiology. PG is counted among the neutrophilic dermatoses because of the massive neutrophilic infiltrates within the skin. It may belong to the autoinflammatory disease spectrum.

CLINICAL MANIFESTATION

THREE TYPES Acute. Acute onset with painful hemorrhagic pustule or painful nodule either de novo or after trauma. *There is the phenomenon of pathergy,* where a needle prick, insect bite, biopsy, or other minimal trauma can trigger a lesion. **Chronic:** Slow progression with granulation and hyperkeratosis. Less painful. **Bullous:** True blisters often hemorrhagic and associated with hematologic disease.
SKIN LESIONS Acute. Superficial hemorrhagic pustule surrounded by erythematous halo; very painful (Fig. 7-1). Breakdown occurs with ulcer formation, whereby ulcer borders are dusky-red or purple, irregular and raised, undermined, boggy with perforations that drain pus (Fig. 7-2). The base of the ulcer is purulent with hemorrhagic exudate, partially covered by necrotic eschar (Fig. 7-3), with or without granulation tissue. Pustules both at the advancing border and in the ulcer base; a halo of erythema spreads centrifugally at the advancing edge of the ulcer (Fig. 7-3). *Chronic:* Lesions may slowly progress, grazing over large areas of the body and exhibiting massive granulation within the ulcer from the outset (Fig. 7-4) with crusting and even hyperkeratosis on the margins (Fig. 7-5). Lesions are usually solitary but may be multiple and form clusters that coalesce. Most common sites: Lower extremities (Figs. 7-2 and 7-5) > buttocks > abdomen (Fig. 7-3) > face (Fig. 7-4). Healing of ulcers results in thin atrophic cribriform scars. *Bullous:* Blisters from the outset, often hemorrhagic, followed by ulceration.
MUCOUS MEMBRANES Rarely, aphthous stomatitis–like lesions; very rarely massive ulceration of oral mucosa and conjunctivae.

General Examination

Patient appears ill.

Associated Systemic Diseases

Up to 50% of cases occur without associated disease. The remainder of cases are associated with arthritis, large- and small-bowel disease (Crohn disease and ulcerative colitis), diverticulosis (diverticulitis), paraproteinemia and myeloma, leukemia, active chronic hepatitis, Behçet syndrome (which is also a disease with pathergy).

LABORATORY EXAMINATIONS

There is no single diagnostic test.
ESR Variably elevated.

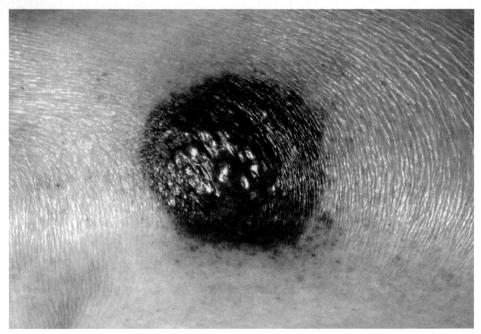

FIGURE 7-1 Pyoderma gangrenosum The initial lesion is a rapidly enlarging hemorrhagic nonfollicular pustule surrounded by an erythematous halo and is very painful.

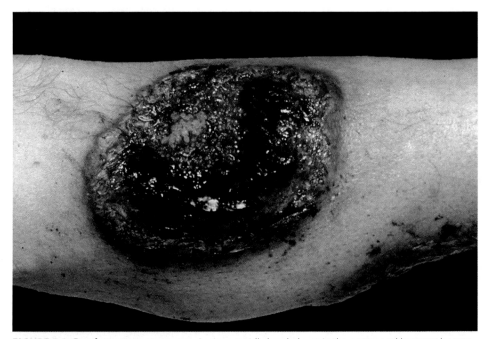

FIGURE 7-2 Pyoderma gangrenosum Lesions rapidly break down in the center and become boggy, hemorrhagic, and purulent ulcers.

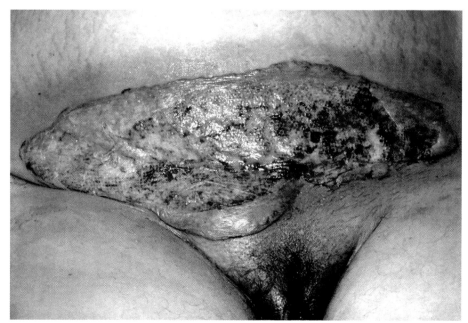

FIGURE 7-3 Pyoderma gangrenosum A very large ulcer with raised bullous undermined borders covered with hemorrhagic and fibrinous exudate. There is erythema surrounding advancing borders of the lesion. When the bullae are opened, pus is drained. This lesion arose acutely and spread rapidly after laparotomy for an ovarian carcinoma.

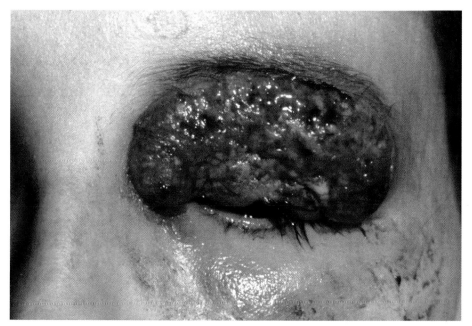

FIGURE 7-4 Pyoderma gangrenosum: chronic type The lesion involves the upper eyelid and represents an ulcer with elevated granulating base with multiple abscesses. The lesion later spread slowly to involve the temporal and zygomatic regions and eventually healed under systemic glucocorticoid treatment, leaving a thin cribriform scar that did not impair the function of the eyelid.

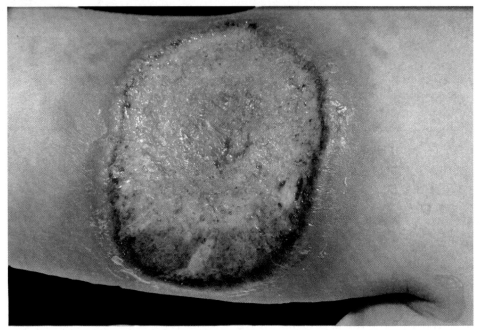

FIGURE 7-5 Pyoderma gangrenosum: chronic type This lesion, which appears like a plaque, spread slowly but was also surrounded by an erythematous border. The lesion is crusted and hyperkeratotic and is less painful than the lesions in acute pyoderma gangrenosum.

DERMATOPATHOLOGY Not diagnostic. Neutrophilic inflammation with abscess formation and necrosis.

DIAGNOSIS AND DIFFERENTIAL DIAGNOSIS

Clinical findings plus history and course; confirmed by compatible dermatopathology. Differential diagnosis: Ecthyma and ecthyma gangrenosum, atypical mycobacterial infection, clostridial infection, deep mycoses, amebiasis, leishmaniasis, bromoderma, pemphigus vegetans, stasis ulcers, and granulomatous vasculitis.

COURSE AND PROGNOSIS

Untreated, course may last months to years, but spontaneous healing can occur. Ulceration may extend rapidly within a few days or slowly. Healing occurs centrally with peripheral extension. New ulcers may appear as older lesions resolve. Pathergy.

MANAGEMENT

WITH ASSOCIATED UNDERLYING DISEASE Treat underlying disease.

SYSTEMIC TREATMENT High doses of oral glucocorticoids or IV glucocorticoid pulse therapy (1 to 2 g/d prednisolone) may be required. Sulfasalazine (particularly in cases associated with Crohn disease), sulfones, cyclosporine, and, more recently, infliximab, etanercept, and adalimumab.

TOPICAL In singular small lesion, topical tacrolimus ointment or intralesional triamcinolone.

BOWEL BYPASS SYNDROME (BOWEL-ASSOCIATED DERMATOSIS-ARTHRITIS SYNDROME) ICD-10: L98.2

- Associated with bowel surgery for obesity or inflammatory bowel disease.
- Serum sickness-like manifestations. Erythematous, purpuric papules, vesiculo pustules, and subcutaneous nodules.
- Associated with polyarthritis and tendosynovitis.

SWEET SYNDROME (SS) ICD-10: L98.2

- An uncommon, acute, and recurrent, cytokine-induced skin reaction associated with various etiologies.
- Painful plaque-forming inflammatory papules, often with massive exudations giving the appearance of vesiculation (pseudovesiculation).
- Accompanied by fever, arthralgia, and peripheral leukocytosis.
- Associated with infection, malignancy, or drugs.
- Treatment: Systemic glucocorticoids, potassium iodide, dapsone, or colchicine.
- *Synonym*: Acute febrile neutrophilic dermatosis.

EPIDEMIOLOGY AND ETIOLOGY

AGE OF ONSET Most often 30 to 60 years.
SEX Women > men.
ETIOLOGY Unknown, possibly hypersensitivity reaction. It belongs to the group of neutrophilic dermatoses and possibly to the spectrum of autoinflammatory diseases.
ASSOCIATED DISORDERS Febrile upper respiratory tract infection. In some cases, associated with *Yersinia* infection. Hematologic malignancy; drugs: granulocyte colony-stimulating factor (G-GSF) and others.

CLINICAL MANIFESTATION

Prodromes are febrile upper respiratory tract infections. Gastrointestinal symptoms (diarrhea), tonsillitis, influenza-like illness, 1 to 3 weeks before skin lesions. Lesions tender/painful. Fever (not always present), headache, arthralgia, and general malaise.
SKIN LESIONS Bright red, smooth, tender papules (2 to 4 mm in diameter) that coalesce to form irregular, sharply bordered, inflammatory plaques (Fig. 7-6A). Pseudovesiculation: Intense edema gives the appearance of vesiculation (Figs. 7-6A and 7-7A). Lesions arise rapidly, and as they evolve, central clearing may lead to annular or arcuate patterns. Tiny, superficial pustules may occur. May present as a single lesion or multiple lesions, asymmetrically or symmetrically distributed. Most common on face (Fig. 7-6A), neck (Fig. 7-6B), and upper extremities but also on lower extremities, where lesions may be deep in the fat and thus mimic panniculitis. Truncal lesions are uncommon but widespread and generalized forms occur. If associated with leukemia, bullous lesions may occur (Fig. 7-7B) and lesions may mimic bullous PG.
MUCOUS MEMBRANES ± Conjunctivitis, episcleritis

General Examination

Patient may appear ill. There may be involvement of cardiovascular, central nervous system, gastrointestinal, hepatic, musculoskeletal, ocular, pulmonary, renal, and splenic organs.

LABORATORY EXAMINATIONS

COMPLETE BLOOD COUNT Leukocytosis with neutrophilia (not always present).
ESR Elevated.
DERMATOPATHOLOGY Diagnostic. Epidermis usually normal, sometimes subcorneal pustulation. Massive edema of papillary body, dense leukocytic infiltrate with starburst pattern in mid-dermis, consisting of neutrophils with occasional eosinophils/lymphoid cells. Leukocytoclasia, nuclear dust, but no vasculitis. ± Neutrophilic infiltrates in subcutaneous tissue.

DIAGNOSIS AND DIFFERENTIAL DIAGNOSIS

Clinical impression and by histopathology.
DIFFERENTIAL DIAGNOSIS Erythema multiforme, erythema nodosum, prevesicular herpes simplex infection, preulcerative PG.

COURSE AND PROGNOSIS

Untreated, lesions enlarge over a period of days or weeks and eventually resolve without scarring. Recurrences occur in 50% of patients, often in previously involved sites. Some cases follow *Yersinia* infection or are associated with acute myelocytic leukemia, transient myeloid proliferation, various malignant tumors, ulcerative colitis, benign monoclonal gammopathy; some follow drug administration, most commonly by GSF.

MANAGEMENT

Rule out sepsis.
PREDNISONE 30 to 50 mg/d, tapering in 2 to 3 weeks lesions resolve within a few days; some, but not all, patients respond to dapsone, 100 mg/d, or to potassium iodide. Some respond to colchicine.
ANTIBIOTIC THERAPY Clears eruption in *Yersinia*-associated cases; in all other cases, antibiotics are ineffective.

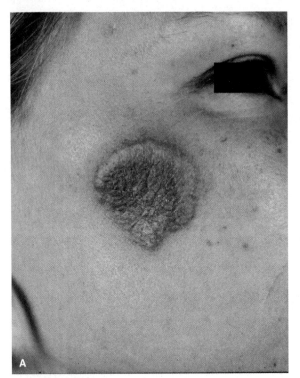

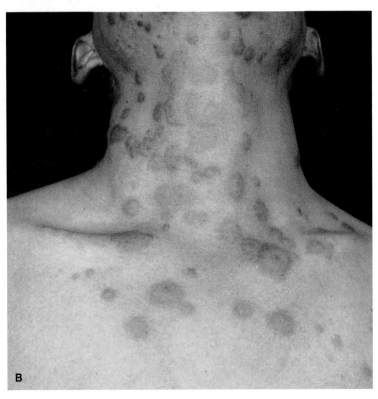

FIGURE 7-6 Sweet syndrome
(A) An erythematous, edematous plaque that has formed from coalescing papules on the right cheek. The border of the plaque looks as if composed of vesicles, but palpation reveals that it is solid (pseudovesiculation). This lesion occurred in a 26-year-old female following an upper respiratory infection, and the patient also had fever and leukocytosis. **(B)** A more exanthematic eruption in a 23-year-old female. There are multiple, coalescing, inflammatory, and very exudative papules with a wheal-like appearance on the neck. This patient also had leukocytosis and fever.

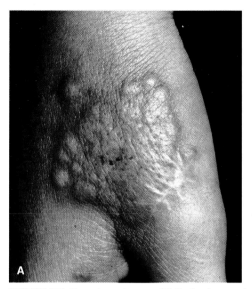
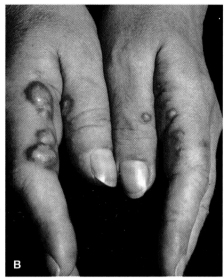

FIGURE 7-7 Sweet syndrome (A) Coalescing exudative papules that look like vesicles. Upon palpation, lesions were solid. **(B)** Bullous type of Sweet syndrome. These are true bullae and pustules. The patient had myelomonocytic leukemia.

GRANULOMA FACIALE (GF)   ICD-10: L92.2

- A rare, localized inflammatory disease of unknown etiology, clinically characterized by reddish-brown papules or small plaques primarily in the face.
- Single or multiple lesions with characteristic orange peel-like surface (Fig. 7-8).
- Histologically, chronic leukocytoclastic vasculitis with eosinophils, fibrin deposition, and fibrosis.
- Therapy: topical glucocorticoids; dapsone.

FIGURE 7-8 Granuloma faciale: classic presentation
A single, sharply defined, brown plaque with a characteristic orange peel-like surface.

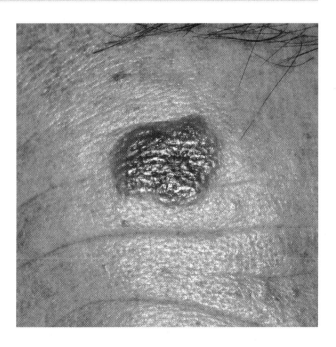

ERYTHEMA NODOSUM (EN) SYNDROME ICD-10: L52

- EN is an important and common acute inflammatory/immunologic reaction pattern of the subcutaneous fat.
- Characterized by the appearance of painful nodules on the lower legs.
- Lesions are bright red and flat but nodular upon palpation.
- Often fever and arthritis.
- Multiple and diverse etiologies.

The most common type of panniculitis, with a peak incidence at 20 to 30 years, but any age may be affected. Three to six times more common in females than in males.

ETIOLOGY EN is cutaneous reaction pattern to various etiologic agents. These include infections, drugs, and other inflammatory/granulomatous diseases, notably sarcoidosis (Table 7-1).

CLINICAL MANIFESTATION

Painful, tender lesions, usually of a few days' duration, accompanied by fever, malaise, and arthralgia (50%), most frequently of ankle joints. Other symptoms depending on etiology.
SKIN LESIONS Indurated, very tender nodules (3 to 20 cm), not sharply marginated (Fig. 7-9), deep seated in the subcutaneous fat, mostly on the anterior lower legs, bilateral but not symmetric. Nodules are bright to deep red and are appreciated as such only upon palpation. The term *erythema nodosum* best describes the

skin lesions: *they look like erythema but feel like nodules* (Fig. 7-9). Lesions are oval, round, and arciform; as they age, they become violaceous, brownish, yellowish, or green, like resolving hematomas. Lesions may also occur on the knees and arms but only rarely on the face and neck.

LABORATORY EXAMINATIONS

HEMATOLOGY Elevated ESR and C-reactive protein; leukocytosis.
BACTERIAL CULTURE Culture throat for group A β-hemolytic streptococcus, stool for *Yersinia*.
IMAGING Radiologic examination of the chest and gallium scan are important to rule out sarcoidosis.
DERMATOPATHOLOGY Acute (polymorphonuclear) and chronic (granulomatous) inflammation in the subcutis, around blood vessels in the septum and adjacent fat. EN is a septal panniculitis.

TABLE 7-1 Causes of Erythema Nodosum[a]

Infections	Other
Bacterial	**Drugs**
Streptococcal infections; tuberculosis, yersiniosis Other: *Salmonella, Campylobacter, Shigella,* brucellosis, psittacosis, *Mycoplasma*	Sulfonamides; bromides and iodides Oral contraceptives Other: minocycline, gold salts, penicillin, salicylates
Fungal	**Malignancies**
Coccidioidomycosis, blastomycosis, histoplasmosis, sporotrichosis, dermatophytosis	Hodgkin and non-Hodgkin lymphoma, leukemia, renal cell carcinoma
Viral	**Other**
Infectious mononucleosis, hepatitis B, orf, herpes simplex	Sarcoidosis Inflammatory bowel disease: ulcerative colitis, Crohn disease
Other Amebiasis, giardiasis, ascariasis	Behçet disease

[a]For a more complete list of etiologic factors in EN, see Aronson IK et al., in Goldsmith LA, Katz SI, Gilchrest BA, Paller AS, Leffell DJ, and Wolff K (eds.): *Fitzpatrick's Dermatology in General Medicine* 8th edition. New York, McGraw-Hill, 2012.

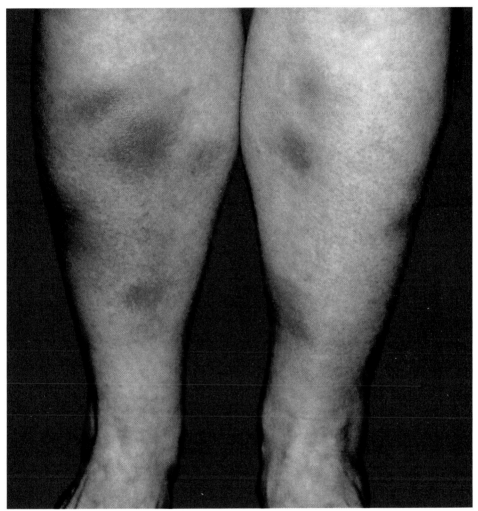

FIGURE 7-9 Erythema nodosum Indurated, very tender, inflammatory nodules mostly in the pretibial region. Lesions are seen as red, ill-defined erythemas but palpated as deep-seated nodules, hence the designation. In this 49-year-old female, there was also fever and arthritis of the ankle joints following an upper respiratory tract infection. The throat cultures yielded β-hemolytic streptococci.

COURSE

Spontaneous resolution occurs in 6 weeks, with new lesions erupting during that time. Course depends on the etiology. Lesions never break down or ulcerate and heal without scarring.

DIAGNOSIS AND DIFFERENTIAL DIAGNOSIS

Diagnosis rests on clinical criteria and histopathology, if needed. Differential diagnosis includes all other forms of panniculitis, panarteritis nodosa, nodular vasculitis, pretibial myxedema, nonulcerated gumma, and lymphoma.

MANAGEMENT

SYMPTOMATIC Bed rest or compressive bandages (lower legs), wet dressings.

ANTI-INFLAMMATORY TREATMENT Salicylates, nonsteroidal anti-inflammatory drugs. Systemic glucocorticoids—response is rapid, but their use is indicated only when the etiology is known and infectious agents are excluded.

OTHER PANNICULITIDES ICD-10: M79.3

- Panniculitis is the term used to describe diseases where the major focus of inflammation is in the subcutaneous tissue. In general, panniculitis presents as an erythematous or violaceous nodule in the subcutaneous fat that may be tender or not, may ulcerate or heal without scarring, and may be soft or hard on palpation. Thus, the term *panniculitis* describes a wide spectrum of disease manifestations.
- An accurate diagnosis requires an ample deep skin biopsy that should reach down to, or even beyond, the fascia. The panniculitides are classified histologically as lobular or septal but a clear separation is often not possible. A simplified classification of panniculitis is given in Table 7-2.
- Only two forms of panniculitis are briefly discussed here.[1] Other diseases in which panniculitis occurs are referred to in Table 7-2.
- *Pancreatic panniculitis* manifests as painful erythematous nodules and plaques that may fluctuate and occur at any site, with a predilection for abdomen, buttocks, and legs (Fig. 7-10). Frequently accompanied by arthritis and polyserositis. Associated with pancreatitis or pancreatic carcinoma. In middle-aged to elderly individuals, males > females. History: alcoholism, abdominal pain, weight loss, or recent-onset diabetes mellitus. Skin biopsy reveals lobular panniculitis; liquefied fat may drain from the biopsy site. General examination may reveal pleural effusion, ascites, and arthritis, particularly of the ankles. *Laboratory:* Eosinophilia, hyperlipasemia, hyperamylasemia, and increased excretion of amylase and/or lipase in the urine. The pathophysiology is probably a breakdown of subcutaneous fat caused by pancreatic enzymes released into the circulation. Course and prognosis depend on the type of pancreatic disease. Treatment is directed at the underlying pancreatic disorder.
- α_1-*Antitrypsin-deficiency panniculitis* is also characterized by recurrent tender, erythematous, subcutaneous nodules ranging from 1 to 5 cm and located predominantly on the trunk and the proximal extremities. Nodules break down and discharge a clear serous or oily fluid. Diagnosis is substantiated by a decrease of serum α_1-antitrypsin, and treatment consists of oral dapsone in doses up to 200 mg/d. The intravenous infusion of human α_1-proteinase inhibitor concentrate has been shown to be very effective.

---

[1]The reader is also referred to Aronson IK et al., in Goldsmith LA, Katz SI, Gilchrest BA, Paller AS, Leffell DJ, and Wolff K (eds.): *Fitzpatrick's Dermatology in General Medicine* 8th edition. New York, McGraw-Hill, 2012.

TABLE 7-2 Simplified Classification of Panniculitis

	Lobular Panniculitis	**Septal Panniculitis**
Neonatal	Sclerema neonatorum, neonatal subcutaneous fat necrosis	
Physical	Cold, trauma	
Drugs	Poststeroid panniculitis	Erythema nodosum
Idiopathic		Eosinophilic fasciitis Eosinophilia myalgia syndrome
Infection-induced panniculitis	Caused by large number of infectious agents: bacteria, fungi, viruses, and parasites	
Pancreatic	With pancreatitis or carcinoma of the pancreas	
Panniculitis with other systemic disease	Lupus erythematosus; sarcoidosis, lymphoma, histiocytic cytophagic panniculitis	Scleroderma
With vasculitis	Nodular vasculitis	
Metabolic deficiency	α_1-Antitrypsin deficiency	Lipodermatosclerosis (see Section 17) Thrombophlebitis, panarteritis nodosa

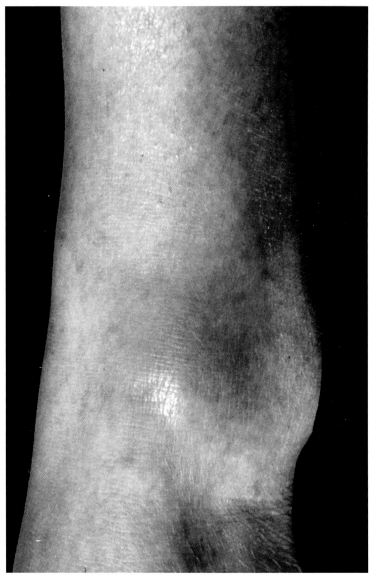

FIGURE 7-10 Pancreatic panniculitis There is a painful, erythematous nodule that fluctuates on the ventral malleolar region but similar lesions were also found on the trunk and on the buttocks.

PERNIOSIS (CHILBLAINS) ICD-10: T69.1

- Localized inflammatory lesions caused by continuous exposure to cold (Fig. 7-11).
- More common in children; women with a low body mass index.
- Single or multiple burning erythematous or purplish swellings on proximal fingers, toes, heels, nose, and ears; also on calves and thighs (e.g., often seen in bicycle or horseback riders).
- Resolves in 2 to 3 weeks.
- Management and prophylaxis: warm, loosely fitting clothes.

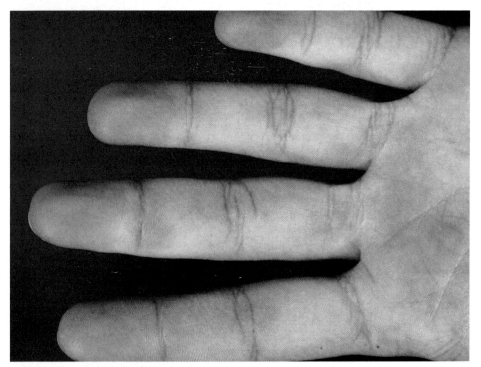

FIGURE 7-11 Perniosis (Chilblains) Erythematous to slightly violaceous swellings on the distal digits and palm There is burning and pain.

THE ACUTELY ILL AND HOSPITALIZED PATIENT

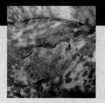

EXFOLIATIVE ERYTHRODERMA SYNDROME (EES) ICD10*

- EES is a serious, at times life-threatening, reaction pattern of the skin characterized by a uniform redness, infiltration, and scaling, which involves practically the entire skin.
- It is associated with fever, malaise, shivers, and generalized lymphadenopathy.
- Two stages, acute and chronic, merge one into the other. In the acute and subacute phases, there is rapid onset of generalized vivid red erythema and fine branny scales; the patient feels hot and cold, shivers, and has a fever. In chronic EES, the skin thickens, and scaling continues and becomes lamellar.
- There may be loss of scalp and body hair, and the nails become thickened and separated from the nail bed (onycholysis).
- There may be hyperpigmentation or patchy loss of pigment in patients whose normal skin pigmentation is brown or black.
- The most frequent preexisting skin disorders are (in order of frequency) psoriasis, atopic dermatitis, adverse cutaneous drug reaction, lymphoma, allergic contact dermatitis, seborrheic dermatitis, and pityriasis rubra pilaris.

[See "Sézary Syndrome" in Section 21 for a special consideration of this form of EES.]

EPIDEMIOLOGY

AGE OF ONSET Usually >50 years; in children, EES usually results from atopic dermatitis.
SEX Males > females.

ETIOLOGY

Some 50% of patients have a history of preexisting dermatosis. Most frequent are psoriasis, atopic dermatitis, adverse cutaneous drug reactions, cutaneous T-cell lymphoma (CTCL), allergic contact dermatitis, seborrheic dermatitis and pityriasis rubra pilaris. Drugs most commonly implicated in EES are shown in Table 8-1. In 20% of patients, it is not possible to identify the cause.

PATHOGENESIS

The metabolic response to EES may be profound. Large amounts of warm blood are

*ICD-10 codes are assigned according to etiology: psoriasis L40.85, atopic dermatitis L20.85, adverse cutaneous drug reaction L27.85, lymphoma I91.72, allergic contact dermatitis L23, pityriasis rubra pilaris L44.4.

TABLE 8-1 The Most Commonly Implicated Drugs In Exfoliative Dermatitis[a]

Allopurinol	Dapsone	Penicillin	Sulfasalazine
Antimalarials	Diphenylhydantoin	Phenothiazines	Sulfonamides
Bactrim	Gold	Phenytoin	Sulfonylureas
Barbiturates	Isoniazid	Quinidine	
Calcium channel blockers	Lithium	Streptomycin	
Carbamazepine			
Cimetidine			

[a]Modified with permission from Grant-Kels JM, Fedeles F, Roth MJ. Exfoliative dermatitis. In: Goldsmith LA, Katz SI, Gilchrest BA, et al, eds. *Fitzpatrick's Dermatology in General Medicine.* 8th ed. New York, NY: McGraw-Hill; 2012, pp. 266–279.

present in the skin caused by dilatation of the capillaries, resulting in considerable heat dissipation. Also, there may be high-output cardiac failure; the loss of scales (and thus proteins) through exfoliation can be considerable, up to 9 g/m² of body surface per day.

CLINICAL MANIFESTATION

Depending on the etiology, the acute phase may develop rapidly, usually in a drug reaction, or psoriasis. At this early acute stage, it is still possible to identify the preexisting dermatosis. There is fever, pruritus, fatigue, weakness, anorexia, weight loss, malaise, feeling cold, and shivers.

APPEARANCE OF PATIENT Frightened, red, "toxic," may be malodorous.

SKIN LESIONS Skin is red, thickened, and scaly. Dermatitis is uniform involving the entire body surface (Figs. 8-1 to 8-3), except for pityriasis rubra pilaris, where EES spares sharply defined areas of normal skin (Fig. 3-16). Thickening leads to exaggerated skin folds (Figs. 8-2 and 8-3); scaling may be fine and branny, and may be barely perceptible (Fig. 8-2) or large, up to 0.5 cm, and lamellar (Fig. 8-1).

Palms and Soles. Usually involved, with massive hyperkeratosis and deep fissures in pityriasis rubra pilaris, Sézary syndrome (CTCL), and psoriasis.

HAIR Telogen effluvium, even alopecia, except for EES arising in eczema or psoriasis.

NAILS Thickening of nail plates, onycholysis, and shedding of nails.

PIGMENTATION In chronic EES, there may be hyperpigmentation or patchy loss of pigment in patients whose normal skin is brown or black.

General Examination

Lymph nodes generalized, rubbery, and usually small; enlarged in Sézary syndrome. Edema of lower legs and ankles.

LABORATORY EXAMINATIONS

CHEMISTRY Low serum albumin and increase in gammaglobulins; electrolyte imbalance; acute-phase proteins increased.

HEMATOLOGY Leukocytosis.

BACTERIAL CULTURE *Skin*: Rule out secondary *Staphylococcus aureus* infection. *Blood*: Rule out sepsis.

DERMATOPATHOLOGY Depends on the type of underlying disease. In all, there is parakeratosis, inter- and intra-cellular edema, acanthosis with

elongation of the rete ridges, exocytosis of cells, edema of the dermis, and an inflammatory infiltrate.

IMAGING CT scans or MRI should be used to find evidence of lymphoma.

LYMPH NODE BIOPSY When there is suspicion of lymphoma.

DIAGNOSIS

The history of the preexisting dermatosis may be the only clue. Also, pathognomonic signs and symptoms of the preexisting dermatosis may help, e.g., dusky-red color in psoriasis (Fig. 8-1) and yellowish red in pityriasis rubra pilaris (see Fig. 3-16); typical nail changes of psoriasis; lichenification, erosions, and excoriations in atopic dermatitis and eczema; diffuse, relatively nonscaling palmar hyperkeratoses with fissures in CTCL and pityriasis rubra pilaris; sharply demarcated patches of noninvolved skin within the erythroderma in pityriasis rubra pilaris; massive hyperkeratotic scale of scalp, usually without hair loss in psoriasis and with hair loss in CTCL and pityriasis rubra pilaris; in the latter and in CTCL, ectropion may occur.

COURSE AND PROGNOSIS

Guarded, depends on underlying etiology. Patients may succumb to infections or, if they have cardiac problems, to cardiac failure (high-output failure) or, as was unfortunately often the case in the past, to the effects of prolonged glucocorticoid therapy.

MANAGEMENT

This important medical problem should be dealt with in a modern inpatient dermatology facility with experienced personnel. The patient should be hospitalized in a single room where conditions (hot and cold) should be adjusted to the patient's needs; most often, these patients need a warm room with many blankets.

TOPICAL Water baths with added bath oils, followed by application of bland emollients.

SYSTEMIC Oral glucocorticoids for remission induction but not for maintenance; *systemic and topical therapy as required by underlying condition.* Antibiotics if there is bacteremia or septicemia.

SUPPORTIVE Supportive cardiac, fluid, electrolyte, and protein replacement therapy as required.

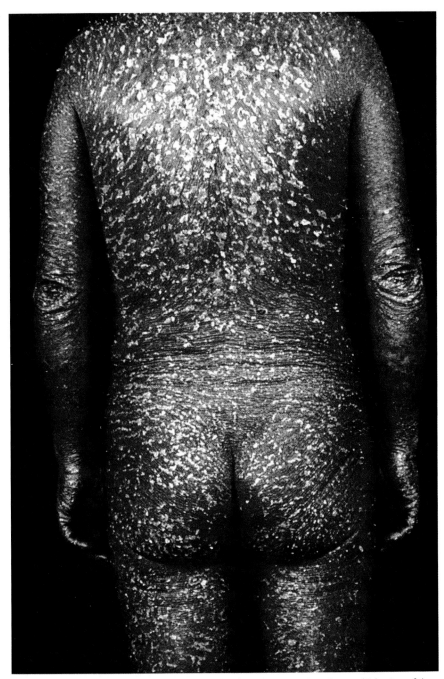

FIGURE 8-1 Exfoliative dermatitis: psoriasis There is universal erythema, thickening of the skin, and heavy scaling. This patient had psoriasis as suggested by the large silvery white scales and the scalp and nail involvement, which is not seen in this illustration. The patient had fatigue, weakness, malaise, and was shivering. It is quite obvious that such massive scaling can lead to protein loss and the maximal dilatation of skin capillaries to considerable heat dissipation and high-output cardiac failure.

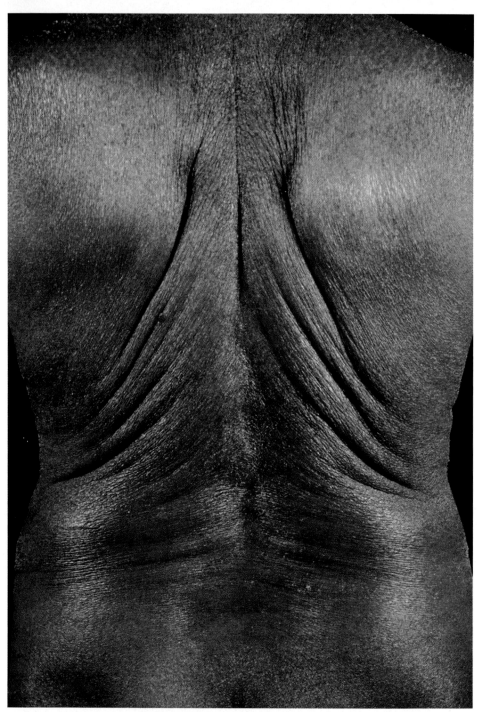

FIGURE 8-2 Exfoliative dermatitis: drug induced This is generalized erythroderma with thickening of skin resulting in increased skin folds, universal redness, a fine brawny scaling. This patient had developed erythroderma following the injection of gold salts for rheumatoid arthritis.

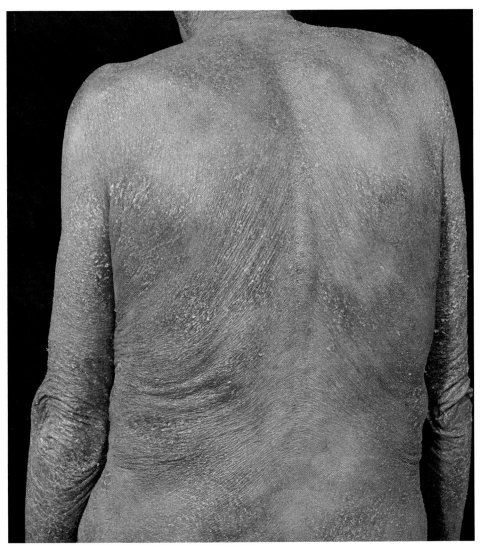

FIGURE 8-3 Exfoliative dermatitis: cutaneous T-cell lymphoma (Sézary syndrome) There is universal erythema, thickening, and scaling. Note that in contrast to erythroderma shown in Figs. 8-1 and 8-2, the degree of erythema and thickness is not uniform and the redness has a brownish hue. In addition, this elderly patient had hair loss, massive involvement of the palms and soles with diffuse hyperkeratoses, cracks, and fissures. Generalized lymphadenopathy was also present.

RASHES IN THE ACUTELY ILL FEBRILE PATIENT (ICD-10 codes based on etiology)

- The sudden appearance of a rash and fever causes anxiety for the patient and medical advice is sought immediately. About 10% of all patients seeking emergency medical care have a dermatologic problem.
- The diagnosis of an acute rash with a fever is a clinical challenge (Figs. 8-4 and 8-5). If a diagnosis is not established promptly in certain patients [e.g., those having septicemia (Fig. 8-6)], lifesaving treatment may be delayed.
- The cutaneous findings alone are often diagnostic before confirmatory laboratory data are available. On the basis of a careful differential diagnosis, appropriate therapy—whether antibiotics or glucocorticoids—may be started. Furthermore, prompt diagnosis and isolation of the patient with a contagious disease, which may have serious consequences, prevents spreading to other persons. Contagious diseases presenting with rash and fever as the major findings include *viral infections* (Fig. 8-5).
- The diagnosis of skin eruptions is based mainly on precise identification of the type of skin lesions and additional morphologic clues such as the *configuration* (annular? iris?) of the individual lesion, the *arrangement* (zosteriform? linear?) and the *distribution pattern* (exposed areas? centripetal or centrifugal? mucous membranes?).
- In the *differential diagnosis* of exanthems, it is important to determine, by history, the *site of first appearance* and temporal evolution (the rash of Rocky Mountain spotted fever characteristically appears first on the wrists and ankles), in measles (see Fig. 8-5) it spreads from head to toe in a period of 3 days, while in rubella it spreads rapidly in 24 to 48 h from head to toe and then sequentially clears—first face, then trunk, followed by limbs. Contrasting this evolution, drug eruptions usually start simultaneously on the whole body (Fig. 8-4) or as fixed drug eruption at preferential sites (see Section 23).
- Although there may be some overlap, the differential diagnostic possibilities may be grouped into five main categories according to the type of lesion (Table 8-2).

LABORATORY TESTS AVAILABLE FOR QUICK DIAGNOSIS

The physician should make use of the following laboratory tests immediately or within 8 hours:

1. *Direct smear from the base of a vesicle.* This procedure, known as the *Tzanck test*, is described in the "Introduction of the book." Smears are examined for acantholytic cells, giant acanthocytes, and/or multinucleated giant cells.
2. *Viral culture*, negative stain (electron microscopy), polymerase chain reaction for infections with herpes viruses, and direct fluorescence (DIF) technique.
3. *Gram stain of aspirates or scraping of pustules.* Organisms can be seen in the lesions of acute meningococcemia, rarely in the skin lesions of gonococcemia and ecthyma gangrenosum.
4. *Touch preparation.* Helpful in deep fungal infections and leishmaniasis. The dermal part of a skin biopsy specimen is touched repeatedly to a glass slide, which is *immediately* fixed in 95% ethyl alcohol. Special stains will reveal organisms.
5. *Biopsy of the skin lesion.* All purpuric lesions, inflammatory dermal nodules, and most ulcers should be biopsied (at the base and margin) and a portion of tissue minced and cultured for bacteria and fungi. In gangrenous cellulitis (see Section 25), frozen sections of a deep biopsy will verify the diagnosis in minutes.
6. *Blood and urine examinations.* Blood culture, rapid serologic tests for syphilis, and serology for lupus erythematosus. Examination of urine sediment may reveal red cell casts in renal involvement in allergic vasculitis.
7. *Dark-field examination.* In the skin lesions of secondary syphilis, repeated examinations of papules show *Treponema pallidum*. Not reliable in the mouth because of resident nonpathogenic organisms but a lymph node aspirate can be subjected to a dark-field examination.

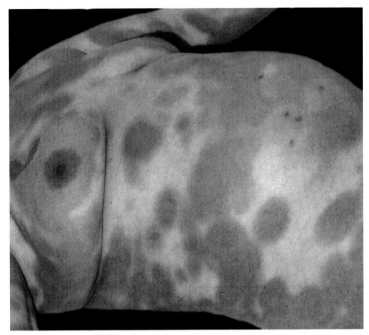

FIGURE 8-4 Generalized fixed drug eruption: tetracycline Prostrated, 59-year-old woman with fever. Multiple confluent violaceous red erythematous areas, some of which later became bullous.

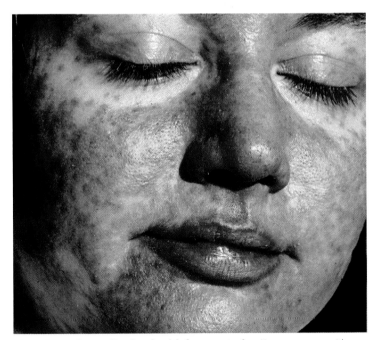

FIGURE 8-5 Generalized rash with fever: measles Young woman with high fever, cough, conjunctivitis, and a confluent maculopapular eruption in the edematous face. The rash also involves the trunk and the extremities. The patient has measles.

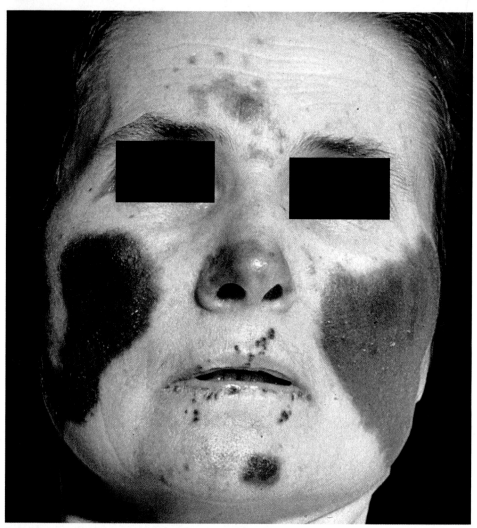

FIGURE 8-6 Generalized purpura, necrosis and fever: DIC A 54-year-old woman with fever, prostration, and extensive geographic infarctions on the face, trunk, and extremities. This is disseminated intravascular coagulation: purpura fulminans following sepsis after abdominal surgery.

TABLE 8-2 Generalized Eruptions in the Acutely Ill Patient: Diagnosis According to Type of Lesion[a]

Generalized Eruptions Manifested by Macules, Papules	Generalized Eruptions Manifested by Wheals, Plaques	Generalized Eruptions Manifested by Vesicles, Bullae, or Pustules	Generalized Eruptions Manifested by Purpuric Macules, Purpuric Papules, or Purpuric Vesicles	Diseases Manifested by Widespread Erythema ± Papules Followed by Desquamation
Drug hypersensitivities	Serum sickness	Drug hypersensitivities	Drug hypersensitivities	Drug hypersensitivities
Acute HIV syndrome	Sweet syndrome	Allergic contact dermatitis from plants	Meningococcemia[b] (acute or chronic)	Staphylococcal scalded-skin syndrome
Erythema infectiosum (parvovirus B19)	Acute urticaria	Rickettsialpox	Gonococcemia[b]	Toxic shock syndrome
Cytomegalovirus, primary infection	Erythema marginatum	Varicella (chickenpox)[c]	Staphylococcemia	Kawasaki syndrome
Epstein-Barr virus, primary infection		Eczema herpeticum[c]	Pseudomonas bacteremia	Exfoliative dermatitis
Exanthem subitum (HHV 6)		Enterovirus infections (Coxsackie), including hand, foot, and mouth disease	Subacute bacterial endocarditis	
Measles (rubeola)			Enterovirus infections (echovirus, Coxsackie)	
German measles (rubella)[d]		Toxic epidermal necrolysis	Rickettsial diseases: Rocky Mountain spotted fever	
Enterovirus infections (echovirus and Coxsackie)		Smallpox or variola	Typhus, louse-borne (epidemic)	
Adenovirus infections		Staphylococcal scalded-skin syndrome	Hypersensitivity vasculitis[b]	
Scarlet fever		Erythema multiforme	Disseminated intravascular coagulation (purpura fulminans[b,e])	
Ehrlichiosis		von Zumbusch pustular psoriasis	Vibrio infections	
Typhoid fever		Acute graft-versus-host reaction		
Secondary syphilis				
Typhus, murine (endemic)				
Rocky Mountain spotted fever (early lesions)[d]				
Other spotted fevers				
Disseminated deep fungal infection in immunocompromised patients				
Erythema multiforme				
Systemic lupus erythematosus				
Acute graft-versus-host reaction				

[a]With regard to the detailed morphologies, the reader is referred to the respective sections.
[b]Often present as infarcts.
[c]Umbilicated vesicles.
[d]May have arthralgia or musculoskeletal pain.
[e]Leading to large areas of black necrosis.

STEVENS–JOHNSON SYNDROME (SJS) AND TOXIC EPIDERMAL NECROLYSIS (TEN) ICD-10: L51.1/51.2

- SJS and TEN are acute life-threatening mucocutaneous reactions characterized by extensive necrosis and detachment of the epidermis.
- They are variants of the same disease and differ only in the percentage of the body surface involved.
- Either "idiopathic" or drug induced.
- Pathomechanism is widespread apoptosis of keratinocytes induced by a cell-mediated cytotoxic reaction.
- Confluent erythematous purpuric and target-like macules evolve into flaccid blisters and epidermal detachment mostly on the trunk and extremities. There is also associated mucous membrane involvement.
- Histopathologically: Full-thickness necrosis of the epidermis and a sparse lymphocytic infiltrate.
- Treatment is symptomatic. Systemic treatment with glucocorticoids and high-dose intravenous immunoglobulin is advocated by some but still controversial.

DEFINITION

There is now consensus that SJS and TEN are different from erythema multiforme (EM).

TEN is a maximal variant of SJS differing only in the extent of body surface involvement. Both can start with macular and target-like lesions. However, about 50% of TEN cases do not start with either, and in these, the condition evolves from diffuse erythema to immediate necrosis and epidermal detachment.

SJS: <10% epidermal detachment.
SJS/TEN overlap: 10 to 30% epidermal detachment.
TEN: >30% epidermal detachment.

EPIDEMIOLOGY

AGE OF ONSET Any age, but most common in adults >40 years. Equal sex incidence.
OVERALL INCIDENCE *TEN*: 0.4 to 1.2 per million person-years. *SJS*: 1.2 to 6 per million person-years.
RISK FACTORS Systemic lupus erythematosus, HLA-B12, HLA-B1502, and HLA-B5801 in Han Chinese, and HIV/AIDS.

ETIOLOGY AND PATHOGENESIS

Polyetiologic reaction pattern, but drugs are clearly the leading causative factor. *TEN*: 80% of cases have strong association with specific medication (Table 8-3); <5% of patients report no drug use. *SJS*: 50% are associated with drug exposure. Also chemicals, *Mycoplasma pneumoniae*, viral infections, immunization. Etiology often not clear.

Pathogenesis of SJS-TEN is only partially understood. It is viewed as a cytotoxic immune reaction aimed at the destruction of keratinocytes expressing foreign (drug-related) antigens. Epidermal injury is based on the induction of apoptosis. Fas and Fas-ligand interactions and/or the proapoptotic protein granulysin are implicated.

CLINICAL MANIFESTATION

Time from first drug exposure to onset of symptoms: 1 to 3 weeks. Occurs more rapidly with rechallenge, often after a few days; a newly added drug is most suspect. Prodromes: fever, malaise, arthralgias 1 to 3 days prior to eruption. Mild to moderate skin tenderness, conjunctival burning or itching, then skin pain, burning sensation, tenderness, paresthesia. Mouth lesions are painful, tender. Impaired alimentation, photophobia, painful micturition, and anxiety.
SKIN LESIONS Prodromal Rash. Morbilliform, can be target-like lesion, with/without purpura (Fig. 8-7); rapid confluence of individual lesions (Fig. 8-8); alternatively, it can start with diffuse erythema and no rash (Fig. 8-9).
Early. Necrotic epidermis first appears as macular areas with a crinkled surface that enlarge and coalesce (Fig. 8-7). Sheetlike loss of epidermis (Fig. 8-8). Raised flaccid blisters that spread with lateral pressure (Nikolsky sign) on erythematous areas. Full-thickness epidermal detachment yields exposed, red, oozing dermis (Fig. 8-9) resembling a second-degree thermal burn.
Distribution. Initial erythema on face, extremities, becoming confluent over a few hours or days. Epidermal sloughing may be generalized, resulting in large denuded areas (Figs. 8-8 and 8-9). The scalp, palms, and soles may be less severely involved.

TABLE 8-3 Medications and the Risk of Toxic Epidermal Necrolysis

High Risk	Lower Risk	Doubtful Risk	No Evidence of Risk
Allopurinol	NSAIDs (e.g., diclofenac)	Paracetamol (acetaminophen)	Aspirin
Sulfamethoxazole	Aminopenicillins	Pyrazolone analgesics	Sulfonylurea
Sulfadiazine	Cephalosporins	Corticosteroids	Thiazide diuretics
Sulfapyridine	Quinolones	Other NSAIDs (except aspirin)	Furosemide
Sulfadoxine	Cyclins	Sertraline	Aldactone
Sulfasalazine	Macrolides		Calcium channel blockers
Carbamazepine			β-Blockers
Lamotrigine			Angiotensin-converting enzyme inhibitors
Phenobarbital			Angiotensin II receptor antagonists
Phenytoin			Statins
Phenylbutazone			Hormones
Nevirapine			Vitamins
Oxicam NSAIDs			
Thiacetazone			

NSAIDs, nonsteroidal anti-inflammatory drugs.

Source: Reproduced with permission from Valeyrie-Allanore L, Roujeau J-C. Epidermal necrolysis. In: Goldsmith LA, Katz SI, Gilchrest BA, et al, eds. *Fitzpatrick's Dermatology in General Medicine*. 8th ed. New York, NY: McGraw-Hill; 2012, Chap. 40.

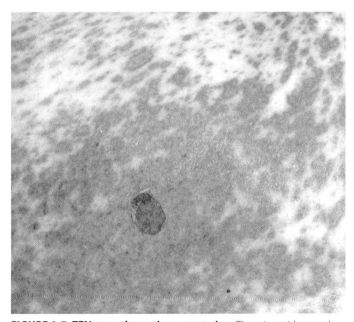

FIGURE 8-7 TEN, exanthematic presentation There is a widespread confluent macular rash with crinkling of the epidermis in some areas. There is detachment of the epidermis at the site of pressure (Nikolsky sign), resulting in a red erosion. This eruption was caused by allopurinol.

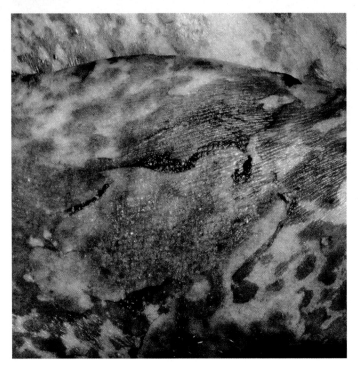

FIGURE 8-8 TEN, exanthematic presentation
A macular rash has started to coalesce. Dislodgment and shedding of the necrotic epidermis has led to a large oozing and extremely painful erosion. The eruption resulted from a sulfonamide.

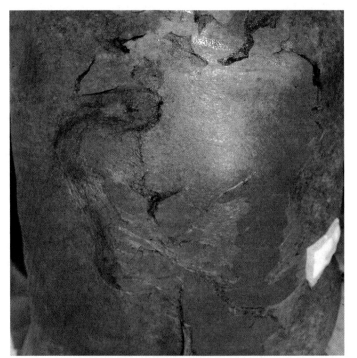

FIGURE 8-9 TEN, nonexanthematic diffuse presentation This 65-year-old woman developed diffuse erythema over almost the entire body, which then resulted in epidermal crinkling, detachment, and shedding of epidermis leaving large erosions. This is reminiscent of extensive scalding.

MUCOUS MEMBRANES Invariably involved, i.e., erythema, painful erosions: lips, buccal mucosa, conjunctiva, genital, and anal skin.
EYES 85% have conjunctival lesions: hyperemia, pseudomembrane formation; keratitis, corneal erosions; later, synechiae between eyelids and bulbar conjunctiva.
Recovery. Regrowth of epidermis begins within days; completed in >3 weeks. Pressure points and periorificial sites exhibit delayed healing. Skin that is not denuded acutely is shed in sheets, especially on the palms/soles. Nails and eyelashes may be shed.

GENERAL FINDINGS

- Fever usually higher in TEN than in SJS.
- Usually mentally alert. Distress caused by severe pain.
- Cardiovascular: Pulse may be >120 beats/min. Blood pressure.
- Renal: Tubular necrosis may occur. Acute renal failure.
- Respiratory and GI tracts: Sloughing of epithelium with erosions.

LABORATORY EXAMINATIONS

HEMATOLOGY Anemia, lymphopenia; eosinophilia uncommon. Neutropenia correlates with poor prognosis. Serum urea increased, serum bicarbonate decreased.
DERMATOPATHOLOGY Early. Vacuolization/necrosis of basal keratinocytes and throughout the epidermis.
Late. Full-thickness epidermal necrosis and detachment with subepidermal split above basement membrane. Sparse lymphocytic infiltrate in dermis. Immunofluorescence studies unremarkable, ruling out other blistering disorders.

DIAGNOSIS AND DIFFERENTIAL DIAGNOSIS

EARLY Exanthematous drug eruptions, EM major, scarlet fever, phototoxic eruptions, toxic shock syndrome, and graft-versus-host disease (GVHD).
FULLY EVOLVED EM major (typical target lesions, acute GVHD (may mimic TEN; less mucosal involvement), thermal burns, phototoxic reactions, staphylococcal scalded-skin syndrome (in young children, rare in adults and no mucosal involvement), generalized bullous fixed drug eruption, and exfoliative dermatitis.

COURSE AND PROGNOSIS

Average duration of progression is <4 days. A prognostic scoring system is shown in Table 8-4. Course similar to that of extensive thermal burns. Prognosis related to the extent of skin necrosis. Transcutaneous fluid loss is large and varies with area of denudation; associated electrolyte abnormalities. Prerenal azotemia is common. Bacterial colonization

TABLE 8-4 Scorten: A Prognostic Scoring System for Patients with Epidermal Necrolysis

Prognostic Factors	Points
Age >40 yr	1
Heart rate >120 beats/min	1
Cancer or hematologic malignancy	1
Body surface area involved >10%	1
Serum urea level >10 mM	1
Serum bicarbonate level <20 mM	1
Serum glucose level >14 mM	1

Scorten	Mortality Rate (%)
0–1	3.2
2	12.1
3	35.8
4	58.3
>5	90

Source: Data from Bastuji-Garin S, et al: SCORTEN: A severity-of-illness score for toxic epidermal necrolysis. *J Invest Dermatol*. 115:149,2000; from Valeyrie-Allanore L, Roujeau J-C. Epidermal necrolysis. In: Goldsmith LA, Katz SI, Gilchrest BA, et al, eds. *Fitzpatrick's Dermatology in General Medicine*. 8th ed. New York, NY: McGraw-Hill; 2012, Chap. 40.

Note: Although it is highly appreciated that this scoring system exists, we do have one reservation with SCORTEN. Only one point is assigned to body surface area involvement (>10%). There is definitely a prognostic difference between 20% and 70% body surface area involvement and this should be reflected in the total score.

is common and associated with sepsis. Other complications include hypermetabolic state and diffuse interstitial pneumonitis. Mortality rate for TEN is 30%, mainly in elderly; for SJS, 5 to 12%. If the patient survives the first episode of SJS/TEN, reexposure to the causative drug may be followed by recurrence within hours to days, more severe than the initial episode.

SEQUELAE

Skin. Scarring, hypo- and hyper-pigmentation, and abnormal regrowth of nails.

Eyes. Common, including Sjögren-like sicca syndrome with deficiency of mucin in tears; entropion, trichiasis, squamous metaplasia, neovascularization of conjunctiva and cornea; synblepharon, punctate keratitis, corneal scarring; persistent photophobia, burning eyes, visual impairment, and blindness.

Anogenitalia: Phimosis, vaginal synechiae.

MANAGEMENT

- Early diagnosis and withdrawal of suspected drug(s).
- Patients are best cared for in an intermediate or intensive care unit.

- Manage replacement of IV fluids and electrolytes as for patient with extensive thermal burn. However, less fluid is usually required as for thermal burn of similar extent.
- Systemic glucocorticoids early in the disease and in high doses are reported helpful in reducing morbidity or mortality (as is also the experience of the authors), but this has been questioned. Late in the disease, they are contraindicated.
- High-dose IV immunoglobulins halt progression of TEN if administered early. This is questioned by some authors; the discrepancy may be explained by the different products and batches used.
- With oropharyngeal involvement, suction to prevent aspiration pneumonitis.
- Surgical debridement is not recommended.
- Diagnose and treat complicating infections, including sepsis (fever, hypotension, and change in mental status).
- Treat eye lesions early with erythromycin ointment.

PREVENTION The patient must be aware of the likely offending drug and that other drugs of the same class can cross-react. These drugs must never be readministered. Patient should wear a medical alert bracelet.

BENIGN NEOPLASMS AND HYPERPLASIAS

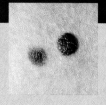

DISORDERS OF MELANOCYTES

ACQUIRED MELANOCYTIC NEVI (MN) ICD-10: D22.L10

- MN, commonly called *moles*, are very common, small (<1 cm), circumscribed, acquired pigmented macules, papules, or nodules.
- Composed of groups of melanocytic nevus cells located in the epidermis, dermis, and, rarely, the subcutaneous tissue.
- They are benign, acquired tumors arising as nevus cell clusters at the dermal–epidermal junction (*junctional MN*), invading the papillary dermis (*compound MN*), and ending their life cycle as *dermal MN* with nevus cells located exclusively in the dermis where, with progressive age, there will be fibrosis.

EPIDEMIOLOGY AND ETIOLOGY

One of the most common acquired new growths in Caucasians (most adults have about 20 nevi), less common in African Americans or darker pigmented persons; sometimes absent in persons with red hair and marked freckling (skin phototype I).

RACE African Americans and Asians have more nevi on the palms, soles, and nail beds.

HEREDITY Common acquired MN occur in family clusters. Dysplastic melanocytic nevi (DN) (see Section 12), which are putative precursor lesions of malignant melanoma, are different from MN. They occur in virtually every patient with familial cutaneous melanoma and in 30 to 50% of patients with sporadic nonfamilial primary melanoma.

SUN EXPOSURE A factor in the induction of nevi on the exposed areas.

SIGNIFICANCE Risk of melanoma is related to the numbers of MN and to DN. In the latter, even if only a few lesions are present.

CLINICAL MANIFESTATION

DURATION AND EVOLUTION OF LESIONS MN appear in early childhood and reach a maximum in young adulthood even though some MN may arise in adulthood. Later on, there is a gradual involution and fibrosis of lesions, but most disappear after the age of 60. In contrast, DN continue to appear throughout life and are believed not to involute (see Section 12).

SKIN SYMPTOMS MN are asymptomatic. However, MN grow and growth is often accompanied by itching. Itching per se is not a sign of malignancy, but if a lesion *persistently* itches or is tender, it should be followed carefully or excised, since *persistent* pruritus may be an early indication of malignant change.

CLASSIFICATION

MN are multiple (Fig. 9-1A) and can be classified according to their state of evolution and thus according to the histologic level of the nevus cell clusters (Fig. 9-1B).

1. *Junctional melanocytic MN*: These arise at the dermal–epidermal junction, on the epidermal side of the basement membrane; in other words, they are intraepidermal (Figs. 9-1B and 9-2).
2. *Compound MN*: Nevus cells invade the papillary dermis, and nevus cell nests are now found both intraepidermally and dermally (Figs. 9-1B and 9-3).
3. *Dermal MN*: These represent the last stage of the evolution of MN. "Dropping off" into the dermis is now completed, and the nevus grows or remains intradermal (Figs. 9-1B and 9-4). With progressive age, there will be gradual fibrosis (Fig. 9-4C).

Thus, melanocytic MN undergo the evolution from junctional → compound → dermal MN (Fig. 9-1B). Since the capacity of MN

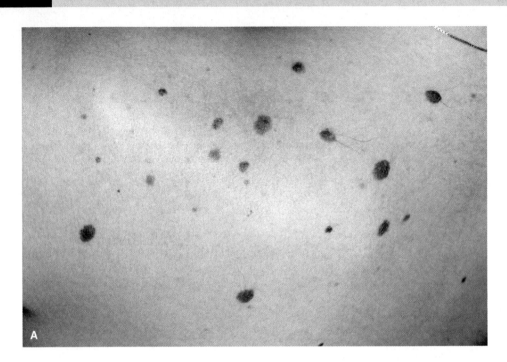

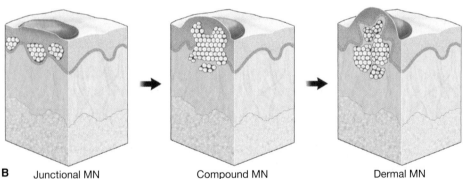

B   Junctional MN   Compound MN   Dermal MN

FIGURE 9-1 (A) Multiple MN on the shoulder of a 32-year-old female Most of these nevi are junctional MN; some are slightly elevated and thus compound MN. Note relatively uniform shape and color of the lesions. Because of different developmental stages, they are of varying size ranging from 1 to 4 mm in diameter. They are regular and have a relatively uniform shape. **(B) Junctional MN** arise at dermal–epidermal junction and are intraepidermal, pigmented, and flat. In *compound MN*, nevus cells have invaded the dermis and are thus both intraepidermal and dermal. Since, as a rule, only junctional nevus cells have the capacity to form melanin, they are still pigmented, but since they continue to grow, they are more elevated than junctional MN. In *dermal* MN, all nevus cells are now in the dermis and have lost the capacity to produce melanin. Dermal MN are thus skin-colored, pink, or only slightly tan. As they still grow and expand into the dermis, they lift the lesion upward and are thus usually dome-shaped or papillomatous.

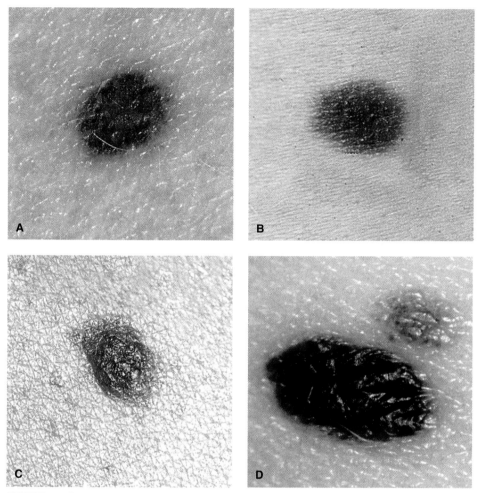

FIGURE 9-2 (A–D) Junctional MN Lesions are completely flat **(A, B)** or minimally elevated as in **(C)** and **(D)** They are symmetric with a regular border and, depending on the skin type of the individuals, have different shades of brown to black **(D)**.

cells to form melanin is greatest when they are located at the dermal–epidermal junction (intraepidermally) and because MN cells lose their capacity for melanization, the further they penetrate into the dermis, the lesser is the intensity of pigmentation with the increase in the dermal proportion of the nevus. Purely dermal MN are therefore almost always without pigment. In a simplified manner, the clinical appearance of MN along this evolutionary path can be characterized as follows: junctional MN is flat and dark, compound MN is raised and dark, and dermal MN is raised and light.

This evolution also reflects the age at which the different types of MN are found. Junctional and compound MN are usually seen in childhood and through the teens, whereas dermal MN start manifesting in the third and fourth decade.

Junctional Melanocytic Nevi

LESIONS Macule, or only very slightly raised (Fig. 9-2). Uniform tan, brown, dark brown, or even black. Round or oval with smooth, regular borders. Scattered discrete lesions. Never >1 cm in diameter; if >1 cm, the "mole" is a

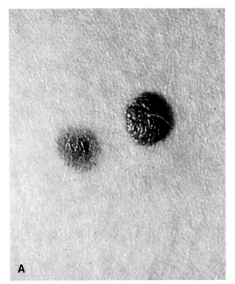 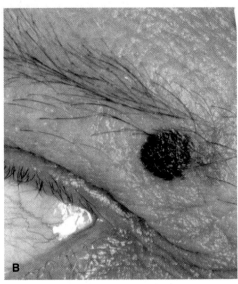

FIGURE 9-3 Compound MN Uniformly pigmented papules and small domed nodules. **(A)** The lesion to the left is flatter and tan with a more elevated darker center; the larger lesion (on the right) is older and chocolate-brown; the left lesion is younger and has a predominantly junctional component at the periphery. **(B)** A heavily pigmented dome-shaped lesion in the eyebrow. It is sharply defined, uniformly black, smooth and slightly cobblestone-like surface, and sharply and regularly defined. It measures less than 5 mm.

congenital nevomelanocytic nevus, a DN, or a melanoma (see Section 12).

Compound Melanocytic Nevi

LESIONS Papules or small nodules (Fig. 9-3). Dark brown, sometimes even black; dome-shaped, smooth, or cobblestone-like surface, regular and sharply defined border, sometimes papillomatous or hyperkeratotic. Never >1 cm in diameter; if >1 cm, the mole is a congenital nevomelanocytic nevus, a DN, or a melanoma. Consistency either firm or soft. Color may become mottled as progressive conversion into dermal MN occurs. May have hairs.

Dermal Melanocytic Nevi

LESIONS Sharply defined papule or nodule. Skin-colored, tan, or flecks of brown, often with telangiectasia. Round, dome-shaped (Fig. 9-4), smooth surface, diameter <1 cm. Usually not present before the second or third decade. Older lesions, mostly on the trunk, may become pedunculated and do not disappear spontaneously. May be hairy.

DISTRIBUTION Face, trunk, extremities, scalp. Random. Occasionally palmar and plantar, in which case these MN usually have the appearance of junctional MN.

DIAGNOSIS AND DIFFERENTIAL DIAGNOSIS

DIAGNOSIS Made clinically. As for all pigmented lesions, the ABCDE rule applies (see Section 12). In case of doubt, apply dermoscopy, and if malignancy cannot be excluded even by this procedure, excise lesions with a narrow margin.

DIFFERENTIAL DIAGNOSIS *Junctional MN:* All flat, deeply pigmented lesions. Solar lentigo, flat atypical nevus, and lentigo maligna. *Compound MN:* All raised pigmented lesions. Seborrheic keratosis, DN, small superficial spreading melanoma, early nodular melanoma, pigmented basal cell carcinoma (BCC), dermatofibroma, Spitz nevus, and blue nevus. *Dermal MN:* All light tan or skin-colored papules. BCC, neurofibroma, trichoepithelioma, dermatofibroma, and sebaceous hyperplasia.

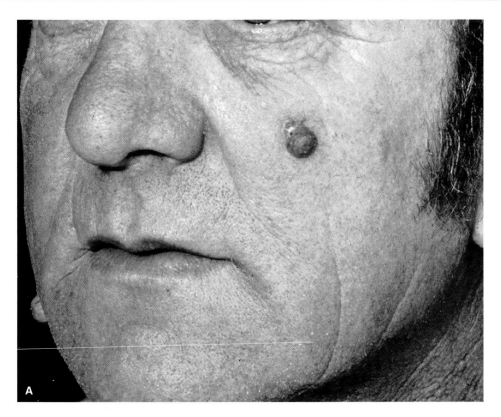

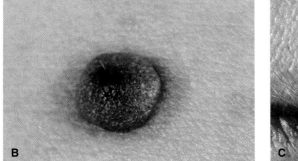

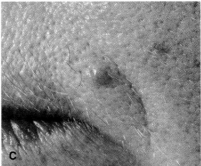

FIGURE 9-4 Dermal melanocytic MN (A) Two dome-shaped, sharply defined relatively soft tan nodules on the left cheek and right lateral mandibular region in a 60-year-old male. These lesions were previously much darker and less elevated. **(B)** A larger magnification of a dermal MN. This lesion is sharply defined, has a reddish color with a central regular pigmented spot where the nevus obviously is still compound in nature. **(C)** Old dermal nevus on the upper lip of a 65-year-old woman. This lesion is relatively hard, has a smooth surface, and a pinkish color. This lesion is fibrosing.

MANAGEMENT

Indications for removal of acquired melanocytic MN are the following:

Site: Lesions on the scalp (only if difficult to follow and not a classic dermal MN); mucous membranes, and anogenital area.

Growth: If there is a rapid change in size.

Color: If color becomes variegated.

Border: If irregular borders are present or develop.

Erosions: If lesion becomes eroded without major trauma.

Symptoms: If lesion begins to *persistently* itch, hurt, or bleed.

Dermoscopy: If criteria for melanoma or a dysplastic nevus are present or appear de novo.

Melanocytic MN *never* become malignant because of manipulation or trauma. In those cases where this was claimed, the lesion was initially a misdiagnosed melanoma. If there is an indication for the removal of an MN, the nevus should always be excised for histologic diagnosis and for definite treatment (particularly applicable to and decisive in ruling out congenital, dysplastic, or blue nevi). Removal of papillomatous, compound, or dermal MN for cosmetic reasons by electrocautery requires that a nevus be unequivocally diagnosed as benign MN and histology be performed. If an early melanoma cannot be excluded with certainty, an excision for histologic examination is obligatory but can be performed with narrow margins.

HALO MELANOCYTIC NEVUS ICD-10: D22-L34

- An NMN that is encircled by a halo of leukoderma or depigmentation. The leukoderma is based on a decrease of melanin in melanocytes and/or disappearance of melanocytes at the dermal–epidermal junction (Fig. 9-5A).
- Mechanism: Autoimmune (cellular, humoral) mechanism leading to apoptosis of nevus cells and melanocytes in surrounding epidermis.
- Prevalence: 1%. Occurs spontaneously or in patients with vitiligo.
- A white halo around a MN indicates regression and halo nevi most often undergo spontaneous involution.
- Usually in children or young adults mostly on the trunk (Fig. 9-5A).
- Three stages: (1) White halo around preexisting MN (Fig. 9-5B), may be preceded by erythema (Fig. 9-5C); (2) disappearance of MN (months to years) (Fig. 9-5A); and (3) repigmentation of halo (years).
- Halo MN may indicate incipient vitiligo.
- Halo around other lesions: Blue nevus, congenital MN, Spitz nevus, malignant melanoma and melanoma metastases, dermatofibroma, neurofibroma.
- *Synonym*: Sutton leukoderma acquisitum centrifugum.

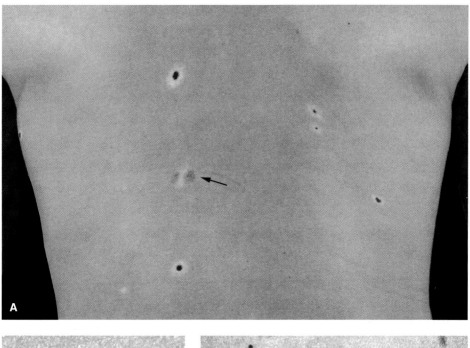

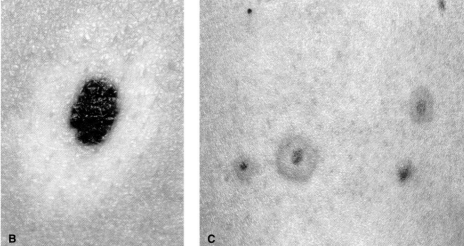

FIGURE 9-5 (A) Halo melanocytic MN on the back of a 22-year-old female There are five halo nevi, all with a pigmented dot-like central junctional or compound MN surrounded by a hypo- or amelanotic halo. The arrow indicates one lesion where the central nevus has completely regressed; the reddish color is caused by telangiectasia. **(B)** Larger magnification of a halo MN. The nevus is a junctional MN (compare with **Fig. 9-2**) that is surrounded by a hypomelanotic almost white halo. **(C)** Several tan junctional MN that are surrounded by an erythematous halo. This is the early stage of halo development but is observed only rarely. The erythematous rim will later turn white.

BLUE NEVUS ICD-10: D22. L42

- A blue nevus is an acquired, firm, dark-blue to gray-to-black, sharply defined papule or nodule representing a localized proliferation of melanin-producing *dermal* melanocytes.
- Three types: Common blue nevus, cellular blue nevus, combined MN/blue nevus.
- Blue nevi and combined MN/blue nevi are benign. Cellular blue nevi are larger and have a very rare tendency to become malignant.
- Ectopic accumulation of melanin-producing melanocytes; derived from melanoblasts arrested during migration from neural crest.
- Papules, nodules, blue-gray, blue-black, <10 mm in diameter (Figs. 9-6 and 9-7A). Cellular blue nevi larger (>1 cm) and irregular (Fig. 9-7B).
- Differential diagnosis: Dermatofibroma, glomus tumor, nodular or metastatic melanoma, traumatic tattoo, pigmented BCC.
- Treatment not necessary. If in doubt, excision.
- Cellular blue nevi should be excised.
- *Synonyms*: Blue neuronevus, dermal melanocytoma.

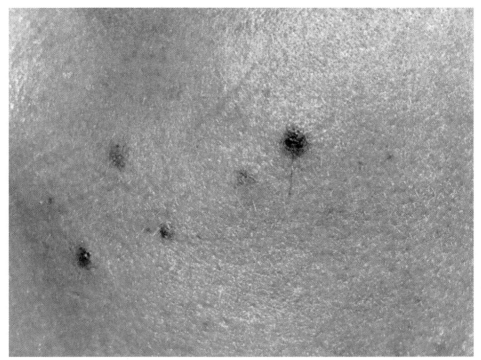

FIGURE 9-6 Blue nevus There are four tan junctional MN and one bluish-black round lesion on the cheek of a 17-year-old girl. In contrast to the junctional MN, the blue nevus is palpable with a relatively high consistency, and upon dermoscopy will appear as an ill-defined uniformly bluish lesion deep in the dermis.

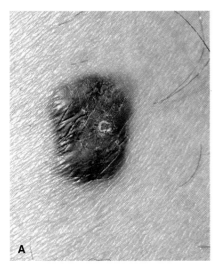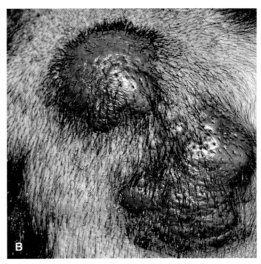

FIGURE 9-7 Blue nevus and cellular blue nevus (A) This blue nevus has regular borders but is not circular and is solidly blue-black in color. The epidermis is smooth, indicating that the lesion is in the dermis. The consistency is increased and the margins are well defined. Differential diagnosis must include nodular melanoma. **(B)** This cellular blue nevus appeared as two large, bluish-black nodules on the scalp. After excision, histology showed that they were contiguous and thus represented one single lesion. Cellular blue nevi are much larger and should always be excised to rule out melanoma, which, albeit rarely, can develop in these lesions.

NEVUS SPILUS ICD-10: L81.48

- Light brown pigmented macule varying from a few centimeters to a large area (>15 cm), and many dark brown small macules (2 to 3 mm) or papules scattered throughout the pigmented background (Fig. 9-8A). The pigment in the macular background may be so faint that it can be recognized only under Wood light (Fig. 9-8B).
- The pathology of the macular pigmented lesion is the same as lentigo simplex, i.e., increased numbers of melanocytes, while the flat or raised lesions scattered throughout are either junctional or compound; rarely, these may be DN.
- The lesions are not as common as junctional or compound MN but are not at all rare. In one series, the nevus spilus was present in 3% of white patients.
- Malignant melanoma very rarely arises in these lesions.

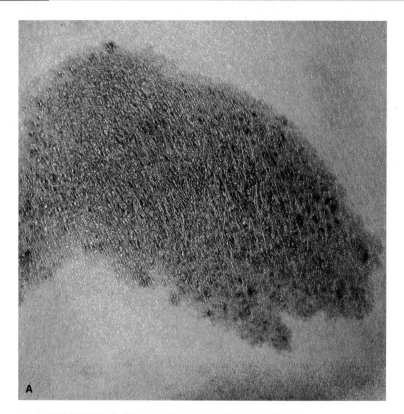

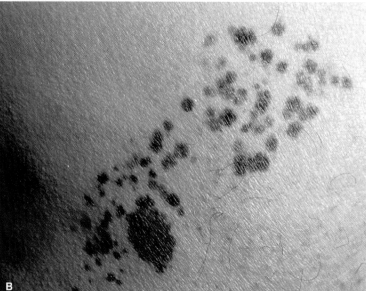

FIGURE 9-8 Nevus spilus (A) This dark brown pigmented macule measuring about 10 cm along the long axis is peppered with many small, dark brown to black macules and papules. **(B)** This is also nevus spilus but the macular background is only slightly pigmented so that it will be revealed only under Wood light. The lesion is peppered with many small dark brown macules and flat papules.

SPITZ NEVUS ICD-10: D22.L30

- Spitz nevus is a benign, dome-shaped, hairless, small (<1 cm in diameter) nodule, most often pink, red, or tan (Fig. 9-9A). There is often a history of recent rapid growth.
- Incidence is 1.4:100,000 (Australia). It occurs at all ages but a third of the patients are children <10 years; rarely seen in persons ≥40 years. *Lesions* arise within months. They are papules, dome-shaped, relatively flat nodules, round, well-circumscribed, smooth-topped, and hairless. They are a uniform pink-red (Fig. 9-9A), tan, brown, dark brown, or even black (Fig. 9-9B); are firm; and usually distributed on the head and neck.
- *Differential diagnosis* includes all pink, tan, or darkly pigmented papules: pyogenic granulom, hemangioma, molluscum contagiosum, juvenile xanthogranuloma, mastocytoma, dermatofibroma, MN, DN (amelanotic), and nodular melanoma.
- *Dermatopathology*: Hyperplasia of the epidermis and melanocytes and dilation of capillaries. Admixed large epithelioid cells, large spindle cells with abundant cytoplasm, and occasional mitotic figures.
- Histologic examination must be done to confirm the clinical diagnosis. Excision in its entirety is important because the condition recurs in 10 to 15% of all cases in lesions that have not been excised completely. Spitz nevi are benign, but there can be a histologic similarity to melanoma and the histopathologic diagnosis requires the help of an experienced dermatopathologist.
- Spitz nevi do not usually involute, as do common acquired MN. However, some lesions have been observed to transform into common compound MN, whereas others undergo fibrosis and in late stages may resemble dermatofibromas.
- *Synonyms*: Pigmented and epithelioid spindle cell nevus. Decades ago, these were called "juvenile melanoma."

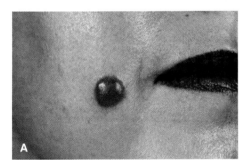 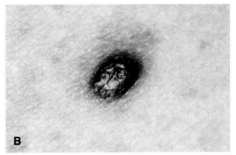

FIGURE 9-9 Spitz nevus (A) Pink dome-shaped nodule on the cheek of a 25-year old woman, developing abruptly within the previous 12 months; the lesion can be mistaken for a hemangioma. **(B)** Pigmented Spitz nevus (also called Reed nevus). A black papule surrounded by a tan macular region developed within a few months on the back of a young female; as such a lesion cannot be distinguished from a nodular melanoma, the lesion was excised and the diagnosis confirmed histologically.

MONGOLIAN SPOT ICD-10:D22.505

- These congenital gray-blue macular lesions are characteristically located on the lumbosacral area (Fig. 9-10) but can also occur on the back, scalp, or anywhere on the skin. There is usually a single lesion, but rarely, several truncal lesions can be present at birth (Fig. 9-11).
- The underlying pathology is dispersed spindle-shaped melanocytes within the dermis (dermal melanocytosis). It is believed that these ectopic melanocytes represent pigment cells that have been interrupted in their migration from the neural crest to the epidermis.
- Mongolian spots may disappear in early childhood, in contrast to nevus of Ota (see Fig. 9-12).
- As the term *Mongolian* implies, these lesions are found almost always (99 to 100%) in infants of Asiatic and Native American origin; however, they have been reported in African American and, rarely, in Caucasian infants.
- No melanomas have been reported to occur in these lesions.

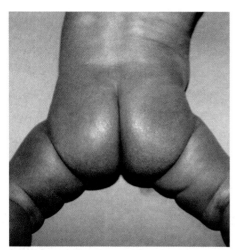

FIGURE 9-10 Mongolian spot A large gray-blue macular lesion involving the entire lumbosacral and gluteal area and the left thigh in a baby from Sri Lanka. Although Mongolian spots are common in Asians, the parents of this baby were alarmed because the lesion was so large.

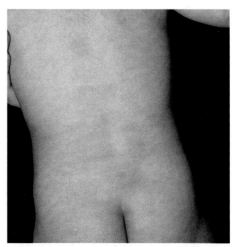

FIGURE 9-11 Mongolian spots Multiple, ill-defined, bluish lesions are scattered on the back of this Japanese child. They were present at birth. Most of these lesions disappeared later in childhood.

NEVUS OF OTA ICD-10: D22.301

- Very common in Asian populations and is said to occur in 1% of dermatologic outpatients in Japan. It has been reported in East Indians, African Americans, and, rarely, Caucasian.
- The pigmentation, which can be quite subtle or markedly disfiguring, consists of a mottled, dusky admixture of blue and brown hyperpigmentation of the skin. It mostly involves the skin and mucous membranes innervated by the first and second branches of the trigeminal nerve (Fig. 9-12).
- The blue hue results from the presence of ectopic melanocytes in the dermis. It can occur in the hard palate and in the conjunctivae (Fig. 9-12), sclerae, and tympanic membranes.
- Nevus of Ota may be bilateral. It may be congenital but is not hereditary; more often, it appears in early childhood or during puberty and remains for life, in contrast to the Mongolian spot, which may disappear in early childhood.
- Treatment with lasers is an effective modality for this disfiguring disorder.
- Malignant melanoma can occur but is very rare.

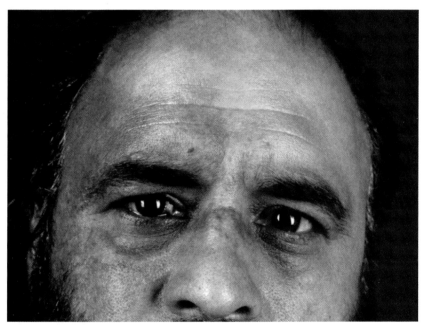

FIGURE 9-12 Nevus of Ota There is an ill-defined, mottled, dusky, gray to bluish hyper-pigmentation in the regions supplied by the first and second branches of the right trigeminal nerve. The lesion was unilateral and there was also hyperpigmentation of the sclera and eyelids.

VASCULAR TUMORS AND MALFORMATIONS

- The present binary biologic classification distinguishes between vascular tumors and vascular malformations. The latter are subclassified according to the structural components into capillary, venous, lymphatic, arterial, or combined forms (Table 9-1).
- *Vascular tumors* (e.g., hemangiomas) show endothelial hyperplasia, whereas *malformations* have a normal endothelial turnover.
- Hemangiomas of infancy are not present at birth but appear postnatally; grow rapidly during the first year (proliferating phase), undergo slow spontaneous regression during childhood (involution phase), and remain stable thereafter.
- Vascular malformations are errors of morphogenesis and are presumed to occur during intrauterine life. Most are present at birth, though some do not appear until years later. Once manifested, they grow proportionally but enlargement can occur as a result of various factors.
- Both vascular tumors and malformations can be separated into slow-flow or fast-flow types.
- Classification of vascular tumors and malformations is shown in Table 9-1, and the distinguishing features of vascular tumors and vascular malformations are shown in Table 9-2.

TABLE 9-1 Classification of Vascular Anomalies

Vascular Tumors	Vascular Malformations

■ Hemangioma
  ■ Hemangioma of infancy
  ■ Congenital
    ■ Rapidly involuting congenital hemangioma
    ■ Noninvoluting congenital hemangioma
■ Hemangioendotheliomas
  ■ Kaposiform hemangioendothelioma
  ■ Tufted angioma
■ Angiosarcoma
	■ Capillary
	  ■ Capillary malformation (port-wine stain)
	  ■ Telangiectasia (hereditary benign telangiectasia; essential telangiectasia)
	  ■ Hereditary hemorrhagic telangiectasia
	  ■ Capillary–arteriovenous malformation
	  ■ Sturge–Weber syndrome
	■ Venous
	  ■ Venous malformation
	  ■ Familial form: Cutaneomucosal venous malformation
	  ■ Glomuvenous malformation
	  ■ Blue rubber bleb nevus or Bean syndrome
	■ Lymphatic
	  ■ Lymphatic malformation
	  ■ Primary lymphoedemas
	■ Arterial
	  ■ Arteriovenous malformation
	  ■ Capillary–arteriovenous malformation
	  ■ Arteriovenous fistula
	■ Syndromic malformations
	  ■ Slow-flow
	    ■ Klippel–Trénaunay syndrome (capillary–lymphaticovenous malformation)
	    ■ Maffucci syndrome
	  ■ Fast-flow
	    ■ Parkes Weber syndrome

Source: Reproduced with permission from Boon LM, Vikkula M. Vascular malformations. In: Wolff K, Goldsmith LA, Katz SI, et al, eds. *Fitzpatrick's Dermatology in General Medicine*. 7th ed. New York: NY: McGraw-Hill; 2008, pp. 1651–1666.

TABLE 9-2 Distinguishing Features of Vascular Tumors (Hemangiomas) and Vascular Malformations

	Tumors	**Malformations**
Presence at birth	Usually postnatal, 30% nascent, rarely full grown	100% (presumably), not always obvious
Male:female ratio	1:3–1:5	1:1
Incidence	1–12.6% at birth; 10–12% at 1 year	0.3–0.5% port-wine stain
Natural history	Phases: proliferating, involuting, and involuted	Proportionate growth; can expand
Cellular	Endothelial hyperplasia	Normal endothelial turnover
Skeletal changes	Occasional mass effect on adjacent bone; rare hypertrophy	Slow-flow: distortion, hypertrophy, or hyperplasia
		Fast-flow: destruction, distortion, or hypertrophy

Source: Reproduced with permission from Virnelli-Grevelink S, Mulliken JB. Vascular anomalies and tumors of skin and subcutaneous tissues. In: Freedberg IM, Eisen AZ, Wolff K, et al, eds. *Fitzpatrick's Dermatology in General Medicine*. 6th ed. New York, NY: McGraw-Hill; 2003:1002–1019.

VASCULAR TUMORS

HEMANGIOMA OF INFANCY (HI) ICD-10: D18.008

Formerly strawberry, cherry, capillary hemangioma.

EPIDEMIOLOGY

The most common tumor of infancy. Incidence in newborns is between 1% and 2.5%; in Caucasian children by 1 year of age, it is 10%. Females to males ratio is 3 to 1.

ETIOLOGY AND PATHOGENESIS

HI is a localized proliferative process of angioblastic mesenchyme. A clonal expansion of endothelial cells resulting from somatic mutations of genes regulating endothelial cell proliferation.

CLINICAL MANIFESTATION

The initial proliferative phase lasts from 3 to 9 months. HIs usually enlarge rapidly during the first year. In a subsequent phase of involution, the HI regresses gradually over 2 to 6 years. Involution is usually completed by the age of 10 and varies greatly between individuals. It is not correlated with size, location, or appearance of the lesion.

SKIN LESIONS Soft, bright red to deep purple, compressible. On diascopy, does not blanch completely. Nodule or plaque, 1 to 8 cm (Figs. 9-13A and 9-14A). With the onset of spontaneous regression, a white-to-gray area appears on the surface of the central part of the lesion (Fig. 9-14A). Ulceration may occur.

Distribution. Lesions are usually solitary and localized or extended over an entire region (Fig. 9-15). They usually cover 50% of the head and neck and 25% of the trunk. Face, trunk, legs, and oral mucous membrane.

SPECIAL PRESENTATIONS

DEEP HI (Formerly, cavernous hemangioma.) In the lower dermis and subcutaneous fat. Localized, firm rubbery mass of bluish or normal skin color with telangiectases in overlying skin (Fig. 9-16). Can be combined with superficial hemangioma (Fig. 9-14A). Does not involute as well as superficial type.

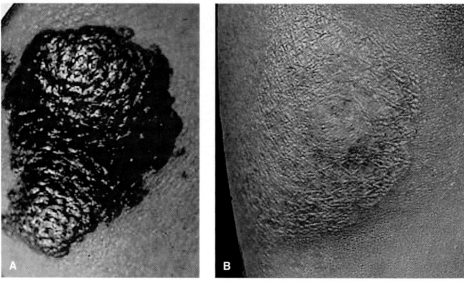

FIGURE 9-13 Hemangioma of infancy (A) This bright red nodular plaque in an infant of African extraction is frightening to the parents, and caution is needed to prevent scarring from the treatment itself. Since most of these lesions disappear spontaneously with only 20% showing residual atrophy or depigmentation, a wait-and-see strategy is recommended. **(B)** The same lesion after 3 years. The hemangioma has faded spontaneously, and there is only slight residual atrophy.

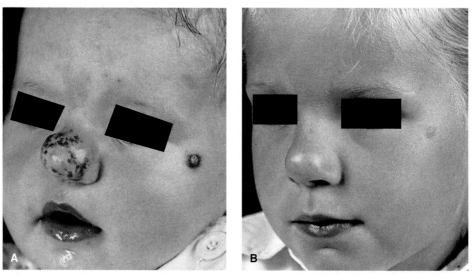

FIGURE 9-14 Hemangioma of infancy (A) This lesion on the nose consists of a superficial and deep portion, and incipient involution is already apparent for the superficial compartment. Note an additional small hemangioma of infancy on the left zygomatic region. **(B)** By the fifth year, the hemangioma on the nose has almost disappeared and so has the lesion on the zygomatic region; the latter, however, has left a small scar.

FIGURE 9-15 Hemangioma of infancy Here, it involves a large segment of skin. While early involution is already apparent on the forehead, the lesion on the upper eyelid and the medial canthus impairs proper function of the lid, and this indicates that vision might be compromised in the future. In this patient, treatment was indicated.

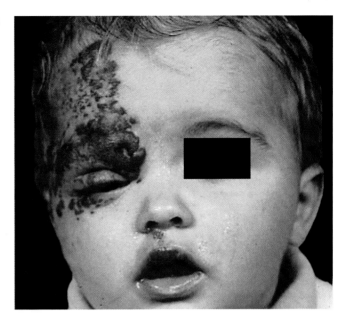

FIGURE 9-16 Hemangioma of infancy, deep lesion There is a rubbery mass in the subcutis associated with a superficial (red) portion. These lesions hardly regress. The hemangioma was removed by surgery.

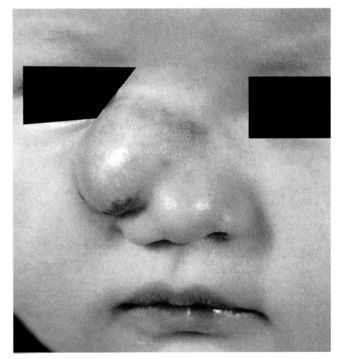

MULTIPLE HIS Multiple small (<2 cm), cherry-red papular lesions involving skin alone (*benign cutaneous hemangiomatosis*) or skin and internal organs (*diffuse neonatal hemangiomatosis*).

CONGENITAL HEMANGIOMAS These develop in utero and are subdivided into rapidly involuting congenital hemangiomas (RICH) and non-involuting congenital hemangiomas (NICH). They present as violaceous tumors with overlying telangiectasia with large veins in periphery or as red-violaceous plaques invading deeper tissues. NICH are fast-flow hemangiomas requiring surgery.

LABORATORY EXAMINATION

DERMATOPATHOLOGY Proliferation of endothelial cells in various amounts in the dermis and/or subcutaneous tissue; there is usually more endothelial proliferation in the superficial type and little in the deep angiomas. *GLUT-1 immunoreactivity is found in all hemangiomas but not in vascular malformations.*

DIAGNOSIS

Made on clinical findings and MRI; Doppler and arteriography to demonstrate fast flow. Determine GLUT-1 immunoreactivity to rule out vascular malformation.

COURSE AND PROGNOSIS

HIs spontaneously involute by the fifth year, with some few percent disappearing only by age 10 (Figs. 9-13B and 9-14B). There is virtually no residual skin change at the site in most lesions (80%); in the rest, there is atrophy, depigmentation, telangiectasia, and scarring. HIs may, however, pose a considerable problem during the growth phase when they interfere with vital functions, such as obstruction of vision (Fig. 9-15) or of larynx, nose, or mouth. Deeper lesions, especially those involving mucous membranes, may not involute completely. Synovial involvement may be associated with hemophilia-like arthropathy. Special forms of HI, *tufted angiomas* and *Kaposiform hemangioendothelioma*, may have platelet entrapment, thrombocytopenia (Kasabach–Merritt syndrome), and even disseminated intravascular coagulation. Rarely, morbidity associated with HI occurs secondary to hemorrhage or high-output heart failure.

MANAGEMENT

Each lesion must be judged individually regarding the decision to treat or not to treat and the selection of a treatment mode. Systemic treatment is difficult, requires experience, and should be performed by an expert. Surgical and medical interventions include continuous wave or pulsed dye laser, cryosurgery, intralesional and systemic high-dose glucocorticoids, interferon-α (IFN-α), and propranolol. For the majority of HIs, active nonintervention is the best approach because spontaneous resolution gives the best cosmetic results (Figs. 9-13B and 9-14B). Treatment is indicated in about a quarter of HIs (5% that ulcerate; 20% that obstruct vital structures, i.e., eyes, ears, and larynx).

PYOGENIC GRANULOMA ICD-10: L98.0

- Pyogenic granuloma is a rapidly developing vascular lesion usually following minor trauma.
- This is a very common solitary eroded vascular nodule that bleeds spontaneously or after minor trauma. The lesion has a smooth surface, with or without crusts and with or without erosion (Fig. 9-17A). It appears as a bright red, dusky red, violaceous, or brown-black papule with a collar of hyperplastic epidermis at the base (Fig. 9-17B) and occurs on the fingers, lips, mouth, trunk, and toes.
- Histopathology: Lobular aggregates of proliferating capillaries with edema and numerous neutrophils. Thus, pyogenic granuloma is neither pyogenic (associated with bacterial infection), nor a granuloma.
- Treatment is surgical excision or curettage with electrodesiccation at the base.
- The importance of pyogenic granuloma is that it can be mistaken for amelanotic nodular melanoma, and vice versa.

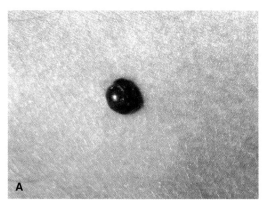
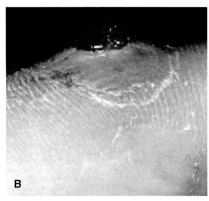

FIGURE 9-17 Pyogenic granuloma (A) This is a solitary vascular nodule of recent onset that bleeds spontaneously or after minor trauma. The lesions usually have a smooth surface, with or without crusts and with or without erosion. **(B)** On palms and soles, they have a typical collar of thickened stratum corneum at the base. This collar can best be seen when viewed from the side.

GLOMUS TUMOR ICD-10: D18.022

- A tumor of the *glomus body*. This is an anatomic and functional unit composed of specialized smooth muscle and *glomus cells* that surround thin-walled endothelial spaces; this anatomic unit functions as an arteriovenous shunt linking arterioles and venules. Glomus bodies are present on the pads and nail beds of the fingers and toes, and also on the volar aspect of hands and feet, in the skin of the ears, and in the center of the face.
- The glomus tumor presents as an exquisitely tender subungual or subcutaneous papule or nodule. Glomus tumors are characterized by paroxysmal painful attacks, especially elicited by exposure to the cold. They are most often present as solitary subungual tumors (Fig. 9-18A) but may rarely occur as multiple papules or nodules. These are noted, especially in children, as discrete papules or sometimes plaques anywhere on the skin surface (Fig. 9-18B).
- Therapy is by excision.

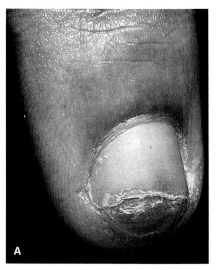
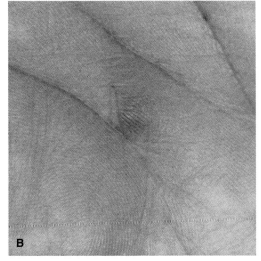

FIGURE 9-18 Glomus tumor (A) This is an exquisitely painful subungual nodule of reddish color; pain becomes paroxysmal upon exposure to cold. **(B)** Glomus tumor on the palm of a 16-year-old boy.

VASCULAR MALFORMATIONS

- These are malformations that do not undergo spontaneous involution.
- *Capillary malformations* (CMs) (e.g., nevus flammeus, or port-wine stain (PWS), according to the old nomenclature), *lymphatic malformation, capillary–lymphatic malformation* (CLM), *venous malformation* (VM), and *arteriovenous malformation* (AVM) are distinguished.
- Histologically, they consist of enlarged, tortuous vessels of various types.
- Only the most common and important are being dealt with here.

CAPILLARY MALFORMATIONS

PORT-WINE STAIN ICD-10: Q82.510

- A PWS is an irregularly shaped, red or violaceous, macular CM that is present at birth and never disappears spontaneously.
- It is common (0.3% of newborns); the malformation is usually confined to the skin.
- May be associated with vascular malformations in the eye and leptomeninges (Sturge–Weber syndrome [SWS]).
- *Synonym*: Nevus flammeus.

SKIN LESIONS Macular (Fig. 9-19) with varying hues of pink to purple. Large lesions follow a dermatomal distribution, usually unilateral (85%), although not always. Most commonly in the face, in the distribution of the trigeminal nerve (Fig. 9-19), and usually the superior and middle branches; mucosal involvement of conjunctiva and mouth may occur. CM may also involve other sites. With increasing age of the patient, papules or rubbery nodules (Fig. 9-20) cause significant disfigurement.

Clinical Variant

Nevus flammeus nuchae ("stork bite," salmon patch, erythema nuchae) occurs in approximately one-third of infants on the nape of the neck and tends to regress spontaneously. Similar lesions may occur on eyelids and glabella. It is not really a CM but rather a transitory vasodilatation phenomenon.

HISTOPATHOLOGY

Reveals ectasia of capillaries and no proliferation of endothelial cells. *GLUT-1 immunoreactivity is negative.*

COURSE AND PROGNOSIS

PWS are CMs that do not regress spontaneously. The area of involvement tends to increase in proportion to the size of the child. In adulthood, PWS usually become raised with papular and nodular areas and are the cause of significant progressive cosmetic disfigurement (Fig. 9-20).

MANAGEMENT

Treatment with tunable dye or copper vapor lasers is highly effective.

SYNDROMIC CM

SWS is the association of PWS in the trigeminal distribution with vascular malformations in the eye and leptomeninges, and superficial calcifications of the brain. May be associated with contralateral hemiparesis, muscular hemiatrophy, epilepsy, mental retardation, and glaucoma and ocular palsy. Characteristic calcifications of vascular malformations or localized linear calcification along cerebral convolutions at x-ray. CT scan should be done. It should, however, be noted that PWS with trigeminal distribution is common and does not necessarily indicate the presence of SWS. *Klippel–Trénaunay–Weber syndrome* may have an associated PWS overlying the deeper vascular malformation of soft tissue and bone. *PWS on the midline back* may be associated with an underlying AVM of the spinal cord.

FIGURE 9-19 Port-wine stain Sharply marginated, port-wine red macule occurring in a distribution of the second branch of the trigeminal nerve in a child.

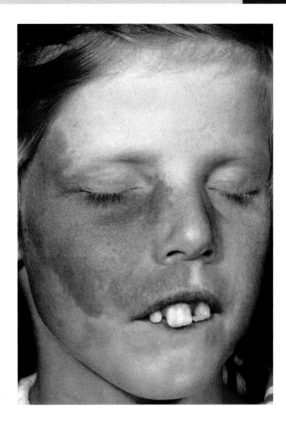

FIGURE 9-20 Port-wine stain With increasing age, the color deepens and papular and nodular vascular lesions develop within the previously macular lesion, causing progressively increasing disfigurement.

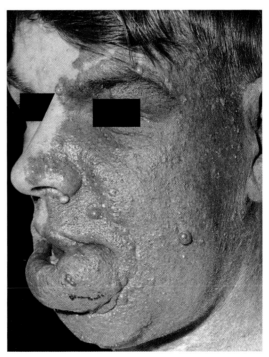

SPIDER ANGIOMA   ICD-10: I78.11

- A very common red focal telangiectatic network of dilated capillaries radiating from a central arteriole (punctum) (Fig. 9-21A). The central papular punctum is the site of the feeding arteriole with macular radiating telangiectatic vessels. Up to 1.5 cm in diameter. Usually solitary.
- On diascopy, the radiating telangiectasia blanches and the central arteriole may pulsate.
- Most commonly occurs on the face, forearms, and hands.
- It frequently occurs in normal persons and is more common in females; occurs in children.
- It may be associated with hyperestrogenic states, such as pregnancy (one or more in two-thirds of pregnant women), in patients receiving estrogen therapy, e.g., oral contraceptives, or in those with hepatocellular disease such as subacute and chronic viral hepatitis and alcoholic cirrhosis (Fig. 9-21B).
- Spider angioma arising in childhood and pregnancy may regress spontaneously.
- The lesion may be confused with *hereditary hemorrhagic telangiectasia, ataxia-telangiectasia,* or *telangiectasia* in systemic scleroderma.
- Lesions may be treated easily with electro- or laser surgery.
- *Synonyms*: Nevus araneus, spider nevus, arterial spider, spider telangiectasia, vascular spider.

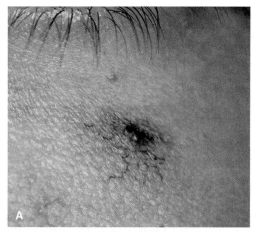 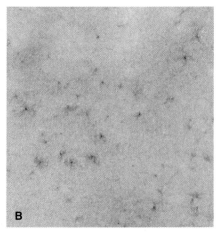

FIGURE 9-21 Spider nevus (A) Two small papules from which telangiectasias radiate. Upon compression the lesion blanches completely. **(B)** Spider nevi on the chest of a patient with cirrhosis.

VENOUS LAKE ICD-10: L98.8

- A venous lake is a dark blue to violaceous, asymptomatic, soft papule resulting from a dilated venule, occurring on the face, lips, and ears of patients >50 years of age (Figs. 9-22A and B).
- Etiology unknown, but it has been related to solar exposure.
- Lesions are few in number and remain for years. A dilated cavity is lined with a single layer of flattened endothelial cells filled with red blood cells and surrounded by a thin wall of fibrous tissue.
- Because of its dark blue or sometimes even black color, the lesion may be confused with nodular melanoma, pigmented BCC, or pyogenic granuloma.
- The lesion can be partially compressed and lightened up by diascopy, and the use of dermoscopy permits its diagnosis as a vascular lesion.
- Management is for cosmetic reasons and can be accomplished with electrosurgery, laser, or, rarely, with surgical excision.

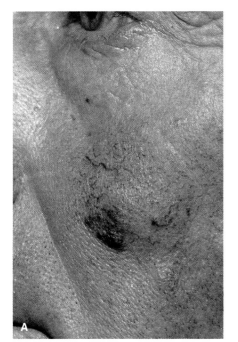 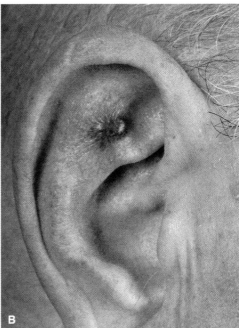

FIGURE 9-22 Venous lake (A) On the cheek of a 70-year-old male. The lesion was almost black and became a matter of concern to the patient, who feared he might have melanoma. However, it blanched completely after compression. **(B)** Venous lake on the auricle of a 75-year-old male. The lesion is dark bluish-red and smooth resembling a basal cell carcinoma. It blanched upon compression.

CHERRY ANGIOMA ICD-10: D18.012

- Cherry angiomas are exceedingly common, asymptomatic, bright red to violaceous or even black, domed vascular lesions (~3 mm) (Fig. 9-23), or occurring as myriads of tiny red papular spots simulating petechiae.
- They are found principally on the trunk. The lesions appear first at about age 30 and increase in number over the years.
- Almost all elderly people have a few lesions.
- The histology consists of numerous moderately dilated capillaries lined by flattened endothelial cells; stroma is edematous with homogenization of collagen.
- They are of no consequence other than their cosmetic appearance. Management is electro- or laser coagulation if indicated cosmetically. Cryosurgery is not effective.
- *Synonyms:* Campbell de Morgan spots, senile (hem)angioma.

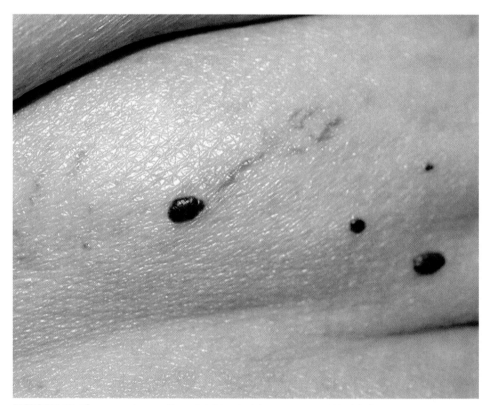

FIGURE 9-23 Cherry angiomas These bright red, violaceous, or even black lesions appear progressively on the trunk with advancing age.

ANGIOKERATOMA ICD-10: code according to type (see text)

- The term *angio* ("blood vessel") *keratoma* would imply a vascular tumor with keratotic elements. But, capillaries and postcapillary venules are packed into the papillary body just beneath and bulging into the epidermis, leading to hyperkeratosis. This and the fact that the lumina are usually at least partially thrombosed impart a firm consistency to the lesions.
- Angiokeratomas are dark violaceous to black, often keratotic papules or small plaques that are hard upon palpation and cannot be compressed by diascopy (Fig. 9-24).
- Angiokeratoma can appear as a solitary lesion (*solitary angiokeratoma*). The most important differential diagnosis is a small nodular or superficial spreading melanoma (Fig. 9-24).
- The most common is *angiokeratoma of Fordyce* [ICD10:D29.420]; this disease involves the scrotum and vulva; the lesions are multiple papules (≤4 mm) that are dark red to black in color and present in quite large numbers (Fig. 9-25).
- *Angiokeratoma of Mibelli* [ICD-10:D23.L74] comprises pink to dark red and even black papules that occur on the elbows, knees, and dorsa of the hands. This autosomal-dominant disease is rare and occurs in young females.
- *Angiokeratoma corporis diffusum (Fabry disease)*[ICD10:E75.250], an X-linked recessive disease, is an inborn error of metabolism in which there is a deficiency of α-galactosidase A leading to an accumulation of neutral glycosphingolipid ceramide trihexoside in endothelial cells, fibrocytes, and pericytes in the dermis, heart, kidneys, and autonomic nervous system. Lesions are numerous dark red, punctate, and tiny (<1 mm) (Fig. 9-26), located on the lower half of the body: lower abdomen, genitalia, and buttocks, although lesions may also occur on the lips. The homozygous males also have symptoms related to involvement of other organ systems: acroparesthesias, excruciating pain, transient ischemic attacks, and myocardial infarction. Heterozygous females may have corneal opacities. Fabry disease is very rare but serious.

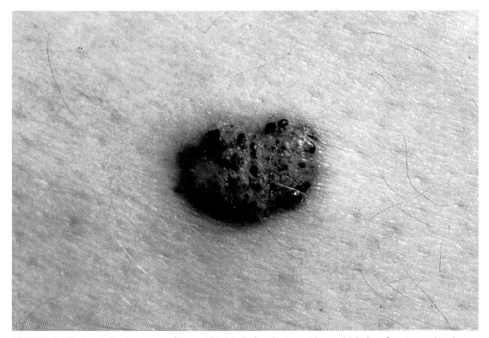

FIGURE 9-24 Angiokeratoma: solitary This black, firm lesion with a pebbled surface immediately sparks the suspicion of superficial spreading melanoma. It is noncompressible, but dermoscopy reveals the typical lacunae of thrombosed vascular spaces. Nonetheless, such lesions should be excised.

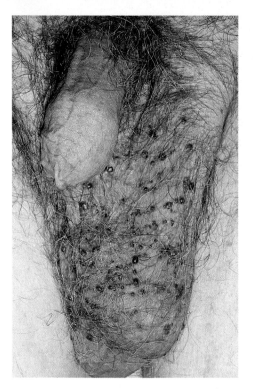

FIGURE 9-25 Angiokeratoma of Fordyce
Reddish, violaceous, and black papules on the scrotum. They blanch upon diascopy and this verifies the diagnosis. *Note*: Thrombosed angiokeratomas do not blanch.

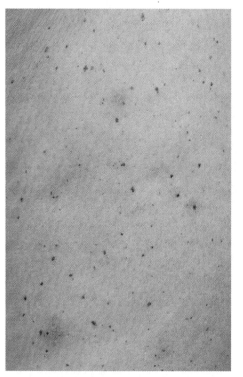

FIGURE 9-26 Angiokeratoma corporis diffusum (Fabry disease) Numerous red, punctate lesions on the lower flank.

LYMPHATIC MALFORMATION

"LYMPHANGIOMA" ICD-10: D18.100O

- The term LYM is now the terminology for what was formerly called "lymphangioma."
- These typical lesions comprise multiple, grouped, small macroscopic vesicles filled with clear or serosanguineous fluid ("frog-spawn") (Fig. 9-27). However, these are not true vesicles but microcystic lesions (lymphangioma) as opposed to a macrocystic lesion (cystic hygroma), which is located deep in the dermis and subcutis, and appears as a large soft subcutaneous tumor often distorting the face or an extremity.
- The microcystic LYM is present at birth or appears in infancy or childhood. It may disappear spontaneously, but this is extremely rare. Bacterial infection may occur.
- LYM may occur as an isolated solitary lesion, as in Figure 9-27, or cover large areas (up to 10 × 20 cm); it may be associated with a capillary venous lymphatic (CVL) malformation.
- The lesion can be excised, if feasible, or treated with sclerotherapy.

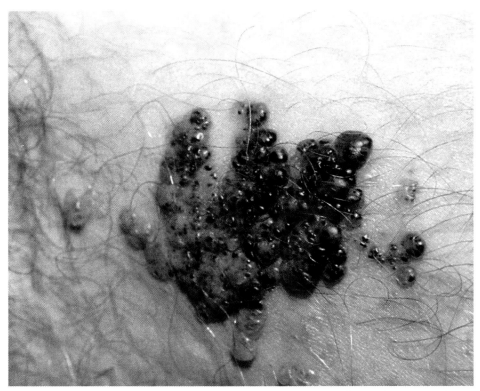

FIGURE 9-27 Lymphatic malformation (lymphangioma) Frog-spawn–like confluent grouped "vesicles" filled with a serosanguineous fluid.

CAPILLARY/VENOUS MALFORMATIONS (CVMs) ICD-10: Q82.9

- CVMs are deep vascular malformations characterized by soft, compressible deep-tissue swelling. Lesions are not apparent at birth but become so during childhood.
- They manifest as soft-tissue swelling, dome-shaped or multinodular (Fig. 9-28), and are slow-flow lesions. When vascular malformation extends to the epidermis, the surface may be verrucous. Borders are poorly defined, and there is considerable variation in size. Often, CVMs are normal skin color, with the nodular portion blue to purple. They are easily compressed and fill promptly when pressure is released. Some types may be tender, and they may be associated with CMs.
- CVMs may be complicated by ulceration and bleeding, scarring, and secondary infection; and, with large lesions, by high-output heart failure.
- CVMs may interfere with food intake or breathing and, if located on the eyelids or in the vicinity of the eyes, will obstruct vision and may lead to blindness.
- There is no satisfactory treatment except compression. In larger lesions—if organ function is compromised—surgical procedures and intravascular coagulation should be performed. High-dose systemic glucocorticoids or IFN-α or propranolol may be effective.

VARIANTS

VASCULAR HAMARTOMAS CVLs with deep soft-tissue involvement and resultant swelling or diffuse enlargement of an extremity. May involve skeletal muscle with muscle atrophy. Cutaneous changes include dilated tortuous veins and arteriovenous fistulas.

KLIPPEL–TRÉNAUNAY SYNDROME A CVM or CVL malformation, slow-flow lesion. Local overgrowth of soft tissue and bone results in enlargement of an extremity. Associated cutaneous changes include phlebectasia, nevus flammeus-like cutaneous CM (Fig. 9-29), lymphatic hypoplasia, and lymphedema.

BLUE RUBBER BLEB NEVUS A CVM, spontaneously painful and/or tender. A compressible, soft, blue swelling in the dermis and subcutaneous tissue. Size ranges from a few millimeters to several centimeters (Fig. 9-30). May exhibit localized hyperhidrosis over CVM malformations and occurs, often multiply, on the trunk and upper arms. Similar vascular lesions can

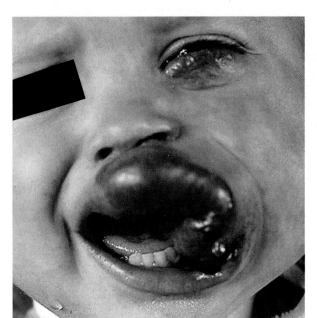

FIGURE 9-28 Capillary–venous malformation In an infant. There is a soft, compressible, and bluish-red tissue swelling distorting the upper lip and lower eyelid. It is a slow-flow lesion but requires therapeutic intervention.

FIGURE 9-29 Capillary–venous malformation In a 31-year-old Thai woman. This nevus flammeus-like lesion was associated with phlebectasia, lymphedema, and an enlarged right lower extremity (Klippel–Trénaunay syndrome).

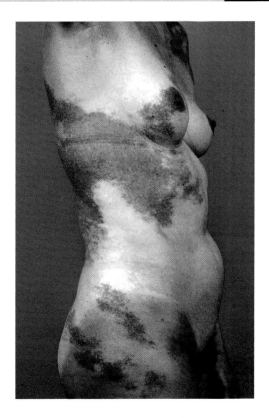

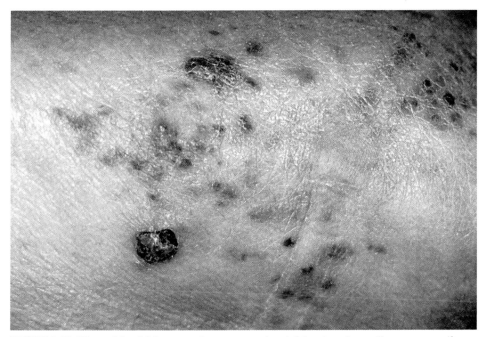

FIGURE 9-30 Blue rubber bleb nevus A spontaneously painful and tender capillary-venous malformation. There are a number of compressible bluish-violaceous papules and nodules on the upper arm.

occur in the gastrointestinal tract and may be a source of hemorrhage.

MAFFUCCI SYNDROME A slow-flow venous or lymphatic/venous malformation associated with enchondromas and manifested as hard nodules on fingers or toes and as bony deformities. Patients may develop chondrosarcoma.

PARKES WEBER SYNDROME A fast-flow capillary arteriovenous malformation (CAVM) or CM, with soft tissue and skeletal hypertrophy.

MISCELLANEOUS CYSTS AND PSEUDOCYSTS

EPIDERMOID CYST ICD-10: L72.010

- An epidermoid cyst is the most common cutaneous cyst, derived from epidermis or the epithelium of the hair follicle, and is formed by cystic enclosure of epithelium within the dermis that becomes filled with keratin and lipid-rich debris.
- It occurs in young to middle-aged adults on the face, neck, upper trunk, and scrotum.
- The lesion, which is usually solitary but may be multiple, is a dermal-to-subcutaneous nodule, 0.5 to 5 cm, which often connects with the surface by keratin-filled pores (Fig. 9-31).
- The cyst has an epidermal-like wall (stratified squamous epithelium with well-formed granular layer); the content of the cyst is keratinaceous material—cream-colored with a pasty consistency and the odor of rancid cheese. Scrotal lesions may calcify.
- The cyst wall is relatively thin. Following rupture of the wall, the cyst contents initiate an inflammatory reaction, enlarging the lesion manifold; the lesion is now associated with a great deal of pain. Ruptured cysts are often misdiagnosed as being infected rather than ruptured.
- *Synonyms*: Wen, sebaceous cyst, infundibular cyst, epidermal cyst.

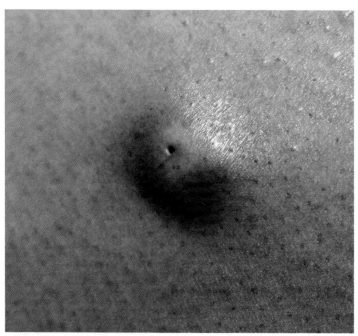

FIGURE 9-31 Epidermoid cyst A rounded nodule within the dermis with an opening (which is not always visible) in which caseous keratinous material can be expressed.

TRICHILEMMAL CYST ICD-10: L72.100

- A trichilemmal cyst is the second most common type of cutaneous cyst and is seen most often in middle age, more frequently in females. It is often familial and occurs frequently as multiple lesions.
- These are smooth, firm, dome-shaped, 0.5- to 5-cm nodules or tumors; they lack the central punctum seen in epidermoid cysts. They are not connected to the epidermis.
- More than 90% occur on the scalp, and the overlying scalp hair is usually normal but may be thinned if the cyst is large (Fig. 9-32).
- The cyst wall is usually thick, and the cyst can be removed intact. The wall is a stratified squamous epithelium with a palisaded outer layer resembling that of the outer root sheath of hair follicles. The inner layer is corrugated without a granular layer.
- The cyst contains keratin—very dense, homogeneous; it is often calcified, with cholesterol clefts. If cyst ruptures, it may be inflamed and very painful.
- *Synonyms*: Pilar cyst, isthmus catagen cyst. *Archaic* terms: Wen, sebaceous cyst.

EPIDERMAL INCLUSION CYST ICD-10: L72.810

- An epidermal inclusion cyst occurs secondary to traumatic implantation of epidermis into the dermis. Traumatically grafted epidermis grows in the dermis, with accumulation of keratin within the cyst cavity, enclosed in a stratified squamous epithelium with a well-formed granular layer.
- The lesion appears as a dermal nodule (Fig. 9-33) and most commonly occurs on the palms, soles, and fingers.
- It should be excised.
- *Synonym*: Traumatic epidermoid cyst.

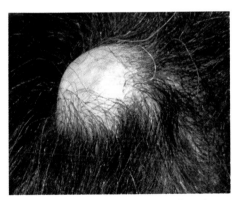

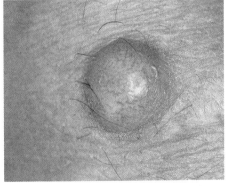

FIGURE 9-32 Trichilemmal cyst A firm, dome-shaped nodule on the scalp. Pressure by the cyst has caused atrophy of hair bulbs, and it thus appears without hairs.

FIGURE 9-33 Epidermal inclusion cyst A small dermal nodule on the knee at the site of the laceration.

MILIUM ICD-10: L72.830

- A milium is a 1- to 2-mm, superficial, white to yellow, keratin-containing epidermal cyst, occurring multiply, located on the eyelids, cheeks, and forehead in pilosebaceous follicles (Figs. 9-34A and B).
- The lesions can occur at any age, even in infants.
- Milia arise either de novo, especially around the eye, or in association with various dermatoses with subepidermal bullae or vesicles (pemphigoid, porphyria cutanea tarda, bullous lichen planus, and epidermolysis bullosa) (Fig. 9-34C) and skin trauma (abrasion, burns, dermabrasion, and radiation therapy).
- Incision and expression of contents are the method of treatment.

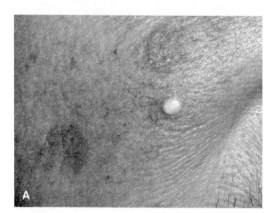

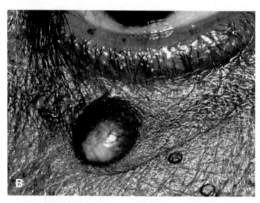

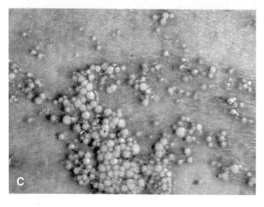

FIGURE 9-34 Milia (A) A small chalk-white or yellowish papule on the cheek; it can be slit with a scalpel, releasing a little ball of horny material. **(B)**. A larger lesion on the lower lid of an African woman. **(C)** Multiple milia on the trunk of a child with hereditary dystrophic epidermolysis bullosa (see Section 6).

DIGITAL MYXOID CYST ICD-10: M25.8

- A digital myxoid cyst is a pseudocyst occurring over the distal interphalangeal joint and the base of the nail of the finger (**Fig. 9-35A**) or toe, often associated with Heberden's (osteophytic) node.
- The lesion occurs in older patients, usually >60 years of age.
- It is usually a solitary cyst, rubbery, translucent. A clear gelatinous viscous fluid may be expressed (**Fig. 9-35B**).
- When the myxoid cyst is over the nail matrix, a nail plate dystrophy occurs in the form of a 1- to 2-mm groove that extends to the length of the nail (**Fig. 9-35A**).
- Various methods of management have been advocated, including surgical excision, incision and drainage, injection of sclerosing material, and injection of a triamcinolone suspension. A simple and most effective method is to make a small incision, express the gelatinous contents, and use a firm compression bandage over the lesion over a period of weeks.
- *Synonyms*: Mucous cyst, synovial cyst, myxoid pseudocyst.

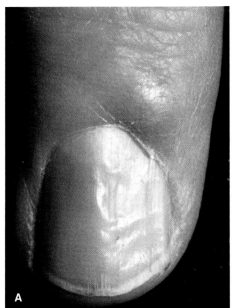 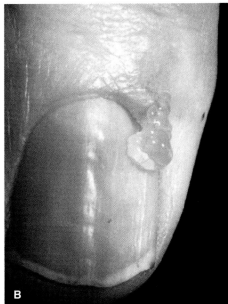

FIGURE 9-35 Digital myxoid cyst (A) The cyst has led to a 3- to 4-mm groove of the nail plate.
(B) Slitting it with a scalpel and pressure releases a gelatinous viscous fluid.

MISCELLANEOUS BENIGN NEOPLASMS AND HYPERPLASIAS

SEBORRHEIC KERATOSIS ICD-10: L82

- The seborrheic keratosis is the most common of the benign epithelial tumors.
- These lesions, which are hereditary, do not appear until age 30 and continue to occur over a lifetime, varying in extent from a few scattered lesions to literally hundreds in some very elderly patients.
- Lesions range from small, barely elevated papules to plaques with a warty surface and a "stuck on" appearance.
- Lesions are benign and do not require treatment except for cosmetic reasons. They can become irritated or traumatized, with pain and bleeding. SCC and melanoma should be ruled out.
- *Synonym*: verruca seborrhoica.

EPIDEMIOLOGY

ONSET Rarely before 30 years.
SEX Slightly more common and more extensive involvement in males.

CLINICAL MANIFESTATION

Evolve over months to years. Rarely pruritic; tender if secondarily infected.
SKIN LESIONS Early. Small, 1- to 3-mm, barely elevated papule, later a larger plaque (Figs. 9-36 and 9-37) with or without pigment. The surface has a greasy feel and often shows, with a hand lens, fine stippling like the surface of a thimble.
Late. Plaque with warty surface and "stuck on" appearance (Fig. 9-38), "greasy." With a hand lens, horn cysts can often be seen; with dermoscopy they can always be seen and are diagnostic. Size from 1 to 6 cm. Flat nodule. Brown, gray, black, skin-colored, round, or oval (Figs. 9-37 and 9-38A, B).
Distribution. Isolated lesion or generalized. Face, trunk (Fig. 9-39), upper extremities. In females, commonly occur in submammary intertriginous skin. In darker-skinned people, multiple, small black lesions in the face are called *dermatosis papulosa nigra* (Fig. 9-37). When numerous and dense, SKs may become confluent.

LABORATORY EXAMINATION

DERMATOPATHOLOGY Proliferation of mono-morphous keratinocytes (with marked papil-lomatosis) and melanocytes, and formation of horn cysts.

DIAGNOSIS AND DIFFERENTIAL DIAGNOSIS

Clinically, the diagnosis is made easily.
"TAN MACULES" Early "flat" lesions may be confused with solar lentigo or spreading pig-mented actinic keratosis (see Figs. 10-22 and 11-13).
SKIN-COLORED/TAN/BLACK VERRUCOUS PAPULES/ PLAQUES Larger pigmented lesions are easily mistaken for pigmented BCC or malignant melanoma (Fig. 9-38) (only biopsy will settle this, or dermoscopy will be of assistance); ver-ruca vulgaris may be similar in clinical appear-ance, but thrombosed capillaries are present in verrucae.

COURSE AND PROGNOSIS

Lesions develop with increasing age; they are benign and do not become malignant.

MANAGEMENT

Light electrocautery permits the whole lesion to be easily rubbed off. However, this precludes histopathologic verification of diagnosis and should be done only by an experienced diag-nostician. Cryosurgery with liquid nitrogen spray works only in flat lesions, and recur-rences are possibly more frequent. The best approach is curettage after slight freezing with cryospray, which also permits histopathologic examination.

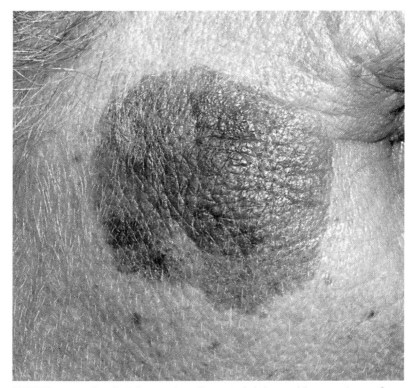

FIGURE 9-36 Seborrheic keratosis, solitary A slightly raised, keratotic, brown, flat plaque on the zygomatic region in an older female. The differential diagnosis includes lentigo maligna and lentigo maligna melanoma.

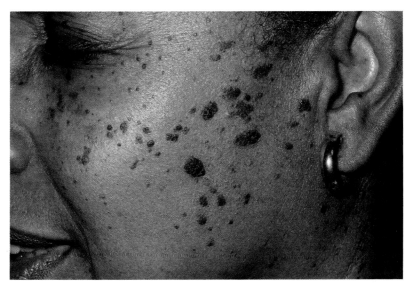

FIGURE 9-37 Seborrheic keratoses (dermatosis papulosa nigra) This consists of a myriad of tiny black lesions, some enlarging to more than a centimeter. This is seen in Black Africans, African Americans, and deeply pigmented South East Asians.

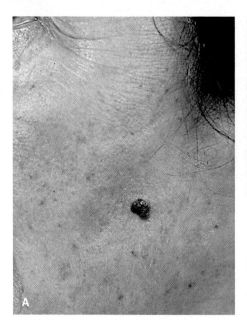
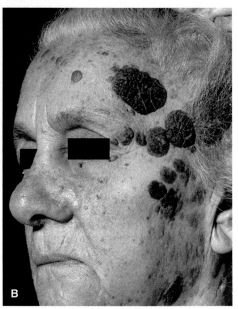

FIGURE 9-38 Seborrheic keratosis (A) Small, heavily pigmented seborrheic keratoses can have a smooth surface and present a differential diagnostic challenge: pigmented basal cell carcinoma and nodular melanoma have to be excluded. **(B)** Large seborrheic keratoses have a "stuck on" appearance and can be very dark and irregular. Because of their multiplicity, they usually do not present a diagnostic problem. As shown here, they can be disfiguring.

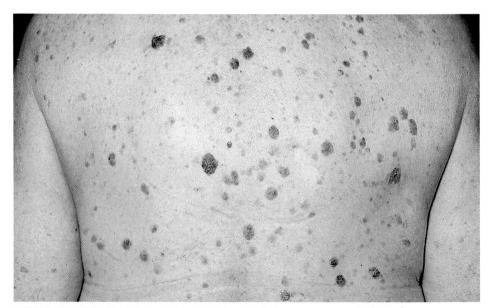

FIGURE 9-39 Seborrheic keratoses, multiple Multiple brown, warty papules and nodules on the back, having a "greasy" feel and "stuck on" appearance. This picture also shows the evolution of the lesions: from small only slightly tan, very thin papules, or plaques to larger, darker nodular lesions with a verrucous surface. Practically all lesions on the back of this elderly patient are seborrheic keratoses; what they have in common is that they give the impression that they could be scraped off easily, which, in fact, they can.

BECKER NEVUS (BN) ICD-10: D22,502

- BN is a distinctive asymptomatic clinical lesion that is a pigmented hamartoma, i.e., a developmental anomaly consisting of changes in pigmentation, hair growth, and a slightly elevated smooth verrucous surface (Fig. 9-40).
- It occurs mostly in males and in all races. It appears not at birth but usually before 15 years of age, although sometimes after this age.
- The lesion is predominantly a macule but with a papular verrucous surface not unlike the lesion of acanthosis nigricans. It is light brown in color and has a geographic pattern with sharply demarcated borders (Fig. 9-40A).
- Commonest locations are the shoulders and the back. The increased hair growth follows the onset of the pigmentation and is localized to the areas that are pigmented (Fig. 9-40B). The pigmentation is related to increased melanin in basal cells and not to an increased number of melanocytes.
- It is differentiated from a hairy congenital melanocytic nevus, because BN is not usually present at birth, and from café au lait macules because these are not hairy.
- The lesion extends for a year or two and then remains stable, only rarely fading.
- There is very rarely hypoplasia of underlying structures, e.g., shortening of the arm or reduced breast development in areas under the lesion.
- Management: The hypertrichosis can be of cosmetic concern to some individuals.

FIGURE 9-40 A and B Becker nevus (A) A slightly raised light-tan plaque with sharply defined and highly irregular border and slight hypertrichosis on the chest of a 16-year-old male patient. **(B)** In this case of Becker nevus, the massive hypertrichosis conceals the tan background plaque.

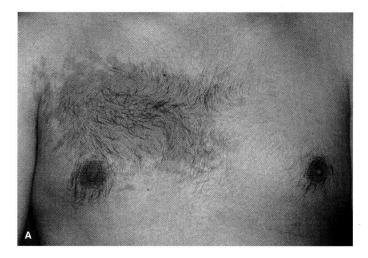

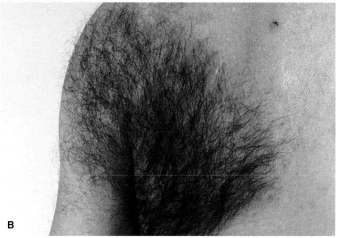

TRICHOEPITHELIOMA ICD-10: D23.L13

- Trichoepitheliomas are benign appendage tumors with hair bulb differentiation.
- The lesions, which appear at puberty, occur on the face (Fig. 9-41) and less often on the scalp, neck, and upper trunk.
- Lesions may be only a few small pink or skin-colored papules. They gradually increase in number and can be confused with BCC (Fig. 9-41A).
- Trichoepitheliomas can also appear as solitary tumors, which may be nodular (Fig. 9-41B), or appear as ill-defined plaques like sclerosing BCC.
- Treatment: Eelectrocautery or excision.

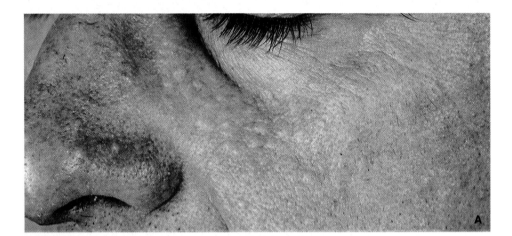

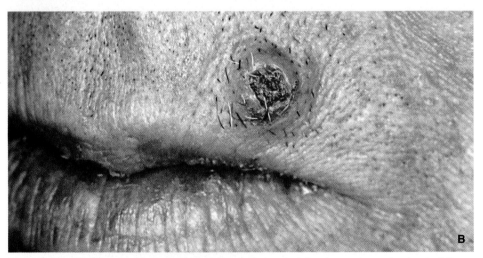

FIGURE 9-41 Trichoepitheliomas (A) Multiple, small, sharply defined smooth papules that look like early BCCs. **(B)** Trichoepithelioma, solitary type. A nodular tumor on the upper lip that can be confused with a basal carcinoma or squamous cell carcinoma.

SYRINGOMA ICD-10: D23.L41

- Syringomas are benign adenomas of the eccrine ducts. They are 1- to 2-mm, skin-colored or yellow, firm papules that occur mostly in women, beginning at puberty; they may be familial.
- Most often multiple rather than solitary, they occur most frequently on the lower periorbital area, usually symmetrically but also on the eyelids (Fig. 9-42), face, axillae, umbilicus, upper chest, and vulva.
- The lesions have a specific histologic pattern: many small ducts in the dermis with comma-like tails with the appearance of "tadpoles."
- The lesions can be disfiguring, and most patients want them removed; this can be done easily with electrosurgery.

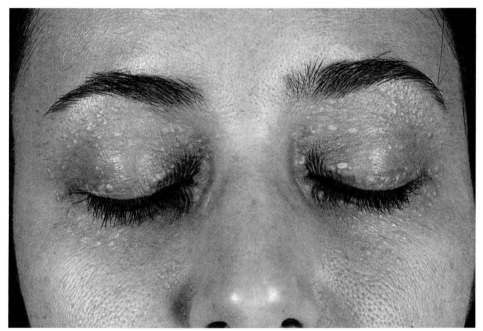

FIGURE 9-42 Syringomas Symmetric eruption of 1- to 2-mm skin-colored, smooth papules on the upper and lower eyelids.

CYLINDROMA ICD-10: 23.L33

- Rare appendage tumor of apocrine, or as some believe, eccrine glands.
- Two forms: Ssolitary or multiple. The latter often familial and inherited as an autosomal dominant trait. Often in the setting of Brooke–Spiegler syndrome, in association with trichoepitheliomas and other hamartomas and basal cell carcinomas.
- Reddish papule or nodule on the scalp. In the multiple phenotype, often densely aggregated "turban" tumors) (Fig. 9-43), also on face and trunk.
- Extremely rarely may turn malignant.
- Therapy: Surgical excision.

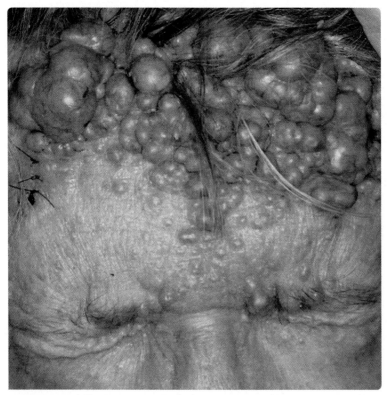

FIGURE 9-43 Cylindroma Cylindromas (turban tumors), familial variant. Closely set papules and nodules of skin to reddish color. (Reproduced, with permission, from Goldsmith LA, Katz SI, Gilchrest BA, et al. *Fitzpatrick's Dermatology in General Medicine.* 8th ed. New York, NY: McGraw-Hill Education, 2012. Figure 119-6A.)

SEBACEOUS HYPERPLASIA ICD-10: D23.L16

- These are very common lesions in older persons and are confused with small BCCs. Also occurs in solid organ transplant recipients treated with cyclosporine. The lesions are 1 to 3 mm in diameter and have both telangiectasia and central umbilication (Fig. 9-44).
- Two features distinguish sebaceous hyperplasia from nodular BCC: (1) Sebaceous hyperplasia is soft to palpation, not firm as in nodular BCC; and (2) with firm lateral compression, it is often possible to elicit a very small globule of sebum in the valley of the umbilicated portion of the lesion.
- Sebaceous hyperplasias can be destroyed with light electrocautery.

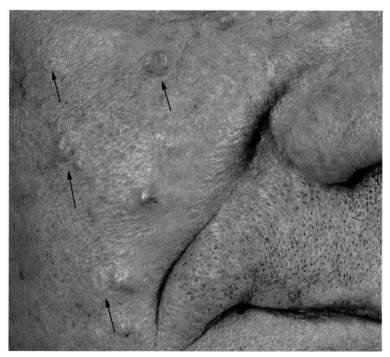

FIGURE 9-44 Sebaceous hyperplasia 1- to 4-mm smooth papules on the cheek of a 65-year-old man. They look like small basal cell carcinomas but have a central umbilication (*arrows*).

NEVUS SEBACEOUS ICD-10: Q82.570

- This congenital malformation of sebaceous differentiation occurs on the scalp or rarely on the face (Fig. 9-45).
- A hairless, thin, elevated, 1- to 2-cm plaque, sometimes larger, with a characteristic orange color and a pebbly or warty surface.
- About 10% of patients can be expected to develop BCC in the lesion.
- Excision is recommended at around puberty for cosmetic reasons and to prevent the occurrence of BCC.
- *Synonym*: Organoid nevus.

EPIDERMAL NEVUS ICD-10: D23.L86

- A developmental (hamartomatous) disorder characterized by hyperplasia of epidermal structures (epidermis and adnexa). There are no melanocytic nevus cells.
- Usually present at birth or occurs in infancy; rarely, it develops in puberty. All epidermal nevi on the head/neck region are present at birth.
- Several variants: The *verrucous epidermal nevus* may be localized or multiple. Lesions are skin-colored, brown, or grayish-brown (**Fig. 9-46**) and are composed of closely set verrucous papules, well circumscribed; they are often in a linear arrangement—especially on the leg—or they may appear in Blaschko lines on the trunk. Excision is the best treatment, if feasible.
- When the lesions are extensive, they are termed *systematized epidermal nevus*, and when they are located on half the body, they are termed *nevus unius lateris*.
- Linear lesions can exhibit erythema, scaling, and crusting, and are then called *inflammatory linear verrucous epidermal nevus* (ILVEN). The lesions gradually enlarge and become stable in adolescence.
- There is also a *noninflammatory linear verrucous epidermal nevus* (NILVEN).
- Extensive epidermal nevi (*epidermal nevus syndrome*) may be multisystem disorders and may be associated with developmental abnormalities (bone cysts, hyperplasia of bone, scoliosis, spina bifida, and kyphosis), vitamin D-resistant rickets, and neurologic problems (mental retardation, seizures, cortical atrophy, and hydrocephalus). These patients require a complete examination, including the eyes (cataracts, optic nerve hypoplasia), and cardiac studies to rule out aneurysms or patent ductus arteriosus.

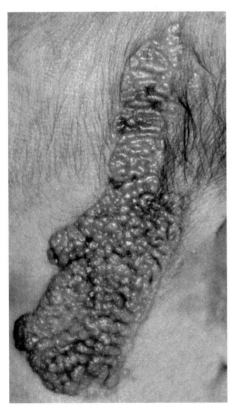

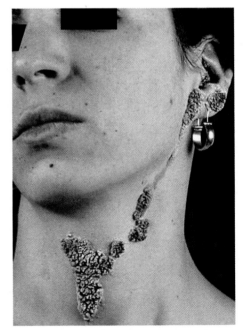

FIGURE 9-45 Nevus sebaceous In a baby an elevated plaque of orange color and pebbly surface in the preauricular region. Note that the lesion is hairless on the scalp.

FIGURE 9-46 Epidermal nevus A grayish irregular plaque with a verrucous surface on the ear extending linearly down to the neck.

BENIGN DERMAL AND SUBCUTANEOUS NEOPLASMS AND HYPERPLASIAS

LIPOMA   ICD-10: D17.910

- Lipomas are single or multiple, benign subcutaneous tumors that are easily recognized because they are soft, rounded, or lobulated and movable against the overlying skin (**Fig. 9-47**).
- Many lipomas are small but may also enlarge to >6 cm.
- They occur mostly on the neck, trunk, and on the extremities (**Fig. 9-47**) but can occur anywhere on the body.
- Lipomas are composed of fat cells that have the same morphology as normal fat cells within a connective tissue framework. Angiolipomas have a vascular component and may be tender in cold ambient temperature and with compression.
- Angiolipomas often require excision, whereas other lipomas should be excised only when considered disfiguring. Liposuction can also be performed when liposomas are soft and thus have only a minor connective tissue component.
- *Familial lipoma syndrome*, an autosomal-dominant trait appearing in early adulthood, consists of hundreds of slowly growing nontender lesions.
- *Adipositas dolorosa*, or *Dercum disease*, occurs in women in middle age; there are multiple tender, not circumscribed but rather diffuse fatty deposits.
- *Benign symmetric lipomatosis*, which affects middle-aged men, consists of many large nontender, coalescent poorly circumscribed lipomas, mostly on the trunk and upper extremities; they coalesce on the neck and may lead to a "horse-collar" appearance.

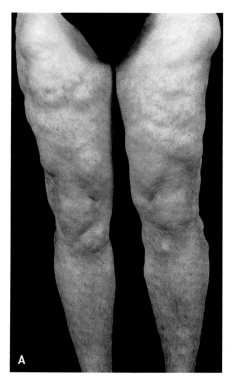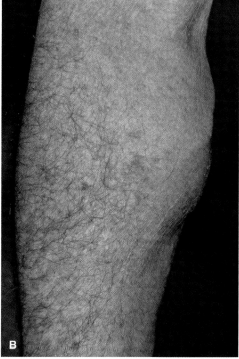

FIGURE 9-47 Lipoma (A) Well-defined, soft, rounded tumors in the subcutis, movable both against the overlying skin and the underlying structures, in a 56-year-old male patient. In this patient, lesions were symmetric and were also found on the trunk and upper extremities. **(B)** Solitary lipoma on the lower arm of a 50-year-old patient.

DERMATOFIBROMA ICD-10: D23-L62

- A dermatofibroma is a very common, button-like dermal nodule, usually occurring on the extremities.
- Important only because of its cosmetic appearance or its being mistaken for other lesions, such as malignant melanoma when it is pigmented.
- Considered to represent late histiocytic reaction to an arthropod bite.
- Asymptomatic nodule (Fig. 9-48), 3 to 10 mm in diameter, domed but also sometimes depressed below surrounding skin. Surface dull, shiny or scaly. Firm, color viarable—skin-colored, pink (Fig. 9-48A), brown or dark chocolate brown (Fig. 9-48B); borders ill defined. Dimple sign: lateral compression produces a "dimple" (Fig. 9-48C).
- Rarely may be tender.
- Appears gradually over several months and persists without further increase in size for years but may regress spontaneously.
- Treatment not necessary. Excision produces scar, cryosurgery with cotton tip applicator usually has to be repeated and produces a cosmetically more acceptable scar.
- *Synonyms*: Solitary histiocytoma, sclerosing hemangioma.

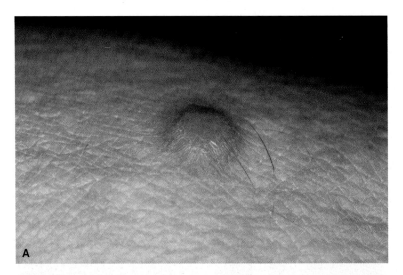

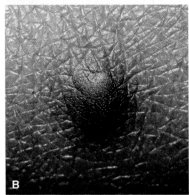
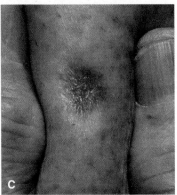

FIGURE 9-48 Dermatofibroma (A) A dome-shaped, slightly erythematous and tan nodule with a button-like, firm consistency. **(B)** This lesion is pigmented. Can be confused with blue nevus or even nodular melanoma. The pigment is melanin and hemosiderin. **(C)** "Dimple sign." Dimpling of the lesion is seen when pinched between two fingers.

HYPERTROPHIC SCARS AND KELOIDS ICD-10: L91.00

- Hypertrophic scars and keloids are exuberant fibrous repair tissues after a cutaneous injury.
- A *hypertrophic scar* remains confined to the site of original injury.
- A *keloid*, however, extends beyond this site, often with claw-like extensions.
- May be cosmetically very unsightly and pose a serious problem for the patient if the lesion is large and on the ear or face or over a joint.

EPIDEMIOLOGY AND ETIOLOGY

AGE OF ONSET Third decade, but all ages.
SEX Equal incidence in males and females.
RACE Much more common in blacks and in persons with blood group A.
ETIOLOGY Unknown. They usually follow injury to skin, i.e., surgical scar, laceration, abrasion, cryosurgery, and electrocoagulation as well as vaccination, acne, etc. *Keloid may also arise spontaneously, without history of injury, usually in presternal site.*

CLINICAL MANIFESTATION

SKIN SYMPTOMS Usually asymptomatic. May be pruritic or painful if touched.
SKIN LESIONS Papules to nodules (Fig. 9-49) to large tuberous lesions. Most often, the color of the normal skin but also bright red or bluish. May be linear after traumatic or surgical injury (Fig. 9-49A) oval or round (Fig. 9-49B). Hypertrophic scars tend to be elevated and are confined to approximately the site of the original injury (Fig. 9-49). Keloids, however, may be nodular (Fig. 9-50) or extend in a claw-like fashion far beyond the original injury (Fig. 9-51A). Firm to hard; may be tender, surface smooth. Spontaneous keloids arise de novo without trauma or surgery, and usually occur on the chest (Fig. 9-51B).
Distribution. Earlobes, shoulders, upper back, chest.

LABORATORY EXAMINATION

DERMATOPATHOLOGY Hypertrophic Scar.
Whorls of young fibrous tissue and fibroblasts in haphazard arrangement.
Keloid. Features of hypertrophic scar with added feature of thick, eosinophilic, acellular bands of collagen.

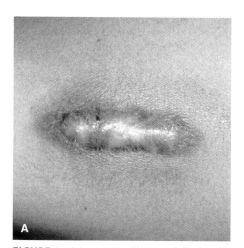
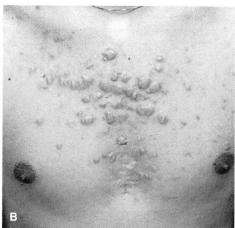

FIGURE 9-49 Hypertrophic scar (A) A broad, raised scar developing at the site of surgical incision with telangiectatic blood vessels and a shiny atrophic epidermis. **(B)** Multiple hypertrophic scars on the chest of a 22-year-old male with a history of severe cystic acne.

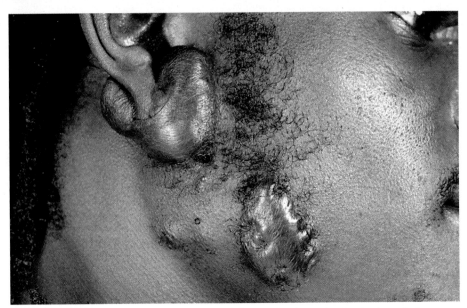

FIGURE 9-50 Keloids Well-defined irregular nodules, very hard on palpation, in the auricular region, and cheek of a 30-year-old man. The lesions on the earlobe arose after piercing and the lesion on the mandibular region after incision of an inflamed cyst.

DIAGNOSIS AND DIFFERENTIAL DIAGNOSIS

Clinical diagnosis; biopsy not warranted unless there is clinical doubt, because this may induce new hypertrophic scarring. Differential diagnosis includes dermatofibroma, dermatofibrosarcoma protuberans, desmoid tumor, scar with sarcoidosis, and foreign-body granuloma.

COURSE AND PROGNOSIS

Hypertrophic scars tend to regress, in time becoming flatter and softer. Keloids, however, may continue to expand in size for decades.

MANAGEMENT

This is a real challenge, as no treatment is highly effective.

INTRALESIONAL GLUCOCORTICOIDS Intralesional injection of triamcinolone (10 to 20 mg/mL) every month may reduce pruritus or sensitivity of lesion, as well as reduce its volume and flatten it. Works quite well in small hypertrophic scars but less well in keloids.

SURGICAL EXCISION Lesions that are excised surgically often recur larger than the original lesion. Excision with immediate postsurgical radiotherapy is beneficial.

SILICONE CREAM AND SILICONE GEL SHEET Reported to be beneficial in keloids and is painless and noninvasive. Not very effective in authors' experience.

PREVENTION Individuals prone to hypertrophic scars or keloids should be advised to avoid cosmetic procedures such as ear piercing. Scars from burns tend to become hypertrophic. Can be prevented by compression garments.

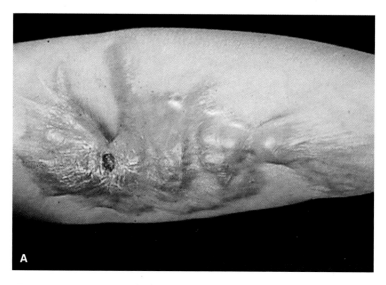

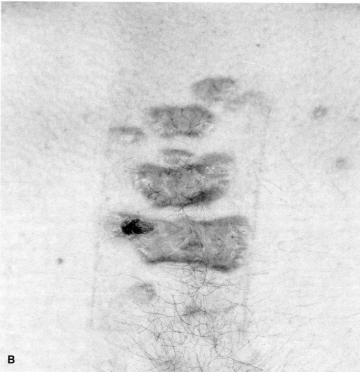

FIGURE 9-51 Keloids (A) Keloid after a deep burn. Note sausage- and clawlike extensions of the keloid into normal skin. **(B)** Spontaneous keloids that arose without apparent cause on the chest of a 19-year-old man.

INFANTILE DIGITAL FIBROMATOSIS ICD-10: M72.850

- A rare form of superficial juvenile fibromatosis.
- Presenting as asymptomatic flesh-colored or pink firm nodule on the fingers and toes (Fig. 9-52).
- Appears in the first year of life, less commonly in childhood.
- Histologically interlacing bundles of myofibroblasts with eosinophilic inclusions.
- Benign. Spontaneous regression is rare. Treatment is surgical
- *Synonym*: Rye tumor.

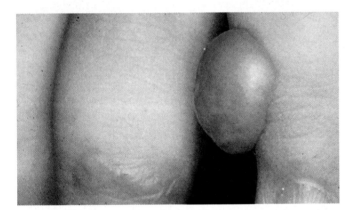

FIGURE 9-52 Infantile digital fibromatosis A well-defined pink nodule on the finger of an infant. Usually the third to fifth digits are affected. Here, the tumor is found on the second digit.

SKIN TAG ICD-10: L91.8

- A skin tag is a very common, soft, skin-colored or tan or brown, round or oval, pedunculated papilloma (polyp) (Fig. 9-53); it is usually constricted at the base and may vary in size from >1 mm to as large as 10 mm. Occurring in the middle aged and elderly.
- Histologic findings include a thinned epidermis and a loose fibrous tissue stroma.
- Usually asymptomatic but occasionally may become tender following trauma or torsion and may become crusted or hemorrhagic.
- More common in females and in obese patients and most often noted in intertriginous areas (axillae, inframammary, groin) and on the neck and eyelids.
- It occurs in acanthosis nigricans and metabolic syndrome.
- May be confused with a pedunculated seborrheic keratosis, dermal or compound melanocytic nevus, solitary neurofibroma, or molluscum contagiosum.
- Lesions tend to become larger and more numerous over time, especially during pregnancy. Following spontaneous torsion, autoamputation can occur.
- Management is accomplished with simple snipping with scissors, electrodesiccation, or cryosurgery.
- *Synonyms*: Acrochordon, cutaneous papilloma, soft fibroma.

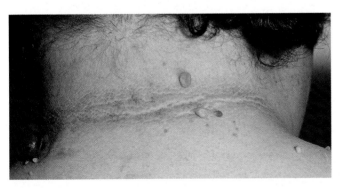

FIGURE 9-53 Skin tags Soft skin-colored and tan pedunculated papillomas. These are very common in the elderly obese and are obligatory lesions in acanthosis nigricans, as in this patient.

PHOTOSENSITIVITY, PHOTO-INDUCED DISORDERS, AND DISORDERS BY IONIZING RADIATION

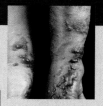

SKIN REACTIONS TO SUNLIGHT ICD-10: L56.8

The term *photosensitivity* describes an abnormal response to sunlight. Cutaneous photosensitivity reactions require absorption of photon energy by molecules in the skin. Energy is either dispersed harmlessly or elicits chemical reactions that lead to clinical disease. Absorbing molecules can be: (1) exogenous agents applied topically or systemically, (2) endogenous molecules either usually present in skin or produced by an abnormal metabolism, or (3) a combination of exogenous and endogenous molecules that acquire antigenic properties and thus elicit a photoradiation-driven immune reaction. *Photosensitivity disorders occur only in body regions exposed to solar radiation* (Fig. 10-1).
Three types of acute photosensitivity:

1. A *sunburn*-type response with skin changes simulating a normal sunburn such as in phototoxic reactions to drugs or phytophotodermatitis (PPD).
2. A *rash* response with macules, papules, or plaques, as in eczematous dermatitis. These are usually photoallergic in nature.
3. *Urticarial* responses are typical for solar urticaria; but urticarial lesions can also occur in erythropoietic porphyria.

Chronic photosensitivity: Chronic repeated sun exposures over time result in polymorphic skin changes that have been termed *dermatoheliosis* (DHe) or photoaging. A classification of skin reactions to sunlight is shown in Table 10-1.

BASICS OF CLINICAL PHOTOMEDICINE

The main culprit of solar radiation-induced skin pathology is the ultraviolet (UV) portion of the solar spectrum. Ultraviolet radiation (UVR) is divided into two principal types: UVB (290 to 320 nm), the "sunburn spectrum," and UVA (320 to 400 nm) that is subdivided into UVA-1 (340 to 400 nm) and UVA-2 (320 to 340 nm). The unit of measurement of sunburn is the *minimum erythema dose* (MED), which is the minimum UV exposure that produces an erythema 24 h after a single exposure. UVB erythema develops in 6 to 24 h and fades within 72 to 120 h. UVA erythema develops in 4 to 16 h and fades within 48 to 120 h.

VARIATIONS IN SUN REACTIVITY IN NORMAL PERSONS: FITZPATRICK SKIN PHOTOTYPES

(Table 10-2) Sunburn is seen most frequently in individuals who have pale white or white skin and a limited capacity to develop inducible, melanin pigmentation (tanning) after exposure to UVR. Basic skin color is divided into white, brown, and black. Not all persons with light skin, such as Caucasians, have the same capacity to develop tanning, and this fact is the principal basis for the classification of "white" persons into four *skin phototypes* (SPT). The SPT is based on the basic skin color and on a *person's own estimate* of sunburning and tanning (Table 10-2).

SPT I persons usually have pale white skin color, blond or red hair, and blue eyes. In fact,

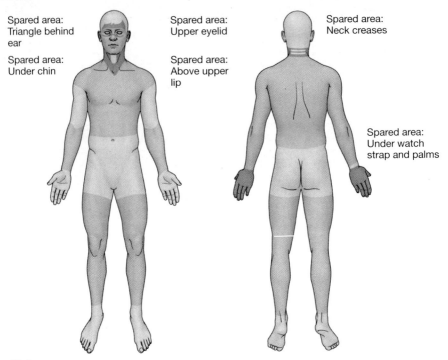

Spared area:
Triangle behind
ear

Spared area:
Under chin

Spared area:
Upper eyelid

Spared area:
Above upper
lip

Spared area:
Neck creases

Spared area:
Under watch
strap and palms

Male

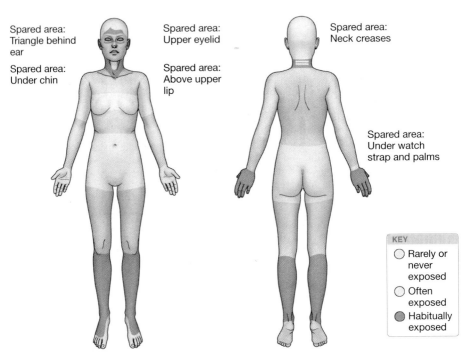

Spared area:
Triangle behind
ear

Spared area:
Under chin

Spared area:
Upper eyelid

Spared area:
Above upper
lip

Spared area:
Neck creases

Spared area:
Under watch
strap and palms

KEY

◯ Rarely or
never
exposed

◯ Often
exposed

⬤ Habitually
exposed

Female

FIGURE 10-1 Variations in solar exposure on different body areas.

TABLE 10-1 Simplified Classification of Skin Reactions to Sunlight

Phototoxicity
  Sunburn
  Drug/chemical induced
  Plant induced (phytophotodermatitis)

Photoallergy
  Drug/chemical induced
  Chronic actinic dermatitis
  Solar urticaria

Idiopathic
  Polymorphous light eruption
  Actinic prurigo[a]
  Hydroa vacciniforme[a]

Metabolic and nutritional
  Porphyria cutanea tarda
  Variegate porphyria
  Erythropoietic protoporphyria
  Pellagra

DNA-deficient photodermatoses
  Xeroderma pigmentosum[a]
  Other rare syndromes[a]

Photo-exacerbated dermatoses

Chronic photodamage
  Dermatoheliosis (photoaging)
  Solar lentigo
  Actinic keratoses
  Skin cancer[b]

[a]Conditions not dealt with here. The reader is referred to Goldsmith LA, Katz SI, Gilchrest BA, et al (eds). *Fitzpatrick's Dermatology in General Medicine*. 8th ed. New York, NY: McGraw-Hill; 2012.
[b]For coverage of skin cancer, see Sections 11 and 12.

TABLE 10-2 Classification of Fitzpatrick's Skin Phototypes (SPT)

SPT	Basic Skin Color	Response to Sun Exposure
I	Pale white	Burn easily, do not tan
II	White	Burn easily, tan with difficulty
III	White	May burn initially but tan easily
IV	Light brown/ olive	Hardly burn, tan easily
V	Brown	Usually do not burn, tan easily
VI	Black	Do not burn, become darker

they can also have dark brown hair and brown eyes. SPT I persons sunburn easily with short exposures and do not tan. SPT II persons sunburn easily but *tan with difficulty*, whereas SPT III persons may have some sunburn with short exposures but can develop marked tanning. SPT IV persons tan with ease and do not sunburn with short exposures. Persons with constitutive brown skin are termed SPT V and with black skin SPT VI. Note that sunburn depends on the amount of UVR energy absorbed. Thus, with excessive sun exposure, even a SPT VI person can have sunburn.

ACUTE SUN DAMAGE (SUNBURN) ICD-10: L55

- Sunburn is an acute, delayed, and transient inflammatory response of normal skin after exposure to UVR from sunlight or artificial sources.
- By nature, it is a phototoxic reaction.
- Sunburn is characterized by erythema (Fig. 10-2) and, if severe, by vesicles and bullae, edema, tenderness, and pain.

EPIDEMIOLOGY

Sunburn depends on the amount of UVR energy delivered and the susceptibility of the individual (SPT). It will therefore occur more often around midday, with decreasing latitude, increasing altitude, and decreasing SPT. Thus, the "ideal" setting for a sunburn to occur would be an SPT I individual (highest susceptibility) on Mount Kenya (high altitude, close to the equator) at noon (UVR is highest). Of course, sunburn can occur at any latitude, but the probability for it to occur decreases with increasing distance from the equator.

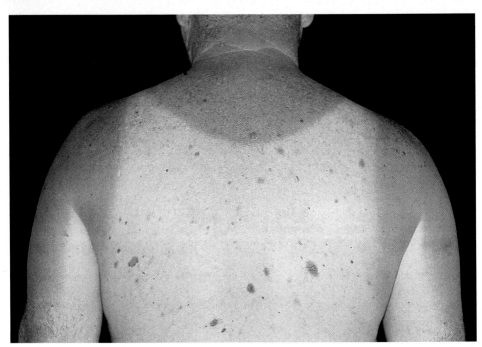

FIGURE 10-2 Acute sunburn Painful, tender, bright erythema with mild edema of the upper back with sharp demarcation between the sun-exposed and sun-protected white areas.

PATHOGENESIS

Molecules that absorb UVR for UVB sunburn erythema are not known, but damage to DNA may be the initiating event. The mediators that cause the erythema include histamine for both UVA and UVB. In UVB erythema, other mediators include TNF-α, serotonin, prostaglandins, nitric oxide, lysosomal enzymes, and kinins. TNF-α can be detected as early as 1 h after exposure.

CLINICAL MANIFESTATION

SKIN SYMPTOMS Onset depends on intensity of exposure. Pruritus may be severe even in mild sunburn; pain and tenderness occur with severe sunburn.

CONSTITUTIONAL SYMPTOMS Some SPT I and II persons develop headache and malaise even after short exposures. In severe sunburn, the patient is "toxic"—with fever, weakness, lassitude, and a rapid pulse rate.

SKIN LESIONS Confluent bright erythema always confined to sun-exposed areas and thus sharply marginated at the border between exposed and covered skin (Fig. 10-2). Develops after 6 h and peaks after 24 h. Edema, vesicles, and even bullae; always uniform erythema and no "rash," as occurs in most photoallergic reactions. As edema and erythema fade vesicles and blisters dry to crusts, which are then shed.

Distribution. Strictly confined to areas of exposure; sunburn can occur in areas covered with clothing, depending on the degree of UV transmission through clothing, the level of exposure, and the SPT of the person.

MUCOUS MEMBRANES Sunburn is frequent on the vermilion border of the lips and can occur on the tongue in mountain climbers who stick their tongue out panting.

LABORATORY EXAMINATIONS

DERMATOPATHOLOGY "Sunburn" cells in the epidermis (apoptotic keratinocytes); exocytosis of lymphocytes, vacuolization of melanocytes, and Langerhans cells. *Dermis*: endothelial cell swelling of superficial blood vessels.

DIAGNOSIS AND DIFFERENTIAL DIAGNOSIS

History of UVR exposure and sites of reaction on exposed areas. *Phototoxic erythema*:

History of medications that induce phototoxic erythema. *SLE* can cause a sunburn-type erythema. *Erythropoietic protoporphyria* (EPP) causes erythema, vesicles, edema, and purpura.

COURSE AND PROGNOSIS

Sunburn, unlike thermal burns, cannot be classified on the basis of depth, i.e., first-, second-, and third-degree because 3° burns after UVR do not occur. Therefore, there is no scarring. A permanent reaction from severe UV burns is mottled depigmentation, probably related to the destruction of melanocytes, and eruptive solar lentigines (Dermatoheliosis: solar lentigines, p. 218).

MANAGEMENT

PREVENTION SPT I or II should avoid sunbathing, especially between 11 am and 2 pm. Clothing: UV-screening cloth garments. There are now many highly effective topical chemical filters (sunscreens) in lotion, gel, and cream formulations.
Topical. Cool wet dressings and topical glucocorticoids.
Systemic. Acetylsalicylic acid, indomethacin, and NSAIDs.
SEVERE SUNBURN Bed rest. If very severe, a "toxic" patient may require hospitalization for fluid replacement, prophylaxis of infection.

DRUG-/CHEMICAL-INDUCED PHOTOSENSITIVITY ICD-10: L56.0

- Interaction of UVR with a chemical or drug within the skin.
- Two mechanisms: *Phototoxic reactions*, which are photochemical reactions and *photoallergic reactions*, where a photoallergen is formed that initiates an immunologic response and manifests in skin as a type IV immunologic reaction.
- The difference between phototoxic and photoallergic eruptions is that the former manifests like an irritant (toxic) contact dermatitis or sunburn and the latter like an allergic eczematous contact dermatitis (see Table 10-3).

TABLE 10-3 Characteristics of Phototoxicity and Photoallergy

	Phototoxicity	Photoallergy
Clinical presentation	Sunburn reaction: erythema, edema, vesicles and bullae burning smarting; frequently resolves with hyperpigmentation	Eczematous lesions, papules, vesicles, scaling, crusting; usually pruritic
Histology	Apoptotic keratinocytes, sparse dermal infiltrate of lymphocytes, macrophages, and neutrophils	Spongiotic dermatitis, dense, dermal lymphohistiocytic infiltrate
Pathophysiology	Direct tissue injury	Type IV delayed hypersensitivity response
Occurrence after first exposure	Yes	No
Onset of eruption after exposure	Minutes to hours	24–48 h
Dosage of agent needed for eruption	Large	Small
Cross-reactivity with other agents	Rare	Common
Diagnosis	Clinical + phototests	Clinical + phototests + photopatch tests

Source: Adapted with permission from Lim HM. Abnormal responses to ultraviolet radiation: photosensitivity induced by exogenous agents. In: Goldsmith LA, Katz SI, Gilchrest BA, et al, eds. *Fitzpatrick's Dermatology in General Medicine*. 8th ed. New York, NY: McGraw-Hill; 2012.

PHOTOTOXIC DRUG-/CHEMICAL-INDUCED PHOTOSENSITIVITY ICD-10: L56.0

- An adverse reaction of the skin that results from simultaneous exposure to certain drugs (via ingestion, injection, or topical application) and to UVR or visible light or chemicals that may be therapeutic, cosmetic, industrial, or agricultural.
- Two types of reaction: (1) Systemic phototoxic dermatitis, occurring in individuals systemically exposed to a photosensitizing agent (drug) and subsequent UVR, and (2) local phototoxic dermatitis, occurring in individuals topically exposed to the photosensitizing agent and subsequent UVR.
- Both are *exaggerated sunburn responses* (erythema, edema, vesicles, and/or bullae).
- Systemic phototoxic dermatitis occurs in *all UVR-exposed sites*; local phototoxic dermatitis only in the *topical application sites*.

SYSTEMIC PHOTOTOXIC DERMATITIS ICD-10:L56.1

EPIDEMIOLOGY

Occurs in everyone after ingestion of a sufficient dose of a photosensitizing drug and subsequent UVR.

ETIOLOGY AND PATHOGENESIS

Toxic photoproducts such as free radicals or reactive oxygen species such as singlet oxygen. Principal sites of damage are nuclear DNA cell membranes (plasma, lysosomal, mitochondrial). The action spectrum is UVA. Drugs eliciting systemic phototoxic dermatitis are listed in Table 10-4. Some drugs causing phototoxic reactions can also elicit photoallergic reactions (see the following discussion).

CLINICAL MANIFESTATION

An "exaggerated sunburn" after solar or UVR exposure that *normally would not elicit a sunburn in that particular individual*. Occurs usually within hours after exposure, with some agents such as psoralens after 24 h, and peaking at 48 h. Skin symptoms: burning, stinging, and pruritus.

SKIN LESIONS Early. The skin lesions are those of an "exaggerated sunburn." Erythema, edema (Fig. 10-3A), and vesicle and bulla formation (Fig. 10-3B) confined to areas exposed to light. An eczematous reaction is *not* seen in phototoxic reactions.

SPECIAL PRESENTATIONS: PSEUDOPORPHYRIA
With some drugs there is little erythema but

TABLE 10-4 The Most Common Systemic Phototoxic Agents[a]

Property	Generic Name	Property	Generic Name
Antimicrobials	**Lomefloxacin** **Nalidixic acid** **Sparfloxacin** **Demeclocycline** **Doxycycline**	Antipsychotic drugs	**Chlorpromazine** **Prochlorperazine**
Furocoumarins	**5-Methoxypsoralen** **8-Methoxypsoralen** **4, 5′, 8-Trimethylpsoralen**	Photodynamic therapy agents	**Porfimer** **Verteporfin**
NSAIDs	**Piroxicam** **Naproxen** **Nabumetone** **Tolbutamide**	Cardiac medications Diuretics	**Amiodarone** **Furosemide** **Chlorothiazide** **Dyazide**

[a]These are the most commonly reported drugs. For a complete list, see Lim HM. In: Goldsmith LA, Katz SI, Gilchrest BA, et al, eds. *Fitzpatrick's Dermatology in General Medicine.* 8th ed. New York, NY: McGraw-Hill; 2012.

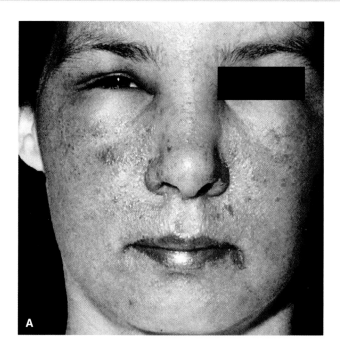

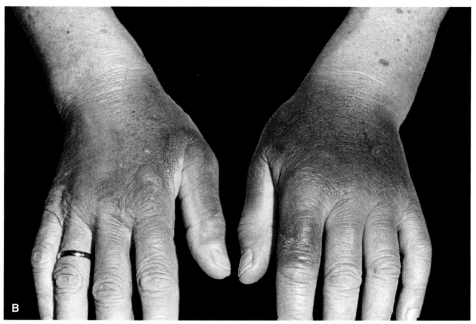

FIGURE 10-3 Phototoxic drug-induced photosensitivity (A) Massive edema and erythema in the face of a 17-year-old girl who was treated with demethylchlortetracycline for acne. **(B)** Dusky erythema with blistering on the dorsa of both hands in a patient treated with piroxicam.

pronounced blistering and skin fragility with erosions (Pseudoporphyria, see Section 23) and, upon repeated exposures, healing with milia, particularly on the dorsa of the hands and lower arms. Clinically indistinguishable from porphyria cutanea tarda (PCT) (see Porphyria cutanea tarda, p. 208) except for the lack of facial hypertrichosis, hence the term *pseudoporphyria* (see Section 23).

NAILS Subungual hemorrhage and photo-onycholysis can occur with certain drugs (psoralens, demethylchlortetracycline, and benoxaprofen).

PIGMENTATION Marked brown epidermal melanin pigmentation may occur in the course. With certain drugs especially, chlorpromazine and amiodarone, a slate gray dermal melanin pigmentation develops (see Drug-induced pigmentation, see Section 23).

LABORATORY EXAMINATIONS

DERMATOPATHOLOGY Inflammation, "sunburn cells" (apoptotic keratinocytes) in the epidermis, epidermal necrobiosis, intraepidermal, and subepidermal vesiculation.

PHOTOTESTING Template test sites are exposed to increasing doses of UVA (*phototoxic reactions are almost always resulting from UVA*)

while the patient is on the drug. The UVA MED will be much lower than that for normal individuals of the same SPT. After the drug has been eliminated from the skin, a repeat UVA phototest will reveal an *increase* in the UVA MED.

DIAGNOSIS AND DIFFERENTIAL DIAGNOSIS

History of exposure to drugs and morphologic changes in the skin characteristic of phototoxic drug eruptions. Differential diagnosis includes regular sunburn, phototoxic reactions caused by excess of endogenous porphyrins, and photosensitivity resulting from other diseases, e.g., SLE.

COURSE AND PROGNOSIS

Phototoxic drug sensitivity seriously limits or excludes the use of important drugs: diuretics, antihypertensive agents, and drugs used in psychiatry. Phototoxic drug reactions disappear after cessation of drug.

MANAGEMENT

As for sunburn.

TOPICAL PHOTOTOXIC DERMATITIS ICD-10: L56.0

- Inadvertent contact with or therapeutic application of a photosensitizer, followed by UVA irradiation (practically all topical photosensitizers have an action spectrum in the UVA range).
- The most common topical phototoxic agents are Rose Bengal used for ophthalmologic examination, the dye fluorescein and furocoumarins that occur in plants (*compositae* spp and *umbiliforme* spp), vegetables and fruits (lime, lemon celery, or parsley), in perfumes and cosmetics (oil of bergamot), and drugs used for topical photochemotherapy (psoralens). The most common route of contact is either therapeutic or occupational exposure.
- Clinical presentation is like acute irritant contact dermatitis (see Section 2), with erythema, swelling, vesiculation, and blistering confined to the sites of contact with the phototoxic agent.
- Symptoms are smarting, stinging, and burning rather than itching.
- Healing usually results in pronounced pigmentation (see Berloque dermatitis, p. 200). The most common and thus important topical phototoxic dermatitis is PPD, which is described as follows.

PHYTOPHOTODERMATITIS (PPD) ICD-10: L56.22

- An inflammation of the skin caused by contact with certain plants during recreational or occupational exposure to sunlight (plant + light = dermatitis).
- The inflammatory response is a phototoxic reaction to photosensitizing chemicals in several plant families.
- Common types of PPD are caused by exposure to limes, celery, and meadow grass.
- *Synonyms*: Berloque dermatitis, lime dermatitis.

EPIDEMIOLOGY AND ETIOLOGY

Common. Usually in spring and summer or all year in tropical climates.

RACE All skin colors; brown- and black-skinned persons may develop only marked spotty dark pigmentation without erythema or bullous lesions.

OCCUPATION Celery pickers, carrot processors, gardeners if exposed to carrot greens or to "gas plant" (*Dictamnus albus*), and bartenders (lime juice) who are exposed to sun in outside bars. Nonoccupational: Housewives and users of perfumes containing oil of bergamot; persons walking and children playing in meadows develop PPD on the legs; meadow grass contains agrimony.

ETIOLOGY Phototoxic reaction caused by photoactive furocoumarins (psoralens) contained in the plants.

CLINICAL MANIFESTATION

The patient gives a history of exposure to certain plants (lime, lemon, wild parsley, celery, giant hogweed, parsnips, carrot greens, and figs). Use of perfumes containing oil of bergamot (which contains bergapten, 5-methoxypsoralen) may develop streaks of pigmentation only in areas where the perfume was applied. This is called *berloque dermatitis* (French: *berloque*, "pendant").

SKIN SYMPTOMS Smarting, sensation of sunburn, pain, and later pruritus.

SKIN LESIONS Acute: Erythema, edema, vesicles, and bullae (Fig. 10-4). Lesions may appear pseudopapular before vesicles are evident (Fig. 10-5). Often bizarre streaks and artificial patterns (Fig. 10-5). On the sites of contact,

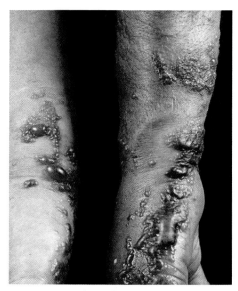

FIGURE 10-4 Phytophotodermatitis (plant + light): acute with blisters These bullae were the result of exposure to umbilliferae and the sun. This 50-year-old housewife was weeding her garden on a sunny day. Umbilliferae contain bergapten (5-methoxypsoralen), which is a potent topical phototoxic chemical.

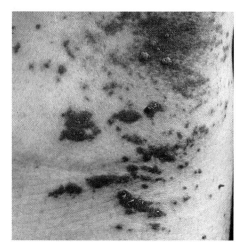

FIGURE 10-5 Phytophotodermatitis In a 48-year-old man who was sunbathing in a meadow. Before vesicles and blisters arise erythematous lesions may appear raised, giving the false impression of being papular. Note streaky pattern.

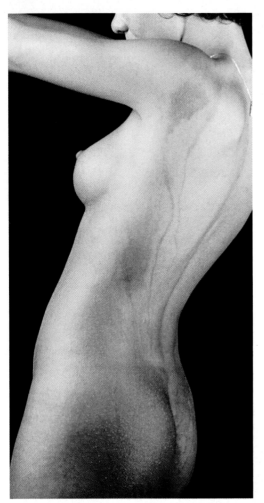

FIGURE 10-6 Berloque dermatitis The patient had applied a fragrant bath oil to her shoulders and chest but showered only the front of her body before going into the sun. The bath oil contained oil of bergamot, and pigmentation is now noted where it trickled down from the shoulders to the buttocks. (Used with permission from Dr. Thomas Schwarz.)

especially the arms, legs, and face. Residual hyperpigmentation in bizarre streaks (berloque dermatitis) (Fig. 10-6).

DIAGNOSIS AND DIFFERENTIAL DIAGNOSIS

By recognition of pattern and careful history. Differential diagnosis is primarily acute irritant contact dermatitis, with streaky pattern. Poison ivy dermatitis (see Fig. 2-8), but this is eczematous.

COURSE

May be an important occupational problem, as in celery pickers. The acute eruption has a short life and fades spontaneously, but the pigmentation may last for many weeks.

MANAGEMENT

Wet dressings may be indicated in the acute vesicular stage. Topical glucocorticoids.

PHOTOALLERGIC DRUG/CHEMICAL-INDUCED PHOTOSENSITIVITY ICD-10: L56.1

- This results from interaction of a photoallergen and UVA radiation.
- In sensitized individuals, exposure to a photoallergen and sunlight results in a pruritic eczematous eruption confined to exposed sites and clinically indistinguishable from allergic contact dermatitis.
- In most patients, the eliciting drug/chemical has been applied topically, but systemic elicitation also occurs.

EPIDEMIOLOGY

AGE OF ONSET More common in adults.
RACE All SPTs and colors.
INCIDENCE Photoallergic drug reactions occur much less frequently than do phototoxic drug reactions.

ETIOLOGY AND PATHOGENESIS

Topically applied chemical/drug plus UVA radiation. The chemicals are disinfectants, antimicrobials, agents in sunscreens, perfumes in aftershaves, or whiteners (Table 10-5). The chemical agent present in the skin absorbs photons and forms a photoproduct. This then binds to a soluble or membrane-bound protein to form an antigen to which a type IV immune response is elicited. Photoallergy is elicited only in those who have been sensitized. It can also be induced by systemic administration of a drug and elicited by topical administration of the same drug and vice versa. UVA is always required.

TABLE 10-5 Topical Photoallergens[a]

Group	Chemical Name
Sunscreens	Para-aminobenzoic acid (PABA)
	Benzophenones
Fragrances	6-Methylcoumarin
	Musk ambrette
Antibacterials	Dibromosalicylanilide
	Tetrachlorosalicylanilide
	Bithionol
	Sulfonamides
Others	Chlorpromazine

[a]These are the commonly reported drugs. For a complete list of topical photoallergens, see Lim HW. In: Goldsmith LA, Katz SI, Gilchrest DA, et al, eds. *Fitzpatrick's Dermatology in General Medicine.* 8th ed. New York, NY: McGraw-Hill; 2012.

CLINICAL MANIFESTATION

SKIN LESIONS Highly pruritic. Acute photoallergic reaction patterns are clinically indistinguishable from allergic contact dermatitis (Fig. 10-7): papular, vesicular, scaling, and crusted. Occasionally, there can also be a lichenoid eruption similar to lichen planus. In chronic drug photoallergy, there is scaling, lichenification, and marked pruritus mimicking atopic dermatitis or, again, chronic allergic contact dermatitis (Fig. 10-8).
Distribution. Confined primarily to areas exposed to light (distribution pattern of photosensitivity), but there may be spreading onto adjacent nonexposed skin. Of diagnostic help is the fact that in the face the upper eyelids, the area under the nose, and a thin strip of skin between the lower lip and the chin are often spared (shaded areas) (Fig. 10-7).

LABORATORY EXAMINATION

DERMATOPATHOLOGY. Epidermal spongiosis with lymphocytic infiltration.

DIAGNOSIS

History of exposure to drug, the allergic contact dermatitis pattern of the eruption, and its confinement to sun-exposed sites. Diagnosis is verified by the photopatch test: Photoallergens are applied in duplicate to the skin and covered. After 24 h, one set of the duplicate test sites is exposed to UVA, while the other set remains covered. Test sites are read for reactions after 48 to 96 h. An eczematous reaction in the irradiated site but not in the nonirradiated site confirms photoallergy to the particular agent tested.

COURSE AND PROGNOSIS

Photoallergic dermatitis can persist for months to years. This is known as *chronic actinic dermatitis* (formerly persistent light reaction)

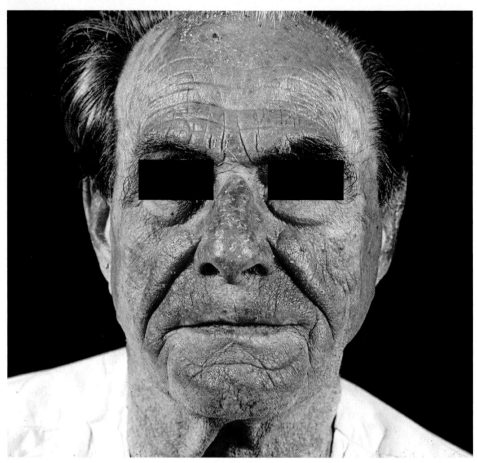

FIGURE 10-7 Photoallergic drug-induced photosensitivity This 60-year-old male shows an eczematous dermatitis in the face. He was taking trimethoprim–sulfamethoxazole. Note relative sparing of eyelids (protected by sunglasses), under the nose, and the area under the lower lip (shaded areas).

(Fig. 10-8). In *chronic actinic dermatitis*, the action spectrum usually broadens to involve UVB, and the condition persists despite discontinuation of the causative photoallergen, with each new UV exposure aggravating the condition. Chronic eczema-like lichenified and extremely itchy confluent plaques result (Fig. 10-8), which lead to disfigurement and a distressing situation for the patient. As the condition is now independent of the original photoallergen and is aggravated by each new solar exposure, avoidance of photoallergen does not cure the disease.

MANAGEMENT

In severe cases, immunosuppression (azathioprine plus glucocorticoids or oral cyclosporine) is required.

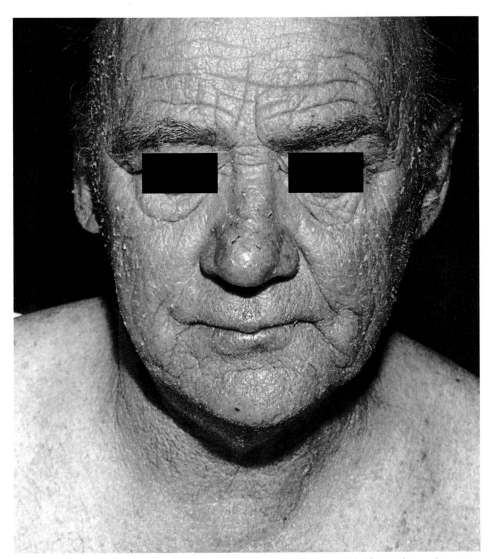

FIGURE 10-8 Drug-induced photosensitivity: chronic actinic dermatitis (formerly persistent light eruption) Erythematous plaques confined to the face and neck, sparing the shoulders. This male has excruciating pruritus.

POLYMORPHOUS LIGHT ERUPTION (PMLE) ICD-10: L56.4

■ PMLE is a term that describes a group of heterogeneous, idiopathic, acquired, and acute recurrent eruptions characterized by delayed abnormal reactions to UVR.
■ Manifested by varied lesions, including erythematous macules, papules, plaques, and vesicles. However, in each patient, the eruption is consistently monomorphous.
■ By far, the most frequent morphologic types are the papular and papulovesicular eruptions.

EPIDEMIOLOGY

INCIDENCE Most common photodermatosis. Prevalence from 10% to 21%. Average age of onset is 23 years and it is much more common in females. All races, but most common in SPT I, II, and III. In American Indians (North and South America), there is a *hereditary* type of PMLE that is called *actinic prurigo*.

PATHOGENESIS

Possibly a delayed-type hypersensitivity reaction to an (auto-) antigen induced by UVR. The action spectrum is UVA and less commonly UVB or UVA and UVB. Since UVA is transmitted through window glass, PMLE can be precipitated while riding in a car.

CLINICAL MANIFESTATION

ONSET AND DURATION OF LESIONS PMLE appears in spring or early summer. It occurs within hours of exposure and once established, it persists for 7 to 10 days. Symptoms are massive pruritus. Scratching is painful.
SKIN LESIONS The papular (Fig. 10-9) and papulovesicular types are the most frequent. Far less common are plaques or urticarial plaques (Fig. 10-10). The lesions are pink to red. In the individual patient, lesions are quite monomorphous, i.e., either papular or papulovesicular or urticarial plaques. Recurrences follow the original pattern.
DISTRIBUTION The eruption often spares habitually exposed areas (face and neck) and appears most frequently on the forearms, upper arms, V area of the neck, and chest (Fig. 10-9). However, lesions may occur on the face (Fig. 10-10), if there has not been previous exposure to the sun.

LABORATORY EXAMINATIONS

DERMATOPATHOLOGY Edema of the epidermis, spongiosis, vesicle formation, and mild liquefaction degeneration of the basal layer with dense lymphocytic infiltrate in the dermis.
IMMUNOFLUORESCENCE Negative ANA.

DIAGNOSIS

Delayed onset of eruption, characteristic morphology, and the history of disappearance of the eruption in days. In plaque-type PMLE, biopsy and immunofluorescence studies are mandatory to rule out LE (Fig. 10-10). *Phototesting* is done with both UVB and UVA. Test sites are exposed daily, starting with two MEDs of UVB and UVA, respectively, for 1 week to 10 days, using increments of the UV dose. In more than 50% of patients, a PMLE-like eruption will occur in the test sites.

COURSE AND PROGNOSIS

The course is chronic and recurrent. Although some patients may develop "tolerance" by the end of the summer, the eruption usually recurs the following spring and/or when the person travels to tropical areas in the winter. Spontaneous improvement or even cessation of eruptions occurs after years.

MANAGEMENT

PREVENTION Sunblocks are not always effective but should be tried first in every patient.
Systemic β-carotene, 60 mg three times a day for 2 weeks, before going in the sun. Oral prednisone 20 mg/day given 2 days before and 2 days during exposure is a good prophylaxis. Also, intramuscular triamcinolone acetonide, 40 mg, will suppress an eruption when administered a few days before a trip to a sunny region.
PUVA (Photochemotherapy) and *narrowband UVB* (311 nm) are very effective when given in early spring by inducing "tolerance" for the summer. Treatments have to be given before the sunny season, be repeated each spring, but are usually not necessary for more than 3 or 4 years.

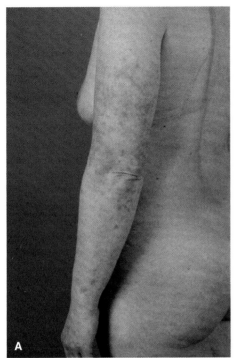
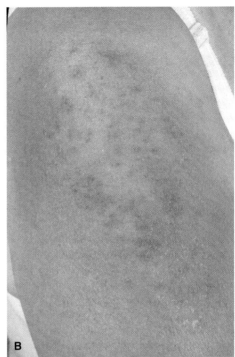

FIGURE 10-9 Polymorphic light eruption, popular variant (A) Clusters of confluent, extremely pruritic papules on the exposed upper and lower arms, occurring in a 35- year- old woman the day following the first sun exposure of the season. The eruption by bilateral but spared face and covered areas of the body. **(B)** Papular and slightly crusted eruption on the shoulders of another patient. There is excruciating pruritus. Scratching causes pain.

FIGURE 10-10 Polymorphic light eruption Erythematous plaques in the face following first sun exposure of the season. The butterfly distribution is very similar to that of lupus erythematosus.

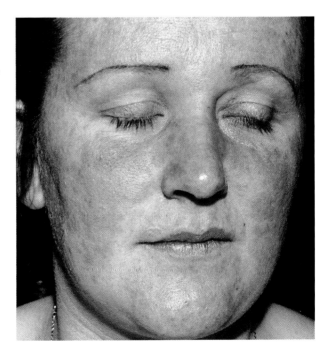

SOLAR URTICARIA ICD-10: L56.3

- Uncommon sunlight-induced healing confined to exposed body sites.
- Eruption occurs within minutes of exposure and resolves in a few hours. Very disabling and sometimes life threatening.
- Action spectrum is UVB, UVA, and visible light or any combination thereof. Most commonly UVA (Fig. 10-11).
- Solar urticaria is an immediate type I hypersensitivity response to cutaneous and/or circulating photoallergens.
- Therapy: Multiple phototherapy sessions in low but increasing doses on the same day ("rush hardening"); oral immunosuppressive agents or plasmapheresis.
- Prevention: Sun avoidance or sunscreens with high protection factors against action spectrum.

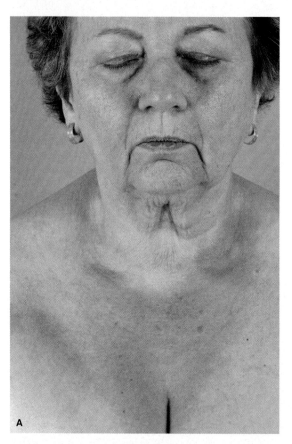

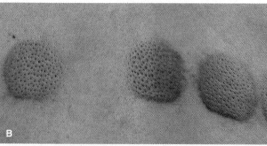

FIGURE 10-11 Solar urticaria
A. Since wheals induced by sun exposure are transient and have usually disappeared when a patient comes to the clinic this 62- year old patient exhibited only residual erythemas on the cheeks and the V of the neck when she was photographed. **B.** The patient was subsequently exposed to various doses of UVA and UVB delivered to template test sites on her back and immediately after exposure this picture was taken. UVA test site shows a massive urticarial reaction verifying UVA-induced solar urticaria.

PHOTO-EXACERBATED DERMATOSES

- Various wavelengths of UVR and/or visible light can elicit or aggravate a number of dermatoses.
- In these cases, the eruption is invariably similar to that of the primary condition.
- An abbreviated list follows, but it should be emphasized that among these disorders SLE is by far the most important.
- Acne, atopic eczema, carcinoid syndrome, cutaneous T-cell lymphoma, Darier disease, dermatomyositis, disseminated superficial actinic porokeratosis, erythema multiforme, Hailey–Hailey disease, herpes labialis, keratosis follicularis (Darier disease) lichen planus, lupus erythematosus, pellagra, pemphigus foliaceus (erythematosus), pityriasis rubra pilaris, psoriasis, reticulate erythematous mucinosis syndrome, rosacea, seborrheic dermatitis, and transient acantholytic dermatosis (Grover disease).

METABOLIC PHOTOSENSITIVITY—THE PORPHYRIAS

For classification of porphyrias, see Table 10-6. Acute intermittent porphyria (AIP) is not dealt with in detail here because it has no skin manifestations.

TABLE 10-6 Classification and Differential Diagnosis of Porphyrias

	Congenital Erythropoietic Porphyrias	Erythropoietic Protoporphyria	Porphyria Cutanea Tarda	Variegate Porphyria	Intermittent Acute Porphyria
Inheritance	Autosomal recessive	Autosomal dominant	Autosomal dominant (familial form)	Autosomal dominant	Autosomal dominant
Signs and symptoms					
Photosensitivity	Yes	Yes	Yes	Yes	No
Cutaneous lesions	Yes	Yes	Yes	Yes	No
Attacks of abdominal pain	No	No	No	Yes	Yes
Neuropsychiatric syndrome	No	No	No	Yes	Yes
Laboratory abnormalities	+	+	+	+	+
Red blood cells					
Fluorescence	+	+	−	−	−
Uroporphyrin	+++	N	N	N	N
Coproporphyrin	++	+	N	N	N
Protoporphyrin	(+)	+++	N	N	N
Plasma					
Fluorescence	+	+	−	+	−
Urine					
Fluorescence	−	−	+	±	−
Porphobilinogen	N	N	N	(+++)	(+++)
Uroporphyrin	+++	N	+++	+++	+++
Feces					
Protoporphyrin	+	++	N	+++	N

Note: N, normal; +, above normal; ++, moderately increased; +++, markedly increased; (+++), frequently increased (depends on whether patient has an attack, or is in remission); (+), increased in some patients.

PORPHYRIA CUTANEA TARDA ICD-10: E80.1

- PCT occurs mostly in adults.
- Patients do not present with characteristic photosensitivity but with complaints of "fragile skin," vesicles, and bullae, particularly on the dorsa of the hands, after minor trauma.
- Purple-red suffusion of central facial skin, brown hypermelanosis, and hypertrichosis of the face.
- Scleroderma-like changes and scars in exposed areas.
- The diagnosis is confirmed by the presence of a pinkish-red fluorescence in the urine when examined with a Wood lamp.
- PCT is distinct from variegate porphyria (VP) and AIP in that patients with PCT do not have acute life-threatening attacks.
- Furthermore, the drugs that induce PCT are fewer than the drugs that induce VP and AIP.

EPIDEMIOLOGY

Onset 30 to 50 years, rarely in children; females on oral contraceptives; males on estrogen therapy for prostate cancer. Equal in males and females.

HEREDITY Most PCT patients have *type I* (*acquired*) induced by drugs or chemicals. *Type II* (*hereditary*), autosomal dominant; possibly these patients actually have VP, but this is not yet resolved. There is also a "dual" type with VP and PCT in the same family.

ETIOLOGY AND PATHOGENESIS

PCT is caused by either an inherited or acquired deficiency of UROGEN decarboxylase. In type I (sporadic, acquired PCT-symptomatic), the enzyme is deficient only in the liver; in type II (PCT-hereditary), it is also deficient in red blood cells (RBCs) and fibroblasts. *Chemicals and drugs that induce PCT*: Ethanol, estrogen, hexachlorobenzene, chlorinated phenols, iron, and tetrachlorodibenzo-*p*-dioxin. High doses of chloroquine lead to clinical manifestations in "latent" cases (low doses are used as treatment). *Other predisposing factors*: Diabetes mellitus (25%), hepatitis C virus, and hemochromatosis.

CLINICAL MANIFESTATION

SKIN LESIONS Gradual onset. Patients present with fragility of skin on exposed sites. Tense bullae and erosions on normal-appearing skin (Fig. 10-12); slowly heal to form pink atrophic scars, milia (1 to 2 mm) on dorsa of hands and feet, nose, forehead, or (bald) scalp. Purple-red suffusion ("heliotrope") of central facial skin (Fig. 10-13A), especially periorbital areas. Brown hypermelanosis, diffuse, on exposed areas. Hypertrichosis of face (Fig. 10-14). Scleroderma-like changes, diffuse or circumscribed, waxy yellowish-white areas on exposed areas of the face (Fig. 10-13B), neck, and trunk.

LABORATORY EXAMINATIONS

DERMATOPATHOLOGY Bullae, subepidermal with "festooned" (undulating) base. PAS staining reveals thickened vascular walls. Paucity of an inflammatory infiltrate.

IMMUNOFLUORESCENCE IgG and other immunoglobulins at the dermal–epidermal junction, in and around blood vessels, and in the sun-exposed areas of the skin.

CHEMISTRY Plasma iron and liver enzymes may be increased. High level of iron stores in the liver. The patient may have hemochromatosis. *Blood glucose* is increased in those patients with diabetes mellitus (25% of patients).

PORPHYRIN STUDIES IN STOOL AND URINE (Table 10-6) Increased uroporphyrin (I isomer, 60%) in urine and plasma. Increased isocoproporphyrin (type III) and 7-carboxylporphyrin but not protoporphyrin in the feces. No increase in δ-aminolevulinic acid or porphobilinogen in the urine.

SIMPLE TEST Wood lamp examination of the urine shows orange-red fluorescence (Fig. 10-15); to enhance, add a few drops of 10% hydrochloric acid.

LIVER BIOPSY Reveals porphyrin fluorescence and often fatty liver. May also show cirrhosis and hemochromatosis.

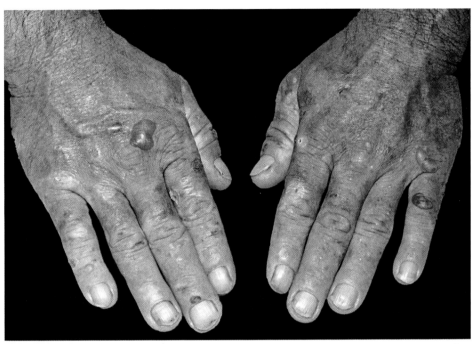

FIGURE 10-12 Porphyria cutanea tarda Bullae and atrophic depigmented scars on the dorsum of both hands. This is not an acute reaction to sun exposure but develops over time with repeated sun exposure and occurs after minor trauma. The patient presents with a history of "fragile" skin bullae and scars.

DIAGNOSIS AND DIFFERENTIAL DIAGNOSIS

By clinical features, pink-red fluorescence of urine and elevated urinary porphyrins. Bullae on dorsa of hands and feet can occur in *pseudo-PCT* (see Section 23) and in chronic renal failure with hemodialysis. *Epidermolysis bullosa acquisita* (see Section 6) has the same clinical picture (increased skin fragility, easy bruising, and light- and trauma-provoked bullae) but no hypertrichosis and hyperpigmentation.

MANAGEMENT

1. Avoid ethanol, stop drugs that could induce PCT, and eliminate exposure to chemicals (chlorinated phenols, tetrachlorodibenzo-*p*-dioxin).

2. Phlebotomy is done by removing 500 mL of blood at weekly or biweekly intervals. Clinical and biochemical remission occurs within 5 to 12 months after regular phlebotomy. Relapse within a year is uncommon (5 to 10%).

3. Low-dose chloroquine is used to induce remission of PCT in patients in who repeated phlebotomies cannot be done because of anemia. Since chloroquine can exacerbate the disease and, in higher doses, may even induce hepatic failure in these patients, this treatment requires considerable experience. However, long-lasting remissions and, in a portion of patients, clinical and biochemical "cure" can be achieved.

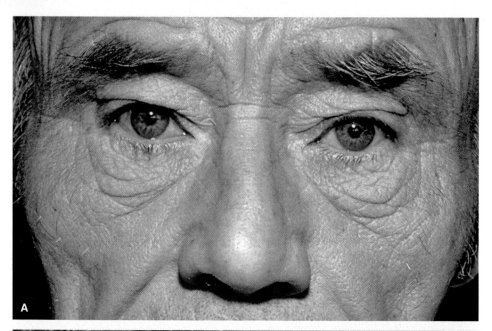

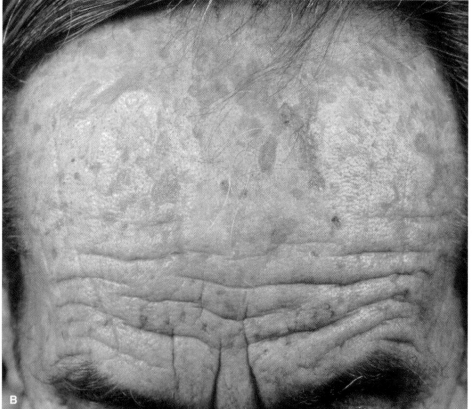

FIGURE 10-13 Porphyria cutanea tarda (A) Very subtle periorbital violaceous coloration.
(B) Sclerodermoid thickening, scars, and erosions on the forehead.

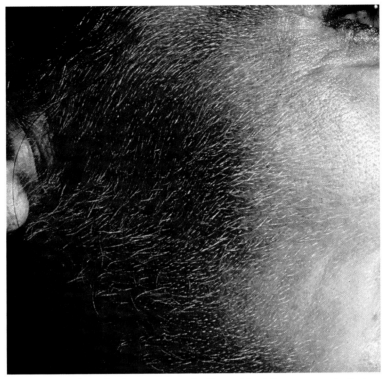

FIGURE 10-14 Porphyria cutanea tarda Hypertrichosis in a woman who had been on a prolonged regimen with estrogens. Under Wood light, her urine showed a bright coral-red fluorescence, as shown in Figure 10-15.

FIGURE 10-15 Porphyria cutanea tarda: Wood light Coral-red fluorescence of the urine of a patient with PCT as compared to that of a normal control.

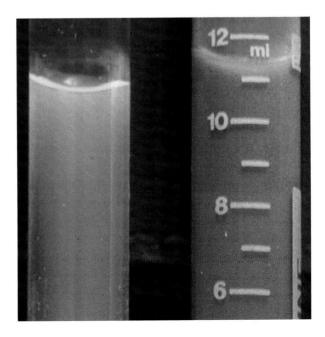

VARIEGATE PORPHYRIA ICD-10: E80.230

- A serious autosomal-dominant disorder of heme biosynthesis. Protogen oxidase defect → accumulation of protoporphyrinogen in the liver → excretion in bile → nonenzymatically converted to protoporphyrin → high fecal protoporphyrin.
- All races; common in *white* South Africans.
- Accentuated by ingestion of drugs (Table 10-7) → precipitation of acute attacks of abdominal pain, nausea, vomiting, delirium, seizures, personality changes, coma, and bulbar paralysis.
- Skin lesions identical to those of PCT such as vesicles and bullae (Fig. 10-16), skin fragility, milia, and scarring of the dorsa of the hands and fingers. Periorbital heliotrope hue, hyperpigmentation, and hypertrichosis in exposed areas. Lesions result from exposure to sunlight.
- Increased excretion of porphyrins; characteristic are high levels of protoporphyrin in the feces (Table 10-6).
- Differential diagnosis: Other porphyrias (Table 10-6); pseudoporphyria, scleroderma, and acquired epidermolysis bullosa.
- Treatment: None, oral β-carotene may prevent or ameliorate skin manifestations.
- Lifetime disease; Prognosis good if exacerbating factors are avoided. Rarely death can occur after ingestion of drugs that increase cytochrome P450.
- *Synonym*: Porphyria variegata.

TABLE 10-7 Drugs Hazardous to Patients with Variegate and Acute Intermittent Porphyria

Anesthetics: barbiturates and halothane
Anticonvulsants: hydantoins, carbamazepine, ethosuximide, methsuximide, phensuximide, primidone
Antimicrobial agents: chloramphenicol, griseofulvin, novobiocin, pyrazinamide, sulfonamides
Ergot preparations
Ethyl alcohol
Hormones: estrogens, progestin, oral contraceptive preparations
Imipramine
Methyldopa
Minor tranquilizers: chlordiazepoxide, diazepam, oxazepam, flurazepam, meprobamate
Pentazocine
Phenylbutazone
Sulfonylureas: chlorpropamide, tolbutamide
Theophylline

FIGURE 10-16 Variegate porphyria
Bullae on the dorsum of the foot and toes, a common site of sun exposure in patients wearing open footwear. This 42-year-old female was initially diagnosed with porphyria cutanea tarda. However, she gave a history of recurrent attacks of abdominal pain, which was a clue to the diagnosis of variegate porphyria; diagnosis was established by the detection of elevated stool protoporphyrins. Variegate porphyria (or South African porphyria) is akin to acute intermittent porphyria, in which there are no skin lesions but a fatal outcome may occur with ingestion of certain drugs (see Table 10-7). In South Africa, every white patient who is scheduled for major surgery must have laboratory tests for porphyrins since variegate porphyria is common in that country.

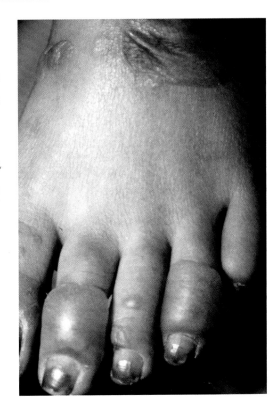

ERYTHROPOIETIC PROTOPORPHYRIA ICD-10: F80.0

- This hereditary metabolic disorder of porphyrin metabolism is unique among the porphyrias in that porphyrins or porphyrin precursors are usually not excreted in the urine.
- Autosomal dominant, variable penetrance. Defective enzyme is ferrochelatase.
- Onset in early childhood or late onset in early adulthood.
- Equal in females and males, within all ethnic groups.
- EPP is characterized by an acute sunburn-like photosensitivity, in contrast to the other common porphyrias (PCT or VP), where obvious acute photosensitivity is *not* a presenting complaint.
- Symptoms occur rapidly within *minutes* of sun exposure and consist of stinging and burning.
- Skin signs are erythema, edema, and purpura on the face and dorsa of the hands (Figs. 10-17 and 10-18).
- Late (chronic) skin signs: Shallow, often linear scars, waxy thickening and wrinkling of the skin on the face, and dorsa of the hands (Fig. 10-19).
- Increased protoporphyrin in RBCs, plasma, and stools (Table 10-6), and decreased ferrochelatase in bone marrow, liver, and skin fibroblasts.
- Test for liver function indicated. Liver biopsy: Portal and periportal fibrosis; brown pigment and birefringent granules in hepatocytes and Kupffer cells. Gallstones may be present, even in children; cirrhosis and liver failure may rarely occur.
- Dermatopathology: Eosinophilic homogenization and thickening of papillary blood vessels.
- Diagnosis: Clinical symptoms (there is no other photosensitivity disorder in which symptoms appear minutes after sun exposure), skin signs, and simple test: RBCs in a blood smear show transient red fluorescence at 400 nm.
- Treatment none. Preventive management is β-carotene PO, which can prevent acute photosensitivity.
- *Synonym:* Erythrohepatic protoporphyria.

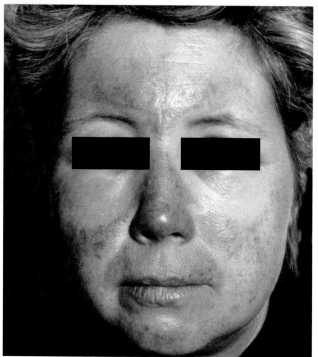

FIGURE 10-17 Erythropoietic protoporphyria Diffuse erythematous swelling of the nose, forehead, and cheeks with petechial hemorrhage and telangiectasia. There are no porphyrins in the urine. A clue to the diagnosis is the history of tingling and burning within 4 to 5 min of sun exposure. The face of this woman appears yellow-orange because she was on β-carotene, which obviously did not protect her sufficiently.

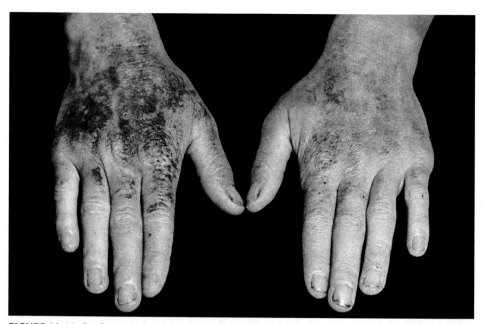

FIGURE 10-18 Erythropoietic protoporphyria Massive petechial, confluent hemorrhage on the dorsa of the hands of a 16-year-old 24 h after exposure to the sun.

FIGURE 10-19 Erythro-poietic protoporphyria, chronic skin changes
Waxy thickening on the upper lip, cheeks, and nose makes the patient look older than he is (27 years). Note waxy thickening on the vermilion of lower lip, deep creases, and tiny shallow scars on the nose.

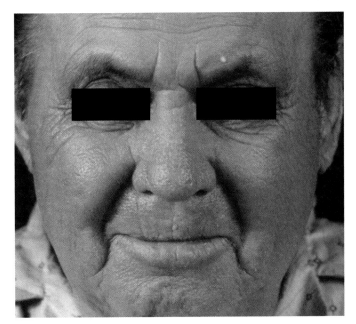

CHRONIC PHOTODAMAGE

DERMATOHELIOSIS ("PHOTOAGING") ICD-10: L57.91

- Repeated solar injuries over many years ultimately can result in the development of a skin syndrome, DHe. Very common.
- It occurs in persons with SPT I–III and in persons with SPT IV who have had heavy cumulative exposure to sunlight, such as lifeguards and outdoor workers, over a lifetime. Most often in persons >40 years.
- Action spectrum UVB but also UVA and possibly infrared.
- Severity depends on the duration and intensity of sun exposure and on the indigenous (constitutive) skin color and the capacity to tan.
- *Note*: If you want to demonstrate to an older patient the role of UVR in photoaging, just have him/her undress and compare the quality of his/her facial skin to that of the suprapubic skin.
- Skin lesions: A combination of atrophy (of epidermis), hypertrophy (of papillary dermis caused by elastosis), telangiectases, spotty depigmentation and hyperpigmentation, and spotty hyperkeratosis in light-exposed areas. Skin appears wrinkled, leathery, and "prematurely aged" (Fig. 10-20). Both fine, cigarette paper-like and deep furrow-like wrinkling; skin is waxy, papular with a yellowish hue, and both glistening and rough (Fig. 10-21). Telangiectasia and bruising (senile purpura) caused by fragility of small vessels. Macular hyperpigmentations: Solar lentigines (see the following discussion); macular hypopigmentations: guttate hypomelanosis, <3 mm in diameter, on the extremities. Comedones, particularly periorbital (termed Favre–Racouchot disease) (Fig. 10-22), particularly in cigarette smokers. Individuals with DHe invariably have actinic keratoses.
- Distribution: Exposed areas, particularly face, periorbital and perioral areas, and scalp (bald males). Nuchal area: Cutis rhomboidalis ("red neck") with rhomboidal furrows; lower arms, dorsa of the hands.
- Current management is to prevent skin cancers and the development of DHe with the use of protective sunblocks, a change of behavior in the sun, and the use of topical chemotherapy (tretinoin) that reverses some of the changes of DHe.

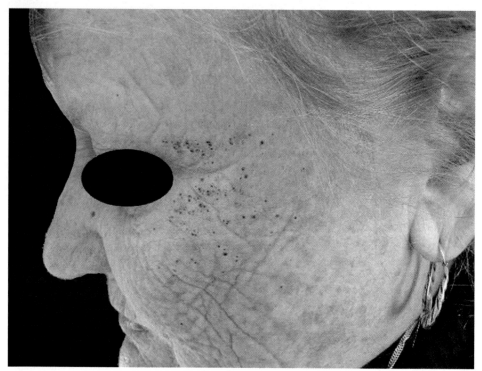

FIGURE 10-20 Dermatoheliosis Severe deep wrinkling. The skin appears waxy, papular with a yellowish hue (solar elastosis). This 68-year-old female mountain farmer lived at an altitude of 1,500 m and had been working outdoors all her life. In addition, she was a heavy smoker and now has multiple black comedones in the zygomatic regions (Favre Racouchot disease). (Used with permission from Dr. Gudrun Ratzinger.)

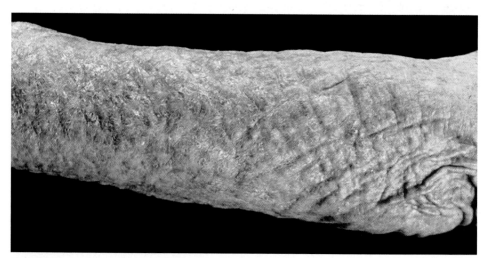

FIGURE 10-21 Severe dermatoheliosis on the forearm of a 70-year-old female farmhand The skin is waxy, deeply wrinkled, and dry. Multiple solar keratoses have been removed from this arm by cryotherapy.

SOLAR LENTIGO ICD-10: L81.416

- Solar lentigo is a circumscribed 1- to 3-cm brown macule resulting from a localized proliferation of melanocytes resulting from acute or chronic exposure to sunlight.
- Onset usually >40 years.
- Multiple lesions usually arise in sun-exposed sites. Most common in Caucasians (SPTs I to II).
- Skin lesions strictly macular, 1 to 3 cm, and as large as 5 cm. Light yellow, light brown, or dark brown; variegated mix of brown (Fig. 10-22). Round, oval, with slightly irregular border, and ill defined. Scattered, discrete lesions, stellate, sharply defined, and roughly the same size after acute sunburn (Fig. 10-23) or overdosage of PUVA.
- Distribution. Exclusively exposed areas: forehead, cheeks, nose, dorsa of the hands and forearms, upper back, chest, and shins.
- Differential diagnosis: "Flat," acquired, brown lesions on the exposed skin of the face, which may on cursory examination appear to be similar and have distinctive features: solar lentigo, freckles, seborrheic keratosis, spreading pigmented actinic keratosis (SPAK), and lentigo maligna (LM).
- Cryosurgery or laser surgery is effective.

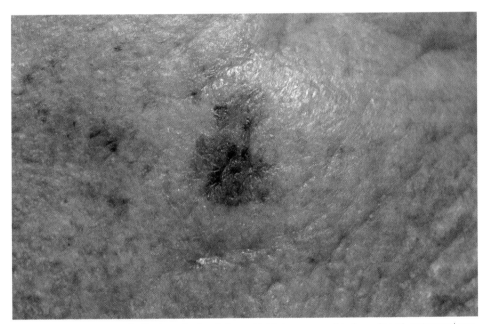

FIGURE 10-22 Dermatoheliosis: solar lentigines Multiple, very small to large (2 cm), variegated, tan-to-dark-brown macules on the cheek. Solar lentigines are not the same as ephelides (freckles). They do not fade in the winter as freckles do. In contrast to the sharply marginated solar lentigines caused by an acute sunburn that have roughly the same size shown in Figure 10-24, the solar lentigines shown here are of different sizes and partially ill defined and confluent, which is characteristic of chronic cumulative solar damage. Note waxy thickening of skin and creases of dermatoheliosis.

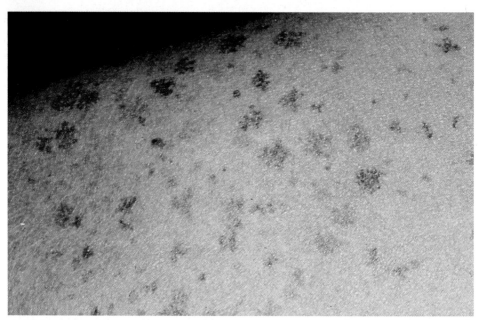

FIGURE 10-23 Dermatoheliosis: solar lentigines Multiple stellate brown macules on the shoulder occurred after a sunburn. They are all of about the same size and sharply marginated, which is characteristic of sunburn-induced solar lentigines.

CHONDRODERMATITIS NODULARIS HELICIS ICD-10: H61.01

- Usually occurs as a single elongated, exquisitely tender nodule, or a "beading" of the free border of helix of the ear. Common, perhaps resulting from constant mechanical trauma but most probably to UV radiation.
- Appears spontaneously, enlarges quickly, measuring less than 1 cm (**Fig. 10-24**), firm, well-defined, round to oval with dome-shaped surface and sloping margins, white-waxy and translucent, and often ulcerated (**Fig. 10-24**).
- More common in males than in females.
- Spontaneous pain or tenderness. Can be intense and stabbing, paroxysmal, or continuous.
- Differential diagnosis: Basal cell carcinoma (BCC), actinic keratosis, in situ or invasive squamous cell carcinoma (SCC), hypertrophic solar keratosis, and keratoacanthoma. Also gouty tophus, rheumatoid and rheumatic nodules, and discoid lupus erythematosus.
- Management includes intralesional injection of triamcinolone acetonide, carbon dioxide laser, and surgery. The definitive treatment is excisional surgery including the underlying cartilage.

FIGURE 10-24 Chondrodermatitis nodularis helicis An extremely painful nodule with central ulceration on the anthelix of a 60-year-old female. The central ulcer is covered with a crust and can be mistaken for a basal cell carcinoma.

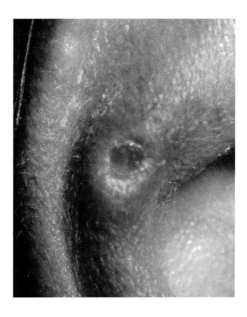

ACTINIC KERATOSIS ICD-10: L57.0

- Single or multiple, discrete, dry, rough, adherent scaly lesions on the habitually sun-exposed skin of adults, usually on a background of DHe.
- Actinic keratoses can progress to squamous cell carcinoma.
- This condition is dealt with in Section 11.
- *Synonym*: Solar keratosis.

SKIN REACTIONS TO IONIZING RADIATION

RADIATION DERMATITIS ICD-10: L58

- Radiation dermatitis is defined as skin changes resulting from exposure to ionizing radiation.
- *Reversible effects* are pain, erythema, epilation, suppression of sebaceous glands, and pigmentation (lasting for weeks to months to years).
- *Irreversible effects* are atrophy, sclerosis, telangiectasias, ulceration, and radiation-induced cancers.

Type of Exposure

Result of therapy (for cancer, formerly also used for acne and psoriasis, and fungal infections of the scalp in children), accidental, or occupational (e.g., formerly, in dentists). The radiation causing radiodermatitis includes superficial and deep x-ray radiation, electron beam therapy, and grenz-ray therapy. It is a prevailing myth that grenz rays are "soft" and not carcinogenic; SCC can appear from >5000 cGy of grenz rays.

Types of Reactions

ACUTE Temporary erythema that lasts 3 days and then persistent erythema, which reaches a peak in 2 weeks and is painful; pigmentation appears around day 20; a late erythema can also occur beginning on day 35 to 40, and usually lasts 2 to 3 weeks. Massive reactions lead to blistering, erosions (Fig. 10-25), and ulceration, also painful; may occur as recall phenomenon. Permanent scarring may result.

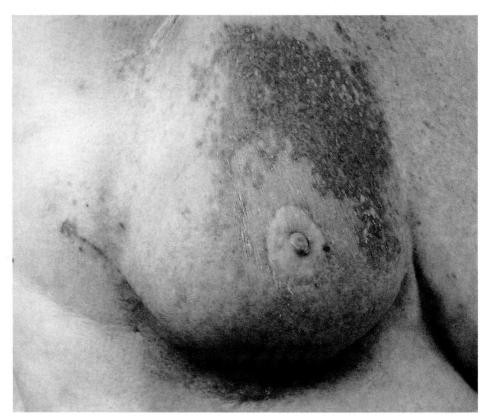

FIGURE 10-25 Radiation dermatitis: acute, recall phenomenon This patient had breast cancer. She had a lumpectomy, methotrexate, and x-ray therapy and developed painful erythema and erosions at the irradiated site.

CHRONIC After *fractional* but relatively intensive therapy with total doses of 3000 to 6000 rad, there develops an epidermolytic reaction in 3 weeks. This is repaired in 3 to 6 weeks, but scars and hypopigmentation develop; there is loss of all skin appendages and atrophy of the epidermis and dermis. During the next 2 to 5 years, the atrophy increases (Fig. 10-26); there is hyper- and hypopigmentation (poikiloderma), telangiectasia (Figs. 10-26 and 10-27). Necrosis and painful ulceration (Fig. 10-28) are rare but occur in accidental exposure or error in dose. Necrosis is leathery, yellow, and adherent and surrounding skin are extremely painful (Fig. 10-28). Ulcerations have a very poor tendency to heal and usually require surgical intervention. Lastly, there may be radiation keratoses and squamous cell carcinoma (Fig. 10-29).

NAILS Longitudinal striations (Fig. 10-29B) show thickening, dystrophy.

COURSE, PROGNOSIS, AND MANAGEMENT

Chronic radiation dermatitis is permanent, progressive, and irreversible. SCC may develop in 4 to 40 years (Fig. 10-29), with a median of 7 to 12 years. Tumors metastasize in about 25%; despite extensive surgery (excision, grafts, etc.), the prognosis is poor, and recurrences are common. BCC may also occur in chronic radiation dermatitis and appears mostly in patients formerly treated with x-rays for acne vulgaris and acne cystica or epilation (tinea capitis) (Fig. 10-27). The tumors may appear 40 to 50 years after exposure. Excision and grafting are often possible before the cancer develops.

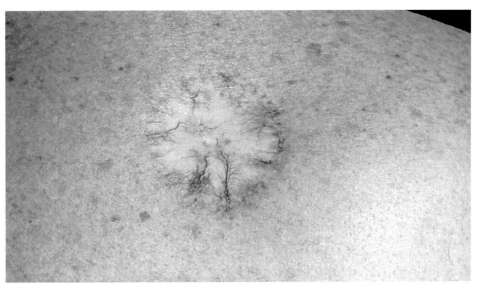

FIGURE 10-26 Radiation dermatitis: chronic There is sclerosis combined with atrophy and telangiectasia. This is the result of the irradiation of an infantile hemangioma in infancy.

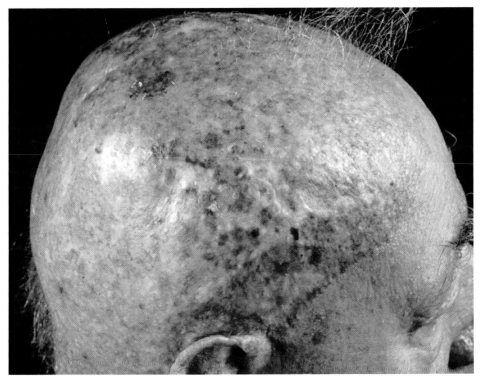

FIGURE 10-27 Radiation dermatitis: chronic There is poikiloderma (brown: hyperpigmentation; white: hypopigmentation; red: telangiectasia) combined with atrophy and sclerosis. Hairs are absent. These massive skin changes are the result of overdosed irradiation that the patient received as a child for fungal infection of the scalp. He is a candidate for SCC in the future.

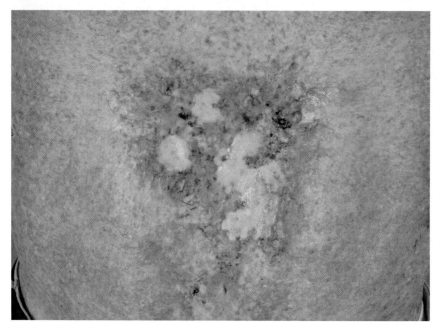

FIGURE 10-28 Radiation dermatitis: chronic An area of severe poikiloderma with telan-giectasias and irregular areas of necrosis that is leathery, yellowish-white, and tightly adherent. The lesion is extremely painful. Occurred after repeated electron beam radiations for mycosis fungoides.

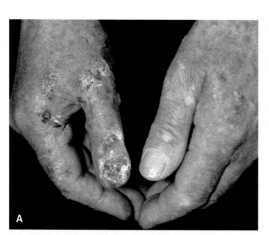
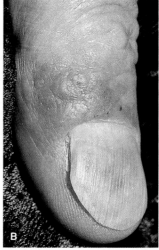

FIGURE 10-29 Radiation-induced squamous cell carcinoma (A) These are the hands of an elderly radiologist who decades ago had disregarded precautionary measures and hardly wore gloves doing fluoroscopic work. There are multiple x-ray keratoses; the hyperkeratotic lesion on the right thumb has destroyed the nail and represents x-ray-induced SCC. **(B)** Nail changes in the site of radiation exposure. Note the linear striations resulting from damage to the nail matrix. At the nailfold and extending proximally on the thumb, there is an irregular ery-thematous plaque that represents mostly SCC in situ but also focally invasive SCC.

PRECANCEROUS LESIONS AND CUTANEOUS CARCINOMAS

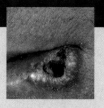

EPIDERMAL PRECANCERS AND CANCERS

Cutaneous epithelial cancers [nonmelanoma skin cancer (NMSC)] originate most commonly in the epidermal germinative keratinocytes or adnexal structures. The two principal NMSCs are basal cell carcinoma (BCC) and squamous cell carcinoma (SCC). SCC often has its origin in an identifiable in situ lesion that can be treated before frank invasion occurs. In contrast, in situ BCC is not known, but minimally invasive "superficial" BCCs are common.

The most common etiology of NMSC in fair-skinned individuals is sunlight, [ultraviolet radiation (UVR)], and human papillomavirus (HPV). Solar actinic keratoses are the most common precursor lesions of SCC in situ (SCCIS) and invasive SCC occurring at sites of chronic sun exposure in individuals of northern European heritage (see Section 10). UVR and HPV cause the spectrum of changes ranging from epithelial dysplasia to SCCIS to invasive SCC. Much less commonly, NMSC can be caused by ionizing radiation (arising in sites of chronic radiation damage), chronic inflammation, hydrocarbons (tar), and chronic ingestion of inorganic arsenic; these tumors can be much more aggressive than those associated with UVR or HPV. In the increasing population of immunosuppressed individuals (those with HIV/AIDS disease, solid organ transplant recipients, etc.), UVR- and HPV-induced SCCs are much more common and can be more aggressive.

ACTINIC KERATOSIS ICD-10: L57.0

- Single or multiple, discrete, dry, rough, or adherent scaly lesions on the habitually sun-exposed skin of adults, usually on a background of DHe.
- Actinic keratoses can progress to squamous cell carcinoma.
- *Synonym*: Solar keratosis.

EPIDEMIOLOGY

AGE OF ONSET Middle age, although in Australia and southwestern United States, solar keratoses may occur in persons <30 years.

SEX More common in males.

RACE SPT I, II, and III; rare in SPT IV; almost never in people with black skin.

OCCUPATION Outdoor workers (especially farmers, ranchers, and sailors) and outdoor sportspersons (tennis, golf, mountain climbing, and deep-sea fishing).

PATHOGENESIS

Prolonged and repeated solar exposure in susceptible persons (SPT I, II, and III) leads to cumulative damage to keratinocytes by the action of UVR, principally, if not exclusively, UVB (290 to 320 nm).

CLINICAL MANIFESTATION

SKIN SYMPTOMS Lesions may be tender. Painful if excoriated with a fingernail.

SKIN LESIONS Takes months to years to develop. Adherent hyperkeratotic scale, which is removed with difficulty and pain (Figs. 11-1 and 11-2). Skin-colored, yellow-brown, or a brown that appears "dirty"; often there is a reddish tinge. Rough, like coarse sandpaper, "better felt than seen" on palpation. Most commonly <1 cm, oval or round (Fig. 11-2).

Special Presentation. SPAK. This lesion is best described as "looks like lentigo maligna (LM) but feels like actinic keratosis" (Fig. 11-3). Uncommon. The distinctive features of SPAK include size (>1.5 cm), pigmentation (brown to black and variegated), and history of slow spreading, especially the verrucous surface. The lesion is important because it can mimic LM.

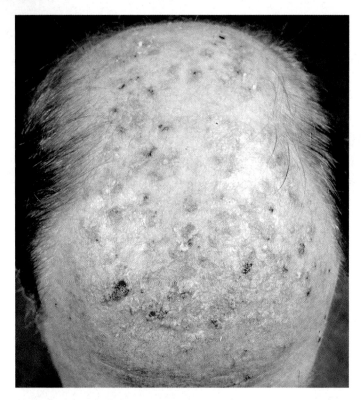

FIGURE 11-1 Erythematous and brownish macules and papules with coarse adherent scale became confluent on the bald scalp with dermatoheliosis These hyperkeratosis are yellowish to grey. Early lesions can be better felt than seen. Gentle abrasion with the fingernail is painful, a helpful diagnostic finding.

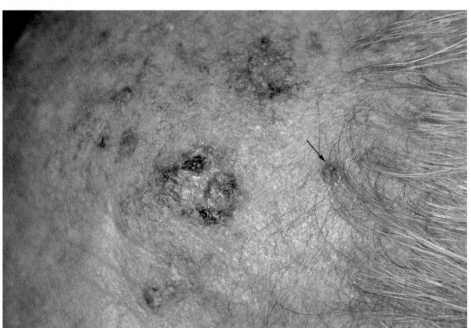

FIGURE 11-2 Actinic keratosis, close up. Greyish, dirty looking, tightly adherent scales
Abrading these hyperkeratosis is painful and leaves erosions. There is a small BCC at the border of the hairy scalp (*arrow*).

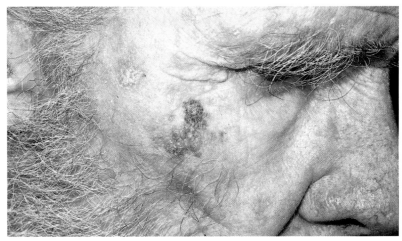

FIGURE 11-3 Spreading pigmented actinic keratosis (SPAK) "Looks like lentigo maligna" (Fig. 12-7) but "feels like actinic keratosis."

Distribution. Isolated single lesion or scattered discrete lesions. Face [forehead (Fig. 11-1), nose, cheeks], temples, vermilion border of lower lip], ears (in males), neck (sides), forearms, and hands (dorsa), shins, and the scalp in bald males (Figs. 11-1 and 11-2). Males with early pattern alopecia are especially prone to severe DHe and solar keratosis on the exposed scalp.

LABORATORY EXAMINATION

DERMATOPATHOLOGY Large bright-staining keratinocytes, with mild-to-moderate pleomorphism in the basal layer extending into follicles, atypical (dyskeratotic) keratinocytes, and parakeratosis.

DIAGNOSIS AND DIFFERENTIAL DIAGNOSIS

Usually made on clinical findings. Differential: Chronic cutaneous lupus erythematosus; seborrheic keratosis, flat warts, SCC (in situ), superficial BCC. Highly hyperkeratotic lesions and SPAK may require a biopsy to rule out SCC (in situ or invasive) or LM.

COURSE AND PROGNOSIS

Solar keratoses may disappear spontaneously, but in general it remains for years. The actual incidence of SCC arising in preexisting solar keratoses (Fig. 11-4) is unknown but is estimated at 1%.

MANAGEMENT

PREVENTION Avoided by use of highly effective UVB/UVA sunscreens.

Topical Therapy of Individual Lesions. *Cryosurgery. Also laser surgery.* Erbium or carbon dioxide lasers. Usually effective for individual lesions. For extensive facial lesions, facial resurfacing is effective. *Photodynamic Therapy.* Effective but painful and cumbersome.

Topical Field Therapy. This treats not only individual lesions but also inapparent early lesions. Therefore, a dermatitis results with many more erosions than there were visible actinic keratoses. The patient has to be warned that this will occur.

5-Fluorouracil (5-FU) Cream 5%. Effective, but difficult for many individuals. Treatment of facial lesions causes significant erythema and erosions, resulting in temporary cosmetic disfigurement. Efficacy can be increased if applied under occlusion and/or combined with topical tretinoin. However, this leads to confluent erosions. Reepithelialization occurs after treatment is discontinued.

Imiquimod (twice weekly for 16 weeks). Causes cytokine dermatitis, also leads to irritation and erosions but is highly effective.

Ingenolmebutat Gel (150 µg/g, 500 µg/g). Daily over three consecutive days leads to massive erosions but is highly effective.

Topical Retinoids. Used chronically, this is effective for prevention and treatment of DHe and superficial solar keratoses.

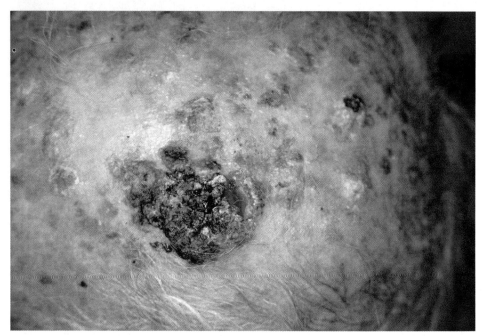

FIGURE 11-4 Solar keratoses and invasive squamous cell carcinoma Multiple, tightly adherent dirty looking solar keratoses. The large nodule shown here is covered by hyperkeratoses and hemorrhagic crusts; it is partially eroded and firm. This nodule is invasive squamous cell carcinoma. The image is shown to demonstrate the transition from precancerous lesions to frank carcinoma.

Diclofenac Gel. Used chronically, this only effective in superficial acting keratoses; also irritating.

Facial Peels. Trichloroacetic acid (5 to 10%) effective for widespread lesions.

EPITHELIAL PRECANCEROUS LESIONS AND SCCIS

Dysplasia of epidermal keratinocytes in epidermis and squamous mucosa can involve the lower portion of the epidermis or the full thickness. Basal cells mature into dysplastic keratinocytes resulting in a hyperkeratotic papule, or plaque, clinically identified as "keratosis." A continuum exists from dysplasia to SCCIS to invasive SCC. These lesions have various associated eponyms such as Bowen disease or erythroplasia of Queyrat, which as descriptive morphologic terms are helpful; terms such as UVR- or HPV-associated SCCIS, however, would be more meaningful but can be used only for those lesions with known etiology.

Epithelial precancerous lesions and SCCIS can be classified into *UV-induced* [solar (actinic) keratoses, lichenoid actinic keratoses, Bowenoid actinic keratoses, and Bowen disease (SCCIS)], *HPV-induced* [low-grade squamous intraepithelial lesions (HSIL) and Bowenoid papulosis (SCCIS)], *arsenical-induced* (palmoplantar keratoses, Bowenoid arsenical) keratosis, and *hydrocarbon (tar) keratoses* and *thermal keratoses.*

SOLAR OR ACTINIC KERATOSIS
(see the preceding discussion)

CUTANEOUS HORN ICD-10: L85.86

- A cutaneous horn (CH) is a *clinical* entity having the appearance of an animal horn with a papular or nodular base and a keratotic cap of various shapes and lengths (Fig. 11-5).
- CHs most commonly represent hypertrophic solar keratoses. Non-precancerous CH formation can also occur in seborrheic keratoses and warts.
- CHs usually arise within areas of dermatoheliosis on the face, ear, dorsum of the hands, or forearms, and shins.
- Clinically, CHs vary in size from a few millimeters to several centimeters (Fig. 11-5). The horn may be white, black, or yellowish in color and straight, curved, or spiral in shape.
- Histologically, there is usually hypertrophic actinic keratosis, SCCIS, or invasive SCC at the base. Because of the possibility of invasive SCC, a CH should always be excised.

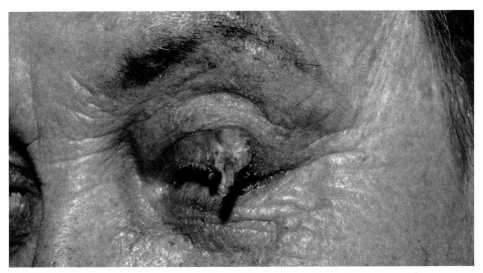

FIGURE 11-5 Cutaneous horn: hypertrophic actinic keratosis A hornlike projection of keratin on a slightly raised base in the setting of advanced dermatoheliosis on the upper eyelid in an 85-year-old female. Excision showed invasive SCC at the base of the lesion.

ARSENICAL KERATOSES ICD-10: L85.810

- Appear decades after chronic arsenic ingestion (medicinal, occupational, or environmental exposure). They have become very rare in industrialized countries but are currently being seen in West Bengal and Bangladesh where drinking water may still contain arsenic.
- Arsenical keratoses have the potential to become SCCIS or invasive SCC.
- Two types: Punctate, yellow papules on palms and soles (Fig. 11-6A); keratoses indistinguishable from actinic keratoses on the trunk and elsewhere. These are often associated with small SCCIS of the Bowen-type and hypopigmented slightly depressed macules ("raindrops in the dust") (Fig. 11-6B).
- Treatment—as for solar keratoses.

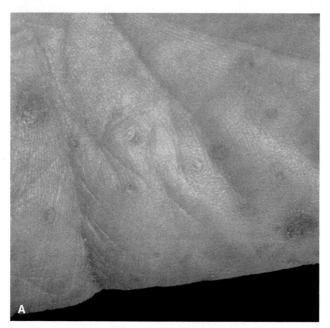

FIGURE 11-6 Arsenical keratoses (A) Multiple punctate, tightly adherent, and very hard keratoses on the palm. **(B)** Arsenical keratoses on the back. Multiple lesions are seen here ranging from red to tan, dark brown, and white. The brown lesions are a mix of arsenical keratoses (hard, rough) and small seborrheic keratoses (soft and smooth). The difference can be better felt than seen. The red lesions are small Bowenoid keratoses and Bowen disease (SCCIS, see Fig. 11-7). The white macular areas are slightly depressed and represent superficial atrophic scars from spontaneously shed or treated arsenical keratoses. The entire picture gives the impression of "rain drops in the dust."

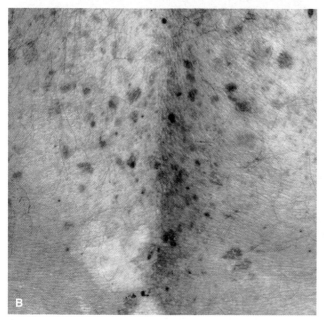

SQUAMOUS CELL CARCINOMA IN SITU ICD-10: C44.L48

- Presents as solitary or multiple macules, papules, or plaques, which may be hyperkeratotic or scaling.
- SCCIS is most often caused by UVR or HPV infection.
- Commonly arises in epithelial dysplastic lesions such as solar keratoses or HPV-induced squamous epithelial lesions (SIL) (see Section 27).
- Pink or red, sharply defined scaly plaques on the skin are called *Bowen disease;* similar but usually non-scaly lesions on the glans and vulva are called *erythroplasia* (see Section 33).
- Anogenital HPV-induced SCCIS is referred to as *Bowenoid papulosis.*
- Untreated SSCIS may progress to invasive SCC. With HPV-induced SCCIS in HIV/AIDS, lesions often resolve completely with successful antiretroviral therapy and immune reconstitution.
- Treatment is topical 5-fluorouracil, imiquimod, cryosurgery, CO_2 laser evaporation, or excision, including Mohs micrographic surgery.

ETIOLOGY

UVR, HPV, arsenic, tar, chronic heat exposure, and chronic radiation dermatitis.

CLINICAL MANIFESTATION

Lesions are most often asymptomatic but may bleed. Nodule formation or onset of pain or tenderness within SCCIS suggests progression to invasive SCC.

SKIN FINDINGS Appears as a sharply demarcated, scaling, or hyperkeratotic macule, papule, or plaque (Fig. 11-7). Pink or red in color, slightly scaling surface or erosions, and can be crusted. Solitary or multiple. Such lesions are called *Bowen disease* (Fig. 11-7).

Red, sharply demarcated, glistening macular or plaque-like SCCIS on the glans penis or labia minora are called *erythroplasia of Queyrat* (see Section 34). Anogenital HPV-induced SCCIS may be red, tan, brown, or black in color and are referred to as *Bowenoid papulosis* (see Section 34). Eroded lesions may have areas of crusting. SCCIS may go undiagnosed for years, resulting in large lesions with annular or polycyclic borders (Fig. 11-8). Once invasion occurs, nodular lesions appear within the plaque and the lesion is then commonly called *Bowen carcinoma* (Fig. 11-8).

Distribution. UVR-induced SCCIS commonly arises within a solar keratosis in the setting of photoaging (dermatoheliosis) (Fig. 11-9); HPV-induced SCCIS, mostly in the genital area but also periungually, most commonly on the thumb or in the nail bed (see Fig. 32-16). X-ray induced SCCIS in chronic radiodermatitis (see Fig. 10 29).

LABORATORY EXAMINATION

DERMATOPATHOLOGY Carcinoma in situ with loss of epidermal architecture and regular differentiation; keratinocyte polymorphism, single cell dyskeratosis, increased mitotic rate, and multinuclear cells. Epidermis may be thickened but basement membrane intact.

DIAGNOSIS AND DIFFERENTIAL DIAGNOSIS

Clinical diagnosis confirmed by dermatopathologic findings. Differential diagnosis includes all well-demarcated pink-red plaque(s): Nummular eczema, psoriasis, seborrheic keratosis, solar keratoses, verruca vulgaris, verruca plana, condyloma acuminatum, superficial BCC, amelanotic melanoma, and Paget disease.

COURSE AND PROGNOSIS

Untreated SCCIS will progress to invasive SCC (Fig. 11-8). In HIV/AIDS, it may resolve with successful antiretroviral therapy (ART). Lymph node metastasis can occur without demonstrable invasion. Metastatic dissemination from lymph nodes.

MANAGEMENT

TOPICAL CHEMOTHERAPY 5-*Fluorouracil* cream applied every day or twice daily, with or without tape occlusion, is effective. *Imiquimod* is also effective but both require considerable time.

CRYOSURGERY Highly effective. Lesions are usually treated more aggressively than solar keratoses, and superficial scarring will result.

PHOTODYNAMIC THERAPY Effective but time consuming and painful.

SURGICAL EXCISION INCLUDING MOHS MICRO-GRAPHIC SURGERY Has the highest cure rate but the greatest chance of causing cosmetically disfiguring scars. It should be done in all lesions where invasion cannot be excluded by biopsy.

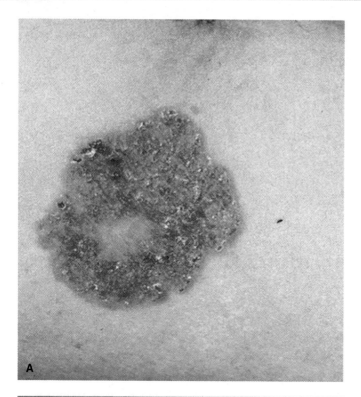

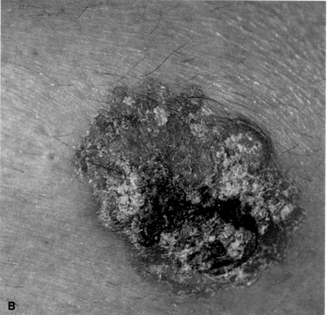

FIGURE 11-7 Squamous cell carcinoma in situ: Bowen disease
(**A**) A large, sharply demarcated, scaly, and erythematous plaque simulating a psoriatic lesion. (**B**) A similar psoriasiform plaque with a mix of
scales, hyperkeratosis, and hemorrhagic crusts on the surface.

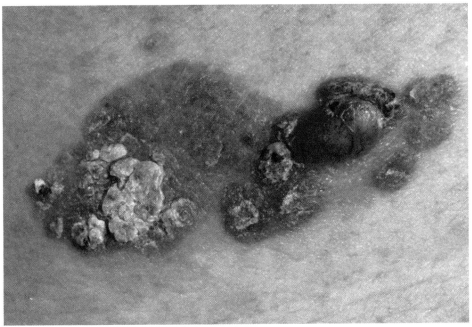

FIGURE 11-8 Squamous cell carcinoma in situ (SCCIS): Bowen disease and invasive SCC: Bowen carcinoma A red to orange plaque on the back, sharply defined, with irregular outlines and psoriasiform scale represents SCCIS, or Bowen disease. The red nodule on this plaque indicates that here the lesion is not anymore an in situ lesion but that invasive carcinoma has developed.

FIGURE 11-9 Squamous cell carcinoma: predilection sites.

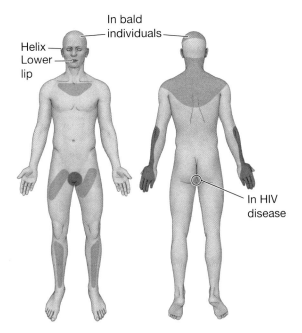

In bald
individuals

Helix
Lower
lip

In HIV
disease

INVASIVE SQUAMOUS CELL CARCINOMA ICD-10: C44.L48

- SCC of the skin is a malignant tumor of keratinocytes, arising in the epidermis.
- SCC usually arises in epidermal precancerous lesions (see the preceding discussion) and, depending on etiology and level of differentiation, varies in its aggressiveness.
- The lesion is a plaque or a nodule with varying degrees of keratinization in the nodule and/or on the surface. Thumb rule: Undifferentiated SCC is soft and has no hyperkeratosis; differentiated SCC is hard on palpation and has hyperkeratosis.
- The majority of UVR-induced lesions are differentiated and have a low rate of distant metastasis in otherwise healthy individuals. Undifferentiated SCC and SCC in immunosuppressed individuals are more aggressive with a greater incidence of metastasis.
- Treatment is by surgery.

EPIDEMIOLOGY AND ETIOLOGY

Ultraviolet Radiation

AGE OF ONSET Older than 55 years of age in Caucasians in the United States and Europe; in Australia, New Zealand, Florida, Southwest and Southern California, particularly Caucasians in their twenties and thirties.

INCIDENCE Continental United States: 12 per 100,000 white men; 7 per 100,000 white women. Hawaii: 62 per 100,000 whites.

SEX Males > females, but SCC can occur more frequently on the legs of females.

EXPOSURE Sunlight. Phototherapy and excessive photochemotherapy can lead to promotion of SCC, particularly in patients with skin phototypes I and II or in patients with history of previous exposure to ionizing radiation.

RACE Persons with white skin and poor tanning capacity (skin phototypes I and II) (see Section 10). Brown- or black-skinned persons can develop SCC from numerous etiologic agents other than UVR.

GEOGRAPHY Most common in areas that have many days of sunshine annually, i.e., in Australia and the Southwestern United States.

OCCUPATION Persons working outdoors—farmers, sailors, lifeguards, telephone line installers, construction workers, and dock workers.

Human Papillomavirus

Most commonly oncogenic HPV type-16, -18, -31 but also type-33, -35, -39, -40, and -51 to -60 are associated with SCCIS and invasive SCC. HPV-5, -8, -9 have also been isolated from SCCs.

Other Etiologic Factors

IMMUNOSUPPRESSION Solid organ transplant recipients, individuals with chronic immunosuppression of inflammatory disorders, and those with HIV disease are associated with an increased incidence of UVR- and HPV-induced SCCIS and invasive SCCs. SCCs in these individuals are more aggressive than in nonimmunosuppressed individuals.

CHRONIC INFLAMMATION Chronic cutaneous lupus erythematosus, chronic ulcers, burn scars, chronic radiation dermatitis, and lichen planus of oral mucosa.

INDUSTRIAL CARCINOGENS Pitch, tar, crude paraffin oil, fuel oil, creosote, lubricating oil, and nitrosoureas.

INORGANIC ARSENIC Trivalent arsenic had been used in the past in medications such as Asiatic pills, Donovan pills, and Fowler solution (used as a treatment for psoriasis or anemia). Arsenic is still present in drinking water in some geographic regions (West Bengal and Bangladesh).

CLINICAL MANIFESTATION

Slowly evolving—any isolated keratotic or eroded papule or plaque in a suspect patient that persists for over a month is considered a carcinoma until proven otherwise. Also, a nodule evolving in a plaque that meets the clinical criteria of SCCIS (Bowen disease), a chronically eroded lesion on the lower lip or on the penis, or nodular lesions evolving in or at the margin of a chronic venous ulcer or within chronic radiation dermatitis. Note that SCC usually is asymptomatic. Potential carcinogens often can be detected only after detailed history.

Rapidly evolving—invasive SCC can erupt within a few weeks and is often painful and/or tender.

For didactic reasons, two types can be distinguished:

1. Highly differentiated SCCs, which practically always show signs of keratinization either within or on the surface (hyperkeratosis) of the tumor. These are firm or hard upon palpation (Figs. 11-10 to 11-13).

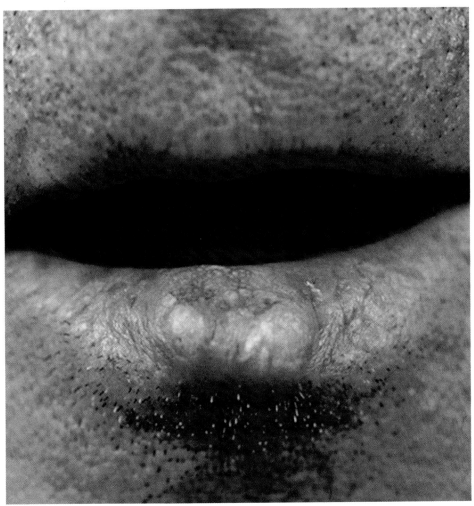

FIGURE 11-10 Squamous cell carcinoma: invasive on the lip A large but subtle nodule, which is better felt than seen, on the vermilion border of the lower lip with areas of yellowish hyperkeratosis. This nodule can be felt to infiltrate the entire lip.

2. Poorly differentiated SCCs, which do not show signs of keratinization and clinically appear fleshy, granulomatous, and consequently are soft upon palpation (Fig. 11-14).

Differentiated SCC

LESIONS Indurated papule, plaque, or nodule (Figs. 11-4, 11-10, and 11-11); adherent thick keratotic scale or hyperkeratosis (Figs. 11-4 and 11-12); when eroded or ulcerated, the lesion may have a crust in the center and a firm, hyperkeratotic, elevated margin (Figs. 11-11 and 11-12). Horny material may be expressed from the margin or the center of the lesion (Figs. 11-11, 11-12, and 11-13). Erythematous, yellowish skin color; hard; polygonal, oval, round, or umbilicated and ulcerated.

Distribution. Usually isolated but may be multiple. Usually exposed areas (Fig. 11-9). Sun-induced keratotic and/or ulcerated lesions especially on the bald scalp, cheeks, nose, lower lips, ears, preauricular area, dorsa of the hands (Fig. 11-13), forearms, trunk, and shins (females).

OTHER PHYSICAL FINDINGS Regional lymphadenopathy resulting from metastases.

SPECIAL FEATURES In UV-related SCC evidence of *dermatoheliosis* and *solar keratoses*. SCCs of the lips develop from leukoplasia or actinic

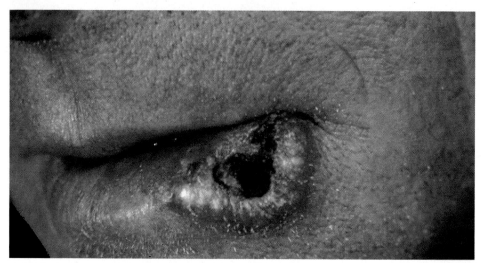

FIGURE 11-11 Squamous cell carcinoma (SCC) A round nodule, firm and indolent with a central black eschar. Note yellowish color in the periphery of the tumor indicating the presence of keratin. The SCC shown in **Figure 11-10** and here is hard and occurs on the lower lip. SCC hardly occurs on the upper lip because this is shaded from the sun. SCC on the lip is easily distinguished from nodular BCC because BCC does not develop hyperkeratosis or keratinization inside the tumor and does not occur on the vermilion lip.

cheilitis. In 90% of cases, they are found on the lower lip (Figs. 11-10 and 11-11). In chronic radiodermatitis, they arise from radiation-induced keratoses; in individuals with a history of chronic intake of arsenic, from arsenical keratoses. Differentiated (i.e., hyperkeratotic) SCC caused by HPV on genitalia; SCC resulting from excessive PUVA therapy on lower extremities (pretibial) or on genitalia. SCCs in scars from burns, in chronic stasis ulcers of long duration, and in sites of chronic inflammation are often difficult to identify. Suspicion is indicated when nodular lesions are hard and show signs of keratinization.

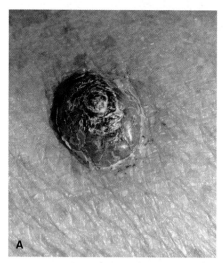

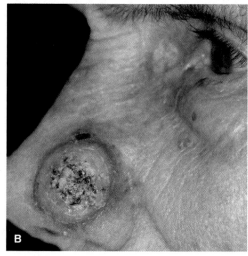

FIGURE 11-12 Squamous cell carcinoma, well differentiated (A) A nodule on the lower arm covered with a dome-shaped black hyperkeratosis. **(B)** A large, round, hard nodule on the nose with central hyperkeratosis. Neither lesion can be clinically distinguished from keratoacanthoma (see **Fig. 11-17**).

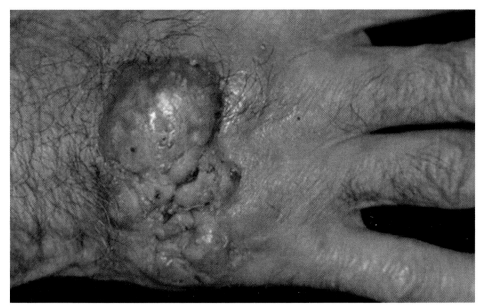

FIGURE 11-13 Squamous cell carcinoma, advanced, well differentiated, on the hand of a 65-year-old farmer The big nodule is smooth, very hard upon palpation, and shows a yellowish color, focally indicating keratin in the body of the nodule. When the lesion was incised in the yellowish areas, a yellowish-white material (keratin) could be expressed.

Special form: *carcinoma cuniculatum*, usually on the soles, highly differentiated, HPV-related but can also occur in other settings (Fig. 11-15); *verrucous carcinoma*, also florid oral papillomatosis, on the oral mucous membranes (see Section 33).

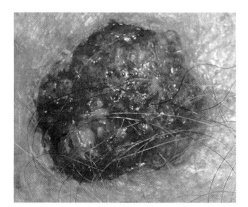

FIGURE 11-14 Squamous cell carcinoma, undifferentiated There is a circular, dome-shaped reddish nodule with partly eroded surface on the temple of a 78-year-old male. The lesion shows no hyperkeratoses and is soft and friable. When scraped, it bleeds easily.

HISTOPATHOLOGY SCCs with various grades of anaplasia and keratinization.

Undifferentiated SCC

LESIONS Fleshy, granulating, easily vulnerable, erosive papules and nodules, and papillomatous vegetations (Fig. 11-14). Ulceration with a necrotic base and soft, fleshy margin. Bleeds easily, crusting; red; soft; polygonal, irregular, often cauliflower-like.
Distribution. Isolated but also multiple, particularly on the genitalia, where they arise from erythroplasia and on the trunk (Fig. 11-8), lower extremities, or face, where they arise from Bowen disease.
MISCELLANEOUS OTHER SKIN CHANGES Lymphadenopathy as evidence of regional metastases is far more common than with differentiated, hyperkeratotic SCCs.
HISTOPATHOLOGY Anaplastic SCC with multiple mitoses and little evidence of differentiation and keratinization.

DIFFERENTIAL DIAGNOSIS

Any persistent nodule, plaque, or ulcer, but especially when these occur in sun-damaged skin, on the lower lips, in areas of radiodermatitis, in old burn scars, or on the genitalia, must

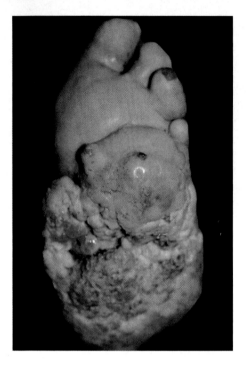

FIGURE 11-15 Squamous cell carcinoma (carcinoma cuniculatum) in a patient with peripheral neuropathy caused by leprosy A large fungating, partially necrotic, and hyperkeratotic tumor on the sole of the foot. The lesion had been considered a neuropathic ulcer, ascribed to leprosy, but continued growing and became elevated and ulcerated.

be examined for SCC. Keratoacanthoma (KA) may be clinically indistinguishable from differentiated SCC (see Keratoacanthoma, p. 238).

MANAGEMENT

SURGERY Depending on localization and extent of lesion, excision with primary closure, skin flaps, or grafting. Mohs micrographic surgery in difficult sites. Radiotherapy should be performed only if surgery is not feasible.

COURSE AND PROGNOSIS

RECURRENCE AND METASTASES SCC causes local tissue destruction and has a potential for metastases. Metastases are directed to regional lymph nodes and appear 1 to 3 years after initial diagnosis. In-transit metastases occur. In solid organ transplant recipients, metastasis can be present when SCC is diagnosed/detected or shortly after. SCC in the skin has an overall metastatic rate of 3 to 4%. High-risk SCCs are defined as having a diameter >2 cm, a level of invasion >4 mm, and Clark levels IV or V[1]; tumor involvement

[1]Clark level I: intraepidermal; level II: tumor invades papillary dermis; level III: tumor fills papillary dermis; level IV: tumor invades reticular dermis; level V: tumor invades subcutis.

of bone, muscle, and nerve (so-called neurotropic SCC, occurs frequently on the forehead and scalp); location on ear, lip, and genitalia; tumors arising in a scar or following ionizing radiation are usually highly undifferentiated. Cancers arising in chronic osteomyelitis sinus tracts, in burn scars, and in sites of radiation dermatitis have a metastatic rate of 31%, 20%, and 18% respectively. SCC arising in solar keratoses has the lowest potential for metastasis.

SCCS IN IMMUNOSUPPRESSION Organ transplant recipients have a markedly increased incidence of NMSCs, primarily high risk SCC, which is 40 to 50 times greater than in the general population. Risk factors include skin type, cumulative sun exposure, age at transplantation, male sex, HPV infections, the degree and length of immunosuppression, and the type of immunosuppressant. Lesions are often multiple, usually in sun-exposed sites but also in the genital, anal, and perigenital regions (Fig. 11-16). These tumors grow rapidly and are aggressive; in one series of heart-transplant patients from Australia, 27% died of skin cancer.

Patients with AIDS have only a slight increased risk of NMSC. In one series, a fourfold increase in their risk of developing lip SCC was noted. However, SCC of the anus is significantly increased in this population (see also Section 27).

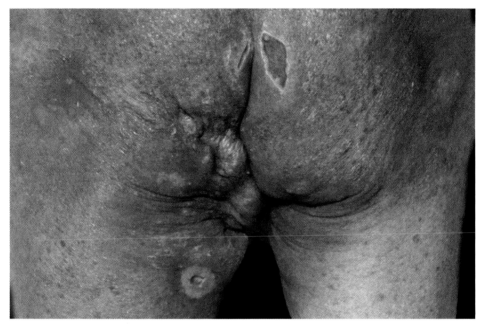

FIGURE 11-16 Squamous cell carcinomas in a renal transplant recipient on the upper thigh and buttocks There are multiple firm nodules, partially ulcerated. The patient had smaller, similar lesions elsewhere on the body. Since he had psoriasis and had spent considerable time in the sun, the lesions in the sun-exposed sides were probably caused by UVR. The lesion shown here was probably initiated by HPV as he had a similar lesion perianally and on the glans. The ulcer on the right buttock is an excision site from which sutures were prematurely removed.

KERATOACANTHOMA ICD-10: D23.L71

- KA is a special lesion; formerly considered a pseudocancer, it is now regarded by most as a variant of SCC.
- A relatively common, rapidly growing epithelial tumor with potential for tissue destruction and (rare) metastasis; however, in most cases there is spontaneous regression.
- HPV 9, -16, -19, -25, -37 have been identified in KAs; other possible etiologic factors include UVR and chemical carcinogens (pitch, tar).
- Age of onset over 40 years. Male: female ratio 2:1.
- A dome-shaped nodule with central keratotic plug (Fig. 11-17). Firm but not hard. Skin-colored, slightly red, brown. Removal of keratotic plaque results in a crater.
- Predilection for sun-exposed sites.
- Multiple KAs occur.
- Spontaneous regression in 6 to 12 months in most cases. However, local or visceral metastases have been detected.
- Histopathology: Not always possible to rule out highly differentiated SCC.
- Treatment is by excision.

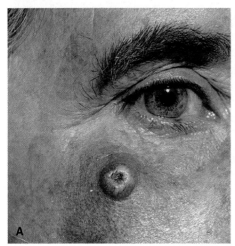
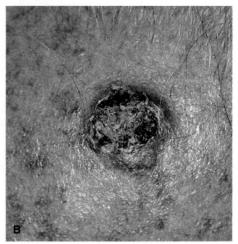

FIGURE 11-17 Keratoacanthoma showing different stages of evolution (A) Initially there is a round dome-shaped, very firm nodule, reddish with a central hyperkeratotic plug. This has been partially shed leaving a central crater. **(B)** Hyperkeratosis has progressed and has now replaced most of the nodule, leaving only a thin rim of tumor tissue in the periphery.

BASAL CELL CARCINOMA (BCC) ICD-10: C44.L21

- BCC is the most common cancer in humans.
- Caused by UVR; *PTCH* gene mutation in many cases.
- Clinically different types: nodular, ulcerating, pigmented, sclerosing, and superficial.
- BCC is locally invasive, aggressive, and destructive but slow growing, and there is very limited (literally no) tendency to metastasize.
- Treatment is by surgical excision, Mohs micrographic surgery, electrodesiccation, and curettage. Also cryosurgery and imiquimod cream.

EPIDEMIOLOGY

AGE OF ONSET Older than 40 years.
SEX Males > females.
INCIDENCE The most common cancer in humans. United States: 500 to 1,000 per 100,000, higher in the sunbelt; >400,000 new patients annually.
RACE Rare in brown- and black-skinned persons.

ETIOLOGY

UVR, mostly of the UVB spectrum (290 to 320 nm) that induces mutations in suppressor genes. The propensity for multiple BCC may be inherited. Associated with mutations in the *PTCH* gene in many cases.
PREDISPOSING FACTORS Skin phototypes I and II and albinos are highly susceptible to develop BCC with prolonged sun exposure.

Also, a history of heavy sun exposure in youth predisposes the skin to the development of BCC later in life. Previous therapy with x-rays for facial acne greatly increased the risk of BCC. Superficial multicentric BCC occurs 30 to 40 years after ingestion of arsenic but also without apparent cause.

CLINICAL MANIFESTATION

Slowly evolving, usually asymptomatic. Erosion or bleeding with minimal trauma may be the first symptom.
SKIN LESIONS There are five *clinical* types: nodular, ulcerating, pigmented, sclerosing (cicatricial), and superficial.

- *Nodular BCC*: Papule or nodule, translucent or "pearly." Skin-colored or reddish, smooth surface with telangiectasia, well defined, firm (Figs. 11-18 and 11-19). Portions of

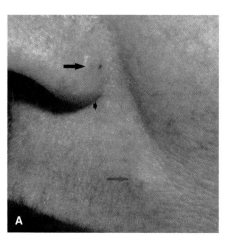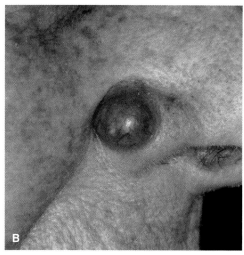

FIGURE 11-18 Basal cell carcinoma: nodular type (A) A small pearly papule (arrow) on the nostril and an even smaller one (small arrow) in the nasolabial fold. These are very early stages of BCC. The gray arrow denotes a dermal MN. **(B)** This is a further advanced nodular BCC. A solitary, shiny reddish nodule with large telangiectatic vessels on the ala nasi, arising on skin with dermatoheliosis.

nodular BCC may have erosions or stipples of melanin pigmentation.

- *Ulcerating BCC*: Ulcer (often covered with a crust) with a rolled border (rodent ulcer), which again is translucent, pearly, smooth with telangiectasia, and firm (Figs. 11-20 and 11-21).
- *Sclerosing BCC*: Appears as a small patch of morphea or a superficial scar, often ill defined, skin-colored, whitish but also with peppery pigmentation (Fig. 11-22). In this infiltrating type of BCC, there is an excessive amount of fibrous stroma. Histologically, finger-like strands of the tumor extend far into the surrounding tissue. Therefore, excision requires wide margins. Sclerosing BCC can progress to nodular or ulcerating BCC (Figs. 11-22B and 11-23).
- *Superficial multicentric BCCs*: Appear as thin plaques (Figs. 11-24 and 11-25). Pink or red; characteristic fine threadlike border and telangiectasia can be seen with the aid of a hand lens. This is the only form of BCC that can exhibit a considerable amount of scaling. This can also give rise to nodular

and ulcerating BCC (Fig. 11-25). BCC often bleeds with minimal excoriation. Solar keratosis, in comparison, does not bleed but is painful with excoriation.

- *Pigmented BCC*: May be brown to blue or black (Fig. 11-26). Smooth, glistening surface; hard, firm; may be indistinguishable from superficial spreading or nodular melanoma but is usually harder. *Cystic* lesions may occur: round, oval shape, depressed center ("umbilicated"). Stippled pigmentation can be seen in any of BCC types.

Distribution (Fig. 11-27). Isolated single lesion; multiple lesions are not infrequent; >90% occur in the face. Search carefully for "danger sites": medial and lateral canthi (Fig. 11-19), nasolabial fold (Fig. 11-18B), and behind the ears (Figs. 11-20B and 11-21). Superficial multicentric BCCs occur on the trunk (Figs. 11-24 and 11-25). BCC arises only from epidermis that has a capacity to develop (hair) follicles. Therefore, BCCs rarely occur on the vermilion border of the lips or on the genital mucous membranes.

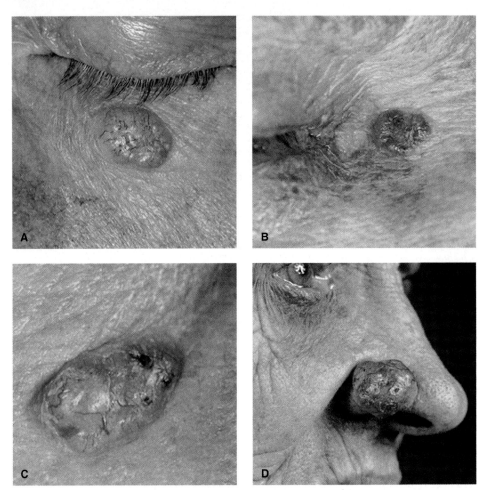

FIGURE 11-19 Basal cell carcinoma: nodular type (A) A glistening, smooth plaque on the lower eyelid with multiple telangiectasias. **(B)** An oval, pearly nodule on the nose close to the inner canthus. **(C)** A smooth, pearly tumor with telangiectasia below the lower eyelid. Tumor feels hard, is well defined, and is asymptomatic. **(D)** A large, firm reddish glistening nodule with small ulcerations on the nose.

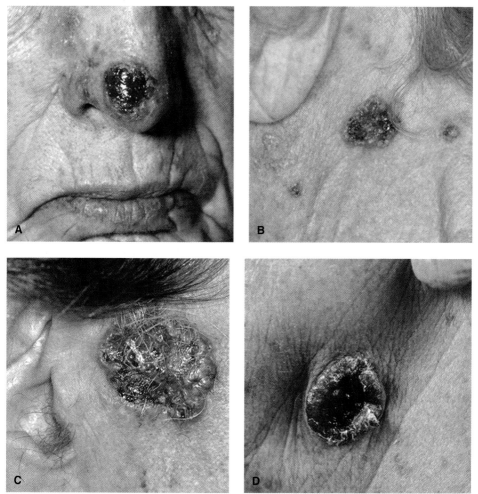

FIGURE 11-20 Basal cell carcinoma, ulcerated: Rodent ulcer (A) A large circular ulcer on the tip of the nose with a wall-like border. **(B)** A similar lesion in the retroauricular region. There is a rolled pearly border surrounding the ulcer. **(C)** Rodent ulcer in the preauricular region. A rolled pearly border surrounds an ulcer with yellow necroses and a tiny black crust. **(D)** A deep ulcer with a surrounding rolled border, smooth, glistening, and partly covered with crusts in the mandibular region. All these lesions are hard upon palpation.

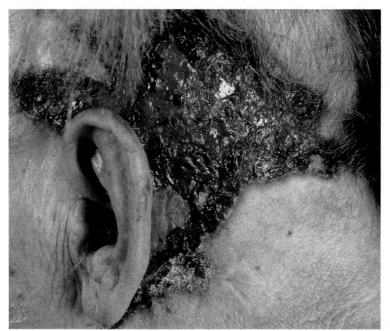

FIGURE 11-21 A large rodent ulcer in the nuchal and retroauricular area extending to the temple The entire lesion consists of a firm granulating tissue, partially covered by hemorrhagic crusts. The diagnosis can be made only by examining the border, which is rolled, elevated, firm, and smooth.

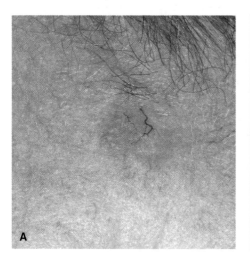

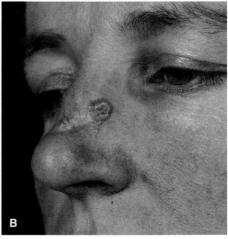

FIGURE 11-22 Basal cell carcinoma: sclerosing type (A) A small inconspicuous area resembling superficial morphea, ill defined, and yellowish with telangiectasia. Upon palpation, however, a platelike induration can be felt and this extends beyond the visible margins of the lesion. After verification of the diagnosis by biopsy, it will require excision with wide margins. **(B)** A large depressed area resembling a scar on the nose; on the right (lateral) and medial margins of this "scar," there is the typical rolled border of a nodular BCC. This lesion is shown to demonstrate that sclerosing and nodular BCC are simply two different growth patterns.

FIGURE 11-23 Basal cell carcinoma (BCC), sclerosing, nodular, and ulcerating A large lesion, which looks like morphea and is whitish and firm upon palpation but within the level of the skin, is found on the temple and in the supraciliary region. Within the lesion and at the margins, there are small nodules of BCCs. On the lateral canthus of the eye, there is a large ulcer with rolled borders representing a rodent ulcer. Again this figure is shown to demonstrate that the different types of BCC are just different growth patterns.

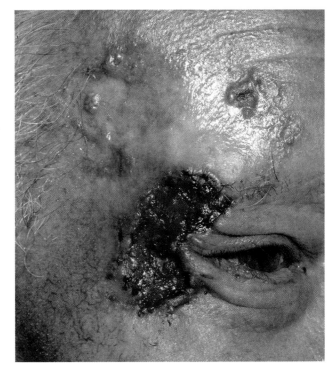

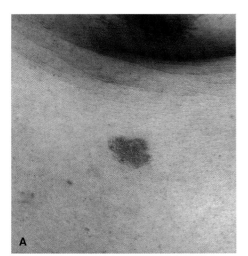

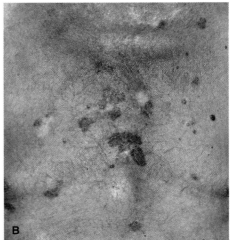

FIGURE 11-24 Superficial basal cell carcinoma (BCC): solitary lesion and multiple lesions
(A) This bright red lesion has a slightly elevated rolled border that can be detected with "side lighting"; although this lesion is typical enough to be diagnosed clinically, a biopsy is necessary to verify the diagnosis. **(B)** Many superficial BCCs on the trunk. They appear as brightly erythematous, often scaling, flat lesions, often without a rolled border. The hypopigmented areas represent superficial scars after cryotherapy of superficial BCCs.

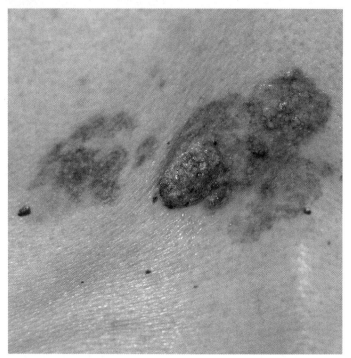

FIGURE 11-25 Superficial basal cell carcinoma (BCC), invasive There are two irregular red areas with rolled borders and central telangiectasia. In the larger lesion, the BCC is elevated with an irregular surface and now assumes the morphology and growth behavior of a nodular BCC; on the right, the lesion is erosive and will progress to an ulcer.

LABORATORY EXAMINATION

DERMATOPATHOLOGY Solid tumor consisting of proliferating atypical basal cells, large, oval, deep-blue staining on H&E, but with little anaplasia and infrequent mitoses; palisading arrangement at periphery; variable amounts of mucinous stroma.

DIAGNOSIS AND DIFFERENTIAL DIAGNOSIS

Serious BCCs occurring in the danger sites (central part of the face, behind the ears) are readily detectable by careful examination with good lighting, a hand lens, and careful palpation and dermoscopy. Diagnosis is made clinically and confirmed microscopically. Differential diagnosis includes all smooth papules such as dermal melanocytic nevi, trichoepithelioma, dermatofibroma, and others; if pigmented, superficial spreading and nodular melanoma; if ulcerated, all nonpainful firm ulcers including SCC and a primary chancre of syphilis.

MANAGEMENT

Excision with primary closure, skin flaps, or grafts. Cryosurgery and electrosurgery are options, but only for very small lesions and not in the danger sites or on the scalp.

For lesions in the danger sites (nasolabial area, around the eyes, in the ear canal, in the posterior auricular sulcus, and on the scalp) and sclerosing BCC, microscopically controlled surgery (Mohs surgery) is the best approach. Radiation therapy is an alternative only when disfigurement may be a problem with surgical excision (e.g., eyelids or large lesions in the nasolabial area) or in very old age.

There are a variety of topical treatments that can be used for superficial BCCs but only for those tumors below the neck; *cryosurgery* is effective but leaves a white scar that remains for life. Electrocautery with curettage is also simple and effective, but it leaves scars and should be used only in small lesions. Topical 5-fluorouracil ointment and imiquimod cream for superficial BCC, 5 times a week for 6 weeks,

FIGURE 11-26 Basal cell carcinoma (BCC), pigmented (A) A nodule with irregular borders and variegation of melanin hues easily confused with a malignant melanoma. Only histology will yield the correct diagnosis. **(B)** A similar black nodule but with central ulceration. This pigmented BCC is clinically also indistinguishable from nodular melanoma.

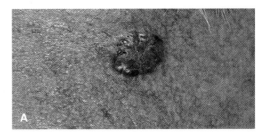

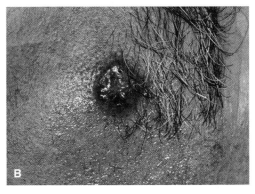

FIGURE 11-27 Basal cell carcinoma (BCC): predilection sites Dots indicate superficial multicentric BCCs.

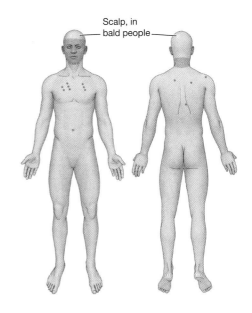

Scalp, in bald people

are effective, do not cause visible scars, but require considerable time and may not radically remove all the tumor tissue. Both require compliance by patient or caregiver. Imiquimod is especially good for young persons who do not want scars. Photodynamic therapy is effective only in very superficial lesions and radiation sessions (photodynamic dye + visible light) are painful.

COURSE AND PROGNOSIS

BCC does not metastasize. The reason for this is the tumor's growth dependency on its stroma, which on invasion of tumor cells into the

vessels is not disseminated with the tumor cells. When tumor cells lodge at distant sites, they do not multiply and grow because of the absence of growth factors derived from their stroma. Exceptions occur when a BCC shows signs of dedifferentiation, for instance, after inadequate radiotherapy. Most lesions are readily controlled by various surgical techniques. Serious problems, however, may occur with BCC arising in the danger sites of the head. In these sites, the tumor may invade deeply, cause extensive destruction of muscle and bone, and even invade to the dura mater. In such cases, death may result from hemorrhage of eroded large vessels or infection but vismodegib is effective.

BASAL CELL NEVUS SYNDROME (BCNS) ICD-10: Q82.804

- This autosomal-dominant disorder is caused by mutations in the patched gene that resides on chromosome 9q (9q22).
- It affects skin with multiple BCCs (Fig. 11-28) and so-called palmoplantar pits (Fig. 11-29) and has a variable expression of abnormalities in a number of systems, including skeletal malformations, soft tissue, eyes, CNS, and endocrine organs.
- Occurs mostly in white pigment skin but also in brown- and black pigments, and there is an equal sex incidence.
- BCCs begin in childhood or early adolescence and continue throughout life.
- There are more BCCs on the sun-exposed areas of the skin, but they also occur in covered areas and there may be hundreds of lesions.
- Characteristic general features are frontal bossing, a broad nasal root, and hypertelorism (Fig. 11-28). Systems review: Congenital anomalies including undescended testes and hydrocephalus, mandibular jaw odontogenic keratocysts, which may be multiple and may be unilateral or bilateral. Defective dentition, bifid or splayed ribs, pectus excavatum, short fourth metacarpals, scoliosis, and kyphosis. Eye lesions include strabismus, hypertelorism, dystopia canthorum, cataracts, glaucoma, and coloboma with blindness. There may be agenesis of the corpus callosum, calcification of the falx, and medulloblastoma. However, mental retardation is rare. Fibrosarcoma of the jaw, ovarian fibromas, teratomas, and cystadenomas have been reported.
- *Skin lesions* are small, pinpoint to larger nodular BCCs (Fig. 11-28), but "regular," nodular, ulcerating, and sclerosing BCCs also occur. Tumors on the eyelids, axillae, and neck tend to be pedunculated and are often symmetric on the face. There are characteristic palmoplantar lesions, which are present in 50% of cases and are small pits that are pinpoint to several millimeters in size and 1 mm deep (Fig. 11-29).
- The significance of the syndrome is that a large number of skin cancers create a lifetime problem of vigilance. The multiple excisions can cause a considerable amount of scarring. The tumors continue throughout life so the patient must be followed carefully.
- *Synonyms*: Gorlin syndrome, nevoid BCC syndrome.

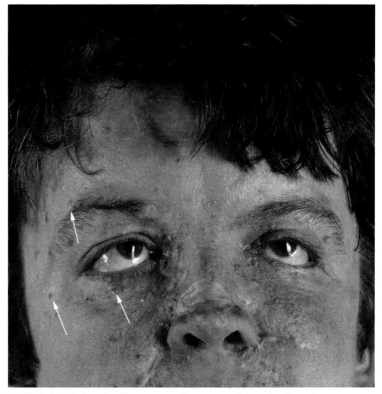

FIGURE 11-28 Basal cell nevus syndrome: small basal cell carcinomas (BCC) Small reddish papular lesions are dispersed over the entire face, three are marked with an arrow. All of these represent small BCCs. Note considerable scarring from removal of previous lesions. Note also frontal bossing and strabism.

FIGURE 11-29 Basal cell nevus syndrome: palmar pits Palmar surface of hand showing 1- to 2-mm, sharply marginated, depressed lesions, i.e., palmar pits.

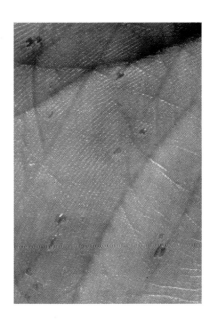

MALIGNANT APPENDAGE TUMORS ICD-10: C44.L6

- Carcinomas of the eccrine sweat gland are rare and include eccrine porocarcinoma, syringoid eccrine carcinoma, mucinous carcinoma, and clear cell eccrine carcinoma.
- Carcinomas of the apocrine glands are also rare, arising in axillae, nipples, vulva, and the eyelids.
- Carcinomas of the sebaceous glands are equally rare, most commonly arising on the eyelids.
- These lesions are clinically indistinguishable from other carcinomas and are usually more aggressive than other invasive cutaneous SCCs.

MERKEL CELL CARCINOMA ICD-10: C44.L44

- Merkel cell carcinoma (MCC) (cutaneous neuroendocrine tumor) is a rare malignant solid tumor thought to be derived from a specialized epithelial cell, the Merkel cell. It is a nonkeratinizing, "clear" cell present in the basal cell layer of the epidermis, free in the dermis, and around hair follicles as the hair disk of Pinkus.
- MCC occurs almost exclusively in white skin.
- MCC is 10 to 30 times as common in immunosuppressed patients as in nonimmunosuppressed patients.
- The etiology is unknown but may be related to chronic UVR damage. Polyoma virus has been found in 80% of MCC.
- The tumor may be solitary or multiple and occurs on the head and on the extremities.
- There is a high rate of recurrence following excision, but, more importantly, it spreads to the regional lymph nodes in >50% of patients and is disseminated to the viscera and CNS.
- MCC presents as a cutaneous to subcutaneous papule, nodule, or tumor (0.5 to 5 cm) (Figs. 11-30 and 11-31), which is pink, red to violet or reddish-brown, dome-shaped, and usually solitary. The overlying skin is intact, but larger lesions may ulcerate.
- They grow rapidly and usually occur in persons >50 years.
- Dermatopathology shows nodular or diffuse patterns of aggregated, deeply blue staining, small basaloid or lymphoma-like-looking cells that can also be arranged in sheets forming nests, cords, and trabeculae.
- Immunocytochemistry shows cytokeratin and neurofilament markers, chromogranin A, and neuron-specific enolase; electron microscopy reveals characteristic organelles.
- Treatment is by excision or Mohs surgery, and sentinel node biopsy or prophylactic regional node dissection is advocated because of the high rate of regional metastases. Radiation therapy to the site of MCC and regional LN is given in most cases except for very small lesions.
- Recurrence rates are high; in one series, even without a local recurrence, about 60% of patients developed regional node metastases, as did 86% of those patients with a local recurrence. Prognosis is guarded.

FIGURE 11-30 Merkel cell carcinoma A small violaceous nodule above the pinna that had been present for about 2 weeks. Sentinel lymph node biopsy revealed metastasis of neuroendocrine carcinoma. Also note actinic keratoses on the helix and concha.

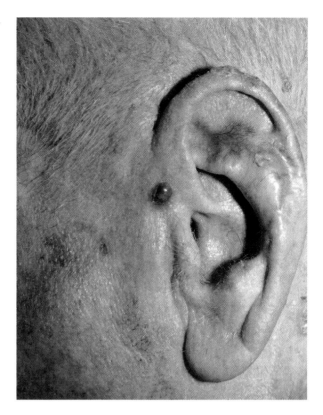

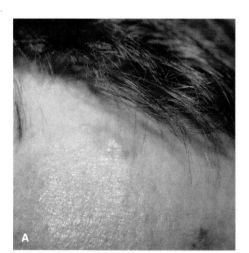

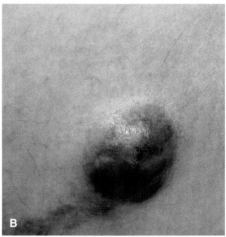

FIGURE 11-31 Merkel cell carcinoma **(A)** A barely noticeable 6-mm slightly dermal nodule below the hairline that had been present for about 6 weeks. Preauricular lymph node metastasis was also present. **(B)** A violaceous dermal nodule, 3 cm in diameter on the forearm of a 60-year-old man. There was metastasis to the axillary lymph nodes.

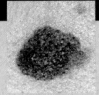

MELANOMA PRECURSORS AND PRIMARY CUTANEOUS MELANOMA

PRECURSORS OF CUTANEOUS MELANOMA

Precursors of melanoma are lesions that are benign per se but have the potential of turning malignant and thus giving rise to melanoma. Two such entities are recognized: (1) dysplastic melanocytic nevi and (2) congenital melanocytic nevi.

DYSPLASTIC MELANOCYTIC NEVUS (DN) ICD-10: D48–54

- Dysplastic nevi (DN) are a special type of acquired, circumscribed, pigmented lesions that represent disordered proliferations of variably atypical melanocytes.
- DN arise de novo or as part of a melanocytic nevus.
- DN are clinically distinctive from common acquired nevi: Larger and more variegated in color, asymmetric in outline, and with irregular borders; they also have characteristic histologic features.
- DN are regarded as potential precursors of superficial spreading melanoma (SSM) and also as markers of persons at risk for developing primary melanoma of the skin, either within the DN or on normal skin.
- DN occur either sporadically or in the context of the *familial DN syndrome*: Kindreds with familial multiple DN and melanomas (formerly FAMMM, or B-K mole syndrome).
- *Synonyms*: atypical melanocytic nevus.

EPIDEMIOLOGY

AGE OF ONSET Children and adults.
PREVALENCE DN are present in 5% of the general white population. They occur in almost every patient with familial cutaneous melanoma and in 30 to 50% of patients with sporadic nonfamilial primary melanomas of the skin.
SEX Equal in males and females.
RACE White persons. Data on persons with brown or black skin are not available; DN are rarely seen in the Japanese population.
TRANSMISSION Autosomal dominant.

PATHOGENESIS

Multiple loci have been implicated in familial melanoma/DN syndrome, and it is likely that DN is a complex heterogeneous trait. It is assumed that an abnormal clone of melanocytes can be activated by exposure to sunlight. Immunosuppressed patients (renal transplantation) with DN have a higher incidence of melanoma. DN favor the exposed areas of the skin, particularly intermittently sun exposed (e.g., back) and this may be related to the degree of sun exposure. However, DN may also occur in completely covered areas.

CLINICAL MANIFESTATION

DURATION OF LESIONS DN usually arises later in childhood than common acquired MN, which first appear in late childhood, just before puberty. New lesions continue to develop over many years in affected persons; in contrast, common acquired MN do not appear after middle age and disappear entirely in older persons. DN are thought not to undergo spontaneous regression at much less than common acquired MN. Also, whereas common MN are usually in a roughly comparable stage of development in a given body region (e.g., junctional, compound, dermal), DN appear "*out of step*," e.g., a mix of large and small, flat and raised, tan, and very dark lesions (Fig. 12-1A).

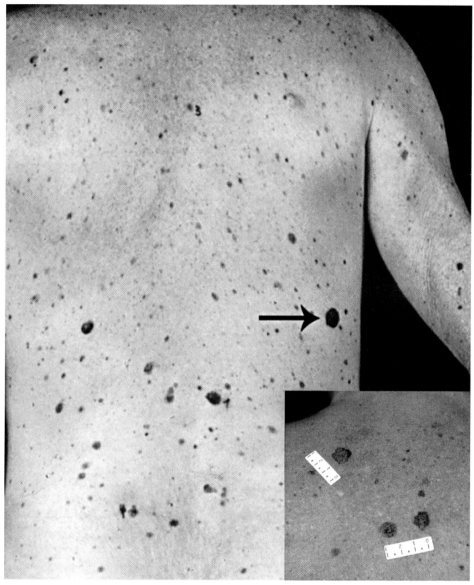

FIGURE 12-1 Dysplastic nevi Overview of the back of a patient with common and dysplastic nevi. Note a number of lesions are of different size and color, "out of step." The lesion marked by an arrow was an SSM. <u>Insert</u>: Larger magnification of three DNs. Note irregularity and variegation of color that are different in the three lesions ("out of step"). Also, the lesions are 1 cm or larger in diameter. The smaller lesions are common MN.

TABLE 12-1 Comparative Features of Common Melanocytic Nevi (MN), Dysplastic Nevi (DN), and Superficial Spreading Melanoma (SSM)

Lesion	MN (Figs. 9-1 to 9-4)	DN (Figs. 12-1 and 12-2)	SSM (Figs. 12-8, 12-12, and 12-13)
Number	Several or many	One or many	Single (1–2% have multiple)
Distribution	Mostly trunk, extremities	Mostly trunk, extremities	Anywhere but predominant upper back, legs
Onset	Childhood, adolescence	Early adolescence	Any age, most in adulthood
Type	Macules (junctional) Papules (compound, dermal)	Macules with raised portions (asymmetrically, maculopapular)	Plaque, irregular
A Asymmetry	Symmetry	Asymmetry	Greater asymmetry
B Border	Regular, well defined	Irregular, ill and well defined	Irregular, well defined
C Color	Tan, brown, dark brown, uniform, orderly pattern	Tan, brown, dark brown, pink, red, not uniform, variegated pattern, "fried egg," "targetoid"	Tan, brown, dark brown, black, pink, red, blue, white, usually a mix, highly variegated, spotted, speckled pattern
D Diameter	<5 mm, rarely up to <10 mm	Up to 15 mm	Most >5 mm (but, of course, starts smaller)
E Enlargement	Stops in adolescence	Continues in adulthood but limited	Growth in size at any age, unlimited

SKIN SYMPTOMS Asymptomatic.

FAMILY HISTORY In the familial setting, family members can develop melanoma without the presence of DN.

CLINICAL FEATURES DN show some of the features of common MN and some of SSM, so that they occupy an intermediary position between these two morphologies (Table 12-1). No single feature is diagnostic; rather there is a constellation of findings. They are more irregular, lighter than common MN, usually maculopapular; have distinct *and* indistinct borders (Figs. 12-1 and 12-2), and a greater complexity of color than common nevi (Figs. 12-1 and 12-2) but less than melanoma. There are "fried-egg" and "targeted" types (Fig. 12-2 and Table 12-1). Melanoma arising in a DN appears initially as a small papule (often of a different color) or change in color pattern and massive color change within the precursor lesion (Fig. 12-3).

DERMOSCOPY This noninvasive technique allows for clinical improvement of diagnostic accuracy in DN by >70%. *Digital dermoscopy* permits computerized follow-up of lesions and immediate detection of any change over time, indicating developing malignancy.

LABORATORY EXAMINATION

DERMATOPATHOLOGY Hyperplasia and proliferation of melanocytes in a single-file, "lentiginous" pattern in the basal cell layer either as spindle cells or as epithelioid cells, and as irregular and dyshesive nests. "Atypical" melanocytes, "bridging" between rete ridges by melanocytic nests; spindle-shaped melanocytes oriented parallel to skin surface. Lamellar fibroplasia and concentric eosinophilic fibrosis (not a constant feature). Histologic atypia do not always correlate with clinical atypia. DN may arise in contiguity with a compound MN (rarely, a junctional nevus) that is centrally located.

DIAGNOSIS AND DIFFERENTIAL DIAGNOSIS

The diagnosis of DN is made by clinical recognition of typical distinctive lesions (see Table 12-1) and diagnostic accuracy is

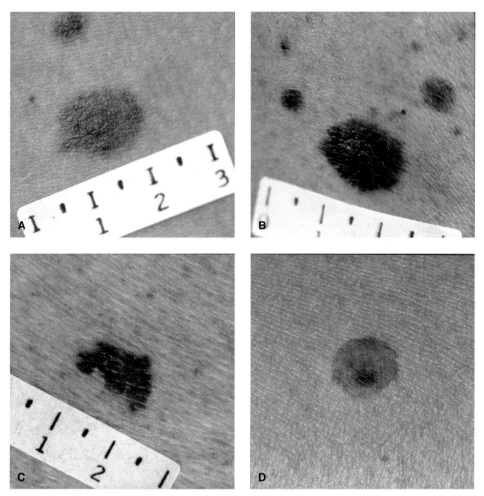

FIGURE 12-2 Dysplastic nevi (A) A large, uniformly tan, very flat macular oval lesion. The notched border on the left and the size (>1 cm) are the only criteria making this suspicious of a DN. **(B)** Though relatively symmetric, this lesion is macular and papular with a variegated color and measures 1.5 cm in diameter. The smaller lesions are common MN. **(C)** A highly asymmetric, both ill- and sharply defined margin, a notched border, and variegated brown to black color. It is clinically indistinguishable from an SSM (see Figs. 12-12A, B) but was histologically a DN. **(D)** A relatively symmetric sharply defined lesion with an eccentric, more heavily pigmented area (targetoid lesion).

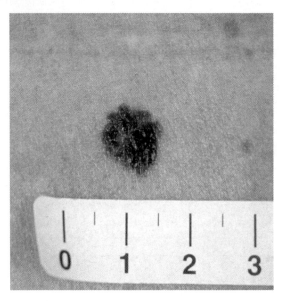

FIGURE 12-3 Superficial spreading melanoma: arising within a dysplastic nevus The entire lesion originally was maculopapular and had the brown color still seen on the upper crescent-like rim. At a follow-up visit 6 years later, the center and lower half of the lesion had become more raised and turned black as shown here. Melanoma had evolved from a DN. Verified by histopathology.

considerably improved by dermoscopy. The clinicopathologic correlations are now well documented. Siblings, children, and parents should also be examined for DN once the diagnosis is established in a family member.

DIFFERENTIAL DIAGNOSIS Congenital MN, common acquired MN, superficial spreading melanoma, melanoma in situ (MIS), lentigo maligna, Spitz nevus, and pigmented basal cell carcinoma.

ASSOCIATION WITH MELANOMA DN are regarded both as markers for persons at risk for melanoma and as precursors of SSM. Anatomic association (in contiguity) of DN has been observed in 36% of sporadic primary melanomas, in about 70% of familial primary melanomas, and in 94% of melanomas with familial melanoma and DN.

Lifetime Risks of Developing Primary Malignant Melanoma

- General population: 1.2%.
- Familial DN syndrome with *two* blood relatives with melanoma: 100%.
- All other patients with DN: 18%.

- The presence of *one* DN doubles the risk for development of melanoma; with ≥10 DN, the risk increases 12-fold.

MANAGEMENT

Surgical excision of lesions with narrow margins. Laser or other types of physical destruction should *never* be used because they do not permit histopathologic verification of diagnosis.

Patients with DN in the familial melanoma setting need to be followed carefully: In familial DN, every 3 months; in sporadic DN, every 6 months to 1 year. Photographic follow-up is important. Most reliable method is digitalized dermoscopy, which should be available in every pigmented lesion and melanoma center. Patients should be given color-illustrated pamphlets that depict the clinical appearance of DN, malignant melanoma, and common acquired MN. Patients with DN (familial and nonfamilial) should not sunbathe and should use sunscreens when outdoors. They should not use tanning parlors. Family members of the patient should also be examined regularly.

CONGENITAL MELANOCYTIC NEVUS (CMN) ICD-10: D22

- CMN are pigmented lesions of the skin usually present at birth; rare varieties of CMN can develop and become clinically apparent during infancy.
- CMN may be any size from very small to very large.
- CMN are benign nevomelanocytic neoplasms.
- However, all CMN, regardless of size, may be precursors of malignant melanoma.

EPIDEMIOLOGY

PREVALENCE Present in 1% of white newborns; the majority <3 cm in diameter. Larger CMN are present in 1:2000 to 1:20,000 newborns. Lesions ≥9.9 cm in diameter have a prevalence of 1:20,000, and giant CMN (occupying a major portion of a major anatomic site) occur in 1:500,000 newborns and are thus very rare.

AGE OF ONSET Present at birth (congenital). Some CMN become visible only after birth (*tardive*), "fading in" as a relatively large lesion over a period of weeks.

SEX Equal prevalence in males and females.

RACE All races.

PATHOGENESIS

Presumably they occur as the result of a developmental defect in neural crest–derived melanoblasts. This defect probably occurs after 10 weeks in utero but before the sixth uterine month; the occurrence of the "split" nevus of the eyelid, i.e., half of the nevus on the upper and half on the lower eyelid, is an indication that melanocytes migrating from the neural crest were in place in this site before the eyelids split (24 weeks).

SMALL AND LARGE CMN CMN have a rather wide range of clinical features, but the following are typical (Figs. 12-4 and 12-5). CMN usually distort the skin surface to some degree and are therefore a plaque with or without coarse terminal dark brown or black hairs (hair growth has a delayed onset) (Figs. 12-4B and 12-5B). Sharply demarcated (Fig. 12-4) or merging imperceptibly with surrounding skin; regular or irregular contours. Large lesions may be "wormy" or soft (Fig. 12-5), rarely firm (desmoplastic type). Skin surface smooth or "pebbly," mamillated, rugose, cerebriform, bulbous, tuberous, or lobular (Fig. 12-5B). These surface changes are observed more frequently in lesions that extend deep into the reticular dermis.

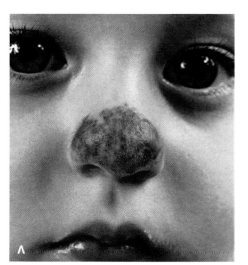 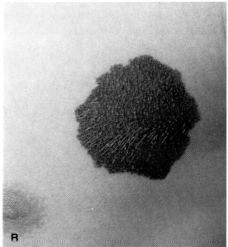

FIGURE 12-4 Congenital nevomelanocytic nevus (A) Small, variegated brown plaque on the nose. The lesion was present at birth. **(B)** Congenital melanocytic nevus, intermediate size. (compare size with mamilla) Sharply demarcated chocolate-brown plaque with sharply defined borders in an infant. With increasing age, lesions may become elevated and hairy and very discrete hairiness is also noted in this lesion.

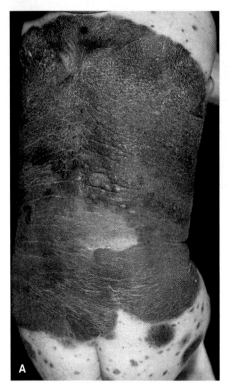
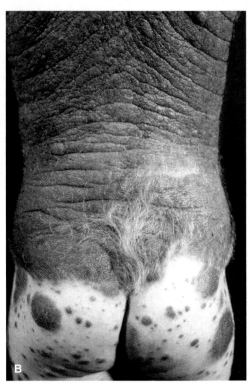

FIGURE 12-5 A Giant congenital nevomelanocytic nevus (A) In this baby the lesion involves the majority of the skin, with complete replacement of normal skin on the back and multiple smaller CMN on the buttocks and thighs. There is hypertrichosis in the lower portion. Melanoma developing in a giant CMN is difficult to diagnose early in a setting of such highly abnormal tissue. **(B)** Giant CMN in the same child 5 years later. The CMN has thickened and has become rugose and more hairy in the sacral region. The lesion is now lighter, i.e. more brown than black and the smaller CMN on the buttocks have increased in size and number.

Color. Light or dark brown, black. With dermoscopy, a fine speckling of a darker hue with a lighter surrounding brown hue is seen; often the pigmentation is follicular. "Halo" CMN are rare.

Size. Small (Fig. 12-4), large (>20 cm), or giant (Fig. 12-5). Acquired MN >1.5 cm in diameter should be regarded as probably tardive CMN or they represent DN.

Shape. Oval or round.

Distribution of Lesions. Isolated, discrete lesion in any site. Fewer than 5% of CMN are multiple. Multiple lesions are more common in association with large CMN. Numerous small CMN occur in patients with giant CNMN, in whom there may be numerous small CMN on the trunk and extremities away from the site of the giant CMN (Fig. 12-5).

Very Large ("Giant") CMN

Giant CNMN of the head and neck may be associated with involvement of the leptomeninges with the same pathologic process; this presentation may be asymptomatic or manifested by seizures, focal neurologic defects, or obstructive hydrocephalus. Giant CMN is usually a plaque with surface distortion, covering entire segments of the trunk, extremities, head, or neck (Fig. 12-5).

Melanoma in CMN

A papule or nodule arises within CMN (Fig. 12-6). Often melanoma arises in dermal or subcutaneous nevomelanocytes and can be far advanced when detected.

DIFFERENTIAL DIAGNOSIS

Common acquired MN, DN, congenital blue nevus, nevus spilus, Becker nevus, pigmented epidermal nevi, and café-au-lait macules should be considered in the differential diagnosis of CMN. Small CMN are virtually indistinguishable

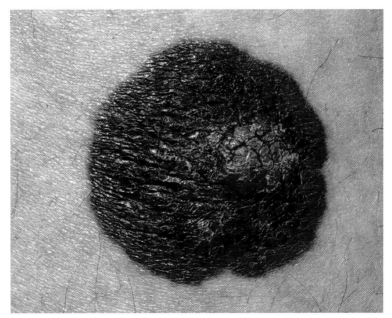

FIGURE 12-6 Melanoma: arising in small CNMN A black plaque on the thigh of a 36-year-old female, which has been present since birth. Recently, a slightly less pigmented excentric nodule had appeared in this lesion. This is a melanoma.

clinically from common acquired MN except for size, and lesions >1.5 cm may be presumed to be either tardive CMN or DN.

LABORATORY EXAMINATION

HISTOPATHOLOGY Nevomelanocytes occur as well-ordered clusters (*theques*) in the epidermis and in the dermis as sheets, nests, or cords. *A diffuse infiltration of strands of nevomelanocytes in the lower one-third of the reticular dermis and subcutis is, when present, quite specific for CMN.* In large and giant CMN, the nevomelanocytes may extend into the muscle, bone, dura mater, and cranium.

COURSE AND PROGNOSIS

By definition, CMN appear at birth, but CMN may arise during infancy (*tardive CMN*). The life history of CMN is not documented, but CMN can be observed in elderly persons, an age when the common acquired MN have disappeared.

Large or Giant CMN. The lifetime risk for development of melanoma in large CMN has been estimated to be at least 6.3%. In 50% of patients who develop melanoma in large CMN, the diagnosis is made between the ages of 3 and 5 years. Melanoma that develops in a large CMN has a poor prognosis because it is detected late.

Small CMN. The lifetime risk of developing malignant melanoma is 1 to 5%. The expected association of small CMN and melanoma is <1:171,000 based on chance alone. Nonetheless, small CMN should be considered for prophylactic excision at puberty if there are no atypical features (variegated color and irregular borders); small CMN with atypical features should be excised immediately.

MANAGEMENT

SURGICAL EXCISION The only acceptable method. *Small and large CMN*: Excision, with full-thickness skin graft, if required; swing flaps, tissue expanders for large lesions. *Giant CMN*: Risk of development of melanoma is significant even in the first 3 to 5 years of age, and thus giant CNMN should be removed as soon as possible. Individual considerations are necessary (size, location, degree of loss of function, or amount of mutilation). New surgical techniques utilizing the patient's own normal skin grown in tissue culture can now be used to facilitate removal of very large CNMN. Also, tissue expanders can be used.

CUTANEOUS MELANOMA ICD-10: C43.L90

- Cutaneous melanoma is the most malignant tumor of the skin. Melanoma arises from the malignant transformation of melanocytes at the dermal–epidermal junction or from the nevomelanocytes of DN or CMN that become invasive and metastasize after various time intervals.

CLASSIFICATION OF MELANOMA

I. De novo melanoma
   A. Melanoma in situ (MIS)
   B. Lentigo maligna melanoma (LMM)
   C. Superficial spreading melanoma (SSM)
   D. Nodular melanoma (NM)
   E. Acral lentiginous melanoma (ALM)
   F. Melanoma of the mucous membranes (MMM)
   G. Desmoplastic melanoma(DM)
II. Melanoma arising from precursors
   A. Melanoma arising in dysplastic MN
   B. Melanoma arising in congenital MN
   C. Melanoma arising in common MN

FOUR IMPORTANT MESSAGES CONCERNING CUTANEOUS MELANOMA

1. Melanoma of the Skin Has Reached Epidemic Proportions

In 2009, it was estimated that in the United States roughly 122,000 men and women were diagnosed with melanoma of which 69,000 were invasive. Melanoma is a common malignancy and its incidence is on the rise. In the United States, the lifetime risk of invasive melanoma in 2010 was 1 in 50. The US surveillance epidemiology and end results (SEER) estimated 8,650 deaths resulting from melanoma in the United States. The number of melanomas in the United States continues to increase by 7% per year. Cutaneous melanoma currently represents 5% of newly diagnosed cancer in men and 6% in women. It is the leading fatal illness arising in the skin and is responsible for 80% of deaths from skin cancer. US cancer statistics show that melanoma had the second highest mortality rate increase among men ≥65 years old. On the other hand, deaths from melanoma occur at a younger age than deaths from most other cancers, and melanoma is among the most common types of cancer in young adults.

2. Early Recognition and Excision of Primary Melanoma Result in Virtual Cure

Current cutaneous melanoma education stresses the detection of early melanoma, with high cure rates after surgical excision. Of all the cancers, melanoma of the skin is the most rewarding for detection of early curable primary tumors, thereby preventing metastatic disease and death. Curability is directly related to size and depth of invasion of the tumor. At present, the most critical tool for conquering this disease is, therefore, the identification of early "thin" melanomas by clinical examination. Total skin examination for melanoma and its precursors should be done routinely.

About 30% of melanomas arise in a preexisting melanocytic lesion; 70% arise in normal skin. Almost all melanomas show an initial radial growth phase followed by a subsequent vertical growth phase. Since metastasis occurs only infrequently during the radial growth phase, detection of early melanomas (i.e., "thin" melanomas) during this phase is essential.

There is the paradox that even with a rising mortality rate, there has been an encouraging improvement in the overall prognosis of melanoma with very high 5-year survival rates (approaching 98%) for thin (<0.75 mm) primary melanoma and an 83% rate for all stages. The favorable prognosis is entirely attributable to early detection.

3. All Physicians and Nurses Have the Responsibility of Detecting Early Melanoma

Early detection of primary melanoma ensures increased survival. The seriousness of this disease thus places the responsibility on the health-care provider in the pivotal role: not to overlook pigmented lesions. Therefore, it is recommended that in clinical practice, no matter what the presenting complaint, total examination of the body should be requested of all Caucasian patients at the time of the first encounter and that all body regions be examined, including the scalp, toe webs, and orifices (mouth, anus, and vulva).

4. Examination of All Acquired Pigmented Lesions According to the ABCDE Rule

This rule analyzes pigmented lesions according to symmetry, border, color, diameter, growth, and elevation (see p. 261 and Table 12-1). While it does not apply to all types of melanoma, it permits differential diagnostic separation of most melanomas from common nevi and other pigmented lesions.

ETIOLOGY AND PATHOGENESIS

The etiology and pathogenesis of cutaneous melanoma are unknown. Epidemiologic studies demonstrate a role for genetic predisposition and sun exposure in melanoma development. The major genes involved in melanoma development reside on chromosome 9p21. Twenty-five to 40% of members of melanoma-prone families have mutations in cyclin-dependent kinase inhibitor 2A (*CDKN2A*) and a few families in the cyclin-dependent kinase 4 (*CDK4*). These are tumor-suppressor genes that provide a rational basis for the link to susceptibility to melanoma. Sixty-six percent of melanomas have a mutation of the *BRAF* gene, others of *MC1R*.

There is convincing evidence from epidemiologic studies that exposure to solar radiation is the major cause of cutaneous melanoma. Cutaneous melanoma is a greater problem in light-skinned whites (skin phototypes I and II). Sunburns during childhood and intermittent burning exposure in fair skin also seem to have a higher impact than cumulative UV exposure over time. Other predisposing and risk factors are the presence of precursor lesions (dysplastic nevi and congenital MN) and a family history of melanoma in parents, children, or siblings. Risk factors for melanoma are listed in Table 12-2.

TABLE 12-2 Risk Factors for the Development of Melanoma

- Genetic markers (*CDKN2a*), *BRAF*, *MC1R*
- Photo skin type I/II
- Family history of dysplastic nevi or melanoma
- Personal history of melanoma
- Ultraviolet irradiation, particularly sunburns during childhood and in termittent burning exposures
- Number (>50) and size (>5 mm) of melanocytic nevi
- Congenltal nevi
- Number of dysplastic nevi (>5)
- Dysplastic melanocytic nevus syndrome

MELANOMA GROWTH PATTERNS

Almost all melanomas show an initial radial growth phase followed by a subsequent vertical growth phase. *Radial growth phase* refers to a mostly intraepidermal, preinvasive, or minimally invasive growth pattern; *vertical growth* refers to growth into the dermis and thus into the vicinity of vessels that serve as avenues for metastasis. Since most melanomas produce melanin pigment, even preinvasive melanomas in their radial growth phase are clinically detectable by their color patterns. The prognostic difference among the clinical types of melanoma relates mainly to the duration of the radial growth phase, which may last from years to decades in LMM, from months to 2 years in SSM, and 6 months or less in NM.

MELANOMA RECOGNITION

Six Signs of Malignant Melanoma (ABCDE Rule)

Note: This does not apply to nodular melanoma.

A. *Asymmetry* in shape—one-half unlike the other half.
B. *Border* is irregular—edges irregularly scalloped, notched, or sharply defined.
C. *Color* is not uniform; mottled—haphazard display of colors; all shades of brown, black, gray, blue, red, and white.
D. *Diameter* is usually large—greater than the tip of a pencil eraser (6.0 mm). D is also used for the "ugly duckling" sign. These lesions are different from other pigmented lesions (nevi) on the body with respect to change in size, shape, and color.
E. *Elevation* is almost always present and is irregular—surface distortion is assessed by side lighting. MIS and acral lentiginous lesions initially macular; E is also used for *Evolving or Enlargement*. A history of an increase in the size of lesion is one of the most important signs of malignant melanoma.

CLINICAL PRESENTATIONS OF MELANOMA

The clinical characteristics of the four major types of melanoma are summarized in Table 12-3. Frequency of melanoma by type of tumor: SSM, 70%; NM, 15%; LMM, 5%; and acral and unclassified melanoma, 10%. MIS and desmoplastic melanoma are also discussed in this section.

TABLE 12-3 Four Major Types of Melanoma

Type	Frequency (%)	Site	Radial Growth	Vertical Growth
Superficial spreading	70	Any site, lower extremities, trunk	Months to 2 years	Delayed
Nodular	15	Any site, trunk, head, neck	No clinically perceptible radial growth	Immediate
Lentigo maligna melanoma	5	Face, neck, dorsa of hands	Years	Much delayed
Acral lentiginous melanoma	5–10	Palms, soles, subungual	Months to years	Early but recognition delayed

MELANOMA IN SITU (MIS) ICD-10: D03.L00

- The clinical features of MIS are not always clearly presented. MIS is primarily a histopathologic definition, and the term is used when melanoma cells are confined to the epidermis, above the basement membrane; basilar melanocytic atypia, hyperplasia, and spread occur either in single-file alignment along the basal membrane or are distributed throughout the epidermis (pagetoid spread). Every melanoma starts as an in situ lesion, but MIS is clinically diagnosable only when the radial growth phase is long enough for it to become visually detectable. Such lesions are flat, within the level of the skin, and thus a *macule* (Fig. 12-7) or a macule with barely perceptible elevation (Fig. 12-8), with irregular borders and marked variegation of color: brown, dark brown, and black or reddish tones but without gray or blue, as this occurs only when melanin (within macrophages), melanocytes, or melanoma cells are located in the dermis. The clinical distinction between MIS and severely atypical DN may not be possible.
- The clinical correlations of MIS are *lentigo maligna* (Fig. 12-7) and flat *SSM* (Fig. 12-8). Both are discussed in the following respective sections.

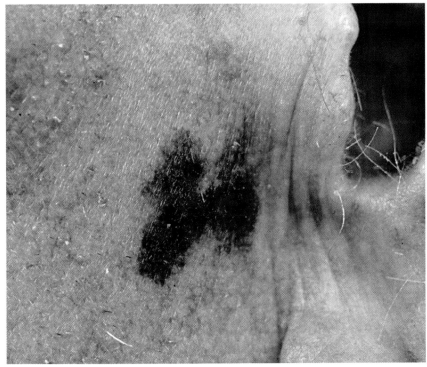

FIGURE 12-7 Melanoma in situ: lentigo maligna A large, very irregular, and asymmetric macule on the preauricular region of a 78-year-old male. There is striking variegation of pigmentation (tan, brown, dark brown, black).

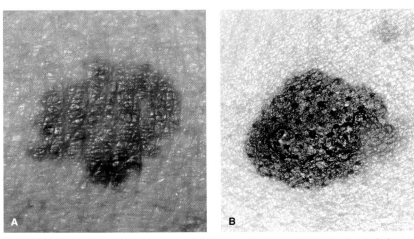

FIGURE 12-8 Melanoma in situ, superficial spreading type (A) Barely elevated plaque on the arm of a 75-year-old white male was first noted 5 years previously, gradually increasing in size. The lesion is asymmetric and there is also asymmetry in the distribution of color that is variegated and shows dark-brown specks against a tan background. Dermatopathology of the lesion showed a superficial spreading melanoma in situ. **(B)** An almost oval, barely elevated small plaque that has a relatively regular border but is striking with regard to the variegation in color: tan, dark brown, and even black with an orange portion on the right. Dermatopathology again showed MIS with a pagetoid growth pattern of intraepidermal melanoma cells.

LENTIGO MALIGNA MELANOMA (LMM) ICD-10: D02

- The least common (<5%) of the four principal melanoma types of Caucasions (Table 12-3).
- It occurs in older persons on their most sun-exposed areas, usually the face and forearms.
- Sunlight is the most important pathogenic factor.
- LMM always starts as *lentigo maligna* (LM), which represents a macular intraepidermal neoplasm and is an MIS (Figs. 12-7 and 12-9). LM is thus not a precursor but an evolving lesion of melanoma.
- Focal papular and nodular areas signal a switch from the radial to the vertical growth phase and thus invasion into the dermis; the lesion is now called LMM (Fig. 12-10).
- For the most important clinical characteristics, see Table 12-3.

EPIDEMIOLOGY

AGE OF ONSET Median age 65.

SEX Equal incidence in males and females.

RACE Rare in brown-skinned persons (e.g., Asians, East Indians) and extremely rare in black-skinned (African Americans and Africans) persons. Highest incidence in whites, skin phototypes I, II, and III.

INCIDENCE 5% of primary cutaneous melanomas.

PREDISPOSING FACTORS Same factors as in sun-induced nonmelanoma skin cancer: Older population and outdoor occupations (farmers, sailors, and construction workers).

PATHOGENESIS

In contrast to SSM and NM, which appear to be related to intermittent high-intensity sun exposure and occur on the intermittently exposed areas (back and legs) of young or middle-aged adults, LM and LMM occur on the face, neck, and dorsa of the forearms or hands (Table 12-3). Furthermore, LM and LMM occur almost always in older persons with evidence of heavily sun-damaged skin (dermatoheliosis). The evolution of the lesion most clearly reveals the transition from the radial to the vertical growth phase and from a clinically recognizable MIS to invasive melanoma (Fig. 12-10).

CLINICAL MANIFESTATION

LMM very slowly evolves from LM over a period of several years, sometimes up to 20 years. There is practically always a background of dermatoheliosis.

SKIN LESIONS Lentigo Maligna. Uniformly *flat*, macule (Fig. 12-7); 0.5 cm or larger, up to 20 cm (Fig. 12-9A). Usually well defined, in some areas also blurred borders or highly irregular borders, often with a notch; "geographic" shape with inlets and peninsulas (Fig. 12-9B). Early lesions tan, advanced lesions: striking variations in hues of brown and black (speckled), appears like a "stain" (Fig. 12-7); haphazard network of black on a background of brown (Fig. 12-9A). *No* hues of red or blue.

Lentigo Maligna Melanoma. The clinical change that indicates the transition of LM to LMM is the appearance of variegated red, white, and blue and also of papules, plaques, or nodules (Fig. 12-10B). Thus, LMM is the same as LM *plus* (1) gray areas (indicate focal regression) and blue areas [indicating dermal pigment (melanocytes or melanin)] and (2) papules or nodules, which may be blue, black, or pink (Fig. 12-9B). Dermoscopy is essential. Rarely, LMM may be nonpigmented. It is then skin colored, patchy red, and clinically not diagnosable (see Amelanotic LMM, p. 277).

Distribution. Single isolated lesion on sun-exposed areas: Forehead, nose, cheeks, neck, forearms, and dorsa of the hands; rarely on the lower legs.

OTHER SKIN CHANGES IN AREAS OF TUMOR Sun-induced changes: Solar keratosis, freckling, telangiectasia, thinning of the skin, i.e., dermatoheliosis.

GENERAL MEDICAL EXAMINATION Check for regional lymphadenopathy.

LABORATORY EXAMINATION

DERMATOPATHOLOGY LM shows increased numbers of atypical melanocytes distributed in a single layer along the basal layer and above the basement membrane of an epidermis that shows elongation of rete ridges (Fig. 12-10). Atypical melanocytes are usually singly dispersed but may also aggregate to small nests and extend into the hair follicles, reaching the middermis, even in the preinvasive stage of LM. In LMM, they invade the dermis (vertical

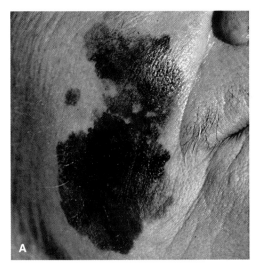
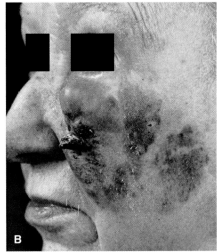

FIGURE 12-9 Lentigo maligna (A) A very large lentigo maligna on the right cheek with the typical variegation in color (tan, brown, black) and highly irregular shape. The lesion is flat, macular, and thus represents an in situ melanoma. **(B)** The classically macular lentigo maligna is highly irregular in shape and variegated in color. However, there is a bluish component and a large pink nodule in the infraorbital region, indicating a switch from the radial to the vertical growth phase and thus invasiveness: the lesion is now called lentigo maligna melanoma.

FIGURE 12-10 Lentigo maligna melanoma
Illustrated on the right of the lesion is a large, variegated, freckle-like macule (not elevated above the plane of the skin) with irregular borders; the tan areas show increased numbers of melanocytes, usually atypical and bizarre, and are distributed single file along the basal layer; at certain places in the dermis, malignant melanocytes have invaded and formed nests (radial growth phase). At the left is a large nodule that is heavily pigmented and composed of epithelioid cells that have invaded the dermis (vertical growth phase); the nodules of all four main subtypes of melanoma are indistinguishable from each other.

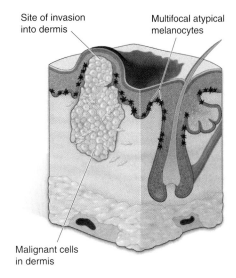

Site of invasion into dermis

Multifocal atypical melanocytes

Malignant cells in dermis

growth phase) and expand into the deeper tissues (Fig. 12-10).

DIFFERENTIAL DIAGNOSIS

VARIEGATE TAN-BROWN MACULE/PAPULE/NODULE
Seborrheic keratoses may be dark but are exclusively papules or plaques and have a characteristic stippled surface, often with a verrucous component, i.e., a "warty" but greasy surface that, when scratched, exhibits fine scales. *Solar lentigo*, although macular, does not exhibit the intensity or variegation of brown, dark brown, and black hues seen in LM. Dermoscopy is essential.

PROGNOSIS

Summarized in Table 12-5.

MANAGEMENT

See also p. 282.

1. Very early LM lesions: Imiquimod.
2. Excise with 1 cm beyond the clinically visible lesion where possible and provided the flat component does not involve a major organ. Use of Wood lamp and dermoscopy help in defining borders.
3. Sentinel node should be done in lesions >1.0 mm in terms of thickness.

SUPERFICIAL SPREADING MELANOMA (SSM) ICD-10: C43.L20

- SSM is the most common melanoma (70%) type in persons with white skin.
- It arises most frequently on the upper back and occurs as a moderately slow-growing lesion over a period of up to 2 years.
- SSM has a distinctive morphology: An elevated, flat lesion (plaque). The pigment variegation of SSM is similar to, but more striking than, the variety of color present in most LMM. The color display is a mixture of brown, dark brown, black, blue, and red, with slate-gray or gray regions in areas of tumor regression.
- For the most important clinical characteristics, see Tables 12-1 and 12-3.

EPIDEMIOLOGY

AGE OF ONSET 30 to 50 (median, 37) years of age.
SEX Slightly higher incidence in females.
RACE Overwhelmingly predominate in white-skinned persons. Only 2% brown or black skinned. Furthermore, brown and black persons have melanomas usually occurring on the extremities; half of brown and black persons have primary melanomas arising on the sole of the foot (see below).
INCIDENCE SSM constitutes 70% of all melanomas arising in white persons.
PREDISPOSING AND RISK FACTORS (see Table 12-2) In order of importance, these are *presence of precursor lesions* (DN, CMN; p. 252 and p. 257); *family history* of melanoma in parents, children, or siblings; *light skin color* (skin phototypes I and II); and sunburns, especially during preadolescence. Especially increased incidence in young urban professionals, with a frequent pattern of intermittent, intense sun exposure ("weekenders") or winter holidays near the equator.

PATHOGENESIS

In the early stages of growth, there is an intraepidermal, or radial, growth phase during which tumorigenic pigment cells are confined to the epidermis and thus cannot metastasize. At this stage, SSM is an MIS (Figs. 12-8 and 12-11). This "grace period" of the radial growth phase, with potential for cure, is followed by the invasive vertical growth phase, in which malignant cells consist of a tumorigenic nodule that vertically invades the dermis with potential for metastasis (Fig. 12-11).

The pathophysiology of SSM is not yet understood. Certainly, in some considerable number of SSMs, sunlight exposure is a factor, and SSM is related to occasional bursts of recreational sun exposure during a susceptible period (<14 years). About 10% of the SSMs occur in high-risk families. The rest of the cases may occur sporadically among persons without a specific genetic risk.

CLINICAL MANIFESTATION

The usual history of SSM is a change in a previously existing pigmented lesion (mostly a DN). It should be noted, however, that 70% of melanomas arise in "normal" skin, but since initial growth is slow and melanomas often occur in persons with many nevi, an early SSM may be mistaken for a preexisting nevus by the patient.

FIGURE 12-11 Superficial spreading melanoma
The border is irregular and elevated throughout its entirety; biopsy of this plaque surrounding the large nodule shows a pagetoid distribution of large melanocytes throughout the epidermis in multiple layers, occurring singly or in nests, and uniformly atypical (radial growth phase). On the left is a large nodule, and scattered throughout the surrounding portion of the plaque are smaller papular and nodular areas (vertical growth phase). The nodules may also show epithelioid, spindle cells, or small malignant melanocytes as in lentigo maligna melanoma and NM.

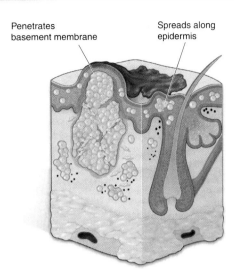

Penetrates basement membrane

Spreads along epidermis

The patient or a close relative may note a gradual darkening in one area of a "mole" (see Figs. 12-3 and 12-8) or a change in shape; and as the dark areas increase, there will develop variegation of color with mixes of brown, dark brown, and black. Also, the borders of a previously regularly shaped lesion may become irregular with pseudopods and a notch.

With the switch from the radial to a vertical growth phase (Fig. 12-11), and thus invasion into the dermis, there is the clinical appearance of a papule and later nodule on top of the slightly elevated plaque of an SSM. Since many SSMs initially have the potential for a tumor-infiltrating lymphocyte (TIL)-mediated regression, albeit only partial, other areas of the SSM plaque may sink to the level of surrounding normal skin and the color mixes of brown to black are expanded by the addition of red, white, and the tell-tale blue and blue-gray.

SKIN LESIONS (Figs. 12-12 and 12-13) SSM is the lesion to which the ABCDE rule (p. 261) best applies. Initially a very flat plaque from 5 to 12 mm or smaller (Fig. 12-8); older lesions, 10 to 25 mm (Fig. 12-12). Asymmetric (one-half unlike the other) (Figs. 12-12A–C) or oval with irregular borders (Fig. 12-12D) and often with one or more indentations (notches) (Figs. 12-12 and 12-13). Sharply defined. Dark brown, black, with admixture of pink, gray, and blue-gray hues—with marked variegation and a haphazard pattern. White areas indicate regressed portions (Figs. 12-12C and D). An SSM is thus a flat plaque with all shades of brown to black plus the American flag or the tricolore (red, blue, white) (Fig. 12-12D). No benign pigmented lesion has these characteristics. As the vertical growth phase progresses, nodules appear (Fig. 12-13B); eventually, erosions and even superficial ulceration develop (Figs. 12-13C and D).

Distribution. Isolated, single lesions; multiple primaries are rare. Back (males and females); legs (females, between knees and ankles); anterior trunk and legs in males; relatively fewer lesions on covered areas, e.g., buttocks, lower abdomen, and bra area.

DERMOSCOPY Increases diagnostic accuracy by more than 70%.

GENERAL EXAMINATION Always search for enlarged regional nodes.

LABORATORY EXAMINATION

DERMATOPATHOLOGY Malignant melanocytes expand in a pagetoid pattern, i.e., in multiple layers within the epidermis (if confined to the epidermis, the lesion is an MIS) and superficial papillary body of the dermis—the radial growth phase. They occur singly and in nests (see Fig. 12-11) and are S-100 and HMB-45 positive. In the vertical growth phase, presenting clinically as small nodules, they expand further into the reticular dermis and beyond (Fig. 12-11). For microstaging, see Table 12-4 and p. 281.

COURSE AND PROGNOSIS

If left untreated, SSM develops deep invasion (vertical growth) over months to years. Prognosis is summarized in Table 12-5.

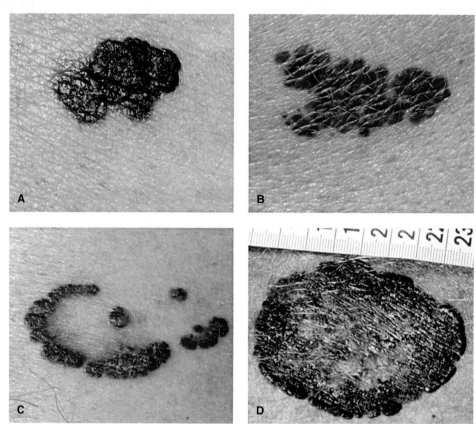

FIGURE 12-12 Superficial spreading melanoma, radial growth phase (A) A flat-topped, elevated, asymmetric, and irregular plaque with variegated color (brown, black) on the trunk with sharply demarcated margins. The surface is also irregular with a cobblestone pattern (see also Fig. 12-3). **(B)** An asymmetric, flat plaque with irregular and sharply defined margins and a cobblestone-like surface. The melanin pigmentation ranges from light brown to dark brown, black, and there are lighter areas interspersed. **(C)** A highly irregular lesion with dark-brown to bluish-black papules forming a ring around a white macular area with a central brownish to bluish papule. This white area marks spontaneous regression. **(D)** A relatively symmetric but large (8 cm) plaque with sharply defined and notched border and a considerable variegation of color: black, blue, red, and white.

DIAGNOSIS

Clinically according to the ABCDE rule, verified by dermoscopy. In case of doubt, *biopsy*; total excisional biopsy with narrow margins is the optimal biopsy procedure. Incisional or punch biopsy is acceptable when total excisional biopsy cannot be performed or when the lesion is large, requiring extensive surgery to remove the entire lesion. Shave biopsy should not be done, as it does not allow assessment of the level of invasion.

MANAGEMENT

SURGICAL TREATMENT See p. 282.

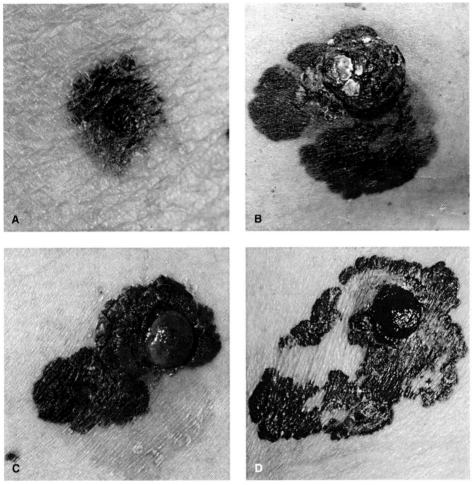

FIGURE 12-13 Superficial spreading melanoma, vertical growth phase (A) An only minimally irregular plaque with variegate color (brown, black). In the center, there is a small black, dome-shaped nodule. This is the switch to the vertical growth phase. **(B)** An irregular very flat plaque with notched borders and highly variegated color (tan, brown, black, and red). Slightly off center there is a large partially crusted nodule (vertical growth phase). **(C)** A highly irregular and asymmetric plaque with a cobblestone-like surface and variegated color (black, brown). On the right there is an excentric, eroded black to blue nodule representing the vertical growth phase. **(D)** A highly irregular, asymmetric bluish to black plaque with brown, red, and white (regression). Off center is an eroded black nodule (vertical growth).

TABLE 12-4 Melanoma TNM Classification

T Classification	Thickness (mm)	Ulceration Status/Mitoses
T1	≤1.0	a: Without ulceration and mitosis $<1/mm^2$ b: With ulceration or mitosis $\geq 1/mm^2$
T2	1.01–2.0	a: Without ulceration b: With ulceration
T3	2.01–4.0	a: Without ulceration b: With ulceration
T4	>4.0	a: Without ulceration b: With ulceration

N Classification	No. of Metastatic Nodes	Nodal Metastatic Mass
N1	1 node	a: Micrometastasis b: Macrometastasis
N2	2–3 nodes	a: Micrometastasis b: Macrometastasis c: In-transit met(s)/satellite(s) without metastatic nodes
N3	4 or more metastatic nodes, or matted nodes, or in-transit met(s)/satellite(s) with metastatic node(s)	

M Classification	Site	Serum Lactate Dehydrogenase
M1a	Distant skin, subcutaneous, or nodal metastases	Normal
M1b	Lung metastases	Normal
M1c	All other visceral metastases Any distant metastasis	Normal Elevated

Source: Reproduced with permission from Balch CM, et al. Update on the melanoma staging system: the importance of sentinel node staging, mitotic rate and primary tumor. *J Surg Oncol* 2011; 104:379–385.

TABLE 12-5 Survival Rates for Melanoma TNM Stages I–III*

Stage	Tumor	Node State	Node Tumor Burden	5-Year Survival Rate (%)
IA	T1a	No	—	97
IB	T1b	No	—	94
IB	T2a	No	—	91
IIA	T2b	No	—	82
IIA	T3a	No	—	79
IIB	T3b	No	—	68
IIB	T4a	No	—	71
IIC	T4b	No	—	53
IIIA	T1–T4a	N1a/N2a	Microscopic	78
IIIB	T1–T4b	N1a/N2a	Microscopic	55
IIIB	T1–T4a	N1b/N2b	Macroscopic	48
IIIC	T1–T4b	N1b/N2b/N3	Macroscopic or 4 + nodes	38
IIIC	T1–T4a	N3	4 + any nodes	47

*From Balch CM, et al. Melanoma of the skin. In: Edge SE, et al. eds. *AJCC, Cancer Staging Manual*. 7th ed. New York, NY: Springer; 2010.

NODULAR MELANOMA (NM) ICD-10: 43.L10

- NM is second in frequency after SSM.
- Occurring largely in middle life in persons with white skin and, as in SSM, on the less commonly exposed areas.
- The tumor from the beginning is in the vertical growth phase (Fig. 12-14).
- NM is uniformly elevated and presents as a thick plaque or an exophytic, polypoid, or dome-shaped lesion.
- The color pattern is usually not variegated and the lesion is uniformly blue or blue-black or, less commonly, can be very lightly pigmented or nonpigmented (amelanotic melanoma).
- NM is the one type of primary melanoma that arises quite rapidly (a few months to 2 years) from normal skin or from a melanocytic nevus as a nodular (vertical) growth without an adjacent epidermal component, as is always present in LMM and SSM.

Note: For the most important clinical characteristics, see Table 12-3.

FIGURE 12-14 Nodular melanoma This arises at the dermal–epidermal junction and extends vertically in the dermis (vertical growth phase). The epidermis lateral to the areas of this invasion does not demonstrate atypical melanocytes. As in lentigo maligna melanoma and superficial spreading melanoma, the tumor may show large epithelioid cells, spindle cells, small malignant melanocytes, or mixtures of all three.

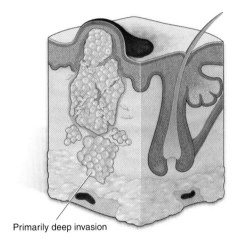

Primarily deep invasion

EPIDEMIOLOGY

AGE OF ONSET Middle life.

SEX Equal incidence in males and females.

RACE NM occurs in all races, but in the Japanese it occurs nine times more frequently (27%) than SSM (3%).

INCIDENCE NM constitutes 15% (up to 30%) of the melanomas in the United States.

PREDISPOSING AND RISK FACTORS See p. 261 and Table 12-2.

PATHOGENESIS

Both NM and SSM occur in approximately the same sites (upper back in males, lower legs in females), and presumably the same pathogenetic factors are operating in NM as were described in SSM. For the growth pattern of NM, see Fig. 12-14. The reason for the high frequency of NM in the Japanese is not known.

CLINICAL MANIFESTATION

This type of melanoma may arise in a preexisting nevus, but more commonly arises de novo from normal skin. In contrast to SSM, NM evolves over a few months and is often noted by the patient as a new "mole" that was not present before.

SKIN LESIONS Uniformly elevated "blueberry-like" nodule (Figs. 12-15A and B) or ulcerated or "thick" plaque; may become polypoid. Uniformly dark blue, black, or "thundercloud" gray (Figs. 12-15A and B); lesions may appear pink with a trace of brown or a black rim (amelanotic NM, see Amelanotic nodular melanoma, p. 277). Surface smooth or scaly, eroded (Fig. 12-15C) or ulcerated (Fig. 12-15D). Early lesions are 1 to 3 cm in size but may grow much larger if undetected. Oval or round, usually with smooth, not irregular, borders, as in all other types of melanoma. Sharply defined, may be pedunculated (Fig. 12-15D).

Distribution. Same as SSM. In the Japanese, NM occurs on the extremities (arms and legs).

GENERAL MEDICAL EXAMINATION Always search for nodes.

LABORATORY EXAMINATIONS

DERMATOPATHOLOGY Malignant melanocytes, which appear as epithelioid, spindle, or small atypical cells, show little lateral (radial) growth within and below the epidermis and invade vertically into the dermis and underlying subcutaneous fat (see Fig. 12-14). They are S-100 and usually HMB-45 positive. For microstaging, see p. 281.

SEROLOGY Serum levels of S-100 beta and melanoma-inhibiting activity (MIA), S-cysteinyl-dopa, and lactate dehydrogenase (LDH) levels are markers for *advanced* melanoma patients. To date, LDH is the only statistically significant marker for *progressive* disease.

DIAGNOSIS

Clinical and with the help of dermoscopy. However, dermoscopy may fail in uniformly black lesions. In case of doubt, *biopsy*. Total excisional biopsy with narrow margins is optimal biopsy procedure, where possible. If biopsy is positive for melanoma, reexcision of site will be necessary (see Management, p. 282). Incisional or punch biopsy acceptable when total excisional biopsy cannot be performed or when lesion is large, requiring extensive surgery to remove the entire lesion.

DIFFERENTIAL DIAGNOSIS

BLUE/BLACK PAPULE/NODULE NM can be confused with *hemangioma* (long history) and *pyogenic granuloma* (short history—weeks) (see Fig. 12-15C) and is sometimes almost indistinguishable from *pigmented basal cell carcinoma*, although it is usually softer. However, any "blueberry-like" nodule of recent origin (6 months to 1 year) should be excised or, if large, an incisional biopsy is mandatory for histologic diagnosis.

PROGNOSIS

Summarized in Table 12-5.

MANAGEMENT

SURGICAL TREATMENT See p. 282.

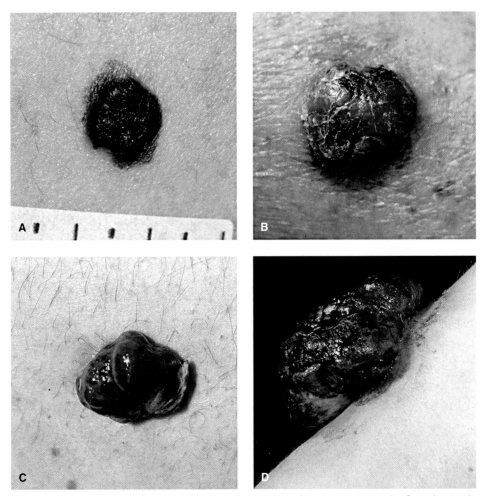

FIGURE 12-15 Nodular melanoma (A) A 9-mm dome-shaped smooth nodule with a flatter brownish rim arising on the back of a 38-year-old male. **(B)** A 1-cm black papule on the posterior thigh of a 60-year-old female. The lesion had been present for less than 1 year. **(C)** An eroded, bleeding, brown nodule having a mushroom-like configuration giving it a stuck-on appearance. Such lesions can be mistaken for a vascular lesion such as a pyogenic granuloma. **(D)** Large (5 cm) irregular, black, bleeding nodule sitting on the skin like a mushroom. The lesion had grown for over a half year and the 56-year-old male patient had not seen a physician out of fear "it might be melanoma."

DESMOPLASTIC MELANOMA (DM)

- The term *desmoplasia* refers to connective tissue proliferation and, when applied to malignant melanoma, describes (1) a dermal fibroblastic component of melanoma with only minimal melanocytic proliferation at the dermal–epidermal junction; (2) nerve-centered superficial malignant melanoma with or without an atypical intraepidermal melanocytic component; or (3) other lesions in which the tumor appears to arise in lentigo maligna or, rarely, in ALM or superficial spreading melanoma.
- Also, DM growth patterns have been noted in recurrent malignant melanoma.
- DM may be a variant of LMM in that most lesions occur on the head and neck in patients with dermatoheliosis.
- DM is more likely to recur locally and metastasize than LMM. DM is rare and occurs more frequently in women and persons >55 years old.
- At diagnosis, DM lesions have been present from months to years. DM is asymptomatic, usually not pigmented and is therefore overlooked by the patient. Early lesions may appear as variegated lentiginous macules or plaques, at times with small blue-gray specks of color. Later, lesions may appear as dermal nodules, and although they commonly lack any melanin pigmentation, they may have gray to blue papular elevations (Fig. 12-16). Borders, when discernible, are irregular as in LM.
- The diagnosis requires an experienced dermatopathologist; S-100 immunoperoxidase-positive spindle cells need to be identified in the matrix collagen. HMB-45 staining may be negative. A typical junctional melanocytic proliferation, either individual or focal nests, occurs, resembling LM. S-100-positive spindle-shaped cells are embedded in matrix collagen that widely separates the spindle cell nuclei. Neurotropism is characteristic, i.e., fibroblast-like tumor cells around or within endoneurium of small nerves.
- There are mixed views about the prognosis of DM. In one series, approximately 50% of patients experienced a local recurrence after primary excision of DM, usually within 3 years of excision; some patients experienced multiple recurrences. Lymph node metastasis occurs less often than local recurrence. In one series, 20% developed metastases, and DM was regarded as a more aggressive tumor than LMM.
- For management, see p. 282.

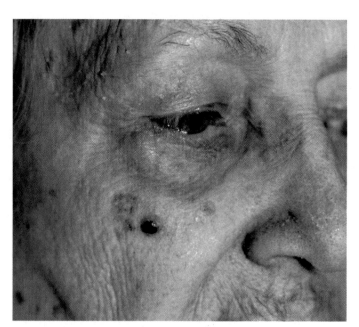

FIGURE 12-16 Desmoplastic melanoma A bluish-black very hard nodule on the cheek of an 85-year-old woman. It recurred 1 year after primary excision: histopathologically, it was a desmoplastic melanoma with a thickness of greater than 3.4 mm and showed neural invasion. Note reddish to bluish tinge of lower eyelid, probably caused by congestion of vessels compressed by the tumor.

ACRAL LENTIGINOUS MELANOMA (ALM) ICD-10: C43.L60

- ALM is a special presentation of cutaneous melanoma arising on the soles, palms, and fingernails or toenail beds.
- ALM occurs most often in Asians, sub-Saharan Africans, and African Americans, comprising 50 to 70% of the melanomas of the skin found in these populations.
- It occurs most often in older males (≥60 years) and often grows slowly over a period of years.
- The delay in development of the tumor is the reason these tumors are often discovered only when nodules appear or, in the case of nail involvement, the nail is shed; therefore, the prognosis is poor.

EPIDEMIOLOGY

AGE OF ONSET Median age is 65.
INCIDENCE AND RACE Seven to 9% of all melanomas; in whites, 2 to 8%; in Asians, Africans, and African Americans, 50% of melanomas; in Japanese 50 to 70% of melanomas.
SEX Male:female ratio, 3:1.

PATHOGENESIS

The pigmented macules that are frequently seen on the soles of African blacks could be comparable with DN. ALM has a similar growth pattern as LMM.

CLINICAL MANIFESTATION

ALM is slow growing (about 2.5 years from appearance to diagnosis). The tumors occur on the volar surface (palm or sole) and in their radial growth phase may appear as a gradually enlarging "stain." ALM as subungual (thumb or great toe) melanoma appears first in the nail bed and involves, over a period of 1 to 2 years, the nail matrix, eponychium, and nail plate. In the vertical growth phase, nodules appear; often there are areas of ulceration, and nail deformity and shedding of the nail may occur.
SKIN LESIONS ACRAL AND PALM/SOLE Macular or slightly raised lesion in the radial growth phase (Fig. 12-17), with focal papules and nodules developing during the vertical growth phase. Marked variegation of color including brown, black, blue, depigmented pale areas (Fig. 12-17). Irregular borders as in LMM; usually well defined but not infrequently ill defined. This type of ALM occurs on the soles, palms, dorsal, and palmar/plantar aspects of the fingers and toes (Fig. 12-17).
SUBUNGUAL Subungual macule beginning at the nail matrix and extending to involve the nail bed and nail plate. Papules, nodules, and destruction of the nail plate may occur

in the vertical growth phase (Fig. 12-17B). Dark brown or black pigmentation that may involve the entire nail and surrounding skin looking like LM (Figs. 12-17A and B). As the lesion switches to the vertical growth phase, a papule or nodule appears and the nail is shed (Figs. 12-17A and B). Often the nodules or papules are unpigmented. Amelanotic ALM is often overlooked for months and, since there are no pigmentary changes, may first present as nail dystrophy.

DIFFERENTIAL DIAGNOSIS

ALM (plantar type) is not infrequently regarded as a "plantar wart" and treated as such. Dermoscopy is of decisive help. Also, often misdiagnosed as tinea nigra.
SUBUNGUAL DISCOLORATION ALM (subungual) is usually considered to be traumatic bleeding under the nail, and subungual hematomas may persist for more than one year. However, usually the whole pigmented area moves gradually forward. Distinction of ALM from subungual hemorrhage can easily be made by dermoscopy. With the destruction of the nail plate, the lesions are most often regarded as "fungal infection." When nonpigmented tumor nodules appear, they are misdiagnosed as pyogenic granuloma.

LABORATORY EXAMINATION

DERMATOPATHOLOGY The histologic diagnosis of the radial growth phase of the volar type of ALM may be difficult and may require large incisional biopsies to provide for multiple sections. There is usually an intense lymphocytic inflammation at the dermal–epidermal junction. Characteristic large melanocytes along the basal cell layer may extend as large nests into the dermis, along eccrine ducts. Invasive malignant melanocytes are often spindle shaped, so that ALM frequently has a desmoplastic appearance histologically.

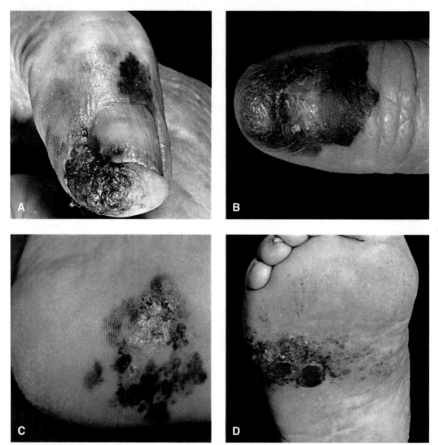

FIGURE 12-17 Acral lentiginous melanoma (A) An ALM arising on the thumb. Lentiginous component on the dorsal skin of the thumb: macular, sharply and ill-defined brown and gray-bluish spots. Subungual and distal ulcerated nodular component. **(B)** The tumor has replaced the entire nail bed and surrounding skin: macular and of variegated color resembling a lentigo maligna. The nail has been shed. This is ALM that has led to destruction of the nail matrix and was first diagnosed as nail dystrophy. **(C)** ALM on the heel. There is a highly variegated macular component—brown to gray and black; the nodular component is hyperkeratotic, reddish, and ulcerated. **(D)** ALM on the sole. This is an advanced lesion with a macular component and a reddish, ulcerated nodule. The lesion measured 10 mm in depth, and there were enlarged inguinal lymph nodes.

PROGNOSIS

The volar type of ALM can be deceptive in its clinical appearance, and "flat" lesions may be quite deeply invasive. Five-year survival rates are <50%. The subungual type of ALM has a better 5-year survival rate (80%) than does the volar type, but the data are probably not accurate. Poor prognosis for the volar type of ALM may be related to inordinate delay in the diagnosis.

MANAGEMENT

In considering surgical excision, it is important that the extent of the lesion be ascertained by viewing the lesion with dermoscopy. Subungual ALM and volar-type ALM: amputation [toe(s), finger(s)]; volar and plantar ALM: wide excision with split skin grafting. Sentinel lymph node procedure necessary in most cases (see "Management of Melanoma," p. 282).

AMELANOTIC MELANOMA ICD-10: C43.L50

- All types of melanoma can be amelanotic.
- Since they do not have the characteristic pigment marker, they are a diagnostic challenge (Fig. 12-18).
- Often there are pigmented clones in the tumor, which reveal its nature as a melanoma (Figs. 12-18B and C).
- In most cases, only a biopsy will reveal the correct diagnosis (Figs. 12-18A and D).

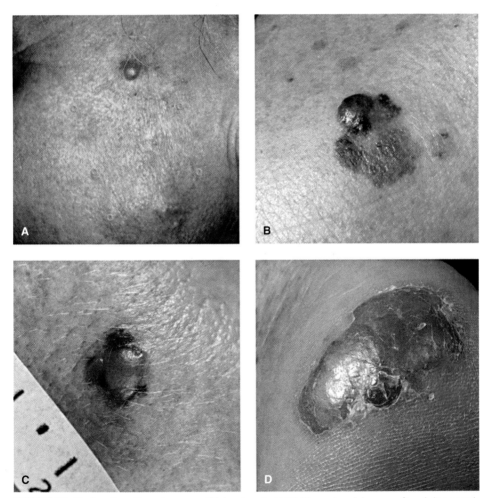

FIGURE 12-18 Amelanotic melanoma (A) Amelanotic LMM. The red nodule was soft and diagnosed as pyogenic granuloma and was excised. Histopathology revealed melanoma and subsequent punch biopsies performed in the erythematous skin of the cheek revealed lentigo maligna (LM). The outlines of the LM lesion as determined by further punch biopsies are marked with green circles. Note that over the mandible lesion is also nodular (vertical) growth. **(B)** Amelanotic superficial spreading melanoma. The true nature of this red nodule is revealed by the blue crescent at its base and the variegated brown-red plaque with which it is contiguous. **(C)** Amelanotic nodular melanoma. This cherry-red nodule has a brown, macular extension at 4, 6, 9 and 12 o'clock, giving away the correct diagnosis. **(D)** Amelanotic ASM on the heel. This cherry-red lesion was clinically diagnosed as eccrine poroma. Biopsy revealed deeply invading ALM.

MALIGNANT MELANOMA OF THE MUCOSA ICD-10: C43.992

- Malignant melanomas arising in the mucosal epithelial lining of the respiratory tract and gastrointestinal and genitourinary tracts are very rare, with an annual incidence of 0.15% per 100,000 individuals.
- Major sites of the mucosal melanomas are the vulva and vagina (45%) as well as the nasal and oral cavity (43%).
- Mucosal melanomas are so rare that there are no large databases compared with those for cutaneous melanoma.
- Therefore, pathologic microstaging has not been possible, and the fine-tuning of the prognosis that has been useful in cutaneous melanoma (Breslow thickness) has so far not been possible in mucosal melanoma.

Melanomas of the Oral Cavity

There is a delay in diagnosis of melanoma of the oral and nasal surfaces. Although melanosis of the mucosa is common in blacks and East Indians, it involves the buccal and gingival mucosa bilaterally (see Section 33). When there is a single area of melanosis, a biopsy should be performed to rule out melanoma; this is also true of pigmented nevi in the oral cavity, which should be excised.

Melanomas in the Genitalia

These melanomas mostly arise on the glans or prepuce (see Section 34) and the labia minora; there are fewer on the clitoris and the labia majora. Most tumors extend to the vagina at the mucocutaneous border. They look and evolve like LM and LMM (see Section 34). Vulva melanomas are often flat like LMM with large areas of MIS. This is important to ascertain in planning excision of all the lesions to prevent recurrence. Dermoscopy should be used to outline the periphery of the lesion, as is done in LMM.

Anorectal Melanoma

Often presents with a localized, often polypoid or nodular primary tumor, but it may also present similarly to LMM.

METASTATIC MELANOMA ICD-10: C77.92/C79.81

- Metastatic melanoma occurs in 15 to 26% of stage I and stage II melanomas (see the following discussion).
- The spread of disease from the primary site usually occurs in a stepwise sequence: primary melanoma → regional metastasis (see Fig. 12-19) → distant metastasis.
- Distant metastasis can occur, skipping the regional lymph nodes and indicating hematogenous spread.
- Distant metastases occur anywhere but usually in the following organs: lungs (18 to 36%), liver (14 to 29%), brain (12 to 20%), bone (11 to 17%), and intestines (1 to 7%).
- Most frequently, melanoma first spreads to distant lymph nodes, skin (Fig. 12-19B), and subcutaneous tissues (42 to 57%) (Fig. 12-19D).
- Local recurrence occurs if excision has not been adequate (Fig. 12-20) or it can involve the skin of an entire region both with and without adequate surgical treatment (Figs. 12-19A and C).
- Widespread metastasis can also lead to single metastatic melanoma cell lodgement in all organs with melanosis of the skin (Fig. 12-21), mucous membranes, liver, kidney, heart muscle, and other tissues.
- *Metastatic melanoma without a detectable primary tumor* is rare, 1 to 6%. It is the result of metastasis from a melanoma that underwent total spontaneous regression.
- *Melanoma may have a late recurrence* (≥10 years). The usual time is 14 years, but there have been "very late" recurrences (>15 years) in one series at the Massachusetts General Hospital, with 0.072% (20 of 2,766 cases).
- *Patients with a solitary metastasis* confined to the subcutaneous, nonregional lymph nodes or lung are most likely to benefit from surgical intervention.

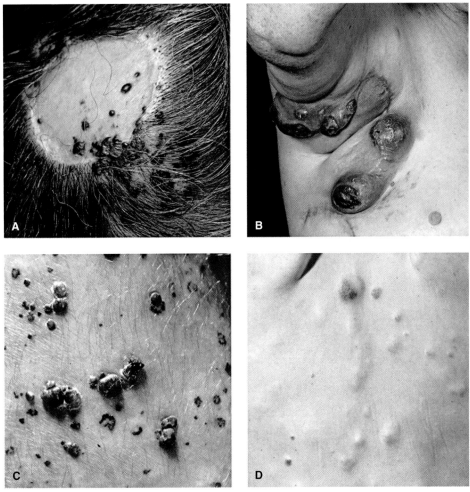

FIGURE 12-19 Metastatic melanoma (A) Local recurrence and in-transit cutaneous metastases after excision of primary melanoma on the scalp and split skin grafting. *Note*: metastases are both in the surrounding skin and the graft. **(B)** Advanced metastases in the axillary lymph nodes and in-transit metastases of the mammary skin. The primary tumor had been a pitch-black nodular melanoma and had been just lateral to the breast (the scar can still be seen). Note that both the in-transit and axillary nodules extending into the skin are amelanotic. **(C)** Multiple melanoma metastases to the skin after hematogenous spread. **(D)** Subcutaneous melanoma metastases by hematogenous spread. Since they are not bluish, they are amelanotic. Primary and metastatic melanoma may differ with regard to pigmentation potential.

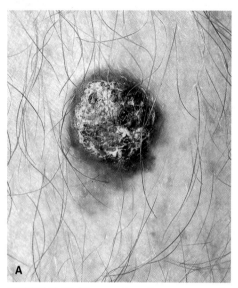 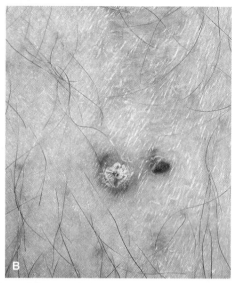

FIGURE 12-20 Metastatic melanoma: recurring in excision scar (A) A pigmented lesion on the shin of a 35-year-old male, present for <2 years. Dermatopathology was initially interpreted as a spindle cell (Spitz) nevus. The primary lesion site was therefore not reexcised. **(B)** Two papules are seen around the excision site scar, one of which has a blue-brown color. The histology from the excised lesion was reviewed and revised as a superficial spreading melanoma, and the histopathology of the two papules seen here was metastatic melanoma.

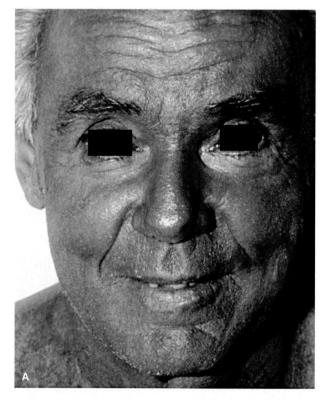

FIGURE 12-21 Universal melanosis caused by metastatic melanoma (A) Single-cell metastases are found throughout the skin and mucous membranes of this white patient and circulating metastatic melanoma cells were found in the blood. The urine was black (melanogenuria), and upon autopsy the internal organs were also black.

FIGURE 12-21 (*continued*)
(B) The patient's hand is shown beside the hand of a nurse to demonstrate the difference in color.

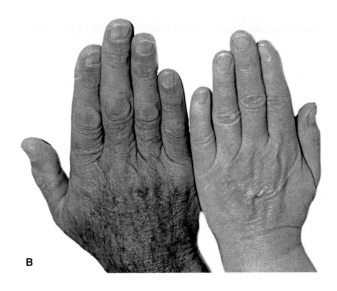

B

STAGING OF MELANOMA

- Staging of melanoma depends on its TNM classification (primary *tumor*, regional *nodes*, *metastases*, Table 12-4).
- *Clinical staging* of melanoma differentiates between local, regional, and distant disease and is based on microstaging of the melanoma and clinical and imaging evaluation for metastases.
- *Pathologic staging* consists of microstaging of the primary tumor and pathologic evaluation of regional lymph nodes (Table 12-5). Staging of melanoma is strongly correlated with survival.

Microstaging

Microstaging is done according to the Breslow method. The thickness of the primary melanoma is measured from the granular layer of the epidermis to the deepest part of the tumor. The thickness of melanoma (level of invasion) is the most important single prognostic variable and thus decisive for therapeutic decisions (Table 12-4). Primary mitotic rate is also a major criterion for melanoma staging (Table 12-4).

According to the tissue level of invasion, Clark microstaging (Clark level I, intraepidermal; level II, invades papillary dermis; level III, fills papillary dermis; level IV, invades reticular dermis; level V, invades subcutaneous fat) is no longer considered a significant prognostic variable.

Sentinel Lymph Node Biopsy

Sentinel lymph node biopsy can predict the presence of clinically nondetectable metastatic melanoma within regional lymph nodes with the identification of malignant cells in H&E sections; staining for S-100 protein, HMB-45, and tyrosinase.

When the nodes are not palpable, it is not certain if there are micrometastases; these can be detected by the *sentinel node technique*. The hypothesis is that the *first* node draining a lymphatic basin, called the *sentinel node*, can predict the presence or absence of metastasis in other nodes in that basin. Either lymphatic mapping (LM) or sentinel lymphadenectomy (SL) is performed on the same day with a single injection of filtered ^{99m}Tc subcutaneously into the site of the primary melanoma for probe-directed LM and SL. Alternatively, one day after lymphoscintigraphy, sentinel node biopsy is performed, guided by a gamma probe and blue dye also injected into the primary site. The sentinel node is subjected to histopathology and immunohistochemistry. LM is very useful in locating the drainage areas, especially in primary tumors on the trunk, which can drain on either side and to both the axillary and inguinal lymph nodes.

Lymph node dissection is performed only if micrometastasis is found in the sentinel node. The sentinel node technique is also essential in making a decision about the use of adjuvant therapy.

PROGNOSIS OF MELANOMA

When regional or distant metastases have occurred, prognosis of melanoma can be either excellent or grave, depending on whether the tumor is diagnosed early or late (Table 12-5). This emphasizes the importance of early diagnosis, of questioning patients for melanoma risks, of screening individuals belonging to risk groups, and of total-body examination of any patient seeing a physician for medical examination. Prognosis relating to stage grouping for cutaneous melanoma is shown in Table 12-5.

MANAGEMENT OF MELANOMA

The only curative treatment of melanoma is early surgical excision.

GUIDELINES FOR BIOPSY AND SURGICAL TREATMENT OF PATIENTS WITH MELANOMA

I. Biopsy
  A. Total excisional biopsy with narrow margins—optimal biopsy procedure, where possible.
  B. Incisional or punch biopsy acceptable when total excisional biopsy cannot be performed or when the lesion is large, requiring extensive surgery to remove the entire lesion.
  C. When sampling the lesion: If raised, remove the most raised area; if flat, remove the darkest area.
II. Melanoma in situ
  A. Excise with an 0.5-cm margin.
III. LMM
  A. Excise with a 1-cm margin beyond the clinically visible lesion or biopsy scar— unless the flat component involves a major organ (e.g., the eyelid), in which case lesser margins are acceptable.
  B. Excise down to the fascia or to the underlying muscle where fascia is absent. Skin flaps or skin grafts may be used for closure.
  C. No node dissection is recommended unless nodes are clinically palpable and suspicious for tumor.
  D. See the recommendation for sentinel node studies for thickness >1 mm (p. 281).
IV. SSM, NM, and ALM
  A. Thickness <1 mm
    1. Excise with a 1-cm margin from the lesion edge.
    2. Excise down to the fascia or to the underlying muscle where fascia is absent. Direct closure without graft is often possible.
    3. Node dissection is not recommended unless nodes are clinically palpable and suspicious for tumor.
  B. Thickness 1 to 4 mm
    1. Excise 2 cm from the edge of the lesion, except on the face, where narrower margins may be necessary.
    2. Excise down to the fascia or to the underlying muscle where fascia is absent. A graft may be required.
    3. The sentinel node procedure for tumors with thickness >1 mm is recommended.
    4. Lymphadenectomy is selectively performed but only for those nodal basins with occult tumor cells (i.e., positive sentinel lymph node). If the sentinel node is negative, then the patient is spared a lymph node dissection.
    5. Therapeutic nodal dissection is recommended if nodes are clinically palpable and suspicious for tumor.
    6. If regional node is positive and completely resected with no evidence of distant disease, adjuvant therapy with interferon-α-2b (IFN-α-2b) is considered.

ADJUVANT THERAPY

This is treatment of a patient after removal of all detectable tumors, but the patient is considered at high risk for recurrence (i.e., stages IIb and III). As previously mentioned, IFN-α-2b (both high and low dose) is subject to intensive investigation. However, despite early promising results to date, no clear benefit on overall survival has been convincingly demonstrated.

Management of Distant Metastases (Stage IV)*

The prospect for patients with unresectable metastatic melanoma has changed dramatically over the last years. While the median survival for these patients was around 6 months in the times of chemotherapy, it has moved up to more than 2 years in recent clinical studies with novel immune checkpoint inhibitors and targeted drugs.

Up to 50% of melanomas harbor a B-RAF V600 mutation, which leads to constitutive activation of the MAP-Kinase signaling pathway. Treatment with mutation-specific B-raf inhibitors leads to, often rapid, responses in more than half of all patients. However, these are often short lived with a median PFS of approximately 7 months. This was significantly improved by combination of B-RAF with MEK inhibitors, which increased the median PFS to more than 12 months, and is the current treatment standard for patients harboring a B-RAF V600 mutation.

_____

*Courtesy of Dr. Christoph Höller.

Immune checkpoints like CTLA-4 or PD1 confer signals that can downmodulate the activity of T-cells. These can be blocked using monoclonal antibodies thereby activating tumor-reactive T-cells. Blocking of CTLA-4 did have modest response rates, but was associated with long-term survival in around 20% of melanoma patients. The PD-1 blocking antibodies have shown response rates of 35 to 40% in clinical studies and seem to be especially efficacious in patients expressing the ligand PD-L1 on the tumor surface. Recently the combination of a CTLA-4 blocking antibody and a PD-1 antibody was approved for the treatment of metastatic melanoma and has shown response rates of around 60%, with complete responses in more than 10% of patients.

Radiation has generally only modest effects and has the best activity when sufficiently high doses can be applied, as for example in stereotactic radiosurgery for brain metastases. Surgery for patients with single- or oligometastatic disease is likewise still a viable strategy, whereas chemotherapy, for which a survival benefit was never demonstrated in a controlled clinical trial, is used increasingly only in later stages of therapy as a palliative measure.

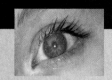

PIGMENTARY DISORDERS

- Normal skin color is composed of a mixture of four biochromes, namely, (1) *reduced hemoglobin* (blue), (2) *oxyhemoglobin* (red), (3) *carotenoids* (yellow; exogenous from diet), and (4) *melanin* (brown).
- The principal determinant of the skin color is melanin pigment, and variations in the amount and distribution of melanin in the skin are the basis of the three principal human skin colors: black, brown, and white.
- These three basic skin colors are genetically determined and are called *constitutive melanin pigmentation*. The normal basic skin color pigmentation can be increased deliberately by exposure to ultraviolet radiation (UVR) or pituitary hormones, and this is called *inducible melanin pigmentation*.
- The combination of the constitutive and inducible melanin pigmentation determines what is called the *skin phototype* (SPT) (see Table 10-2). Ethnicity is not necessarily a part of the definition, e.g., African "black" ethnic persons can be SPT III and an East Indian Caucasian can be SPT IV or even V. *The SPT is a marker for skin cancer risk and should be recorded at the first patient visit .*
- Increase of melanin in the epidermis results in a state known as *hypermelanosis*. This reflects one of two types of changes:
  - An increase in the number of melanocytes in the epidermis producing increased levels of melanin, which is called *melanocytic hypermelanosis* (an example is *lentigo*).
  - No increase of melanocytes but an increase in the production of melanin only, which is called *melanotic hypermelanosis* (an example is *melasma*).
- Hypermelanosis of both types can result from three factors: genetic, hormonal (as in Addison disease), and UVR (as in tanning).
- Hypomelanosis is a decrease of melanin in the epidermis. This reflects mainly two types of changes:
  - A decrease of the production of melanin only, which is called *melanopenic hypomelanosis* (an example is albinism).
  - A decrease in the number or absence of melanocytes in the epidermis producing no or decreased levels of melanin. This is called *melanocytopenic hypomelanosis* (an example is vitiligo).
- Hypomelanosis also results from genetic (as in albinism), from autoimmune (as in vitiligo), or other inflammatory processes (as in postinflammatory leukoderma in psoriasis).

VITILIGO ICD-10: L80

- Worldwide occurrence; 1% of population affected.
- A major psychological problem for brown or black persons, resulting in severe difficulties in social adjustment.
- A chronic disorder with multifactional predisposition and triggering factors.
- Clinically characterized by totally white macules, which enlarge and can affect the entire skin.
- Microscopically: complete absence of melanocytes.
- Rarely associated with systemic autoimmune and/or endocrine disease.

EPIDEMIOLOGY

SEX Equal in both sexes. The predominance in women suggested by the literature likely reflects the greater concern of women about cosmetic appearance.

AGE OF ONSET May begin at any age, but in 50% of cases it begins between the ages of 10 and 30 years.

INCIDENCE Common worldwide. Affects up to 1% of the population.

RACE All races. The apparently increased prevalence reported in some countries and among darker-skinned persons results from a dramatic contrast between white vitiligo macules and dark skin and from marked social stigma in countries such as India.

INHERITANCE Vitiligo has a genetic background; >30% of affected individuals have reported vitiligo in a parent, sibling, or child. Vitiligo in identical twins has also been reported. Transmission is most likely polygenic with variable expression. The risk of vitiligo for children of affected individuals is unknown but may be <10%. Individuals from families with an increased prevalence of thyroid disease, diabetes mellitus, alopecia areata and vitiligo appear to be at increased risk for development of vitiligo.

PATHOGENESIS

Three principal theories have been presented about the mechanism of destruction of melanocytes in vitiligo:

1. The *autoimmune theory* holds that selected melanocytes are destroyed by cytotoxic lymphocytes that have somehow been activated.
2. The *self-destruct hypothesis* suggests that melanocytes are destroyed by toxic substances formed as part of normal melanin biosynthesis. This could then activate mechanisms mentioned in the autoimmune hypothesis.
3. The *neurogenic hypothesis* is based on an interaction of the melanocytes and nerve cells. This probably holds only for segmental vitiligo.

CLINICAL MANIFESTATION

Many patients attribute the onset of their vitiligo to physical trauma (where vitiligo appears at the site of trauma—Koebner phenomenon), illness, or emotional stress. Vitiligo also appears after occupational exposure to phenolic compounds, most often 4-tertiary butyl phenol. A sunburn reaction may precipitate vitiligo.

SKIN LESIONS Macules, 5 mm to 5 cm *or more* in diameter (Figs. 13-1 and 13-2). "Chalk" or pale white, sharply marginated. The disease progresses by gradual enlargement of the old macules or by development of new ones. Margins are *convex*. Trichrome vitiligo (three colors: white, light brown, and dark brown) represents different stages in the evolution of vitiligo. Pigmentation around a hair follicle in a white macule represents residual pigmentation or return of pigmentation.

Distribution. Two general patterns. The *focal* type is characterized by one or several macules in a single site; this may be an early evolutionary stage of one of the other types in some cases. *Generalized* vitiligo is more common and is characterized by widespread distribution of depigmented macules, often in a remarkable symmetry (Fig. 13-2). Typical macules occur around the eyes (Fig. 13-1) and mouth, and on digits, elbows, and knees, as well as on the low back and in genital areas (Fig. 13-3). The *"lip-tip"* pattern involves the skin around the mouth as well as on distal fingers and toes; lips, nipples, genitalia, and anus may be involved. Confluence of vitiligo results in large white areas, and extensive generalized vitiligo may leave only a few normally pigmented areas of skin—*vitiligo universalis* (Fig. 13-4).

SEGMENTAL VITILIGO This is a special subset that usually develops in one unilateral region; usually does not extend beyond that initial one-sided region (though not always). Once present, is very stable. It may have a different pathogenesis than generalized vitiligo but can be associated with vitiligo elsewhere.

ASSOCIATED CUTANEOUS FINDINGS White hair and prematurely gray hair. Circumscribed areas of white hair, analogous to vitiligo macules, are called *poliosis*. Alopecia areata (see Section 31) and halo nevi (see Section 9). In older patients, photoaging as well as solar keratoses may occur in vitiligo macules in those with history of long exposures to sunlight but squamous cell carcinoma, limited to the white macules, is very rare.

GENERAL EXAMINATION Rarely associated with thyroid disease, Hashimoto thyroiditis (Graves disease); also diabetes mellitus—probably <5%; pernicious anemia (uncommon, but increased risk); Addison disease (very uncommon); and multiple endocrinopathy syndrome (rare). Ophthalmologic examination may reveal evidence of healed chorioretinitis or iritis. Vision is unaffected. Hearing is normal. The *Vogt–Koyanagi–Harada syndrome* is vitiligo + poliosis + uveitis + dysacusis + alopecia areata.

LABORATORY EXAMINATIONS

WOOD LAMP EXAMINATION For identification of vitiligo macules in very light skin.
DERMATOPATHOLOGY In certain difficult cases, a skin biopsy may be required. Vitiligo macules show normal skin except for an absence of melanocytes.

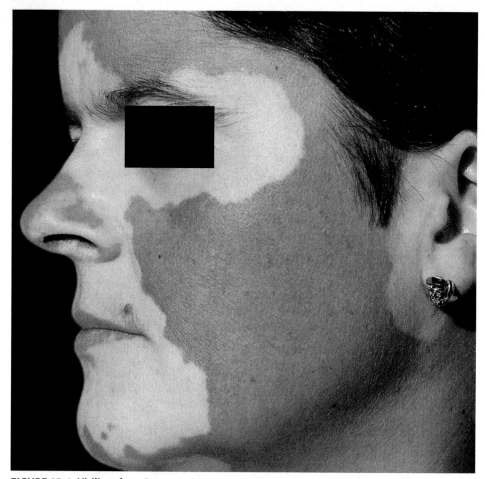

FIGURE 13-1 Vitiligo: face Extensive depigmentation of the central face. Involved vitiliginous skin has convex borders, extending into the normal pigmented skin. Note the chalk-white color and sharp margination. *Note also that the dermal melanocytic nevus on the upper lip has retained its pigmentation.*

ELECTRON MICROSCOPY Absence of melanocytes and of melanosomes in keratinocytes.

LABORATORY STUDIES To rule out associated endocrine or autoimmune diseases.

DIAGNOSIS

Normally, diagnosis of vitiligo can be made readily on clinical examination of a patient with progressive, acquired, chalk-white, bilateral (usually symmetric), sharply defined macules in typical sites.

DIFFERENTIAL DIAGNOSIS OF VITILIGO

- *Pityriasis alba* (slight scaling, fuzzy margins, off-white color) (see Pityriasis alba, p. 300).
- *Pityriasis versicolor alba* (fine scales with greenish-yellow fluorescence under Wood lamp, positive KOH (see Pityriasis versicolor, p. 297 and Section 26).
- *Leprosy* (endemic areas, off-white color, usually ill-defined *anesthetic* macules) (see Section 25).

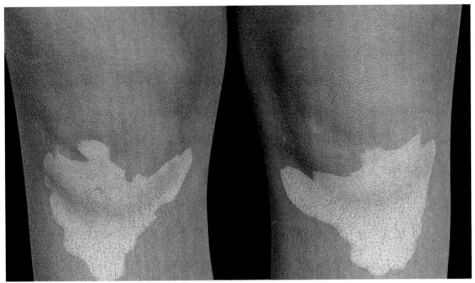

FIGURE 13-2 Vitiligo: knees Depigmented, sharply demarcated macules on the knees. Apart from the loss of pigment, vitiliginous skin appears normal. There is striking symmetry. Note tiny follicular pigmented spots within the vitiligo areas that represent repigmentation.

■ *Postinflammatory leukoderma* (off-white macules; usually a history of psoriasis or eczema in the same macular area, see Postinflammatory hypomelanosis (psoriasis), p. 298).

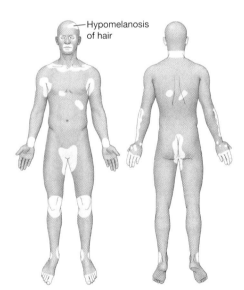

FIGURE 13-3 Vitiligo: predilection sites.

■ *Mycosis fungoides* (may be confusing as only depigmentation may be present and biopsy is necessary) (see Postinflammatory hypopigmentation, p. 300 and Section 21).
■ *Chemical leukoderma* (history of exposure to certain phenolic compounds). This is a difficult differential diagnosis, as melanocytes are absent as in vitiligo. It most probably is vitiligo.
■ *Nevus anemicus* (does not enhance with Wood lamp; does not show erythema after rubbing).
■ *Nevus depigmentosus* (stable, congenital, off-white macules, and unilateral).
■ *Hypomelanosis of Ito* (bilateral, Blaschko lines, marble cake pattern; 60 to 75% have systemic involvement—central nervous system, eyes, and musculoskeletal system).
■ *Tuberous sclerosis* (stable, congenital off-white macules polygonal, ash-leaf shape, occasional segmental macules, and confetti macules) (see Section 16).
■ *Leukoderma associated with melanoma* (is probably also vitiligo).
■ *Vogt–Koyanagi–Harada syndrome* (vision problems, photophobia, and bilateral dysacusis).
■ *Waardenburg syndrome* (commonest cause of congenital deafness, white macules and white forelock, and iris heterochromia).

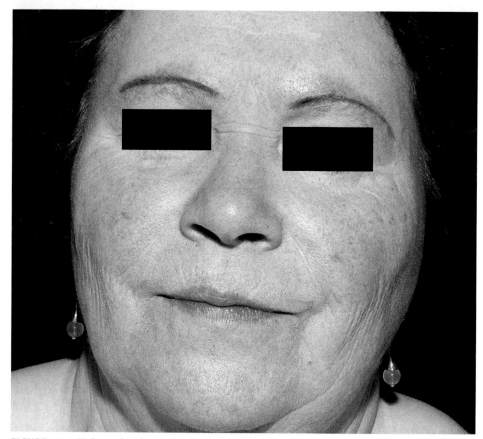

FIGURE 13-4 Universal vitiligo Vitiliginous macules have coalesced to involve all skin sites with complete depigmentation of skin and hair in a female. The patient is wearing a black wig and has darkened the brows with eyebrow pencil and eyelid margins with eye liner.

- *Piebaldism* (congenital, white forelock, stable, dorsal pigmented stripe on back, and distinctive pattern with large hyperpigmented macules in the center of the hypomelanotic areas).

COURSE AND PROGNOSIS

Vitiligo is a chronic disease. The course is highly variable, but rapid onset followed by a period of stability or slow progression is most characteristic. Up to 30% of patients may report some spontaneous repigmentation in a few areas, particularly areas that are exposed to the sun. Rapidly progressive, or "galloping," vitiligo may quickly lead to extensive depigmentation with a total loss of pigment in skin and hair, but not eyes.

The treatment of vitiligo-associated disease (i.e., thyroid disease) has no impact on the course of vitiligo.

MANAGEMENT

The approaches to the management of vitiligo are as follows:

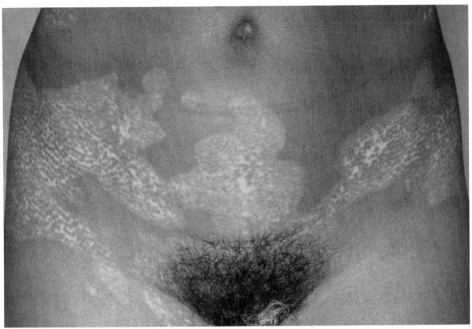

FIGURE 13-5 Vitiligo repigmentation A follicular pattern of repigmentation caused by PUVA therapy occurring in a large vitiliginous macule on the lower abdomen. By confluence of the macules, the vitiliginous areas have almost filled in but are still lighter than the surrounding normal skin. Melanocytes may persist in the hair follicle epithelium and serve to repopulate involved skin, spontaneously, with photochemotherapy, or with 312 nm phototherapy.

Sunscreens

The dual objectives of sunscreens are protection of involved skin from acute sunburn reaction and limitation of tanning of normally pigmented skin.

Cosmetic Coverup

The objective of coverup with dyes or makeup is to hide the white macules so that the vitiligo is not apparent.

Repigmentation

The objective of repigmentation (Figs. 13-5 and 13-6) is the permanent return of normal melanin pigmentation.

LOCALIZED MACULES

- *Topical glucocorticoids:* Monitor for signs of early steroid atrophy.
- *Topical calcineurin inhibitors:* Tacrolimus and pimecrolimus. They are reported to be most effective when combined with UVB or excimer laser therapy.
- *Topical photochemotherapy:* topical 8-methoxypsoralen (8-MOP) and UVA.
- *Excimer laser* (308 nm): Best results in the face.

GENERALIZED VITILIGO

- *Systemic photochemotherapy:* Oral PUVA may be done with sunlight or artificial UVA and either 5-MOP (available in Europe) or 8-MOP. Is up to 85% effective in >70% of patients with vitiligo of the head, neck, upper arms and legs, and trunk (Figs. 13-5 and 13-6). However, at least 1 year of treatment is required to achieve this result. Distal hands and feet, and the "lip-tip" variant of vitiligo are only poorly responsive.
- *Narrow-band UVB, 312 nm:* This is just as effective as PUVA and does not require psoralens. It is the treatment of choice in children <6 years of age.

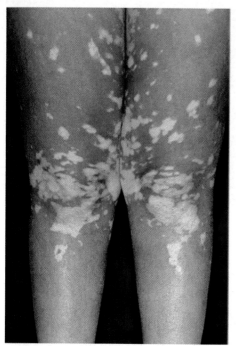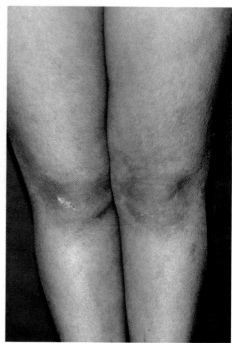

FIGURE 13-6 Vitiligo: therapy-induced repigmentation This 20-year-old Indian female has been treated with photochemotherapy (PUVA). There is slight erythema in the vitiliginous macules in the early phases (left) of therapy that will be followed by follicular pigmentation as in **Figure 13-5**. After 1 year of treatment, vitiligo has completely repigmented, but there is now hyperpigmentation of the knees (right). This, however, will fade with time and the color of the repigmented areas will blend with that of the surrounding skin.

Note: Response to all treatments is slow. When it occurs, it is signaled by tiny, usually follicular macules of pigmentation (Fig. 13-5).

Minigrafting

Minigrafting (autologous Thiersch grafts, suction blister grafts, autologous mini-punch grafts, and transplantation of cultured autologous melanocytes) may be a useful technique for refractory and stable segmental vitiligo macules. "Pebbling" of the grafted site may occur.

Depigmentation

The objective of depigmentation is "one" skin color in patients with extensive vitiligo or in those who have failed or reject other treatments.

TREATMENTS Bleaching of *normally pigmented skin* with monobenzylether of hydroquinone 20% (MEH) cream is a permanent, irreversible process. The success rate is >90%. The end-stage color of depigmentation with MEH is chalk-white, as in vitiligo macules.

OCULOCUTANEOUS ALBINISM ICD-10: E70.390

- Classification, see Table 13-1.
- Prevalence estimated 1:20,000 OCA1 and OCA2 account for 40 to 50%.
- Mutations in the tyrosinase gene are responsible for deficient tyrosinase activity in melanocytes (Table 13-1).
- Present at birth.
- Skin varied depending on type. "Snow white," creamy white (Fig. 13-7; Table 13-1), light tan.
- Hair: White (tyrosinase negative; Fig. 13-7A); yellow, cream, light brown (tyrosinase positive); red, platinum (Table 13-1).
- Eyes: Nystagmus, reduction of visual activity, iris translucency (Fig. 13-7B), decreased retinal pigment, foveal hyperplasia, and strabismus.
- Dermatopathology: Melanocytes are present but tyrosinase reduced depending on type.
- Molecular testing. Available to classify specific gene alterations.
- Significance: Reduction of visual activity; development of dermatoheliosis, and skin cancer without sun protection. Especially important for albinos living in Africa (Fig. 13-8).
- Management: No treatment available. Albinos should be under care of an ophthalmologist (vision problems) and a dermatologist (sun protection and detection of skin cancer).
- National volunteer group of albinos [in the United States: NOAH—*National Organization for Albinism and Hypomelanosis* (Noah of the Old Testament was alleged to be an Albino)].

TABLE 13-1 Classification of Albinism

Type	Subtypes	Gene Locus	Includes	Clinical Findings
OCA1	OCA1A	TYR	Tyrosinase-negative OCA	White hair and skin, eyes (pink at birth → blue)
	OCA1B	TYR	Minimal pigment OCA	
			Platinum OCA	White to near-normal skin and hair pigmentation
			Yellow OCA	Yellow (pheomelanin) hair, light red or brown hair
			Temperature-sensitive OCA Autosomal-recessive OCA (some)	May have near-normal pigment but not in axilla
OCA2		P	Tyrosinase-positive OCA	Yellow hair, skin "creamy" white (Africa)
			Brown OCA	Light brown/tan skin (Africa)
OCA3		TYRP1	Autosomal-recessive OCA (some)	
			Rufous OCA	Red and red-brown skin and brown eyes (Africa) Similar to OCA2 phenotype
OCA4		MATP		
HPS		HPS	Hermansky–Pudlak syndrome Types 1-8	Skin/hair as in OCA1A or OCA1B or OCA2, bleeding diathesis (Puerto Rico)
CHS		LYST	Chédiak–Higashi syndrome	Silver hair/hypopigmentation/ serious medical problems
OA1		OA1	X-linked OA	Normal pigmentation of skin and hair

OCA, oculocutaneous albinism; TYR, tyrosinase; P, pink protein; TYRP1, tyrosinase-related protein 1; OA, ocular albinism; MATP, membrane-associated transporter protein; LYST, lysosome trafficking.

Source: Modified with permission from Bahadoran P, et al. Albinism. In: Freedberg IM, Eisen AZ, Wolff K, et al, eds. *Fitzpatrick's Dermatology in General Medicine*. 6th ed. New York, NY: McGraw-Hill; 2003.

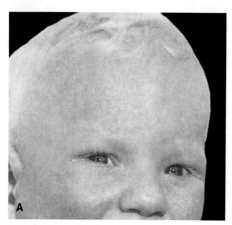
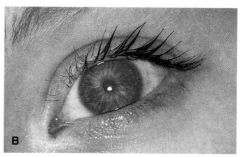

FIGURE 13-7 (A) Oculocutaneous albinism White skin, white eyelashes, eyebrows, and scalp hair. The irises appear translucent. Heme pigment gives the face a pinkish hue. There is squinting resulting from photophobia and nystagmus. **(B) Iris translucency** is a sine qua non in all types of oculocutaneous albinism, even in those patients in whom the iris is brown. The iris is rarely pink except in infants, and the diagnosis of albinism depends on the detection of iris translucency. This is best done in a dark room with a pointed flashlight placed on the sclera.

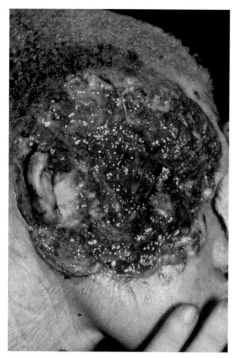

FIGURE 13-8 Squamous cell carcinoma in an Albino from Tanzania This 32-year-old African was completely white and thus unprotected from solar exposure. The carcinoma started at the age of 28 and has destroyed most of the right face including the eye. There were smaller tumors on the left side of the face and the hands and lower arms. The patient succumbed to metastatic carcinoma.

MELASMA ICD-10: L81.1

- Melasma (Greek: "a black spot") is an acquired light- or dark-brown hyperpigmentation that occurs in exposed areas, most often on the face, and results from exposure to sunlight.
- It may be associated with pregnancy, ingestion of contraceptive hormones, or possibly with certain medications such as diphenylhydantoin, or it may be idiopathic.
- Very common, especially among persons with constitutive brown skin taking contraceptive pills and living in sunny climates; 10% of patients are men.
- Macular hyperpigmentation mostly sharply defined in the malar and frontal areas of the face (Fig. 13-9). Usually uniform but also blotchy.
- Management: Commercially available preparations include hydroquinone 3% solution and 4% cream; azelaic acid 20% cream; and a combination of fluocinolone 0.01%, hydroquinone 4%, and tretinoin 0.05%. Hydroquinone 4% cream can be compounded with 0.05% tretinoin cream or glycolic acid by the pharmacist. *Under no circumstances should MEH or the other ethers of hydroquinone (monomethyl or monoethyl) be used in the treatment of melasma because these drugs can lead to a permanent loss of melanocytes with the development of a disfiguring spotty leukoderma.*
- *Prevention: Opaque sun blocks.*
- *Synonyms*: Chloasma (Greek: "a green spot"), mask of pregnancy.

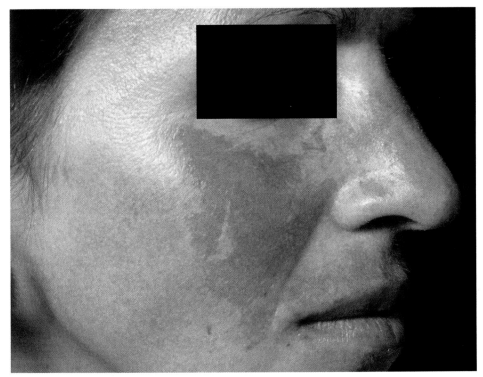

FIGURE 13-9 Melasma Well-demarcated, hyperpigmented macules are seen on the cheek, nose, and upper lip.

PIGMENTARY CHANGES FOLLOWING INFLAMMATION OF THE SKIN

HYPERPIGMENTATION ICD-10: L81.010

- *Postinflammatory epidermal melanin hyperpigmentation* is a major problem for patients with skin phototypes IV, V, and VI (Figs. 13-10 and 13-11). This disfiguring pigmentation can develop with acne (Fig. 13-10), psoriasis, lichen planus (Fig. 13-11), atopic dermatitis, contact dermatitis, or after any type of trauma to the skin. It may persist for weeks to months and does not always respond to topical hydroquinone, which may accelerate its disappearance. Lesions are characteristically limited to the site of the preceding inflammation and usually have indistinct, feathered borders.
- Ashy dermatosis is a slate grey macular hyperpigmentation in skin phototype IV individuals. This is dermal hyperpigmentation and is indistinguishable from hyperpigmentation following lichen planus.
- Some drug eruptions may be associated with *dermal* melanin hyperpigmentation (Fig. 13-12). Dermal and epidermal hyperpigmentation may occur in macular amyloidosis (see Macular amyloidosis, Section 14).
- *Riehl melanosis* (melanodermatitis toxica) is a reticular, confluent black to brown-violet pigmentation of the face and neck (Fig. 13-13). It may be a result of contact sensitivity or photocontact sensitivity related to chemicals, particularly fragrance in cosmetics.

For hypermelanosis caused by phototoxic reactions induced by psoralens (Berloque dermatitis), see Section 10 and for *nonmelanin-based hyperpigmentation* resulting from drugs, see Section 23.

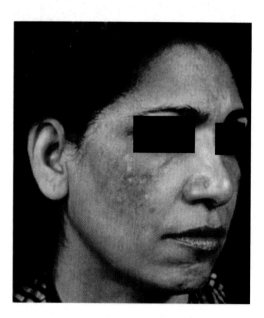

FIGURE 13-10 Hypermelanosis with acne In this 30-year-old Pakistani woman, hypermelanosis due to acne, combined with melasma and hypopigmented acne scars, was considered a cosmetic disaster, not only by the patient but also by her husband. She was successfully treated with 3% hydroquinone incorporated into a 0.05% tretinoin cream.

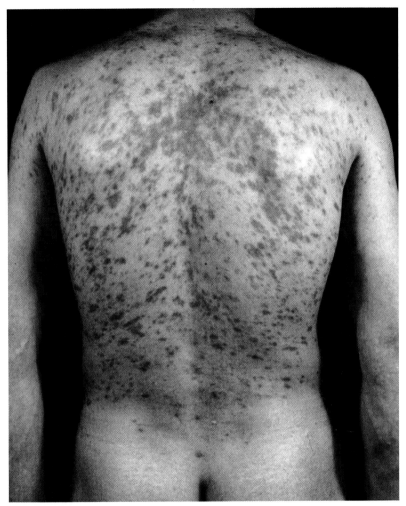

FIGURE 13-11 Postinflammatory hyperpigmentation This may follow a drug eruption, or lichen planus, especially in skin phototypes IV, V and VI, as was the case in this middle-aged East Indian man. There is a condition described as *Ashy dermatosis*, which is clinically indistinguishable from postinflammatory hyperpigmentation following lichen planus as shown here. Postinflammatory hyperpigmentation is a major problem in young females with skin phototypes IV and V.

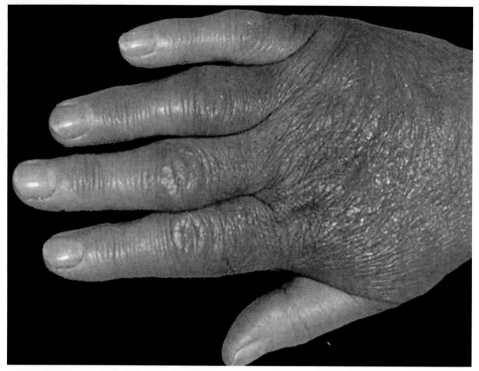

FIGURE 13-12 Postinflammatory dermal hyperpigmentation This appeared on the hand of a skin phototype IV African woman following a fixed drug eruption.

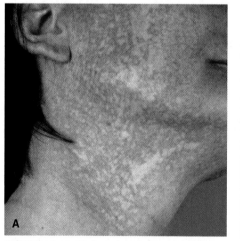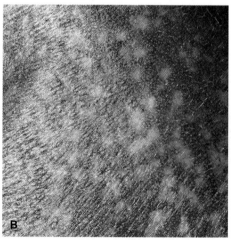

FIGURE 13-13 Melanodermatitis toxica (A) A reticular confluent pigmentation on the face and neck of a 42-year-old female chemist who worked for a cosmetic industry and had applied, over years, most of the scented products she was involved in producing to her own skin. Since she lived in a sunny climate, this increases the suspicion of a chronic photocontact sensitivity. **(B)** In this Indian woman, the mottled hyperpigmentation has coalesced to dark brown mottled hyperpigmentation of the cheeks. This patient had also excessively used cosmetics for professional reasons. Such cases are not so rare in India and are called Indian lichen planus; however, the relationship to common lichen planus is not clear.

HYPOPIGMENTATION ICD-10: L81.89

- Postinflammatory hypomelanosis is always related to loss of melanin. It is a special feature of pityriasis versicolor (Fig. 13-14, see also Section 26), in which the hypopigmentation may also remain for weeks after the active infection has disappeared.
- Hypomelanosis is not uncommonly seen in atopic dermatitis, psoriasis (Fig. 13-15), guttate parapsoriasis, and pityriasis lichenoides chronica.
- It may also be present in cutaneous lupus erythematosus (Fig. 13-16), alopecia mucinosa, mycosis fungoides (Fig. 13-17), lichen striatus, seborrheic dermatitis, and leprosy (see Hansen Disease [Leprosy], Section 25).
- Hypomelanosis may follow dermabrasion and chemical peels. In these conditions, there is a "transfer block," in which melanosomes are present in melanocytes but are not transferred to keratinocytes, resulting in hypomelanosis. The lesions are usually not chalk-white, as in vitiligo, but "off" white and have indiscrete margins.
- A common type of hypopigmentation is associated with *pityriasis alba* (Fig. 13-18). This is a macular hypopigmentation mostly on the face of children, off-white with a powdery scale. Relatively indistinct margins under Wood light and scaling distinguish this eczematous dermatitis from vitiligo. It is self-limited.
- Hypomelanosis not uncommonly follows intralesional glucocorticoid injections. When the injections are stopped, a normal pigmentation develops in the areas.
- Depending on the associated disorder, postinflammatory hypomelanosis may respond to oral PUVA photochemotherapy.

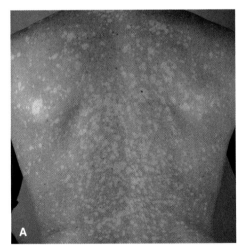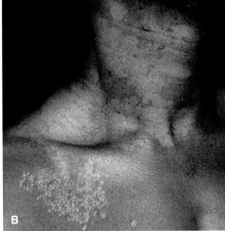

FIGURE 13-14 Pityriasis versicolor (A) Hypopigmented, sharply marginated, scaling macules on the back of an individual with skin phototype III. Gentle abrasion of the surface will accentuate the scaling. This type of hypomelanosis can remain long after the eruption has been treated and the primary process has resolved. **(B) Pityriasis versicolor in African skin** Lesions are perifollicular on the chest and coalesce to large confluent patches on the neck where the fine scaling can best be seen.

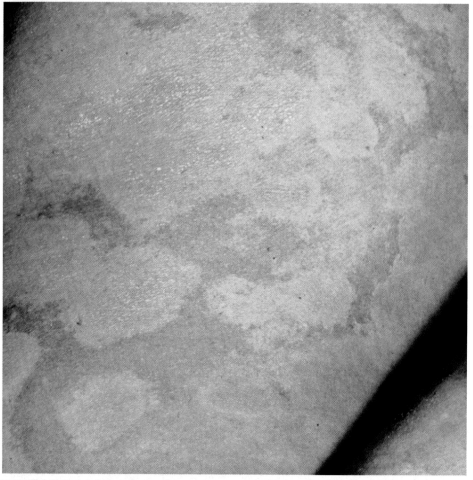

FIGURE 13-15 Postinflammatory hypomelanosis (psoriasis) The hypomelanotic lesions correspond exactly to the antecedent eruption. There is some residual psoriasis within the lesions.

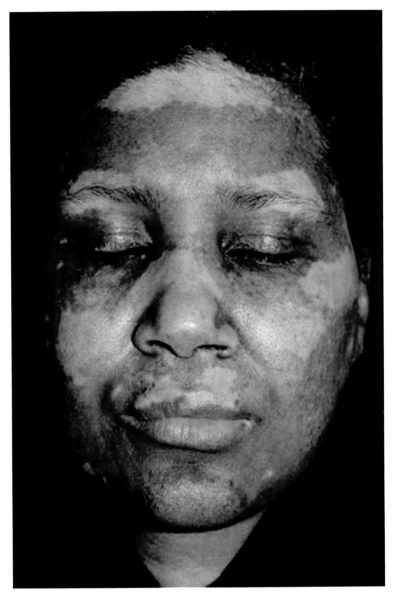

FIGURE 13-16 Postinflammatory hypopigmentation in a 33-year-old Vietnamese female. The patient had had chronic cutaneous lupus erythematosus. Residual inflammation of lupus is still seen on the upper lip.

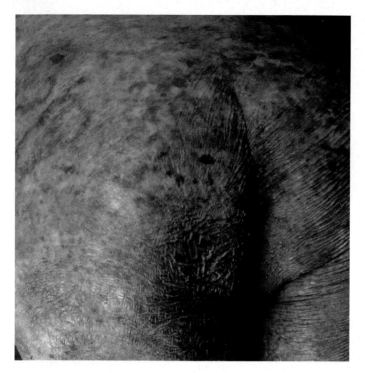

FIGURE 13-17 Mottled hypopigmentation, but also hyperpigmentation in mycosis fungoides. This patient had been treated with electron beam therapy.

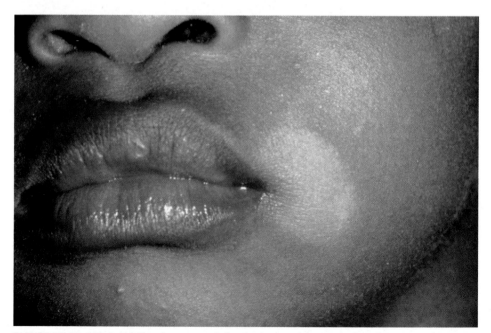

FIGURE 13-18 Pityriasis alba A common disfiguring hypomelanosis, which, as the name indicates, is a white area (alba) with very mild scaling (pityriasis). It is observed in a large number of children in the summer in temperate climates. It is mostly a cosmetic problem in persons with brown or black skin and commonly occurs on the face, as in this child. Among 200 patients with pityriasis alba, 90% ranged from 6 to 12 years of age. In young adults, PA quite often occurs on the arms and trunk.

PART II

Dermatology and Internal Medicine

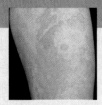

THE SKIN IN IMMUNE, AUTOIMMUNE, AUTOINFLAMMATORY, AND RHEUMATIC DISORDERS

URTICARIA AND ANGIOEDEMA ICD-10: L50

- Urticaria is composed of wheals (transient edematous papules and plaques, usually pruritic and caused by edema of the papillary body) (Fig. 14-1; also see Fig. 14-2). The wheals are superficial and well defined.
- Angioedema is a larger edematous area that involves the dermis *and* subcutaneous tissue (Fig. 14-3) and is deep and ill defined. Urticaria and angioedema are thus the same edematous process but involve different levels of the cutaneous vascular plexus: papillary and deep.
- Urticaria and/or angioedema may be acute recurrent or chronic recurrent.
- Different forms of urticaria/angioedema are recognized: IgE and IgE receptor dependent, physical, contact, mast cell degranulation related, and idiopathic.
- In addition, angioedema/urticaria can be mediated by bradykinin, the complement system, and other effector mechanisms.
- Urticarial vasculitis is a special form of cutaneous necrotizing venulitis (see p. 360).
- There are some syndromes with angioedema in which urticarial wheals are rarely present (e.g., hereditary angioedema).

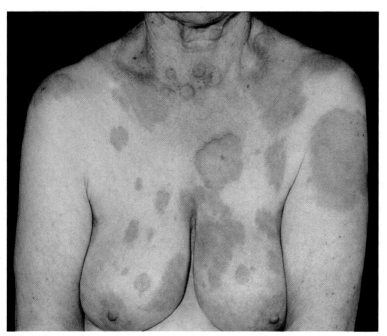

FIGURE 14-1 **Acute urticaria** Small and large wheals with erythematous borders and a lighter color centrally. Well defined. The lesion on the left upper arm is ill defined at its lower border where it is regressing.

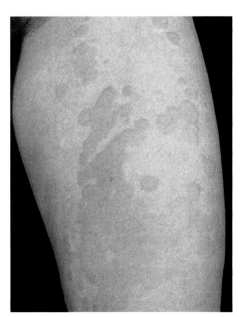

FIGURE 14-2 Chronic urticaria Chronic urticaria of 5-year duration in an otherwise healthy 35-year-old female. Eruptions occur on an almost daily basis and, as they are highly pruritic, greatly impair the patient's quality of life. Although suppressed by antihistamines, there is an immediate recurrence after treatment is stopped. Repeated laboratory and clinical examinations have not revealed an apparent cause. This condition is therefore called chronic idiopathic urticaria.

EPIDEMIOLOGY AND ETIOLOGY

INCIDENCE Fifteen to 23% of the population may have had this condition during their lifetime.

ETIOLOGY Urticaria/angioedema is not a disease but a cutaneous reaction pattern. For classification and etiology, see Table 14-1.

CLINICAL TYPES

ACUTE URTICARIA Acute onset and recurring over <30 days. Usually large wheals are often associated with angioedema (Figs. 14-1 and 14-3); often IgE dependent with atopic diathesis; related to foods, parasites, and penicillin. Also, complement mediated in serum sickness–like reactions (whole blood, immunoglobulins, and penicillin). Often accompanied by angioedema. Common. (See also "Drug-Induced Acute Urticaria" in Section 23.)

CHRONIC URTICARIA Recurring over <30 days. Small and large wheals (Fig. 14-2). Rarely IgE

TABLE 14-1 Etiology and Classification of Urticaria/Angioedema

Immunologic
IgE-mediated urticaria
Complement-mediated urticaria
Autoimmune urticaria
Immune contact urticaria

Physical
Dermographism
Cold urticaria
Solar urticaria
Cholinergic urticaria
Pressure angioedema
Vibratory angioedema

Urticaria due to mast cell–releasing agents, pseudoallergens, ACE inhibitors

Idiopathic urticaria

Nonimmune contact urticaria

Urticaria associated with vascular/connective tissue autoimmune disease

Distinct angioedema (± urticaria) syndromes
Hereditary angioedema
Angioedema–urticaria–eosinophilia syndrome

dependent but often resulting from anti-FcεR autoantibodies; etiology unknown in 80% and therefore considered idiopathic. Intolerance to salicylates and benzoates. Common. Chronic idiopathic urticaria affects adults predominantly and is approximately twice as common in women as in men. Up to 40% of patients with chronic urticaria of >6 months' duration still have urticaria 10 years later.

SYMPTOMS **Pruritus.** In angioedema of palms and soles pain. Angioedema of tongue, pharynx interferes with speech, food intake, and breathing. Angioedema of larynx may lead to asphyxia.

CLINICAL MANIFESTATION

SKIN LESIONS Sharply defined *wheals* (Fig. 14-1), small (<1 cm) to large (>8 cm), erythematous or white with an erythematous rim, round, oval, acriform, annular, serpiginous (Figs. 14-1 and 14-2), caused by confluence and resolution in one area and progression in another (Fig. 14-2). Lesions are pruritic and transient.

Angioedema—skin colored, transient enlargement of portion of face (eyelids, lips, or tongue) (Fig. 14-3 and **Drug-induced**

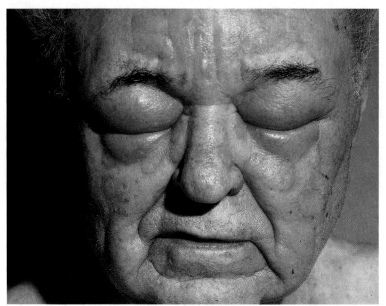

FIGURE 14-3 Acute urticaria and angioedema Note that there are both superficial wheals and deep, diffuse edema. Occurred after the patient had eaten shellfish. He had similar episodes previously but never considered seafood as the cause.

angioedema, Section 23), extremity, or other sites resulting from subcutaneous edema.
Distribution. Usually regional or generalized. Localized in solar, pressure, vibration, and cold urticaria/angioedema and confined to the site of the trigger mechanism (see below).

SPECIAL FEATURES/AS RELATED TO PATHOGENESIS

Immunologic Urticaria. IgE Mediated.
Lesions in acute IgE-mediated urticaria result from antigen-induced release of biologically active molecules from mast cells or basophilic leukocytes sensitized with specific IgE antibodies (type I anaphylactic hypersensitivity). Released mediators increase venular permeability and modulate the release of biologically active molecules from other cell types. Often with atopic background. Antigens: food (milk, eggs, wheat, shellfish, nuts), therapeutic agents, drugs (penicillin) (see also "Drug-Induced Acute Urticaria, Angioedema, Edema, and Anaphylaxis" in Section 23), helminths. Most often acute (Fig. 14-1 and **Drug-induced angioedema**, Section 23).
Complement Mediated. *Acute.* By way of immune complexes activating complement and

releasing anaphylatoxins that induce mast cell degranulation. Serum sickness, administration of whole blood, and immunoglobulins.
Autoimmune. Common, chronic. Autoantibodies against FcεRI and/or IgE. Positive autologous serum skin test. Clinically, patients with these autoantibodies (up to 40% of patients with chronic urticaria) are indistinguishable from those without them (Fig. 14-2). These autoantibodies may explain why plasmapheresis, intravenous immunoglobulins, and cyclosporine induce remission of disease activity in these patients.
Immunologic Contact Urticaria. Usually in children with atopic dermatitis sensitized to environmental allergens (grass and animals) or individuals sensitized to wearing latex rubber gloves; can be accompanied by anaphylaxis.
PHYSICAL URTICARIAS Dermographism.
Linear urticarial lesions occur after stroking or scratching the skin; they itch and fade in 30 min (Fig. 14-4); 4.2% of the normal population have it; symptomatic dermographism is a nuisance.
Cold Urticaria. Usually in children or young adults; urticarial lesions confined to sites exposed to cold occurring within minutes after rewarming. "Ice cube" test (application of

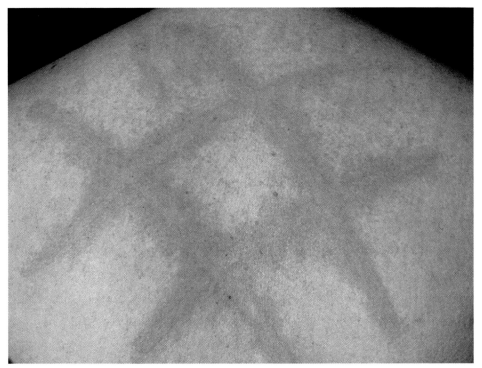

FIGURE 14-4 Urticaria: dermographism Urticaria as it appeared 5 min after the patient was scratched on the back. The patient had experienced generalized pruritus for several months with no spontaneously occurring urticaria.

an ice cube for a few minutes to skin) causes wheal.

Solar Urticaria. Urticaria after solar exposure. Action spectrum from 290 to 500 nm; whealing lasts for <1 h, may be accompanied by syncope; histamine is one of the mediators (see Section 10 and Fig. 10-11).

Cholinergic Urticaria. Exercise to the point of sweating provokes typical small, papular, highly pruritic urticarial lesions (Fig. 14-5). May be accompanied by wheezing.

Aquagenic Urticaria. Very rare. Contact with water of any temperature induces eruption similar to cholinergic urticaria.

Pressure Angioedema. Erythematous swelling induced by sustained pressure (buttock swelling when seated, hand swelling after hammering, foot swelling after walking). Delayed (30 min to 12 h). Painful, may persist for several days, and interferes with quality of life. No laboratory abnormalities; fever may occur.

Vibration Angioedema. May be familial (autosomal dominant) or sporadic. Rare. It is

believed to result from histamine release from mast cells caused by a "vibrating" stimulus— rubbing a towel across the back produces lesions, but direct pressure (without movements) does not.

URTICARIA CAUSED BY MAST CELL–RELEASING AGENTS AND PSEUDOALLERGENS AND CHRONIC IDIOPATHIC URTICARIA Urticaria/angioedema and even anaphylaxis-like symptoms may occur with radiocontrast media and as a consequence of intolerance to salicylates, food preservatives and additives (e.g., benzoic acid and sodium benzoate), several azo dyes, including tartrazine and sunset yellow (pseudoallergens) (Fig. 14-2); also to ACE inhibitors. May be acute and chronic. In chronic idiopathic urticaria, histamine derived from mast cells in the skin is considered the major mediator, also eicosanoids and neuropeptides.

Nonimmune Contact Urticaria. Caused by direct effects of exogenous urticants penetrating into skin or blood vessels. Localized to the site of contact. Sorbic acid, benzoic acid in eye solutions and foods, cinnamic aldehydes in

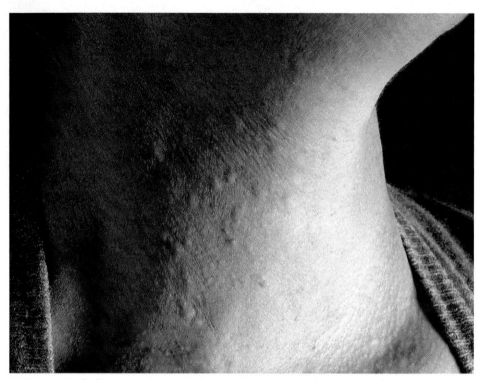

FIGURE 14-5 Cholinergic urticaria Small urticarial papules on neck occurring within 30 min of vigorous exercise. Papular urticarial lesions are best seen under side lighting.

cosmetics, histamine, acetylcholine, serotonin in nettle stings.

URTICARIA ASSOCIATED WITH VASCULAR/ CONNECTIVE TISSUE AUTOIMMUNE DISEASE
Urticarial lesions may be associated with systemic lupus erythematosus (SLE) and Sjögren syndrome. However, in most instances, they represent urticarial vasculitis (see p. 360).

DISTINCT ANGIOEDEMA (± URTICARIA) SYNDROMES
Hereditary Angioedema (HAE). A serious autosomal-dominant disorder; may follow trauma (physical and emotional). Angioedema of the face (Fig. 14-6) and extremities, episodes of laryngeal edema, and acute abdominal pain caused by angioedema of the bowel wall presenting as surgical emergency. Urticaria rarely occurs. Laboratory abnormalities involve the complement system: decreased levels of C1-esterase inhibitor (85%) or dysfunctional inhibitor (15%), low C4 value in the presence of normal C1 and C3 levels. Angioedema results from bradykinin formation, since C1-esterase inhibitor is also the major inhibitor of the Hageman factor and kallikrein, the two enzymes required for kinin formation. Episodes can be life threatening.

Angioedema–Urticaria–Eosinophilia Syndrome. Severe angioedema, only occasionally with pruritic urticaria, involving the face, neck, extremities, and the trunk that lasts for 7 to 10 days. There is fever and marked increase in normal weight (increased by 10 to 18%) owing to fluid retention. No other organs are involved. Laboratory abnormalities include striking leukocytosis (20,000 to 70,000/µL) and eosinophilia (60 to 80% eosinophils), which are related to the severity of attack. There is no family history. This condition is rare and prognosis is good.

LABORATORY EXAMINATIONS

SEROLOGY Search for hepatitis B–associated antigen, assessment of the complement system, assessment of specific IgE antibodies by radioallergosorbent test (RAST), anti-FcεRI autoantibodies. Serology for lupus and Sjögren syndrome. Autologous serum skin test for autoimmune urticaria.

HEMATOLOGY The erythrocyte sedimentation rate (ESR) is often elevated in urticarial vasculitis, and there may be hypocomplementemia;

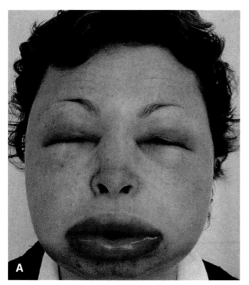
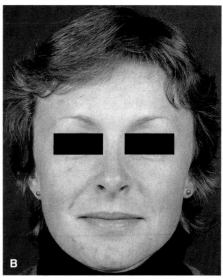

FIGURE 14-6 Hereditary angioedema (A) Severe edema of the face during an episode leading to grotesque disfigurement. **(B)** Angioedema will subside within hours. These are the normal features of the patient. The patient had a positive family history and had multiple similar episodes including colicky abdominal pain.

transient eosinophilia in urticaria from reactions to foods, parasites, and drugs; high levels of eosinophilia in the angioedema–urticaria–eosinophilia syndrome.

COMPLEMENT STUDIES Screening for functional C1 inhibitor in HAE.

ULTRASONOGRAPHY For early diagnosis of bowel involvement in HAE; if abdominal pain is present, this may indicate edema of the bowel.

PARASITOLOGY Stool specimen for presence of parasites.

DIAGNOSIS

A detailed history (previous diseases, drugs, foods, parasites, physical exertion, and solar exposure) is of utmost importance. History should differentiate between *type of lesions*—urticaria, angioedema, or urticaria + angioedema; *duration of lesions* (<1 h or ≥1 h), *pruritus; pain* on walking (in foot involvement), *flushing, burning*, and *wheezing* (in cholinergic urticaria). *Fever* in serum sickness and in the angioedema–urticaria–eosinophilia syndrome; in angioedema, *hoarseness, stridor*, and *dyspnea Arthralgia* (serum sickness, urticarial vasculitis), *abdominal colicky pain* in HAE. A careful history of medications including penicillin, aspirin, nonsteroidal anti-inflammatory drugs, and ACE inhibitors should be obtained.

Dermographism is evoked by stroking the skin; pressure urticaria is tested by application of pressure (weight) perpendicular to the skin; vibration angioedema by a vibratory stimulus, like rubbing the back with a towel. *Cholinergic urticaria* can best be diagnosed by exercise to sweating and intracutaneous injection of acetylcholine or mecholyl, which will produce micropapular whealing. *Solar urticaria* is verified by testing with UVB, UVA, and visible light (see Solar urticarial, Section 10). *Cold urticaria* is verified by a wheal response to the application of an ice cube to the skin or a test tube containing ice water. Autoimmune urticaria is tested by the autologous serum skin test and determination of anti-FcεRI antibody. If urticarial wheals do not disappear in ≤24 h, urticarial vasculitis should be suspected and a biopsy done. The person with *angioedema–urticaria–eosinophilia syndrome* has high fever, high leukocytosis (mostly eosinophils), a striking increase in body weight caused by retention of water, and a cyclic pattern that may occur and recur over a period of years. *HAE* has a positive family history and is characterized by angioedema as the result of trauma, abdominal pain, and decreased levels of C4 and C1-esterase inhibitor.

A practical approach to the diagnosis of urticaria/angioedema is shown in Fig. 14-7 and to angioedema alone in Fig. 14-8.

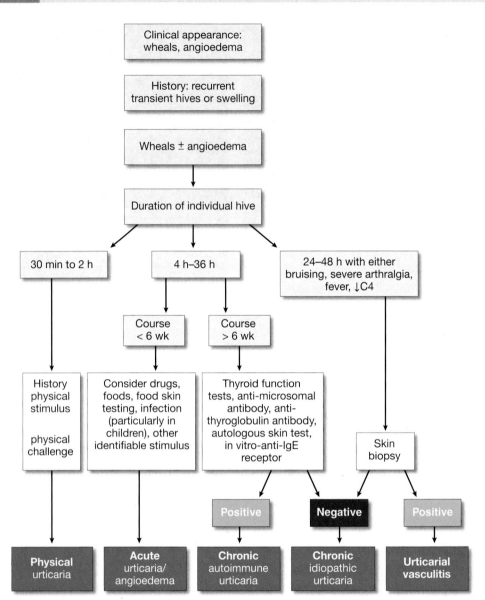

FIGURE 14-7 Approach to the patient with urticaria/angioedema. (Modified with permission from Kaplan AP. Urticaria and angioedema. In: Wolff K, Goldsmith LA, Katz SI, et al, eds. *Fitzpatrick's Dermatology in General Medicine*. 7th ed. New York, NY: McGraw-Hill; 2008, p. 339.)

FIGURE 14-8 Approach to the patient with angioedema (without urticaria). (Modified with permission from Kaplan AP. Urticaria and angioedema. In: Wolff K, Goldsmith LA, Katz SI, et al, eds. *Fitzpatrick's Dermatology in General Medicine*. 7th ed. New York, NY: McGraw-Hill; 2008, p. 339.)

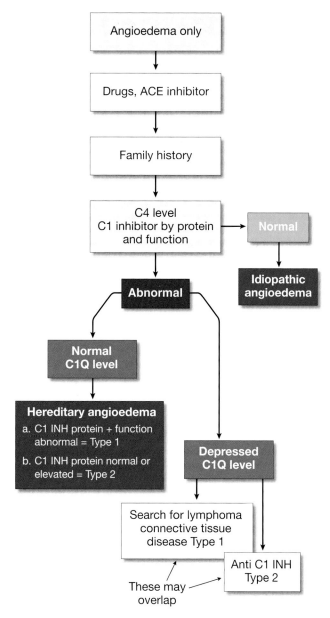

COURSE AND PROGNOSIS

Half of the patients with urticaria alone are free of lesions within 1 year, but 20% have lesions for >20 years. Prognosis is good in most syndromes except HAE, which may be fatal if untreated.

MANAGEMENT

Prevention by elimination of etiologic chemicals or drugs: aspirin and food additives, especially in chronic recurrent urticaria—rarely successful; prevent trigger in physical urticarias.
ANTIHISTAMINES H$_1$-blockers, e.g., hydroxyzine, terfenadine; or loratadine, cetirizine, fexofenadine; 180 mg/d of fexofenadine or 10 to 20 mg/d of loratadine usually controls most cases of chronic urticaria, but cessation of therapy usually results in a recurrence; if they fail, H$_1$ and H$_2$ blockers (cimetidine) and/or mast cell–stabilizing agents (ketotifen). Doxepin, a tricyclic antidepressant with marked H$_1$ antihistaminic activity, is valuable when severe urticaria is associated with anxiety and depression.
PREDNISONE In *acute* urticaria with angioedema; also for angioedema–urticaria–eosinophilia syndrome.
DANAZOL OR STANOZOLOL Long-term therapy for HAE; watch out for hirsutism, irregular menses; whole fresh plasma or C1-esterase inhibitor in the acute attack. Icatibant, a very effective bradikin-B$_2$-receptor antagonist for subcutaneous application, is now available.
OTHER In *chronic idiopathic* or *autoimmune* urticaria, if no response to antihistamines: switch to cyclosporine and taper gradually, if glucocorticoids are contraindicated or if side effects occur.
OMALIZUMAB Chronic idiopathic urticaria that is not controlled by antihistamines (double the conventional dose) will respond to Omalizumab 300 mg SC every 4 weeks. Very expensive.

ERYTHEMA MULTIFORME (EM) SYNDROME ICD-10: L51.1

- A common reaction pattern of blood vessels in the dermis with secondary epidermal changes.
- Manifests clinically as characteristic erythematous iris-shaped papular and vesiculobullous lesions.
- Typically involving the extremities (especially the palms and soles) and the mucous membranes.
- Benign course with frequent recurrences.
- Most cases related to herpes simplex virus (HSV) infection.
- Recurrences can be prevented by long-term anti-HSV medication.
- More severe course in EM *major*.

EPIDEMIOLOGY

AGE OF ONSET 50% under 20 years.
SEX More frequent in males than in females.

ETIOLOGY

A cutaneous reaction to a variety of antigenic stimuli, most commonly to herpes simplex.
INFECTION Herpes simplex, *Mycoplasma*.
DRUGS Sulfonamides, phenytoin, barbiturates, phenylbutazone, penicillin, or allopurinol.
IDIOPATHIC Probably also caused by undetected herpes simplex or *Mycoplasma*.

CLINICAL MANIFESTATION

Evolution of lesions over several days. May have history of prior EM. May be pruritic or painful, particularly mouth lesions. In severe forms constitutional symptoms such as fever, weakness, malaise.
SKIN LESIONS Lesions may develop over ≥10 days. Macule → papule (1 to 2 cm) → vesicles and bullae in the center of the papule. Dull red. *Iris* or *target-like lesions* result and are typical (Figs. 14-9 and 14-10). Localized to hands and face or generalized (Figs. 14-11 and 14-12). Bilateral and often symmetric.

Sites of Predilection. Dorsa of the hands, palms, and soles; forearms, feet, face, elbows and knees; penis (50%) and vulva (see Fig. 14-13).

MUCOUS MEMBRANES Erosions with fibrin membranes; occasionally ulcerations: lips (Figs. 14-10, 14-11, see also Section 33), oropharynx, nasal, conjunctival (Fig. 14-11), vulvar, and anal.

OTHER ORGANS Eyes, with corneal ulcers, anterior uveitis.

COURSE

MILD FORMS (EM MINOR) Little or no mucous membrane involvement; vesicles but no bullae or systemic symptoms. Eruption usually confined to extremities, face, classic target lesions (Figs. 14-9 and 14-10). Recurrent EM minor is usually associated with an outbreak of herpes simplex preceding it by several days.

SEVERE FORMS (EM MAJOR) Most often occurs as a drug reaction, always with mucous membrane involvement; severe, extensive, tendency to become confluent and bullous, positive Nikolsky sign in erythematous lesions (Figs. 14-11 and 14-12). Systemic symptoms: fever and prostration. Cheilitis and stomatitis interfere with eating; vulvitis and balanitis with micturition. Conjunctivitis can lead to keratitis and ulceration; lesions also in pharynx and larynx.

LABORATORY EXAMINATION

DERMATOPATHOLOGY Inflammation characterized by perivascular mononuclear infiltrate, edema of the upper dermis; apoptosis of keratinocytes with focal epidermal necrosis and subepidermal bulla formation. In severe cases, complete necrosis of epidermis similar to toxic epidermal necrolysis (see Section 8).

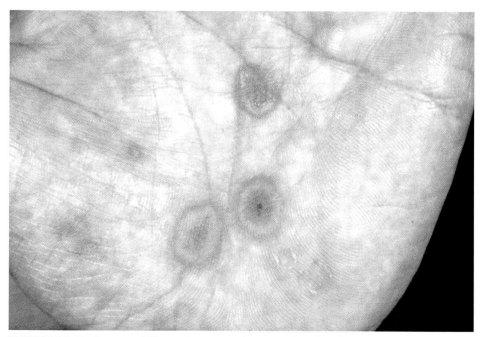

FIGURE 14-9 Erythema multiforme Iris or target lesions on the palm of a 16-year-old. The lesions are very flat papules with a red rim, a violaceous ring, and a red center.

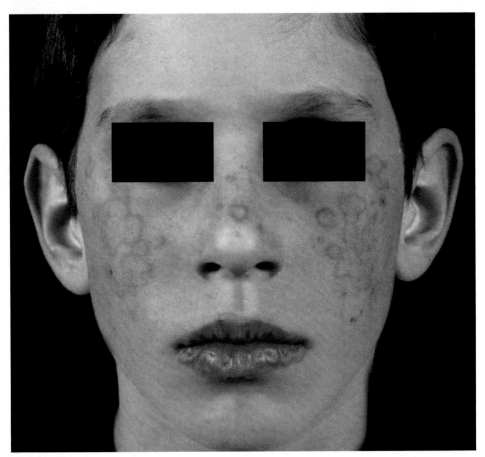

FIGURE 14-10 Erythema multiforme: minor Multiple, confluent, target-like papules on the face of a 12-year-old boy. The target morphology of the lesions is best seen on the lips.

DIAGNOSIS AND DIFFERENTIAL DIAGNOSIS

The target-like lesion and the symmetry are quite typical, and the diagnosis is not difficult. ACUTE EXANTHEMATIC ERUPTIONS Drug eruption, psoriasis, secondary syphilis, urticaria, and generalized Sweet syndrome. Mucous membrane lesions may present a difficult differential diagnosis: bullous diseases, fixed drug eruption, acute lupus erythematosus, or primary herpetic gingivostomatitis.

MANAGEMENT

PREVENTION Control of herpes simplex using oral valaciclovir or famciclovir may prevent development of recurrent EM.
GLUCOCORTICOIDS In severely ill patients, systemic glucocorticoids are usually given (prednisone, 50 to 80 mg/d in divided doses, quickly tapered), but their effectiveness has not been established by controlled studies.

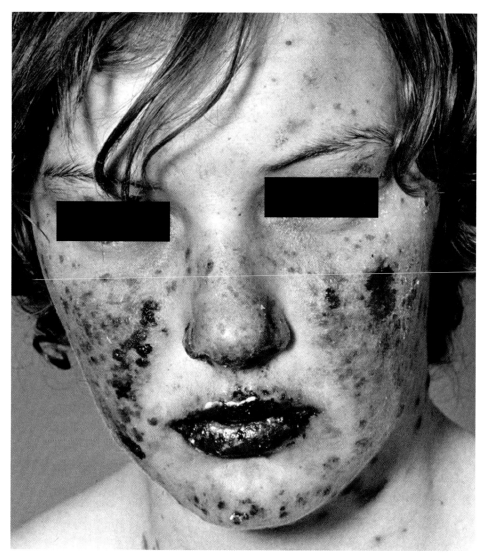

FIGURE 14-11 Erythema multiforme: major Erythematous, confluent, target-like papules, erosions, and crusts on the face. There is erosive and crusted cheilitis indicating mucosal involvement, and there is conjunctivitis with erosions on the eyelids. The patient also had a generalized rash consisting of iris lesions.

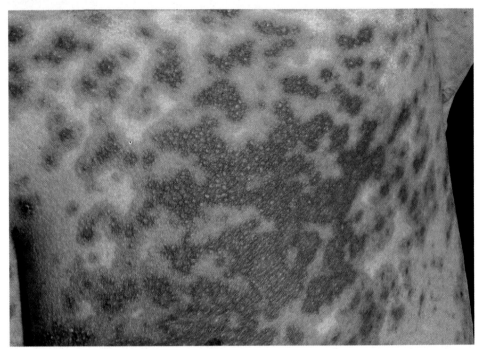

FIGURE 14-12 Erythema multiforme: major Multiple, target lesions have coalesced, and erosions will develop. This patient had fever and mucosal involvement of the mouth, conjunctiva, and genitalia.

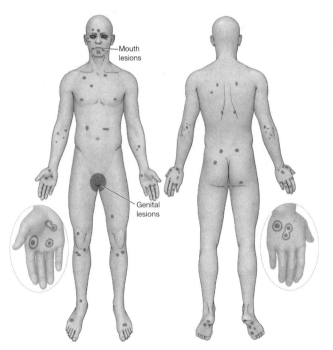

Mouth lesions

Genital lesions

FIGURE 14-13 Erythema multiforme Predilection sites and distribution.

CRYOPYRINOPATHIES (CAPS)* ICD-10: E85.0, L50.8

- Are rare systemic autoinflammatory diseases, autosomal dominant.
- Includes familial cold autoinflammatory syndrome (FCAS), Muckle–Wells syndrome (MWS) (Fig. 14-14), and neonatal-onset multisystem inflammatory disease (NOMID).
- Most have mutations in NLRP3.
- Urticaria-like eruptions (Fig. 14-14), fever (periodic or continuous), conjunctivitis, arthralgia and elevation of acute phase reactants. Untreated develop progressive hearing loss, progressive vision loss (MWS, NOMID), mental retardation, hydrocephalus, bony overgrowth (NOMID), and amyloidosis.
- Histopathology of lesional skin shows edema, dilatation of superficial capillaries, and perivascular and perieccrine neutrophilic infiltrates.
- Anti-IL-1 therapy is effective.

Source: Lee CCR and Goldbach-Mansky R. Systemic autoinflammatory diseases. In: Goldsmith LA, Katz SI, Gilchrest BA, Paller AS, Leffell DJ, and Wolff K (eds.). *Fitzpatrick's Dermatology in General Medicine*, 8th ed. New York, NY: McGraw-Hill; 2012:1584–1599.

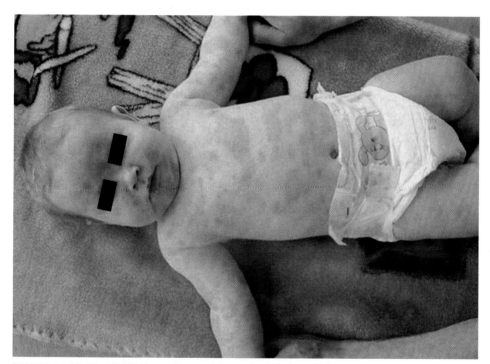

FIGURE 14-14 Muckle-Wells syndrome A 2-month-old baby with fever and arthralgia and an urticarial rash. (Used with permission from Drs. Klemens Rappersberger and Christian Posch.)

LICHEN PLANUS (LP) ICD-10: L43

- Worldwide occurrence; incidence less than 1%, all races.
- LP is an acute or chronic inflammatory dermatosis involving skin and/or mucous membranes.
- Characterized by flat-topped (Latin *planus*, "flat"), pink to violaceous, shiny, and pruritic polygonal papules. The features of the lesions have been designated as the four P's—papule, purple, polygonal, pruritic.
- Distribution: Predilection for flexural aspects of arms and legs, which can become generalized.
- In the mouth, milky-white reticulated papules; may become erosive and even ulcerate.
- Main symptom: Pruritus; in the mouth, pain.
- Therapy: Topical and systemic glucocorticoids, cyclosporine.

EPIDEMIOLOGY AND ETIOLOGY

AGE OF ONSET 30 to 60 years.

SEX Females > males.

ETIOLOGY Idiopathic in most cases but cell-mediated immunity plays a major role. Majority of lymphocytes in the infiltrate are CD8+ and CD45Ro+ (memory) cells. Drugs, metals (gold or mercury), or infection (hepatitis C virus) result in alteration in cell-mediated immunity. There could be HLA-associated genetic susceptibility that would explain a predisposition in certain persons. Lichenoid lesions of chronic graft-versus-host disease (GVHD) of skin are indistinguishable from those of LP (see Section 22).

CLINICAL MANIFESTATION

ONSET Acute (days) or insidious (over weeks). Lesions last months to years, asymptomatic or pruritic; sometimes severe pruritus. Mucous membrane lesions are painful, especially when ulcerated.

SKIN LESIONS Papules, flat-topped, 1 to 10 mm, sharply defined, shiny (Fig. 14-15). Violaceous, with white lines (Wickham striae) (Fig. 14-15A), seen best with hand lens after application of a drop of mineral oil. Polygonal or oval (Fig. 14-15B). Grouped (Figs. 14-15 and 14-16), annular, or disseminated scattered discrete lesions when generalized (Fig. 14-17). In dark-skinned individuals, postinflammatory hyperpigmentation is common. May present on lips (Fig. 14-18A) and in a linear arrangement after trauma (Koebner or isomorphic phenomenon (Fig. 14-18B).

Sites of Predilection. Wrists (flexor), lumbar region, shins (thicker, hyperkeratotic lesions), scalp, glans penis (see Section 34), and mouth (see Section 33).

Variants

Hypertrophic. Large thick plaques arise on the foot (Fig. 14-16B), dorsum of hands (Fig. 14-16A), and shins; more common in black males. Although typical LP papule is smooth, hypertrophic lesions may become hyperkeratotic.

Atrophic. White-bluish, well-demarcated papules and plaques with central atrophy.

Follicular. Individual keratotic-follicular papules and plaques that lead to cicatricial alopecia. Spinous follicular lesions, typical skin and mucous membrane LP, and cicatricial alopecia of the scalp are called *Graham Little syndrome* (see Section 31).

Vesicular. Vesicular or bullous lesions may develop within LP patches or independent of them within normal-appearing skin. There are direct immunofluorescence findings consistent with bullous pemphigoid, and the sera of these patients contain bullous pemphigoid IgG autoantibodies (see Section 6).

Pigmentosus. Hyperpigmented, dark-brown macules in sun-exposed areas and flexural folds. In Latin Americans and other dark-skinned populations. Significant similarity or perhaps identity with ashy dermatosis (see Fig. 13-11).

Actinicus. Papular LP lesions arise in sun-exposed sites, especially the dorsa of the hands and arms.

Ulcerative. LP may lead to therapy-resistant ulcers, particularly on the soles, requiring skin grafting.

MUCOUS MEMBRANES Some 40 to 60% of individuals with LP have oropharyngeal involvement (see Section 33).

Reticular LP. Reticulate (netlike) pattern of lacy white hyperkeratosis on buccal mucosa (see Section 33), lips (Fig. 14-18A), and tongue, gingiva.

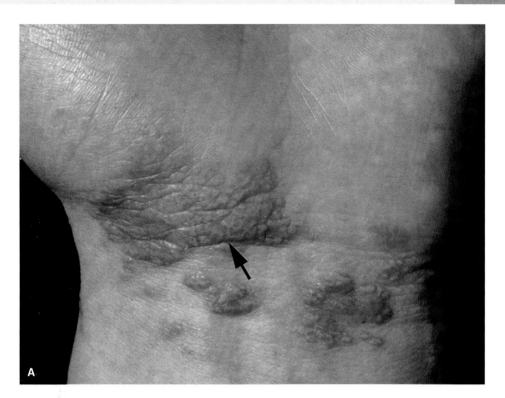

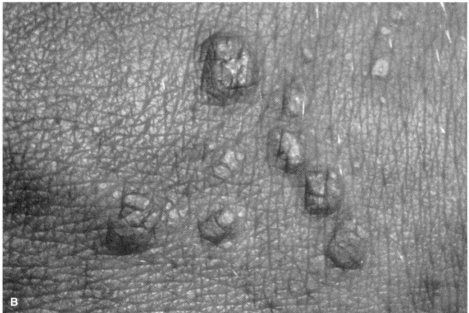

FIGURE 14-15 Lichen planus (A) Flat-topped, polygonal, sharply defined papules of violaceous color, grouped and confluent. Surface is shiny and, upon close inspection with a hand lens, fine white lines are revealed (Wickham striae, *arrow*). **(B)** Close up of flat-topped shiny violaceous papules that are polygonal.

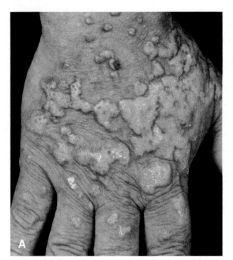
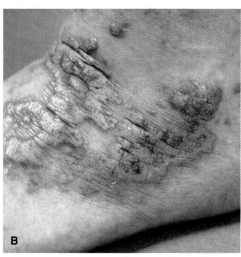

FIGURE 14-16 **Hypertrophic lichen planus** **(A)** Confluent hyperkeratotic papules and plaques on the dorsum of the hand of a light-colored man of African descent. Hyperkeratosis covers Wickham striae, and the characteristic violaceous color of the lesions can be seen only at the very margins. **(B)** Hypertrophic lichen planus on the dorsum of the foot. Lesions form thick plaques with a hyperkeratotic surface and a violaceous border.

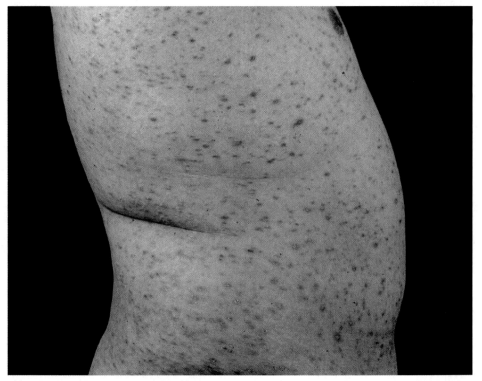

FIGURE 14-17 **Disseminated lichen planus** A shower of disseminated papules on the trunk and the extremities (not shown) in a 45-year-old Filipino. Resulting from the ethnic color of the skin, the papules are not as violaceous as in Caucasians but have a brownish hue.

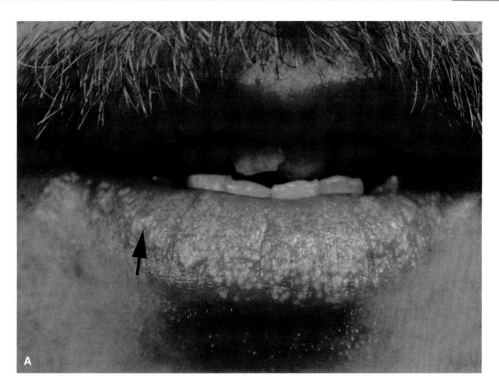

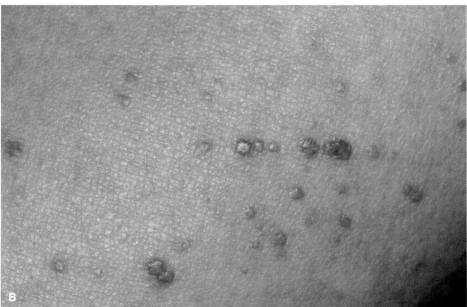

FIGURE 14-18 Lichen planus (A) Silvery-white, confluent, flat-topped papules on the lips. *Note*: Wickham striae (*arrow*). **(B)** Lichen planus, Koebner phenomenon. Linear arrangement of flat-topped, shiny papules that erupted after scratching.

Erosive or Ulcerative LP. Superficial erosion with/without overlying fibrin clot; occurs on tongue and buccal mucosa (see Section 33); shiny red painful erosion of gingiva (desquamative gingivitis) (see Section 33) or lips (Fig. 14-18A). Carcinoma may very rarely develop in mouth lesions.

GENITALIA Papular (see Section 34) agminated, annular, or erosive lesions arise on the penis (especially glans), scrotum, labia majora, labia minora, and vagina.

HAIR AND NAILS **Scalp.** Follicular LP or atrophic scalp skin with scarring alopecia. (See Sections 31 and 32.)

Nails. Destruction of nail fold and nail bed with longitudinal splintering (see Section 32).

LICHEN PLANUS–LIKE ERUPTIONS

LP-like eruptions closely mimic typical LP, both clinically and histologically. They occur as a clinical manifestation of chronic GVHD, in dermatomyositis (DM), and as cutaneous manifestations of malignant lymphoma but may also develop as the result of therapy with certain drugs and after industrial use of certain compounds (see Section 23).

DIAGNOSIS AND DIFFERENTIAL DIAGNOSIS

Clinical findings confirmed by histopathology.
Papular LP. Chronic cutaneous lupus erythematosus, psoriasis, pityriasis rosea, eczematous dermatitis, and lichenoid GVHD; single lesions: superficial basal cell carcinoma or Bowen disease (in situ squamous cell carcinoma).
Hypertrophic LP. Psoriasis vulgaris, lichen simplex chronicus, prurigo nodularis, stasis dermatitis, and Kaposi sarcoma.
MUCOUS MEMBRANES Leukoplakia, pseudomembranous candidiasis (thrush), HIV-associated hairy leukoplakia, lupus erythematosus, bite trauma, mucous patches of secondary syphilis, pemphigus vulgaris, or bullous pemphigoid (see Section 33).
Drug-Induced LP. See Section 23.

LABORATORY EXAMINATION

DERMATOPATHOLOGY Inflammation with hyperkeratosis, increased granular layer, irregular acanthosis, liquefaction degeneration of the basal cell layer, and band-like mononuclear infiltrate that hugs the epidermis. Keratinocyte apoptosis (colloid, Civatte bodies) found at the dermal–epidermal junction. Direct immunofluorescence reveals heavy deposits of fibrin at the junction and IgM and, less frequently, IgA, IgG, and C3 in the colloid bodies.

COURSE

Cutaneous LP usually persists for months, but in some cases for years; hypertrophic LP on the shins and oral LP often persists for decades. The incidence of oral squamous cell carcinoma in individuals with oral LP is increased (5%).

MANAGEMENT

Local Therapy

Glucocorticoids. Topical glucocorticoids with occlusion for cutaneous lesions. Intralesional triamcinolone (3 mg/mL) is helpful for symptomatic cutaneous or oral mucosal lesions and lips.
Cyclosporine and Tacrolimus Solutions. Retention "mouthwash" for severely symptomatic oral LP.

Systemic Therapy

Cyclosporine. In very resistant and generalized cases, 5 mg/kg per day will induce rapid remission, quite often not followed by recurrence.
Glucocorticoids. Oral prednisone is effective for individuals with symptomatic pruritus, painful erosions, dysphagia, or cosmetic disfigurement. A short, tapered course is preferred: 70 mg initially, tapered by 5 mg/d.
Systemic Retinoids (Acitretin). 1 mg/kg per day is helpful as adjunctive measure in severe (oral, hypertrophic) cases, but usually additional topical treatment is required.

PUVA Photochemotherapy

In individuals with generalized LP or cases resistant to topical therapy.

Other Treatments

Mycophenolate mofetil, heparin analogues (enoxaparin) in low doses have antiproliferative and immunomodulatory properties; azathioprine.

BEHÇET DISEASE ICD-10: M35.2

- Rare; worldwide occurrence, but strongly variable ethnic prevalence.
- It is a perplexing multisystem vasculitic disease with multiorgan involvement.
- Main symptoms are recurrent oral aphthous ulcers, genital ulcers, erythema nodosum, superficial thrombophlebitis, skin pustules, iridocyclitis, and posterior uveitis.
- Additional symptoms may be arthritis, epididymitis, ileocecal ulcerations, vascular, and central nervous system (CNS) lesions.
- Chronic relapsing progressive course with potentially poor prognosis.

EPIDEMIOLOGY

AGE OF ONSET Third and fourth decades.
PREVALENCE Highest in Turkey (80 to 420 patients in 100,000), Japan, Korea, Southeast Asia, the Middle East, southern Europe. Rare in northern Europe, United States (0.12 to 0.33 in 100,000).
SEX Males > females, but dependent on ethnic background.

PATHOGENESIS

Etiology unknown. In the eastern Mediterranean and East Asia, HLA-B5 and HLA-B51 association; in the United States and Europe, no consistent HLA association. The lesions are the result of leukocytoclastic (acute) and lymphocytic (late) vasculitis.

CLINICAL MANIFESTATION

Painful ulcers erupt in a cyclic fashion in the oral cavity and/or genital mucous membranes.

Orodynophagia and oral ulcers may persist/recur weeks to months before other symptoms appear.
SKIN AND MUCOUS MEMBRANES **Aphthous Ulcers.** Punched-out ulcers (3 to >10 mm) with rolled or overhanging borders and necrotic base (Fig. 14-19); red rim; occur in crops (2 to 10) on oral mucous membrane (100%) (Fig. 14-19), vulva, penis, and scrotum (Figs. 14-20 and 14-21); very painful.
Erythema Nodosum-Like Lesions. Painful inflammatory nodules on the arms and legs (40%) (see Section 7).
Other. Inflammatory pustules, superficial thrombophlebitis, *inflammatory plaques* resembling those in Sweet syndrome (see Section 7), *pyoderma gangrenosum-like lesions* (see Section 7), *palpable purpuric lesions* of necrotizing vasculitis (see p. 353).
SYSTEMIC FINDINGS **Eyes.** Leading cause of morbidity. Posterior uveitis, anterior uveitis, retinal vasculitis, vitritis, hypopyon, secondary cataracts, glaucoma, and neovascularization.

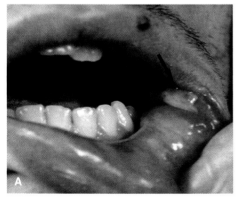
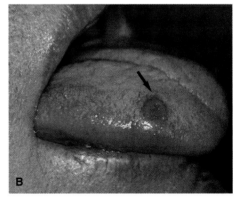

FIGURE 14-19 Behçet disease Oral aphthous ulcers. **(A)** These are highly painful, punched-out ulcers with a necrotic base on the buccal mucosa and lower and upper fornix in this 28-year-old Turkish male (*arrow*). **(B)** A punched-out ulcer on the tongue of another patient (*arrow*).

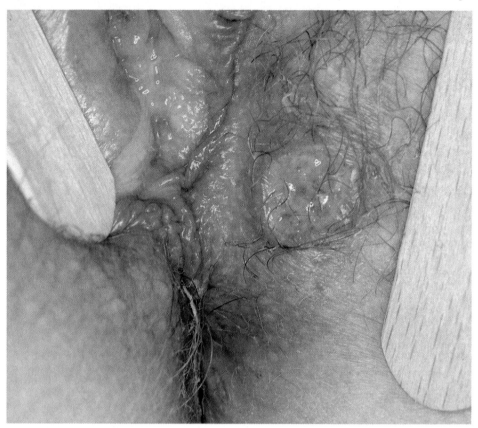

FIGURE 14-20 **Behçet disease: genital ulcers** Multiple large aphthous-type ulcers on the labial and perineal skin. In addition, this 25-year-old patient of Turkish extraction had aphthous ulcers in the mouth and previously experienced an episode of uveitis.

Musculoskeletal. Nonerosive, asymmetric oligoarthritis.

Neurologic. Onset delayed, occurring in one-quarter of patients. Meningoencephalitis, benign intracranial hypertension, cranial nerve palsies, brainstem lesions, pyramidal/extrapyramidal lesions, and psychosis.

Vascular. Aneurysms, arterial occlusions, venous thrombosis, varices; hemoptysis. Coronary vasculitis: myocarditis, coronary arteritis, endocarditis, and valvular disease.

GI Tract. Aphthous ulcers throughout.

LABORATORY EXAMINATIONS

DERMATOPATHOLOGY Leukocytoclastic vasculitis with fibrinoid necrosis of blood vessel walls in acute early lesions; lymphocytic vasculitis in late lesions.

PATHERGY TEST Positive pathergy test read by physician at 24 or 48 h, after skin puncture with a sterile needle. Often leads to inflammatory pustule.

HLA TYPING Significant association with HLA-B5 and HLA-B51, in Japanese, Koreans, and Turks, as well as in the Middle East.

DIAGNOSIS AND DIFFERENTIAL DIAGNOSIS

Diagnosis is made according to the Revised International Criteria for Behçet disease (Fig. 14-22).

DIFFERENTIAL DIAGNOSIS *Oral and genital ulcers*: Viral infection [HSV, varicella-zoster virus (VZV)], hand-foot-and-mouth disease, herpangina, chancre, histoplasmosis, and squamous cell carcinoma.

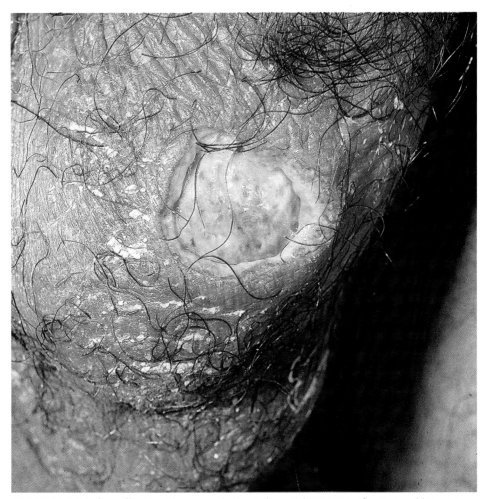

FIGURE 14-21 **Behçet disease** A large, punched-out ulcer on the scrotum of a 40-year-old Korean. The patient also had aphthous ulcers in the mouth and pustules on the thighs and buttocks.

COURSE AND PROGNOSIS

Highly variable course, with recurrences and remissions; the mouth lesions are always present; remissions may last for weeks, months, or years. In the eastern Mediterranean and East Asia, it tends to have a severe course and is one of the leading causes of blindness. With CNS involvement, there is a higher mortality rate.

MANAGEMENT

APHTHOUS ULCERS Potent topical glucocorticoids. Intralesional triamcinolone, 3 to 10 mg/mL, injected into ulcer base. Thalidomide, 50 to 100 mg po in the evening. Colchicine, 0.6 mg po two to three times a day. Dapsone, 50 to 100 mg/d po.

SYSTEMIC INVOLVEMENT Prednisone with or without azathioprine, cyclophosphamide, azathioprine alone, chlorambucil, and cyclosporine.

A

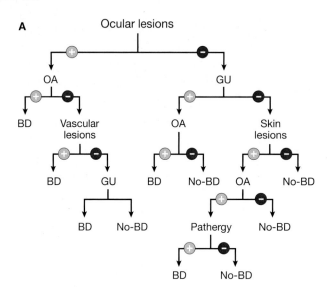

FIGURE 14-22 Revised International Criteria for Behçet Disease (International Team for the Revision of ICBD; coordinator, F. Davatchi) **(A)** The classification tree format and **(B)** the traditional format. BD, Behçet disease; GU, genital ulcer; OA, oral aphthous ulcer. (Modified with permission from Zouboulis CC. Adamantiades-Behçet disease. In: Wolff K, Goldsmith LA, Katz SI, et al, eds. *Fitzpatrick's Dermatology in General Medicine.* 7th ed. New York, NY: McGraw-Hill; 2008, pp. 1620–1622.)

B

Diagnosis of Behçet Disease is made with a score of 3 points:	
1 point	Oral aphthosis
1 point	Skin manifestations (pseudofolliculitis, skin aphthosis)
1 point	Vascular lesions (phlebitis, superficial phlebitis, large vein thrombosis aneurysm, arterial thrombosis)
1 point	Positive pathergy test
2 points	Genital aphthosis
2 points	Ocular lesions

DERMATOMYOSITIS ICD-10: M33.0

- Dermatomyositis (DM) is a systemic disease belonging to the idiopathic inflammatory myopathies, a heterogeneous group of genetically determined autoimmune diseases targeting the skin and/or skeletal muscles.
- DM is characterized by violaceous (heliotrope) inflammatory changes +/− edema of the eyelids and periorbital area; erythema of the face, neck, and upper trunk; and flat-topped violaceous papules over the knuckles.
- It is associated with polymyositis, interstitial pneumonitis, and myocardial involvement.
- There is also a DM without myopathy (amyopathic DM) and polymyositis without skin involvement.
- Juvenile DM runs a different course and is associated with vasculitis and calcinosis.
- Adult-onset DM may be associated with internal malignancy.
- Prognosis is guarded.

EPIDEMIOLOGY AND ETIOLOGY

RARE Incidence >6 cases per million, but this is based on hospitalized patients and does not include individuals without muscle involvement. Juvenile and adult (>40 years) onset.

ETIOLOGY Unknown. In persons >55 years of age, may be associated with malignancy.

CLINICAL SPECTRUM Ranges from DM with only cutaneous inflammation (amyopathic DM) to polymyositis with only muscle inflammation. Cutaneous involvement occurs in 30 to 40% of adults and 95% of children with DM/polymyositis. For classification, see Table 14-2.

CLINICAL MANIFESTATION

SYMPTOMS + PHOTOSENSITIVITY Manifestations of skin disease may precede myositis or vice versa; often, both are detected at the same time. Muscle weakness, difficulty in rising from supine position, climbing stairs, raising arms over head, or turning in bed. Dysphagia; burning and pruritus of the scalp.

SKIN LESIONS Periorbital heliotrope (reddish purple) flush, usually associated with some degree of edema (Fig. 14-23). May extend to involve scalp (+ nonscarring alopecia), entire face, upper chest, and arms (Fig. 14-24A).

TABLE 14-2 Comprehensive Classification of Idiopathic Inflammatory Dermatomyopathies

Dermatomyositis (DM)
- Adult onset
  - Classic DM: alone; with malignancy; as part of an overlap connective tissue disorder
  - Clinically amyopathic DM: amyopathic DM: hypomyopathic DM
- Juvenile onset
  - Classic DM
  - Clinically amyopathic DM: amyopathic DM; hypomyopathic DM

Polymyositis (PM)
- PM alone
- PM as part of an overlap connective tissue disorder
- PM associated with internal malignancy*

Inclusion body myositis

Other clinical–pathologic subgroups of myositis
- Focal myositis
- Proliferative myositis
- Orbital myositis
- Eosinophilic myositis
- Granulomatous myositis

*Although population-based European studies have now clearly confirmed that adult-onset classic DM is associated with a significant risk for internal malignancy, the evidence that such a relationship exists for PM, is much weaker.

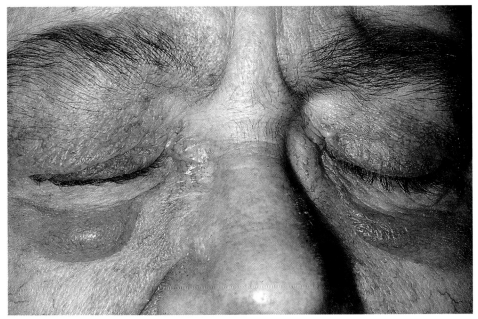

FIGURE 14-23 **Dermatomyositis** Heliotrope (reddish purple) erythema of upper eyelids and edema of the lower lids. This 55-year-old female had experienced severe muscle weakness of the shoulder girdle and presented with a lump in the breast that proved to be carcinoma.

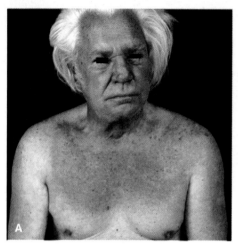
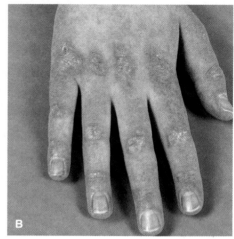

FIGURE 14-24 Dermatomyositis (A) Violaceous erythema and edema on the face, particularly in the periorbital and malar regions and on the chest. The patient could barely lift his arms and could not climb stairs. **(B)** Violaceous erythema and Gottron papules on the dorsa of the hands and fingers, especially over the interphalangeal joints. Periungual erythema and telangiectasias.

In addition, papular dermatitis with varying degrees of violaceous erythema in the same sites. Flat-topped, violaceous papules (Gottron papules) with various degrees of atrophy on the nape of the neck and shoulders and over the knuckles and interphalangeal joints (Fig. 14-24B). *Note*: In lupus, lesions usually occur in the interarticular region of the fingers (see p. 332). Periungual erythema with telangiectasia, thrombosis of capillary loops, and infarctions. Lesions over elbows and knuckles may evolve into erosions and ulcers that heal with stellate scarring (particularly in juvenile DM with vasculitis). Long-lasting lesions may evolve into poikiloderma (mottled discoloration with red, white, and brown) (Fig. 14-25). Calcification in subcutaneous/fascial tissues common later in the course of juvenile DM (Fig. 14-26), particularly around the elbows, trochanteric, and iliac region (calcinosis cutis); may evolve into calcinosis universalis.

MUSCLE ± Muscle tenderness, ± muscle atrophy. Progressive muscle weakness affecting proximal/limb girdle muscles.

Occasional involvement of facial/bulbar, pharyngeal, and esophageal muscles. Deep tendon reflexes within normal limits.

OTHER ORGANS Interstitial pneumonitis, cardiomyopathy, arthritis, particularly in juvenile DM (20 to 65%).

DISEASE ASSOCIATION Patients >50 years of age with DM have a higher than expected risk for malignancy, particularly ovarian cancer in females. Also carcinoma of the breast, bronchopulmonary, and GI tract.

LABORATORY EXAMINATIONS

CHEMISTRY Elevation of creatine phosphokinase (65%), aldolase (40%), lactate dehydrogenase, and glutamic oxaloacetic transaminase.

AUTOANTIBODIES Autoantibodies to 155 kDa and/or Se in 80% to 140 kDa in 58% and to Jo-1 in 20% and to (low specificity) antinuclear antibodies (ANA) in 40%.

URINE Elevated 24-h creatine excretion (>200 mg/ 24 h).

ELECTROMYOGRAPHY Increased irritability on insertion of electrodes, spontaneous fibrillations, pseudomyotonic discharges, and positive sharp waves.

MRI MRI of muscles reveals focal lesions.

ECG Evidence of myocarditis; atrial and ventricular irritability; atrioventricular block.

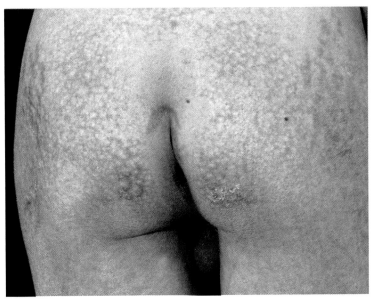

FIGURE 14-25 Dermatomyositis, juvenile onset, poikiloderma There is mottled, reticular brownish pigmentation and telangiectasia plus small white scars. Note striae on trochanteric areas caused by systemic glucocorticoid therapy.

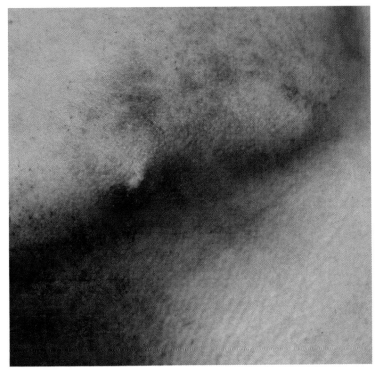

FIGURE 14-26 Dermatomyositis Calcinosis over the mandible. There are two stone hard nodules, which may later ulcerate and reveal a chalk white mass at the base. Upon squeezing, they will exude a white paste.

X-RAY **Chest:** ± interstitial fibrosis. *Esophagus:* reduced peristalsis.

PATHOLOGY **Skin.** Flattening of epidermis, hydropic degeneration of basal cell layer, edema of upper dermis, scattered inflammatory infiltrate, PAS-positive fibrinoid deposits at dermalepidermal junction, accumulation of acid mucopolysaccharides in dermis (all these are compatible with DM but are not diagnostic).

Muscle. Biopsy shoulder/pelvic girdle; one that is weak or tender. Histology—segmental necrosis within muscle fibers with loss of cross striations; myositis. Vasculitis is seen in juvenile DM.

DIAGNOSIS AND DIFFERENTIAL DIAGNOSIS

Skin signs plus proximal muscle weakness with two of three laboratory criteria, i.e., elevated serum "muscle enzyme" levels, characteristic electromyographic changes, and diagnostic muscle biopsy. Differential diagnosis is to lupus erythematosus, mixed connective tissue disease, steroid myopathy, trichinosis, and toxoplasmosis.

COURSE AND PROGNOSIS

Prognosis guarded but with treatment, it is relatively good except in patients with malignancy and those with pulmonary involvement. With aggressive immunosuppressive treatment, the 8-year survival rate is 70 to 80%. A better prognosis is seen in individuals who receive early systemic treatment. The most common causes of death are malignancy, infection, cardiac, and pulmonary disease. Successful treatment of an associated neoplasm is often followed by improvement/resolution of DM.

MANAGEMENT

PREDNISONE 0.5 to 1 mg/kg body weight per day. Taper when "muscle enzyme" levels approach normal. Best if combined with azathioprine, 2 to 3 mg/kg per day. *Note:* Steroid myopathy may occur after 4 to 6 weeks of therapy.

ALTERNATIVES Methotrexate, cyclophosphamide, cyclosporine, anti-tumor necrosis factor (TNF) α agents. High-dose IV immunoglobulin bolus therapy (2 g/kg body weight given over 2 days) at monthly intervals spares glucocorticoid doses to achieve or maintain remissions.

LUPUS ERYTHEMATOSUS (LE) ICD-10: L93

- LE is the designation of a spectrum of disease patterns that are linked by distinct clinical findings and distinct patterns of cellular and humoral autoimmunity.
- LE occurs more commonly in women (male to female ratio 1:9).
- LE ranges from life-threatening manifestations of acute systemic LE (SLE) to the limited and exclusive skin involvement in chronic cutaneous LE (CCLE) (**Fig. 14-27**). More than 85% of patients with LE have skin lesions, which can be classified into LE specific and nonspecific.
- An abbreviated version of Gilliam classification of LE-specific skin lesions is given in **Table 14-3**.
- Acute cutaneous LE (ACLE) is practically always associated with SLE, subacute cutaneous LE (SCLE) in about 50%, and CCLE most often has only skin disease. However, CCLE lesions can occur in SLE.
- ACLE and SCLE are highly photosensitive.

FIGURE 14-27 The spectrum of lupus erythematosus, as envisaged by the late Dr. James N. Gilliam The left comprises conditions that define cutaneous disease only and it can be seen that chronic cutaneous lupus extends into the systemic disease section. This is also true for lupus profundus (lupus panniculitis) and subacute cutaneous lupus, whereas acute cutaneous lupus is characteristic for systemic disease only. The bottom shows that immune complex disease dominates systemic disease and cell-mediated immunity (CMI) is predominant in the cutaneous disease manifestations.

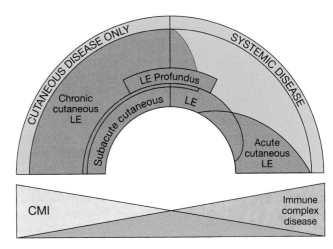

TABLE 14-3 Abbreviated Gilliam Classification of Skin Lesions of LE

I. LE-specific skin disease [cutaneous LE* (CLE)]
  A. Acute cutaneous LE [ACLE]
    1. Localized ACLE (malar rash; butterfly rash)
    2. Generalized ACLE (maculopapular lupus rash, malar rash, photosensitive lupus dermatitis)
  B. Subacute cutaneous LE [SCLE]
    1. Annular SCLE
    2. Papulosquamous SCLE (disseminated DLE, subacute disseminated LE, maculopapular photosensitive LE)
  C. Chronic cutaneous LE [CCLE]
    1. Classic discoid LE [DLE]: (a) localized DLE; (b) generalized DLE
    2. Hypertrophic/verrucous DLE
    3. Lupus profundus
    4. Mucosal DLE: (a) oral DLE; (b) conjunctival DLE
    5. Lupus tumidus (urticarial plaque of LE)
    6. Chilblains LE (chilblains lupus)
    7. Lichenoid DLE (LE/lichen planus overlap)

II. LE-nonspecific skin disease
  These range from necrotizing and urticarial vasculitis to livedo reticularis, Raynaud phenomenon, dermal mucinosis, and bullous lesions in LE.

*Alternative or synonymous terms are listed in parentheses; abbreviations are indicated in brackets.

Source: Sontheimer RD. Lupus 1997;6(2):84–95. Reprinted with permission of Sage. Copyright 1997 by Stockton Press.

SYSTEMIC LUPUS ERYTHEMATOSUS (SLE) ICD-10: M32

- This serious multisystem autoimmune disease is based on polyclonal B cell immunity, which involves connective tissue and blood vessels.
- More common in persons with black African heritage; male to female ratio 1:9.
- The clinical manifestations include fever (90%), skin lesions (85%), arthritis, CNS, renal, cardiac, and pulmonary disease.
- Skin lesions are those of ACLE and SCLE; not uncommonly also of CCLE.
- SLE may uncommonly develop in patients with CCLE; on the other hand, lesions of CCLE are common in SLE (Fig. 14-27).

EPIDEMIOLOGY

PREVALENCE Ranges from 40 cases/100,000 northern Europeans to more than 200/100,000 among people of African descent.
AGE OF ONSET 30 (females), 40 (males).
SEX Male:female ratio 1:9.
RACE More common in people of African descent.
PRECIPITATING FACTORS Family history (<5%); sunlight (UVR) is the most effective precipitating factor (occurs in 36%). An SLE syndrome can be induced by drugs (hydralazine, certain anticonvulsants, and procainamide), but a rash is a relatively uncommon feature of drug-induced SLE.

CLINICAL MANIFESTATIONS

Lesions present for weeks (acute) or months (chronic). Pruritus, burning of skin lesions. Fatigue (100%), fever (100%), weight loss, and malaise. Arthralgia or arthritis, abdominal pain, and CNS symptoms.
SKIN LESIONS Comprise ACLE lesions (Table 14-3) in the acute phases of the disease and SCLE and CCLE lesions. ACLE lesions occur only in acute or subacute SLE; SCLE and CCLE lesions are present in subacute and chronic SLE but may also occur in acute SLE. ACLE lesions are typically precipitated by sunlight.
ACLE. Butterfly Rash Erythematous, confluent, macular butterfly eruption on the face (Fig. 14-28), sharply defined, +/- fine scaling; erosions (acute flares) and crusts.
Generalized. Erythematous, discrete, papular, or urticarial lesions on the face, as well as on the dorsa of the hands (Fig. 14-29A), arms, and V of the neck.
Others. *Bullae*, often hemorrhagic (acute flares). *Papules* and *scaly plaques* as in SCLE (see Subacute cutaneous lupus erythematosus, p. 334) and *discoid plaques* as in CCLE (see Chronic cutaneous lupus erythematosus,

p. 336), predominantly on the face and on the arms and scalp. Erythematous, sometimes violaceous, slightly scaling, densely set and *confluent papules* on the dorsa of the finger, usually with sparing of the articular regions (Fig. 14-29A). Note the difference to DM (Fig. 14-24B). *Palmar erythema*, mostly on fingertips (Fig. 14-29B), *nailfold telangiectasias*, microthrombi, erythema, edema of the periungual skin, (see Section 32). "Palpable" purpura (vasculitis), lower extremities (see Hypersensitivity vasculitis, p. 353). *Urticarial lesions* with purpura (urticarial vasculitis) (see Urticarial vasculitis, p. 360).
HAIR Diffuse alopecia or discoid lesions associated with patchy alopecia (see Fig. 14-34; see Section 31).
MUCOUS MEMBRANES Ulcers arising in purpuric necrotic lesions on palate (80%), buccal mucosa, or gums (see Section 33).
Sites of Predilection (Fig. 14-30). Localized or generalized, preferentially in light-exposed sites. Face (80%); scalp (Fig. 14-34) (discoid lesions); presternal, shoulders; dorsa of the forearms, hands, fingers, and fingertips (Fig. 14-29B).
EXTRACUTANEOUS MULTISYSTEM INVOLVEMENT Arthralgia or arthritis (80%), renal disease (50%), pericarditis (20%), pneumonitis (20%), gastrointestinal (resulting from arteritis and sterile peritonitis), hepatomegaly (30%), myopathy (30%), splenomegaly (20%), lymphadenopathy (50%), peripheral neuropathy (14%), CNS disease (10%), seizures, or organic brain disease (14%).

LABORATORY EXAMINATIONS

PATHOLOGY **Skin.** Atrophy of epidermis, liquefaction degeneration of the dermal–epidermal junction, edema of the dermis, dermal lymphocytic infiltrate, and fibrinoid degeneration of the connective tissue and walls of the blood vessels.

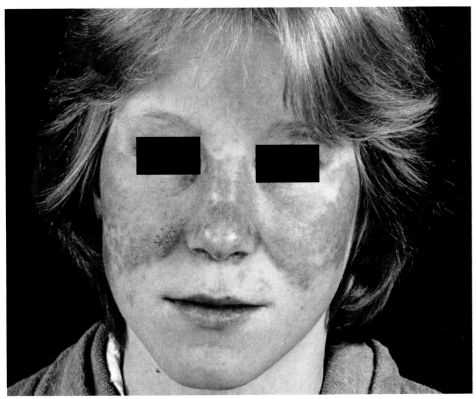

FIGURE 14-28 Acute systemic lupus erythematosus Bright red, sharply defined erythema with slight edema and minimal scaling in a "butterfly pattern" on the face. This is the typical "malar rash." Note also that the patient is female and young.

Immunofluorescence of Skin. The lupus band test (LBT, direct immunofluorescence) shows granular or globular deposits of IgG, IgM, C3 in a band-like pattern along the dermal–epidermal junction. Positive in lesional skin in 90% and in the clinically normal skin (sun exposed, 70 to 80%; non-sun exposed, 50%).

SEROLOGY ANA positive (>95%); peripheral pattern of nuclear fluorescence. Anti–double-strand DNA antibodies, anti-Sm antibodies, and rRNP antibodies specific for SLE; low levels of complement (especially with renal involvement). Anticardiolipin autoantibodies (lupus anticoagulant) in a specific subset (anticardiolipin syndrome); SS-A(Ro) autoantibodies have a low specificity for SLE but are specific in the subset of SCLE (Table 14-4).

HEMATOLOGY Anemia [normocytic, normochromic, or, rarely, hemolytic Coombs-positive,

TABLE 14-4 Pathogenic Autoantibodies in Systemic Lupus Erythematosus

Skin	Anti-double-strand DNA (70–80%) Nucleosome (60–90%) Ro (30–40%)
Brain	NMDA receptor (33–50%)
Kidney	Anti-double-strand DNA (70–80%) Nucleosome (60–90%) C1q (40–50%) Ro (30–40%) Sm (10–30%) Alpha-actinin (20–30%)
Thrombosis	Phospholipids (20–30%)
Fetal cardiac abnormalities	Ro (30–40%) La (15–20%)
Pregnancy loss	Phospholipids (20–30%)

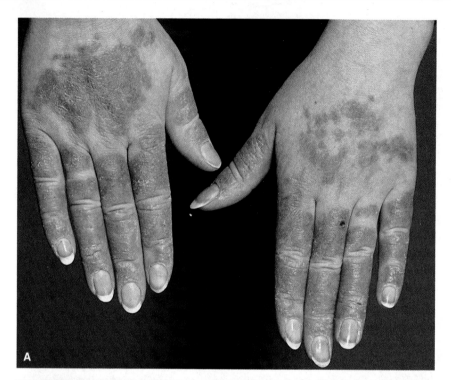

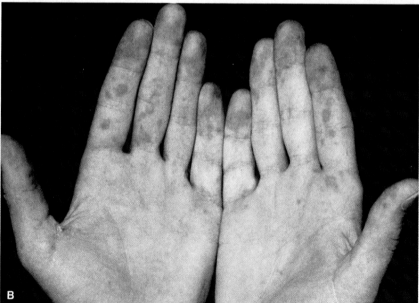

FIGURE 14-29 Acute SLE (A) Red-to-violaceous, well-demarcated papules and plaques on the dorsa of the fingers and hands, characteristically sparing the skin overlying the joints. This is an important differential diagnostic sign when considering dermatomyositis, which characteristically involves the skin over the joints (compare with **Fig. 14-24B**). **(B)** Palmar erythema mainly on the fingertips. This is pathognomonic.

leukopenia (>4000/µL)], lymphopenia, thrombocytopenia, elevated ESR.
URINALYSIS Persistent proteinuria, casts.

DIAGNOSIS

Made on the basis of clinical findings, histopathology, LBT, and serology within the framework of the revised American Rheumatism
Association (ARA) criteria for classification of
SLE (Table 14-5).

PROGNOSIS

Five-year survival is 93%.

MANAGEMENT

GENERAL MEASURES Rest, avoidance of sun
exposure.
INDICATIONS FOR PREDNISONE (60 mg/d in
divided doses): (1) CNS involvement, (2) renal
involvement, (3) severely ill patients without

TABLE 14-5 1982 Revised ARA Criteria for Classification of Systemic Lupus Erythematosus*

Criterion	Definition
1. Malar rash	Fixed erythema, flat or raised, over the malar eminences, tending to spare the nasolabial folds.
2. Discoid rash	Erythematous raised patches with adherent keratotic scaling and follicular plugging; atrophic scarring may occur in older lesions.
3. Photosensitivity	Skin rashes as a result of unusual reaction to sunlight, by patient history or physician observation.
4. Oral ulcers	Oral or nasopharyngeal ulceration, usually painless, observed by a physician.
5. Arthritis	Nonerosive arthritis involving two or more peripheral joints, characterized by tenderness, swelling, or effusion.
6. Serositis	a. Pleuritis—convincing history of pleuritic pain or rub heard by a physician or evidence of pleural effusion *or* b. Pericarditis—documented by ECG or rub or evidence of pericardial effusion.
7. Renal disorder	a. Persistent proteinuria—0.5g/d or 3+ if quantitation not performed *or* b. Cellular casts—may be red cell, hemoglobin, granular, tubular, or mixed.
8. Neurologic disorder	a. Seizures—in the absence of offending drugs or known metabolic derangements, e.g., uremia, ketoacidosis, or electrolyte imbalance *or* b. Psychosis—in the absence of offending drugs or known metabolic derangements, e.g., uremia, ketoacidosis, or electrolyte imbalance.
9. Hematologic disorder	a. Hemolytic anemia—with reticulocytosis *or* b. Leukopenia— <4000/µL total on two or more occasions *or* c. Lymphopenia— <1500/µL on two or more occasions *or* d. Thrombocytopenia— <100,000/µL in the absence of offending drugs.
10. Immunologic disorder	a. Anti-DNA—antibody to native DNA in abnormal titer *or* b. Anti-Sm—presence of antibody to Sm nuclear antigen *or* c. Positive finding of antiphospholipid antibodies based on (1) an abnormal serum level of IgG or IgM anticardiolipin antibodies, (2) a positive test result for lupus anticoagulant using a standard method, or (3) a false-positive serologic test for syphilis known to be positive for at least 6 months and confirmed by negative *Treponema pallidum* immobilization or fluorescent treponemal antibody absorption test.
11. Antinuclear antibody	An abnormal titer of antinuclear antibody by immunofluorescence of an equivalent assay at any point in time and in the absence of drugs known to be associated with "drug-induced lupus" syndrome.

*The proposed classification is based on 11 criteria. For the purpose of identifying patients in clinical studies, a person shall be said to have SLE if any 4 or more of the 11 criteria are present, serially or simultaneously, during any interval of observation. *Source*: Reproduced with permission from Tan EM, et al. The 1982 revised criteria for the classification of systemic lupus erythematosus. *Arthritis Rheum*. 1982;25:1271. ©1982 American College of Rheumatology.

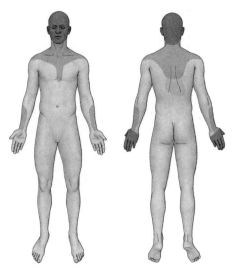

CNS involvement, (4) hemolytic crisis, and (5) thrombocytopenia.

CONCOMITANT IMMUNOSUPPRESSIVE DRUGS Azathioprine, mycophenolate mofetil, methotrexate, cyclophosphamide, depending on organ involvement and activity of disease. In renal disease, cyclophosphamide IV bolus therapy. **ANTIMALARIALS** Hydroxychloroquine is useful for treatment of the skin lesions in subacute and chronic SLE but does not reduce the need for prednisone. Observe precautions in the use of hydroxychloroquine. Alternative: chloroquine, quinacrine.

INVESTIGATIONAL Anti-TNF agents like efalizumab, rituximab, leflunomide, anti-interferon-α agents, belimumab.

FIGURE 14-30 Predilection sites of cutaneous lupus erythematosus.

SUBACUTE CUTANEOUS LUPUS ERYTHEMATOSUS (SCLE) ICD-10: L93.1

- About 10% of the LE population.
- Young and middle age, uncommon in blacks or Hispanics. Females > males.
- *Precipitating factors:* Sunlight exposure.
- Rather sudden onset with annular or psoriasiform plaques erupting mainly on the upper trunk, arms, dorsa of the hands, usually after exposure to sunlight; mild fatigue, malaise; some arthralgia, fever of unknown origin.
- *Two types of skin lesions:* (1) *Psoriasiform papulosquamous*, sharply defined, with slight delicate scaling, evolving into bright red confluent plaques that are oval, arciform, or polycyclic, just as in psoriasis and (2) *annular*, bright red annular lesions with central regression and little scaling (Fig. 14-31). In both, there may be telangiectasia, but there is no follicular plugging and less induration than in CCLE. Lesions resolve with slight atrophy (no scarring) and hypopigmentation. Periungual telangiectasia, diffuse nonscarring alopecia.
- *Distribution:* Scattered, disseminated in light-exposed areas—shoulders, extensor surface of the arms, dorsal surface of the hands, upper back, V-neck area of the upper chest.
- Patients have some criteria of SLE, including photosensitivity, arthralgias, serositis, renal disease; 50% have SLE; LBT positive in 60%. All have anti-Ro (SS-A) and most have anti-La (SS-B) autoantibodies.
- UV testing: Lower than normal UVB minimal erythema dose (see Section 10). Lesions may develop in test sites.
- Better prognosis than for SLE in general but some with renal disease have guardes prognosis. Women with Ro- (SS-A) positive SCLE may give birth to babies with neonatal lupus and congenital heart block.
- Management: Topical glucocorticosteroids, pimecrolimus, and tacrolimus only partially helpful for skin lesions. Systemic thalidomide (100 to 300 mg/d) very effective for skin lesions but not for systemic disease (beware of teratogenicity). Hydroxychloroquine 400 mg/d, quinacrine hydrochloride 100 mg/d. In systemic involvement prednisone ± immunosuppressants.

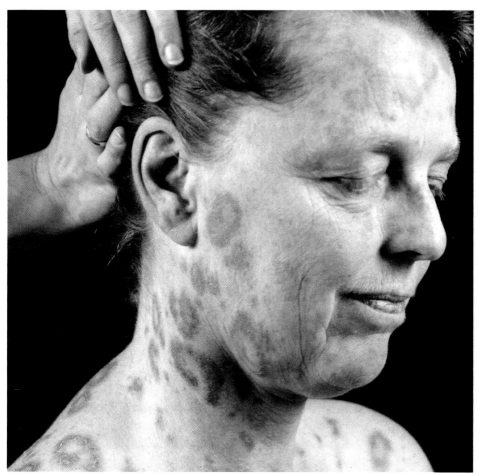

FIGURE 14-31 **Subacute cutaneous lupus erythematosus** Round, oval, and annular red plaques on the forehead, cheeks, neck, and upper trunk that show, but minimal, scaling in a 56-year-old woman. The eruption occurred after solar exposure. This is the annular type of SCLE.

CHRONIC CUTANEOUS LUPUS ERYTHEMATOSUS (CCLE) ICD-10: L93.0

- **Age of Onset:** Twenty to 45 years. Females > males. More severe in blacks.
- This disorder, in most cases, is purely cutaneous without systemic involvement (**Fig. 14-27**). However, CCLE lesions occur in SLE.
- Can be precipitated by sunlight but to a lesser extent than ACLE or SCLE. Lesions last for months to years. Usually no symptoms, sometimes slightly pruritic or smarting. No general symptoms.
- CCLE may manifest as chronic discoid LE (CDLE) or LE panniculitis (see **Table 14-3**).
- CDLE lesions start as bright red papules evolving into plaques, sharply marginated, with adherent scaling (**Fig. 14-32**). Scales are difficult to remove and show spines on the undersurface (magnifying lens) resembling carpet tacks. Plaques are round or oval, annular or polycyclic, with irregular borders and expand in the periphery and regress in the center, resulting in atrophy, and scarring (**Fig. 14-33**). "Burned out" lesions may be pink or white macules and scars (**Fig. 14-34**), but may also be hyperpigmented, especially in persons with brown or black skin (**Fig. 14-35**).
- *CDLE* may be localized or generalized, occurring predominantly on the face and scalp; dorsa of forearms, hands, fingers, toes, and, less frequently, the trunk (**Fig. 14-30**).
- **Mucous Membranes:** <5% of patients have lip involvement (hyperkeratosis, hypermelanotic scarring, erythema) and atrophic erythematous or whitish areas with or without ulceration on the buccal mucosa, tongue, and palate (see Section 33). *Nail apparatus:* Nail dystrophy if nail matrix is involved.
- **Dermatopathology:** Hyperkeratosis, atrophy of the epidermis, follicular plugging, liquefaction degeneration of the basal cell layer lymphocytic inflammatory infiltrate. Strong PAS reaction of the subepidermal, thickened basement zone. LBT positive in 90% of active lesions and negative in burned-out (scarred) lesions and in the normal skin, both sun exposed and nonexposed. Low incidence of ANA with titers >1:16.
- Differential diagnosis of CDLE: actinic keratosis, psoriasis, polymorphous light eruption, LP, tinea facialis, lupus vulgaris.
- Only 1 to 5% may develop SLE; with localized lesions, complete remission occurs in 50%; with generalized lesions, remissions are less frequent (<10%). *Note again*: CCLE lesions may be the presenting cutaneous sign of SLE.
- Management:
  - **Local Glucocorticoids and Calcineurin Inhibitors:** Usually not very effective; topical fluorinated glucocorticoids with caution because of atrophy. Intralesional triamcinolone acetonide, 3 to 5 mg/mL, for small lesions.
  - **Antimalarials:** Hydroxychloroquine, ≤6.5 mg/kg body weight per day. If hydroxychloroquine is ineffective, add quinacrine, 100 mg three times a day. Monitor for ocular side effects.
  - **Retinoids:** Hyperkeratotic CDLE lesions respond well to systemic acitretin (0.5 mg/kg body weight).
  - **Thalidomide:** 100 to 300 mg/d is effective. Observe contraindications.

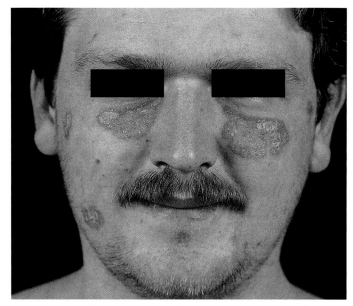

FIGURE 14-32 Chronic cutaneous lupus erythematosus Well-demarcated, erythematous, hyperkeratotic plaques with atrophy, follicular plugging, and adherent scale on both cheeks. This is the classic presentation of chronic discoid LE.

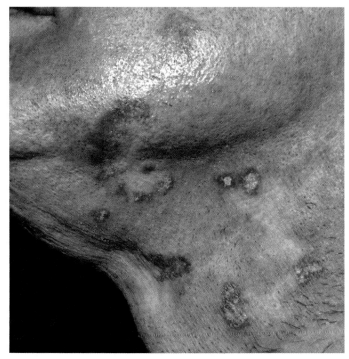

FIGURE 14-33 Chronic cutaneous lupus erythematosus: scarring There are multiple scarred lesions that are white and depressed and at their margins have active erythematous and scaly lesions. This can be quite disfiguring.

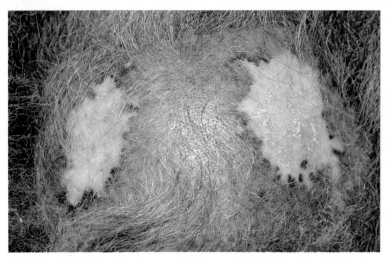

FIGURE 14-34 Chronic cutaneous lupus erythematosus Involvement of the scalp has led to complete hair loss with residual erythema, atrophy, and white scarring in this black male. Sharp demarcation of the lesions in the periphery indicates that these lesions originally were CDLE plaques.

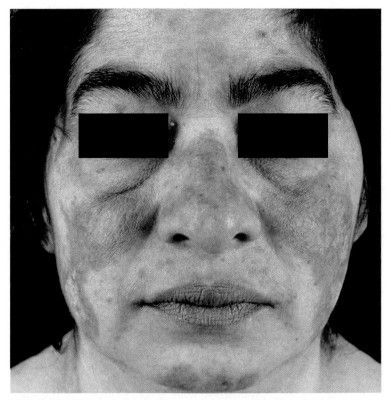

FIGURE 14-35 Chronic cutaneous lupus erythematosus: hyperpigmentation As inflammatory lesions resolve, there may be hyperpigmentation of the atrophic and partially scarred lesional skin, particularly in SPT III and IV patients. Although the skin lesions were CCLE, the patient had SLE.

CHRONIC LUPUS PANNICULITIS (CLP) ICD-10: L93.21

- Chronic lupus panniculitis is a form of CCLE in which there are firm, circumscribed subcutaneous nodules or plate-like infiltrations. May precede or follow onset of CDLE lesions. CDLE lesions may also be absent.
- Subcutaneous nodules occur both with and without CDLE lesions of overlying skin.
- Lead to subcutaneous atrophy and scarring, resulting in sunken areas (**Fig. 14-36**).
- Face, scalp, upper arms, trunk, thigh, and buttocks.
- Usually a form of cutaneous lupus, but 35% of patients have mild SLE (see **Fig. 14-27**).
- Differential diagnosis: Morphea, erythema nodosum, sarcoidosis, other types of panniculitis.
- Management: Antimalarials, thalidomide (beware of contraindications), systemic corticosteroids.
- *Synonym*: Lupus erythematosus profundus.

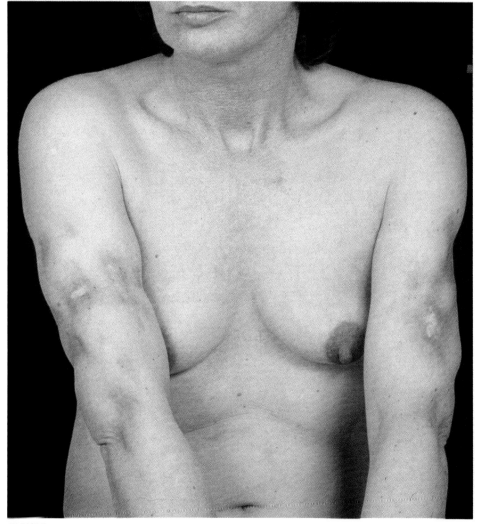

FIGURE 14-36 Lupus panniculitis Chronic panniculitis with atrophy of the subcutaneous tissue, resulting in large sunken areas of overlying skin, representing resolving lesions. Where erythema is still visible, palpation reveals firm subcutaneous nodules and plaques. Also, some lesions reveal scarring in the center.

LIVEDO RETICULARIS ICD-10: L 95.0

- Livedo reticularis (LR) is a mottled bluish (livid) discoloration of the skin that occurs in a netlike pattern. It is not a diagnosis in itself but a reaction pattern.
- Classification distinguishes between:
  - *Idiopathic livedo reticularis* (ILR): A purple/livid discoloration of the skin in a netlike pattern disappearing after warming. A physiologic phenomenon. (*Synonym*: cutis marmorata.)
  - *Secondary (symptomatic) livedo reticularis* (SLR): A purple discoloration occurring in a starburst or lightning-like pattern, netlike but with open (not annular) meshes; mostly, but not always, confined to the lower extremities and buttocks (**Fig. 14-37**). A reaction pattern often indicative of serious systemic disease (**Table 14-6**). (*Synonym*: livedo racemosa.)
  - *Sneddon syndrome* is a potentially life-threatening disease occurring more often in women than in men and manifesting in the skin as SLR (**Fig. 14-37**) and in the CNS as transient ischemic attacks and cerebrovascular insults. May be associated with livedoid vasculitis with ulcerations on ankles and acrally (see Section 27).
  - Management: No treatment necessary for ILR; for SLR, keep from chilling, pentoxifylline, low-dose aspirin, and heparin.

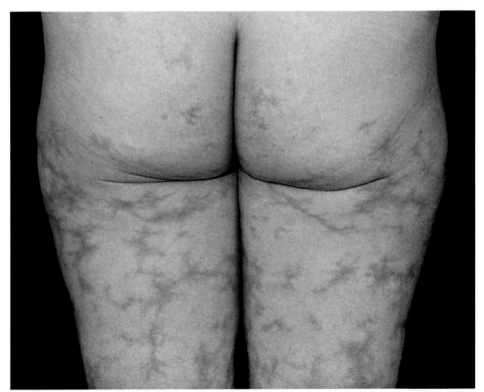

FIGURE 14-37 Symptomatic livedo reticularis A netlike, arborizing pattern on the posterior thighs and buttocks defined by violaceous, erythematous streaks resembling lightning. The skin within the erythematous areas is normally pale. This occurred in a patient with labile hypertension and multiple cerebrovascular attacks and was thus pathognomonic for Sneddon syndrome.

TABLE 14-6 Disorders Associated with Symptomatic Livedo Reticularis

Vascular Obstruction	Viscosity Changes	Drugs
Atheroemboli	Thrombocythemia	Amantadine
Arteriosclerosis	Polyglobulinemia	Quinine
Polyarteritis nodosa	Cryoglobulinemia	Quinidine
Cutaneous polyarteritis nodosa	Cold agglutinemia	
Rheumatoid vasculitis	Disseminated intravascular coagulation.	
Livedoid vasculitis		
Sneddon syndrome	Lupus erythematosus Anticardiolipin syndrome Leukemia/lymphoma	

RAYNAUD PHENOMENON ICD-9: 443.0 ∘ ICD-10: I73

- Raynaud phenomenon (RP) is digital ischemia that occurs on exposure to cold and/or as a result of emotional stress. May occur in persons using vibratory tools (chain sawers, meat cutters), typists, pianists.
- Primary RP is a condition where no etiology is found; secondary RP is the designation for RP and underlying disease.
- The various causes of secondary RP are listed in Table 14-7. *Rheumatic disorders* [systemic scleroderma (85%), SLE (35%), DM (30%), Sjögren syndrome, rheumatoid arthritis, polyarteritis nodosa], *diseases with abnormal blood proteins* (cryoproteins, cold agglutinins, macroglobulins), drugs (β-adrenergic blockers, nicotine), and *arterial diseases* (arteriosclerosis obliterans, thromboangiitis obliterans) are the most common.
- *The Episodic Attack:* There is blanching or cyanosis of the fingers or toes, extending from the tip to various levels of the digits. The finger distal to the line of ischemia is white and/or blue and cold (Fig. 14-38); the proximal skin is pink and warm. When the digits are rewarmed, the blanching may be replaced by cyanosis because of slow blood flow. At the end of the attack, the normal color or a red color reflects the reactive hyperemic phase.
- *Repeated or Persistent Vascular Vasospasm:* Patients with RP often have a persistent vasospasm rather than episodic attacks. Skin changes include trophic changes with development of taut, atrophic skin, pterygium, clubbing, and shortening of the terminal phalanges, sclerodactyly like in limited systemic scleroderma (lSSc) (see Scleroderma). Acral gangrene is rare in RD (<1%), but common in RP associated with scleroderma, painful ulcers. Sequestration of the terminal phalanges or the development of gangrene (Fig. 14-39) may lead to autoamputation of the fingertips.
- Rule out scleroderma and other conditions (Table 14-7).
- Therapy: Calcium channel blockers, anti-adrenergic drugs, IV prostacyclin, bosentan (an endothelin receptor antagonist), or local botox injections.

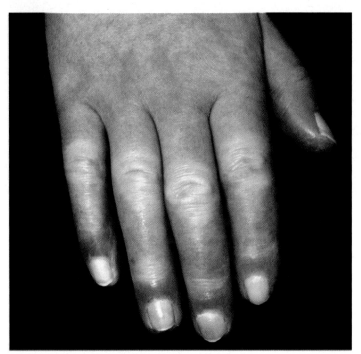

FIGURE 14-38 **Raynaud phenomenon** The hand exhibits a distal cyanosis; it is seen especially well in the nailbeds; proximally the skin is white resulting from vasospasm. Episodes such as this one may occur after contact with cold water.

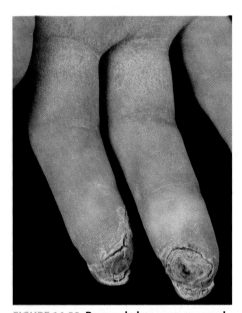

FIGURE 14-39 **Raynaud phenomenon: acral gangrene** Persistent vasospasm of medium-sized arterioles can sometimes lead to gangrene of the terminal digits as illustrated in this patient with scleroderma.

TABLE 14-7 Causes or Disorders Associated with Secondary Raynaud Phenomenon*

- Connective tissue disease
  - Scleroderma, SLE, dermatomyositis, vasculitis
- Obstructive arterial disease
  - Atherosclerosis, thromboembolism
- Drugs and toxins
  - β-Adrenergic blockers, ergotamines, bleomycin
- Neurologic disorders
  - Carpal tunnel syndrome
- Occupation/environmental exposure
  - Vibration injury, vinyl chloride
- Hyperviscosity disorders
  - Cryoproteins, cold agglutinins
- Miscellaneous

*For more detailed information, see Kippel JH. Raynaud phenomenon, in, Wolff K et al. (eds.): *Fitzpatrick's Dermatology in General Medicine*, 7th ed. New York, McGraw-Hill, 2008:1646.

SCLERODERMA ICD-10: M34

- ▦ Scleroderma is a not so rare multisystem disorder characterized by inflammatory, vascular, and sclerotic changes of the skin and various internal organs, especially the lungs, heart, and GI tract.
- ▦ Limited systemic scleroderma (lSSc) (60%) and diffuse systemic scleroderma (dSSc) are recognized.
- ▦ Clinical features always present are skin sclerosis and Raynaud phenomenon.
- ▦ Considerable morbidity; high mortality of dSSc.
- ▦ *Synonyms*: Progressive systemic sclerosis, systemic sclerosis, and systemic scleroderma.

EPIDEMIOLOGY

PREVALENCE 20 per million of US population.
AGE OF ONSET 30 to 50 years.
SEX Female:male ratio, 4:1.

CLASSIFICATION

Systemic scleroderma can be divided into two subsets: lSSc and dSSc. lSSc patients comprise 60%; patients are usually female; older than those with dSSc; and have a long history of Raynaud phenomenon with skin involvement limited to hands, feet, face, and forearms (acrosclerosis) and a high incidence of anticentromeric antibodies. lSSc includes the CREST syndrome, and systemic involvement may not appear for years; patients usually die of other causes. dSSc patients have a relatively rapid onset and diffuse involvement, not only of hands and feet but also of the trunk and face, synovitis, tendosynovitis, and early onset of internal involvement. Anticentromere antibodies are uncommon, but Scl-70 (antitopoisomerase I) antibodies are present in 33%.

ETIOLOGY AND PATHOGENESIS

Unknown. Primary event might be endothelial cell injury in blood vessels. Edema occurs, followed by fibrosis; cutaneous capillaries are reduced in number; remainder dilate and proliferate, becoming visible telangiectasia.

CLINICAL MANIFESTATION

Raynaud phenomenon (see p. 341) with digital pain, coldness. Pain/stiffness of fingers and knees. Migratory polyarthritis. Heartburn, dysphagia, especially with solid foods. Constipation, diarrhea, abdominal bloating, malabsorption, and weight loss. Exertional dyspnea and dry cough.

SKIN **Hands/Feet.** *Early*: Raynaud phenomenon with triphasic color changes, i.e., pallor, cyanosis, and rubor (Fig. 14-40B, see also

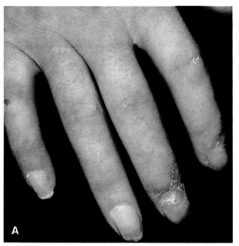 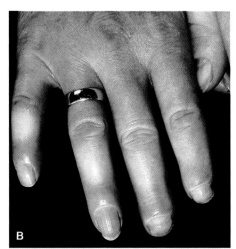

A

B

FIGURE 14-40 **Scleroderma (lSSc): acrosclerosis (A)** Hands and fingers are edematous (nonpitting); skin is without skin folds and bound down. Distal fingers are tapered (Madonna fingers) **(B)** Fingers show both bluish erythema and vasoconstriction (blue and white): Raynaud phenomenon. Fingers are edematous, the skin is bound down. Distal phalanges (index and third finger) are shortened, which is associated with bony resorption.

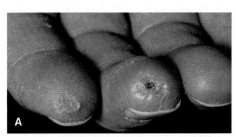
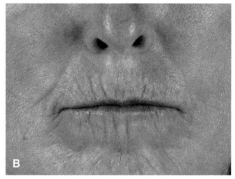

FIGURE 14-41 Scleroderma (lSSc): acrosclerosis (A) Typical "rat bite" necroses and ulcerations of fingertips. **(B)** Thinning of lips—microstomia (which would show better when patient attempts to open her mouth), radial perioral furrowing. Beaklike sharp nose.

Fig. 14-38). Precedes sclerosis by months and years. Nonpitting edema of hands/feet. Painful ulcerations at fingertips ("rat bite necrosis") (Fig. 14-41A), knuckles; heal with pitted scars. *Late*: Scleroidactyly with tapering of fingers (Madonna fingers) (Fig. 14-40A) with waxy, shiny, hardened skin, which is tightly bound down and does not permit folding or wrinkling; leathery crepitation over joints, flexion contractures; periungual telangiectasia, nails grow clawlike over shortened distal phalanges (Fig. 14-40B). Bony resorption and ulceration results in loss of distal phalanges. Loss of sweat glands with anhidrosis; thinning and complete loss of hair on distal extremities.

Face. *Early*: Periorbital edema. *Late*: Edema and fibrosis result in loss of normal facial lines, mask-like (patients look younger than they are) (Fig. 14-42), thinning of lips, microstomia, radial perioral furrowing (Fig. 14-41B), and beak-like sharp nose. Telangiectasia (Fig. 14-43) and diffuse hyperpigmentation.

Trunk. In dSSc, the chest and proximal upper and lower extremities are involved early. Tense, stiff, and waxy appearing skin that cannot be folded. Impairment of respiratory movement of chest wall and of joint mobility.

OTHER CHANGES **Cutaneous Calcification.** Occurs on fingertips or over bony prominences or any sclerodermatous site; may ulcerate and exude white paste.

Color Changes. Hyperpigmentation that may be generalized and on the extremities may be accompanied by perifollicular hypopigmentation.

Mucous Membranes. Sclerosis of sublingual ligament; uncommonly, painful induration of gums, and tongue.

Distribution of Lesions. *Early*: In lSSc, early involvement is seen on the fingers, hands, and face, and in many patients scleroderma remains confined to these regions. *Late*: The distal upper and lower extremities may be involved and occasionally the trunk. In dSSc, sclerosis of the extremities and the trunk may start soon after or concomitant with acral involvement.

CLINICAL VARIANT CREST syndrome, i.e., *c*alcinosis cutis + *R*aynaud phenomenon + *e*sophageal dysfunction + *s*clerodactyly + *t*elangiectasia. Macular, mat-like telangiectasia, especially the face (Fig. 14-43), upper trunk, and hands; also in the entire GI tract. Calcinosis over bony prominences, fingertips, elbows, and trochanteric regions (similar to DM, see Fig. 14-26).

GENERAL EXAMINATION

Esophagus. Dysphagia, diminished peristalsis, and reflux esophagitis.

GASTROINTESTINAL SYSTEM Small intestine involvement may produce constipation, diarrhea, bloating, and malabsorption.

LUNG Pulmonary fibrosis and alveolitis. Reduction in pulmonary function resulting from restricted movement of chest wall.

HEART Cardiac conduction defects, heart failure, and pericarditis.

KIDNEY Renal involvement in 45%. Slowly progressive uremia, malignant hypertension.

MUSCULOSKELETAL SYSTEM Carpal tunnel syndrome. Muscle weakness.

LABORATORY EXAMINATIONS

DERMATOPATHOLOGY *Early*: Mild cellular infiltrate around dermal blood vessels, eccrine

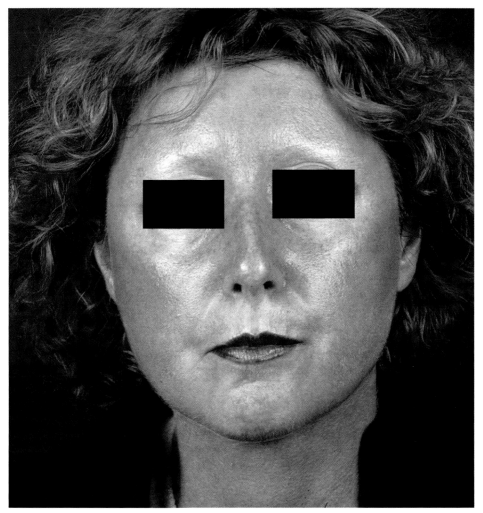

FIGURE 14-42 Scleroderma (dSSc) Mask-like facies with stretched, shiny skin and loss of normal facial lines giving a younger appearance than actual age; the hair is dyed. Thinning of the lips and perioral sclerosis result in a small mouth. Sclerosis (whitish, glistening areas) and multiple telangiectases (not visible at this magnification) are also present.

coils, and at the dermal subcutaneous interphase. *Late*: Broadening and homogenization of collagen bundles, obliteration and decrease of interbundle spaces, thickening of dermis with replacement of upper or total subcutaneous fat by hyalinized collagen. Paucity of blood vessels, thickening/hyalinization of vessel walls. AUTOANTIBODIES Patients with dSSc have circulating ANA. Autoantibodies react with centromere proteins or DNA topoisomerase I; fewer patients have antinuclear antibodies. Anticentromeric autoantibodies occur in 21% of dSSc and 71% of CREST patients, DNA

topoisomerase I (Scl-70) antibodies in 33% of dSSc and 18% of CREST patients.

DIAGNOSIS AND DIFFERENTIAL DIAGNOSIS

Clinical findings confirmed by dermatopathology. DIFFERENTIAL DIAGNOSIS *Diffuse sclerosis*: Mixed connective tissue disease, eosinophilic fasciitis, scleromyxedema, morphea, porphyria cutanea tarda, chronic GVHD, lichen sclerosus et atrophicus, polyvinyl chloride exposure, adverse drug reaction (pentazocine, bleomycin).

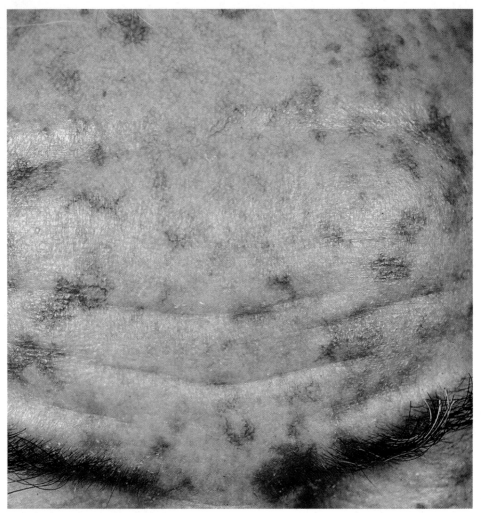

FIGURE 14-43 **Scleroderma: CREST syndrome** Numerous macular or matlike telangiectases on the forehead. Complete features include calcinosis cutis, Raynaud phenomenon, esophageal dysmotility, sclerosis, and telangiectasia.

Gadolinium and nephrogenic systemic fibrosis (see Section 18).

COURSE AND PROGNOSIS

Course of dSSc is characterized by slow, relentless progression of skin and/or visceral sclerosis; the 10-year survival rate is >50%. Renal disease is the leading cause of death, followed by cardiac and pulmonary involvement. Spontaneous remissions do occur. lSSc, including the CREST syndrome, progresses more slowly and has a more favorable prognosis; some cases do not develop visceral involvement.

MANAGEMENT

Systemic glucocorticoids may be of benefit for limited periods early in the disease. All other systemic treatments (EDTA, aminocaproic acid, d-penicillamine, *para*-aminobenzoate, and colchicine) have not been shown to be of lasting benefit. Immunosuppressive drugs (cyclosporine, methotrexate, cyclophosphamide, and mycophenolate mofetil) have shown improvement of skin score but only limited benefit for systemic involvement. Photopheresis: improvement in one-third of patients. Immunoablation/stem cell transplantation: ongoing studies.

SCLERODERMA-LIKE CONDITIONS

- A dSSc-like condition occurs in persons exposed to polyvinyl chloride.
- Bleomycin also produces pulmonary fibrosis and Raynaud phenomenon but not skin sclerosis.
- Cutaneous changes indistinguishable from dSSc-like sclerosis of skin, accompanied by myalgia, pneumonitis, myocarditis, neuropathy, and encephalopathy, are related to the ingestion of certain lots of L-tryptophan (*eosinophilia–myalgia syndrome*).
- The *toxic oil syndrome* that occurred in an epidemic in Spain in 1981 affecting 25,000 people was caused by the consumption of denatured rapeseed oil. After an acute phase, with rash, fever, pneumonitis, and myalgia, the syndrome progressed to a condition with neuromuscular abnormalities and scleroderma-like skin lesions.
- Scleromyxedema and scleredema of Buschke are very rare, separate entities with guarded prognosis.
- lSSc-like sclerosis also occurs in porphyria cutanea tarda (see Section 10) and GVHD (see Section 22).

MORPHEA ICD-10: L94.0

- A localized and circumscribed cutaneous sclerosis characterized by early violaceous, later ivory-colored, hardened skin.
- May be solitary, linear, generalized, and, rarely, accompanied by atrophy of underlying structures.
- It is unrelated to systemic scleroderma.
- *Synonyms*: Localized scleroderma, circumscribed scleroderma.

EPIDEMIOLOGY AND ETIOLOGY

INCIDENCE Rare between the ages of 20 and 50; in linear morphea, earlier. Pansclerotic morphea, a disabling disorder, usually starts before age 14.

SEX Women are affected about three times as often as men, including children. Linear scleroderma is the same in males and females.

Etiology. Unknown. At least some patients (predominantly in Europe) with classic morphea have sclerosis resulting from *Borrelia burgdorferi* infection. Morphea has been noted after x-irradiation for breast cancer. *Morphea is not related to systemic scleroderma.*

CLASSIFICATION OF VARIOUS TYPES OF MORPHEA

- *Circumscribed:* Plaques or bands.
- *Macular:* Small, confluent patches.
- *Linear scleroderma:* Upper or lower extremity.
- *Frontoparietal (en coup de sabre).*
- *Generalized morphea.*
- *Pansclerotic:* Involvement of dermis, fat, fascia, muscle, and bone.

CLINICAL MANIFESTATION

SYMPTOMS Usually none. No Raynaud phenomenon. Linear and pansclerotic morphea can result in major facial or limb asymmetry, flexion contractures, and disability. It san cause severe disfigurement.

SKIN FINDINGS *Plaques*—circumscribed, indurated, hard, but poorly defined areas of skin; 2 to 15 cm in diameter, round or oval, often better felt than seen. Initially, purplish or mauve. In time, surface becomes smooth and shiny after months to years, ivory with lilac-colored edge "lilac ring" (Fig. 14-44). May have hyper- and hypopigmentation in involved sclerotic areas (Fig. 14-45). Rarely, lesions become atrophic and hyperpigmented without going through a sclerotic stage (atrophoderma of Pasini and Pierini) (see Macular form of morphea, atrophic; p. 349).

Distribution

Circumscribed: Trunk (Fig. 14-44), limbs, face, and genitalia; less commonly, axillae, perineum, and areolae.
Generalized: Initially on trunk (upper, breasts, and abdomen) (Fig. 14-45) then thighs.

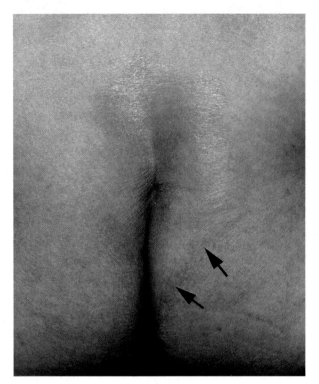

FIGURE 14-44 Morphea This is an indurated ivory-colored, shiny plaque with a lilac-colored, ill-defined border (*arrows*). Most lesions are better felt than seen because they are indurated.

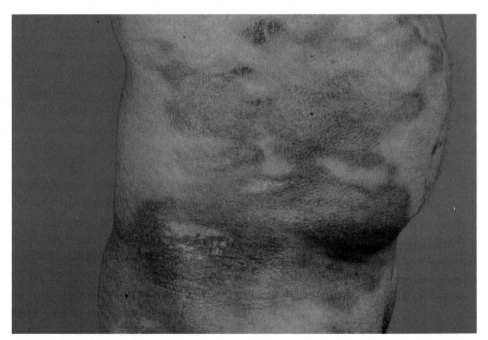

FIGURE 14-45 Morphea Irregular, brownish, indurated lesions with focal ivory-colored macular lesions on the left flank and abdomen. Similar lesions were also found on the back.

Linear: Usually on extremities (Fig. 14-46) or *frontoparietal*—scalp and face (Fig. 14-47); here, it may resemble a scar from a strike with a saber (*en coup de sabre*).

Macular: Small (<3 mm) macular patches, confluent (Fig. 14-48A); clinically indistinguishable from lichen sclerosus et atrophicus (see p. 351).

Atrophic: Atrophoderma of Pasini and Pierini (Fig. 14-48B).

Pansclerotic: On trunk (Fig. 14-49) or extremities.

MOUTH With linear morphea of head, the patient may have associated hemiatrophy of tongue.

HAIR AND NAILS Scarring alopecia with scalp plaque. Particularly with linear morphea of the head. Nail dystrophy in linear lesions of extremity or in pansclerotic morphea.

General Examination

Morphea around joints and linear morphea may lead to flexion contractures. Pansclerotic morphea is associated with atrophy and fibrosis of muscle. Extensive involvement of the trunk may result in restricted respiration. With linear morphea of the head (Fig. 14-47), there may be associated atrophy of ocular structures and atrophy of bone. *Note:* Morphea may be associated with lichen sclerosus et atrophicus.

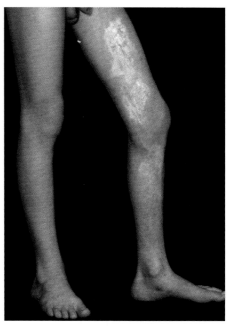

FIGURE 14-46 Linear Morphea Indurated, ivory-white lesion extending from upper thigh to the dorsum of the foot. Induration is pronounced, and in the region above the knee it extends to the fascia (pansclerotic morphea). If progressive, it will limit the movement of the joint.

FIGURE 14-47 Linear morphea, "en coup de sabre" Two linear, partially ivory-white (on the scalp) and hyperpigmented (on the forehead) depressed lesions extending from the crown of the head, where they have led to alopecia, over the forehead to the orbita. They look like scars after strikes with a saber, hence the French designation. These lesions can extend to the bone and rarely to the dura mater.

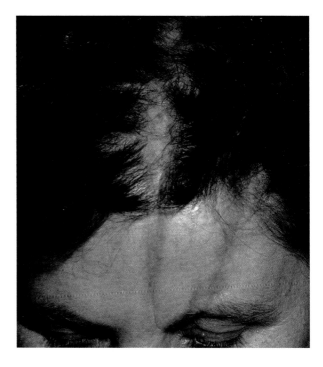

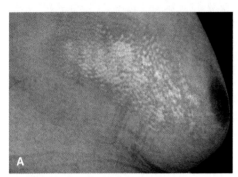
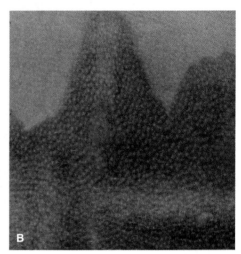

FIGURE 14-48 Macular form of morphea (A) There are multiple, shining, ivory-white macules with confluence leading to a reticulated pattern. These lesions are rather superficial and therefore less indurated. An important differential diagnosis is lichen sclerosus et atrophicus. **(B)** Atrophic, hyperpigmented form of morphea (called atrophoderma of Pasini and Pierini). There is a diffuse brown and sharply defined hyperpigmentation with a less pigmented follicular pattern. These lesions are atrophic and not indurated.

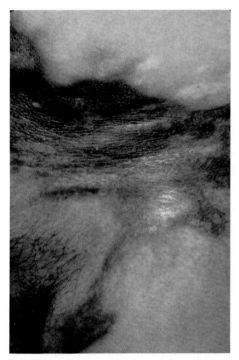

FIGURE 14-49 Pansclerotic morphea This type affects all layers of the skin including the fascia and even muscle. The skin is glistening, hyperpigmented, and hard as wood. It is obvious that pansclerotic morphea leads to considerable functional impairment. If these lesions occur on the upper trunk, they can impair excursion of the chest and thus breathing.

DIAGNOSIS AND DIFFERENTIAL DIAGNOSIS

Clinical, confirmed by biopsy. Sclerotic plaque associated with *B. burgdorferi* infection, acrodermatitis chronica atrophicans, progressive systemic sclerosis, lichen sclerosus et atrophicus, and scleroderma-like conditions (p. 347).

LABORATORY EXAMINATIONS

SEROLOGY Appropriate serologic testing to rule out *B. burgdorferi* infection.

DERMATOPATHOLOGY Epidermis appears normal to atrophic with loss of rete ridges. Dermis edematous with homogeneous and eosinophilic collagen. Slight mixed infiltrate, perivascular or diffuse. Later, dermis thickened with few fibroblasts and dense collagen; inflammatory infiltrate at dermal–subcutis junction; dermal appendages disappear progressively. Histopathology distinct from that of lichen sclerosus et atrophicus.

DIAGNOSIS

Clinical diagnosis, usually confirmed by skin biopsy.

COURSE

May be slowly progressive; "burn out" and spontaneous remissions can rarely occur.

MANAGEMENT

There is no effective treatment for morphea. Some report amelioration of early lesions with several 4-week cycles of prednisone (20 mg/d) interrupted by 2 months intervals of no treatment.

MORPHEA-LIKE LESIONS ASSOCIATED WITH LYME BORRELIOSIS In patients with early involvement, there may be a reversal of sclerosis with high-dose parenteral penicillin or ceftriaxone; treatment given in several courses over a time span of several months. Best response if combined with oral glucocorticoids.

PHOTOTHERAPY WITH UVA-1 (340 TO 400 NM) Somewhat effective, but results in hyperpigmentation.

LICHEN SCLEROSUS ET ATROPHICUS (LSA) ICD-10: L90.0

- LSA is a chronic atrophic disorder mainly of the anogenital skin of females but also of males. Females are 10 times more often affected than males.
- A disease of adults, but also occurring in children 1 to 13 years of age.
- Whitish, ivory or porcelain-white, sharply demarcated, individual papules may become confluent, forming *plaques* (Fig. 14-50). Surface of lesions may be elevated or in the same plane as normal skin; older lesions may be depressed. Dilated pilosebaceous or sweat duct orifices filled with keratin plugs (dells); if plugging is marked, surface appears hyperkeratotic (Fig. 14-50).
- *Bullae* and *erosions* occur and *purpura* is often a characteristic and identifying feature (Fig. 14-50); *telangiectasia.*
- Lesions occur on the genitalia and less commonly also on general skin. On vulva, hyperkeratotic plaques may become erosive, macerated; vulva may become atrophic, shrunken, especially clitoris and labia minora, with vaginal introitus reduced in size (Fig. 14-50, see also Section 34). Fusion of labia minora and majora. May extend to perineum and anus.
- In uncircumcised males, prepuce first shows ivory white confluent papules (see Section 34) but then becomes sclerotic and cannot be retracted (*phimosis*). Glans appears ivory or porcelain-white, semitransparent, resembling mother of pearl with admixed purpuric hemorrhages.
- Nongenital LSA usually asymptomatic; genital symptomatic. In women, vulvar lesions may be sensitive, especially while walking; pruritus; painful, especially if erosions are present; dysuria; dyspareunia. In males, recurrent balanitis, acquired phimosis.
- The histopathology is diagnostic with a dense lymphocytic infiltrate hugging the initially hypertrophic and later, atrophic epidermis and then sinking down into the dermis, being separated from the epidermis by an edematous, structureless subepidermal zone.
- The etiology of LSA is unknown, but reports from Europe have documented an association of DNA of *Borrelia* spp. with LSA in cases from Germany and Japan; DNA of the spirochetes detected in these patients was not found in any of the American samples.
- The course of LSA waxes and wanes. In girls, it may undergo spontaneous resolution; in women, it leads to atrophy of the vulva and in men to phimosis. Patients should be checked for the occurrence of squamous cell carcinoma of the vulva and penis.
- Management is very important, as this disease can cause a devastating atrophy of the labia minora and clitoral hood. Potent topical *glucocorticoid preparations* (clobetasol propionate) have proved effective for genital LSA and should be used for 6 to 8 weeks only. Patients should be monitored for signs of glucocorticoid-induced atrophy. *Pimecrolimus* and *tacrolimus* are almost as effective. *Topical androgens* are less used now because they can sometimes cause a clitoral hypertrophy. *Systemic therapy*: hydroxychloroquine, 125 to 150 mg/d, for weeks to a few months (monitor for ocular side effects).
- In males, *circumcision* relieves symptoms of phimosis and in some cases can result in remission.

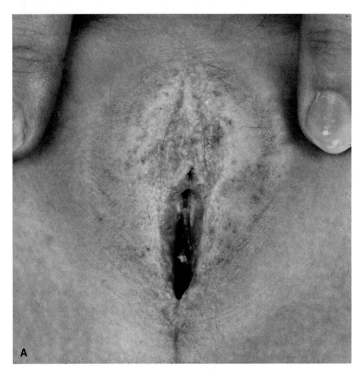

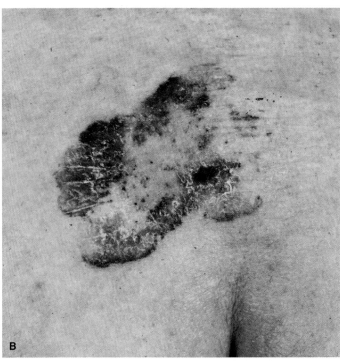

FIGURE 14-50 Lichen sclerosus et atrophicus (A) Lichen sclerosus on the vulva of a 6-year-old girl. The labia minora and majora have fused, are white, sclerotic, and focally hyperkeratotic and there are pinpoint hemorrhages. **(B)** Multiple, ivory-white, indurated, and slightly hyperkeratotic papules coalescing to a white plaque most of which, however, appears bright red caused by pinpoint hemorrhages. Chest of a 42-year-old woman.

VASCULITIS

Vessels are involved in most inflammatory processes in the human body. *Vasculitis* denotes conditions where vessels are the target of inflammation. The vasculitides can best be classified according to the size of vessels involved (Fig. 14-51).

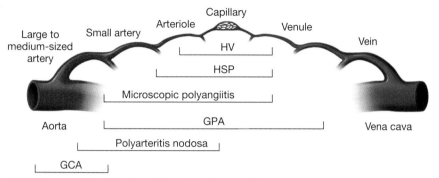

FIGURE 14-51 Classification scheme for the vasculitides HV, hypersensitivity vasculitis; HSP, Henoch–Schönlein purpura; GPA: granulomatosis with polyangitis; GCA, giant cell arteritis. (Modified with permission from Jennette JC, et al. Nomenclature of systemic vasculitides. Proposal of an international consensus conference. *Arthritis Rheum.* 1994;37:187. ©1994 American College of Rheumatology.)

HYPERSENSITIVITY VASCULITIS ICD-10: D69

- Hypersensitivity vasculitis (HV) encompasses a heterogeneous group of vasculitides associated with hypersensitivity to antigens from infectious agents, drugs, or other exogenous or endogenous sources.
- It is characterized pathologically by involvement of postcapillary venules and inflammation and fibrinoid necrosis (necrotizing vasculitis).
- Clinically, skin involvement is characteristic, manifested by "palpable purpura."
- Systemic vascular involvement occurs, chiefly in the kidney, muscles, joints, GI tract, and peripheral nerves.
- Henoch–Schönlein purpura is a type of HV associated with IgA deposits in the skin and involvement of the GI tract, kidneys and joints.
- *Synonyms*: Allergic cutaneous vasculitis, necrotizing vasculitis.

EPIDEMIOLOGY AND ETIOLOGY

AGE OF ONSET All ages.
SEX Equal incidence in males and females.
ETIOLOGY Idiopathic 50%.

PATHOGENESIS

A postulated mechanism for necrotizing vasculitis is the deposition in postcapillary venules of circulating immune complexes. Initial alterations in venular permeability, caused by the release of vasoactive amines from platelets, basophils, and/or mast cells, facilitate the deposition of immune complexes and these may

activate the complement system or may interact directly with Fc receptors on endothelial cell membranes. When the complement system is activated, the generation of anaphylatoxins C3a and C5a can degranulate mast cells. Also, C5a can attract neutrophils that release lysosomal enzymes during phagocytosis of complexes and subsequently damage vascular tissue.

CLINICAL MANIFESTATION

A new drug taken during the few weeks before the onset of HV is a likely etiologic agent, as may be an infection, a known vascular/connective tissue disease, or paraproteinemia.

Onset and course: Acute (days, as in drug induced or idiopathic), subacute (weeks, especially urticarial types), chronic (recurrent over years). Symptoms are pruritus, burning pain; there may be no symptoms or there may be fever, malaise; symptoms of peripheral neuritis, abdominal pain (bowel ischemia), arthralgia, myalgia, kidney involvement (microhematuria), or CNS involvement.

SKIN LESIONS The hallmark is *palpable purpura*. This term describes palpable petechiae that present as bright red, well-demarcated macules and papules with a central, dot-like hemorrhage (Fig. 14-52) (petechiae caused by coagulation defects or thrombocytopenia are strictly macular and, therefore, not palpable).

Lesions are scattered, discrete or confluent, and are primarily localized to the lower legs and the ankles (Figs. 14-52A and B) but may spread to the buttocks and arms. Stasis aggravates or precipitates lesions. Purpuric lesions do not blanch (with a glass slide). Red initially, they turn purple and even black in the center (Fig. 14-52B). In the case of massive inflammation, purpuric papules convert to hemorrhagic blisters, become necrotic (Fig. 14-52B), and even ulcerate.

LABORATORY EXAMINATIONS

HEMATOLOGY Rule out thrombocytopenic purpura.

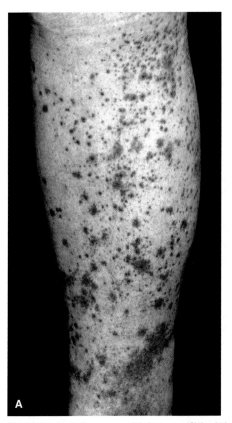 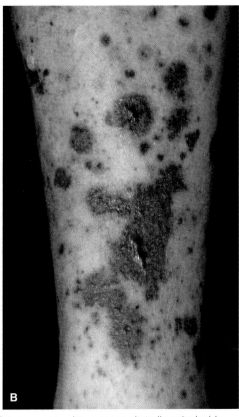

FIGURE 14-52 Hypersensitivity vasculitis (A) Cutaneous vasculitis presents clinically as "palpable purpura" on the lower extremities. Although appearing to the eye as macules, the lesions can be palpated, and this contrasts with petechiae, for instance, in thrombocytopenic purpura. The lesions shown here have central punctum that is a darker red and do not blanch with a glass slide, indicating hemorrhage. **(B)** This is a more advanced stage. Lesions have progressed to hemorrhagic bullae and some have become necrotic. The lesions may progress to ulceration.

ESR Elevated.

SEROLOGY Serum complement is reduced or normal in some patients, depending on associated disorders.

URINALYSIS RBC casts, albuminuria.

OTHERS Depending on underlying disease.

DERMATOPATHOLOGY *Necrotizing Venulitis.* Deposition of eosinophilic material (fibrinoid) in the walls of postcapillary venules in the upper dermis, and perivenular and intramural inflammatory infiltrate consisting predominantly of neutrophils. Extravasated RBC and fragmented neutrophils ("nuclear dust"). Frank necrosis of vessel walls. Intramural C3 and immunoglobulin deposition is seen with immunofluorescent techniques.

DIAGNOSIS AND DIFFERENTIAL DIAGNOSIS

Based on clinical appearance and histopathology. DIFFERENTIAL DIAGNOSIS Thrombocytopenic purpura, rash such as exanthematous drug eruption in setting of thrombocytopenia, disseminated intravascular coagulation (DIC) with purpura fulminans, septic vasculitis (rickettsial spotted fevers), septic emboli (infective endocarditis), bacteremia [disseminated gonococcal infection, meningococcemia (acute/chronic)], pigmented purpura, and other noninfectious vasculitides.

COURSE AND PROGNOSIS

Depends on underlying disease. In the idiopathic variant, multiple episodes can occur over the course of years. Usually self-limited, but irreversible damage to kidneys can occur.

MANAGEMENT

ANTIBIOTICS Antibiotics for patients in whom vasculitis follows bacterial infection.

PREDNISONE For patients with moderate to severe disease.

CYTOTOXIC IMMUNOSUPPRESSIVES Cyclophosphamide, azathioprine usually in combination with prednisone. Cyclosporine and intravenous high-dose immunoglobulin. Infliximab and Rituximab.

HENOCH-SCHÖNLEIN PURPURA ICD-10: 69.0

- This is a specific subtype of hypersensitivity vasculitis that occurs mainly in children but also affects adults.
- There is a history of upper respiratory tract infection (75%), by group A streptococci.
- The disorder consists of palpable purpura (as in Fig. 14-52) accompanied by bowel angina (diffuse abdominal pain that is worse after meals), bowel ischemia, usually including bloody diarrhea, kidney involvement (hematuria and red cell casts), and arthritis.
- Histopathologically, there is necrotizing vasculitis and the immunoreactants deposited in skin are IgA.
- Long-term morbidity may result from progressive renal disease (5%).

POLYARTERITIS NODOSA ICD-10: M30.01

- Polyarteritis nodosa (PAN) is a multisystem, necrotizing vasculitis of small- and medium-sized muscular arteries with involvement of the renal and visceral arteries.
- Microscopic polyangitis (MPA) may be different from PAN, but this is not proven and therefore included in this discussion.
- *Cutaneous PAN* is a rare variant with symptomatic vasculitis limited to skin and at times peripheral nerves.
- Necrotizing inflammation of small- and medium-sized muscular arteries; may spread circumferentially to involve adjacent veins. Lesions segmental, tend to involve bifurcations. About 30% of cases associated with hepatitis B and C antigenemia, i.e., immune complex formation.
- Constitutional symptoms: Fever, asthma, myalgia. Skin symptoms: pain, paresthesia.
- **Skin Lesions:** Occur in 15% of cases. Subcutaneous inflammatory, bright red to bluish nodules (0.5 to 2 cm) that follow the course of involved arteries. Violaceous, become confluent to form painful subcutaneous plaques (Fig. 14-53), and accompanied by livedo reticularis; "starburst" livedo is pathognomonic and marks a cluster of nodular lesions. Ulcers follow ischemia of nodules (Fig. 14-53B). Usually bilaterally on lower legs and thighs. Other areas: Arms, trunk, head, neck, buttocks. Livedo reticularis may extend to trunk. Duration—days to months. Resolves with residual violaceous or postinflammatory hyperpigmentation. Skin lesions in systemic and cutaneous PAN are identical
- Systems review:
  - **Cardiovascular:** Hypertension, congestive heart failure, pericarditis, conduction system defects, and myocardial infarction.
  - **Neurologic:** Cerebrovascular accident. Peripheral nerves: Mixed motor/sensory involvement with mononeuritis multiplex pattern.
  - **Muscles:** Diffuse myalgias (excluding shoulder and hip girdle) and lower extremities.
  - **GI System:** Nausea, vomiting, abdominal pain, hemorrhage, and infarction.
  - **Eyes:** Hypertensive changes, ocular vasculitis, retinal artery aneurysm, and optic disc edema/atrophy.
  - **Kidney:** Renal failure and edema.
  - **Testes:** Pain and tenderness.
- **Dermatopathology:** Polymorphonuclear neutrophils infiltrate all layers of muscular vessel wall and perivascular areas. Fibrinoid necrosis of vessel wall with compromise of lumen, thrombosis, infarction of tissues supplied by involved vessel, with or without hemorrhage.
- **CBC:** Commonly neutrophilic leukocytosis; rarely, eosinophilia; anemia of chronic disease. ± Elevated ESR, serum creatinine, and BUN.
- **Serology:** Antineutrophil cytoplasmic autoantibodies (p-ANCA) in some cases. In 60% of MPA patients, hepatitis B surface antigenemia; in 30% of cases, hepatitis C.
- Untreated, very high morbidity and mortality rates characterized by fulminant deterioration or by relentless progression associated with intermittent acute exacerbations. Death from renal failure, bowel infarction and perforation, cardiovascular complications, and intractable hypertension. *Cutaneous PAN*: Chronic relapsing benign course.
- Management: *Combined therapy*: prednisone, 1 mg/kg body weight per day and cyclophosphamide, 2 mg/kg per day.
- Rituximab as effective as cyclophosphamide.

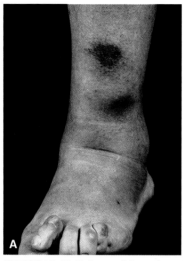 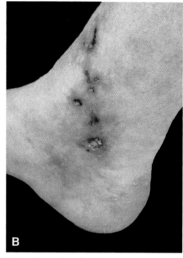

FIGURE 14-53 Polyarteritis nodosa (A) Two dermal and subcutaneous nodules occurring on the pretibial aspects of the lower leg. **(B)** A starburst pattern can be seen in the supra- and retromalleolar region of the right leg in another patient. These lesions represent cutaneous infarction with ulceration.

GRANULOMATOSIS WITH POLYANGITIS ICD-10: M31.3

- Formerly Wegener granulomatosis. It is a systemic vasculitis, defined by a clinical triad of manifestations comprising involvement of the upper airways, lungs, and kidneys.
- A pathologic triad consisting of necrotizing granulomas in the upper respiratory tract and lungs, vasculitis involving both arteries and veins, and glomerulonephritis.
- Skin manifestations are those of hypersensitivity vasculitis, noduloulcerative lesions, and oral/nasal ulcerations. Overall in 50% of patients but in only 13% of patients at initial presentation. *Ulcers with jagged, undermined borders* are most typical; resemble pyoderma gangrenosum (Fig. 14-54). *Papules, vesicles, palpable purpura* as in hypersensitivity (necrotizing) vasculitis (Fig. 14-55), subcutaneous nodules, plaques, noduloulcerative lesions as in PAN. Most common on lower extremities. Also, face, trunk, and upper limbs.
- *Mucous Membranes:* Oral ulcerations (Fig. 14-56). Often first symptom. ± Nasal mucosal ulceration, crusting, blood clots; nasal septal perforation; saddle-nose deformity. Eustachian tube occlusion with serous otitis media; ± pain. External auditory canal: pain, erythema, and swelling. Marked gingival hyperplasia.
- *Eyes:* 65%. Mild conjunctivitis, episcleritis, scleritis, granulomatous sclerouveitis, ciliary vessel vasculitis, and retroorbital mass lesion with proptosis.
- *Nervous System:* Cranial neuritis, mononeuritis multiplex, and cerebral vasculitis.
- *Renal Disease:* 85%. Signs of renal failure in advanced GPA.
- *Pulmonary:* Multiple, bilateral nodular infiltrates. Similar infiltrates in paranasal sinus and nasopharynx.
- Chronic disease syndrome. Fever. Paranasal sinus pain, purulent, or bloody nasal discharge. Cough, hemoptysis, dyspnea, and chest discomfort.
- **Hematology:** Mild anemia. Leukocytosis. ± Thrombocytosis.
- **ESR:** Markedly elevated.
- **Chemistry:** Impaired renal function.
- **Urinalysis:** Proteinuria, hematuria, and RBC casts.
- **Serology:** Antineutrophil cytoplasmic autoantibodies (c-ANCA) are seromarkers for GPA. A 29-kDa protease (PR-3) is the major antigen for c-ANCA; titers correlate with disease activity. Hypergammaglobulinemia and particularly IgA class.
- **Pathology:** All involved tissues including skin—necrotizing vasculitis of small arteries/veins with intra- or extravascular granuloma formation. Kidneys: Focal/segmental glomerulonephritis.
- Untreated, usually fatal because of rapidly progressive renal failure. With combination cyclophosphamide plus prednisone therapy, long-term remission is achieved in 90% of cases.
- **Treatment of Choice: Cyclophosphamide plus prednisone.** *Rituximab:* In refractory patients. *Trimethoprim–Sulfamethoxazole:* As adjunctive therapy and/or prevention of upper airway bacterial infections that promote disease flare.

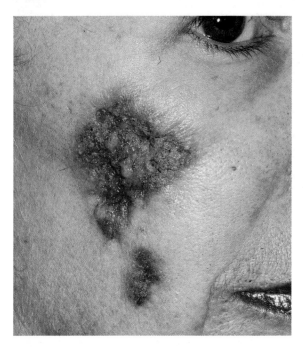

FIGURE 14-54 Granulomatosis with Polyangitis (formerly Wegener granulomatosis) A pyoderma gangrenosum-like irregular ulceration on the cheek with jagged and undermined borders is often the first manifestation of GPA.

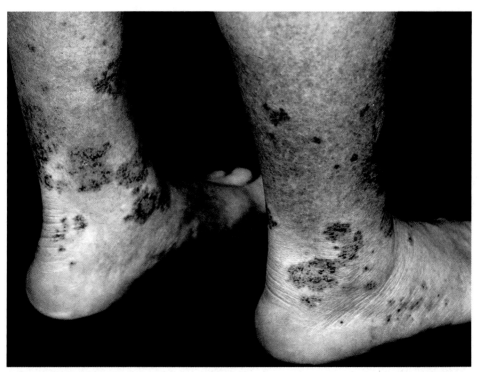

FIGURE 14-55 GPA Palpable purpura with hemorrhagic and necrotic lesions on the legs as in hypersensitivity vasculitis.

FIGURE 14-56 GPA A large ulcer on the palate covered by a dense, adherent, necrotic mass; note accompanying edema of the upper lip. Similar lesions occur in the sinuses and tracheobronchial tree.

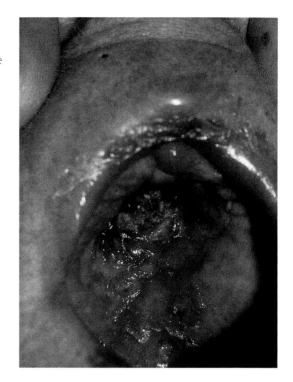

GIANT CELL ARTERITIS ICD-10: M31.610

- Giant cell arteritis is a systemic granulomatous vasculitis of medium- and large-sized arteries, most notably the temporal artery and other branches of the carotid artery in oldpatients (**Fig. 14-57**).
- Cutaneous manifestations: Superficial temporal arteries are swollen, prominent, tortuous, and ± nodular thickenings. Tender. Initially, involved artery pulsates; later, occluded with loss of pulsation. ± Erythema of overlying skin. Gangrene, i.e., skin infarction of the area supplied by affected artery in the temporal/parietal scalp with sharp, irregular borders (**Fig. 14-57A**); ulceration with exposure of bone (**Fig. 14-57B**). Scars at sites of old ulcerations. Postinflammatory hyperpigmentation over involved artery.
- Other symptoms: Chronic disease syndrome. Severe headache usually bilateral, scalp pain, fatigue, anemia, high ESR. Claudication of jaw/tongue while talking/chewing. Eye involvement: Transient impairment of vision, ischemic optic neuritis, retrobulbar neuritis, and persistent blindness. Systemic vasculitis: Claudication of extremities, stroke, myocardial infarction, aortic aneurysms/dissections, and visceral organ infarction. *Polymyalgia rheumatica syndrome*: Stiffness, aching, pain in the muscles of the neck, shoulders, lower back, hips, and thighs.
- **Temporal Artery Biopsy:** Biopsy tender nodule of involved artery after Doppler flow examination. Lesions focal. Panarteritis with inflammatory mononuclear cell infiltrates within the vessel wall with frequent giant cell granuloma formation. Intimal proliferation with vascular occlusion, fragmentation of internal elastic lamina, extensive necrosis of intima and media.
- Untreated, can result in blindness secondary to ischemic optic neuritis. Excellent response to glucocorticoid therapy. Remission after several years.
- Management:
  - **Prednisone:** First-line therapy. Initially, 40 to 60 mg/d; taper when symptoms abate; continue 7.5 to 10 mg/d for 1 to 2 years.
  - **Methotrexate:** Low-dose (15 to 20 mg) methotrexate, once a week, has a considerable glucocorticoid-sparing effect.
  - Rituximab.

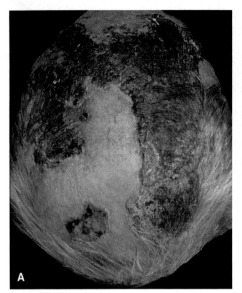 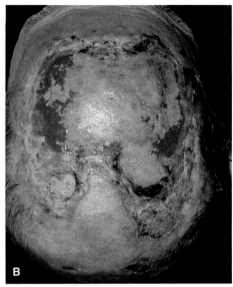

FIGURE 14-57 Giant cell arteritis (A) This elderly male had excruciating headaches and progressive impairment of vision. Necrosis developed bilaterally on the scalp. **(B)** In this patient, the necrotic tissue has been shed, revealing the bare bone of the skull. Both patients survived with high dose prednisone and the ulcers healed.

URTICARIAL VASCULITIS ICD-10: L95.810

- Urticarial vasculitis is a multisystem disease characterized by cutaneous lesions resembling urticaria, except that wheals persist for >24 h. Urticaria like (i.e., edematous plaques and wheals), occasionally indurated, erythematous, circumscribed (Fig. 14-58); lesions may be associated with itching, burning, stinging sensation, pain, tenderness. occasionally with angioedema. Eruption occurs in transient crops, usually lasting >24 h and up to 3 to 4 days. They change shape slowly, often reveal purpura on blanching (glass slide), and resolve with a yellowish-green color and hyperpigmentation.
- Fever, arthralgia, and elevated ESR. Other symptoms: Nausea, abdominal pain. Cough, dyspnea, chest pain, and hemoptysis. Pseudotumor cerebri. Cold sensitivity. Renal involvement: diffuse glomerulonephritis.
- The syndrome is often accompanied by various degrees of extracutaneous involvement. Extracutaneous manifestations: joints (70%), GI tract (20 to 30%), CNS (>10%), ocular system (>10%), kidneys (10 to 20%), lymphadenopathy (5%).
- Thought to be an immune complex disease, similar to hypersensitivity vasculitis (see p. 353). May be symptom of SLE; in serum sickness, hepatitis B; idiopathic.
- Laboratory: Leukocytoclastic vasculitis; microhematuria, proteinuria (10%); hypocomplementemia (70%).
- Most often this syndrome has a chronic (months to years) but benign course. Episodes recur over periods ranging from months to years. Renal disease recur over periods ranging from months to years. Renal disease occurs only in hypocomplementemic patients.
- Management: H_1 and H_2 blockers [doxepin (10 mg twice daily to 25 mg three times daily) *plus* cimetidine (300 mg three times daily)/ranitidine (150 mg twice daily)] *plus* a nonsteroidal anti-inflammatory agent [indomethacin (75 to 200 mg/d)/ibuprofen (1600 to 2400 mg/d)/naprosyn (500 to 1000 mg/d)]. Colchicine, 0.6 mg two or three times daily *or* dapsone, 50 to 150 mg/d. Prednisone; azathioprine, cyclophosphamide; plasmapheresis. TNF-α blockers.

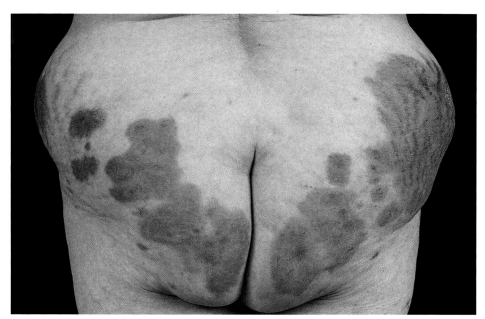

FIGURE 14-58 Urticarial vasculitis Erythematous plaques and wheals on the buttocks that, in part, do not blanch on diascopy (compression of the lesional skin with glass), which indicates hemorrhage. This contrasts with urticaria. Also, in contrast to lesions of urticaria, which usually resolve within 24 h, those of urticarial vasculitis persist for up to 3 days before resolving with residual hyperpigmentation (hemosiderin deposition). Lesions of urticaria change shape in a short time, while those of urticarial vasculitis change slowly.

NODULAR VASCULITIS ICD-10: L95.830

- Nodular vasculitis is a form of lobular panniculitis associated with subcutaneous blood vessel vasculitis with subsequent ischemic changes that produce lipocyte injury, necrosis, inflammation, and granulation.
- Synonyms are *erythema induratum* and *Bazin disease*, but these terms are now reserved for those cases of nodular vasculitis that are associated with *Mycobacterium tuberculosis*.
- Middle aged to older women.
- **Etiology:** Immune complex–mediated vascular injury caused by bacterial antigens has been implicated. Immunoglobulins, complement, and bacterial antigens have been found by immunofluorescence and in some cases mycobacterial DNA sequences by polymerase chain reaction. Bacterial cultures are invariably negative.
- **Skin Lesions:** Initially erythematous, tender, or asymptomatic subcutaneous nodules or plaques (Fig. 14-59) on the calves, rarely on shins and thighs. Lesions become bluish red in color, are firm, and fluctuate before ulcerating. Ulcers drain serous/oily fluid, are ragged, punched-out, and have violaceous or brown margins (Fig. 14-59). They persist for prolonged periods before healing with atrophic scars.
- **Associated Findings:** Follicular perniosis, livedo, varicose veins, thick, stubby lower leg, and a cool, edematous skin.
- **General Examination:** Patients are usually healthy.
- **Dermatopathology:** Tuberculoid granulomas, foreign-body giant cell reaction, and necrosis of fat lobules. Medium-sized vessel vasculitis, predominantly venular but sometimes arterial, in the septal areas.
- **Course:** Chronic recurrent and scarring.
- **Management:** Antituberculous therapy in those cases where *M. tuberculosis* etiology is proved. In other cases, bed rest, compression stockings, tetracyclines, and potassium iodide have proved effective. Systemic glucocorticoids are sometimes necessary for remission. In some cases, dapsone is effective.

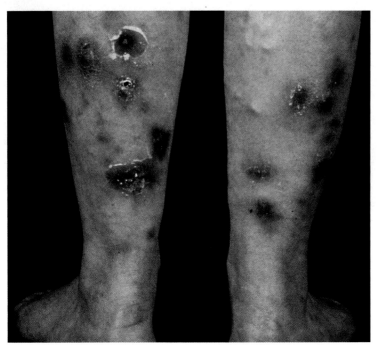

FIGURE 14-59 Nodular vasculitis Multiple, deep-seated, brown to bluish nodules, particularly on the posterior aspects of both lower legs. The lesions, which are relatively asymptomatic, may undergo necrosis forming slowly healing ulcers. Varicose veins are also seen on the right calf.

PIGMENTED PURPURIC DERMATOSES (PPD) ICD-10: L81.7

- PPD are distinguished by their clinical characteristics, having identical dermatopathologic findings, and include:
  - Schamberg disease, also known as progressive pigmented purpuric dermatosis or progressive pigmentary purpura (**Fig. 14-60A**).
  - Majocchi disease, also known as purpura annularis telangiectodes (**Fig. 14-60B**).
  - Gougerot-Blum disease, also known as pigmented purpuric lichenoid dermatitis or purpura pigmentosa chronica.
  - Lichen aureus, also known as lichen purpuricus.
- Clinically, each entity shows recent pinpoint cayenne pepper–colored hemorrhages associated with older hemorrhages and hemosiderin deposition. Capillaritis histologically. Results in spotty hyperpigmentations.
- PPD are significant only if they are a cosmetic concern to the patient; they are important because they are often mistaken as manifestations of vasculitis or thrombocytopenia.
- **Etiology:** Unknown. Primary process believed to be cell-mediated immune injury with subsequent vascular damage and erythrocyte extravasation. Other etiologic factors: Pressure, trauma, and drugs (acetaminophen, ampicillin-carbromal, diuretics, meprobamate, nonsteroidal anti-inflammatory drugs, and zomepirac sodium).
- **Onset and Duration:** Insidious, slow to evolve except drug-induced variant, which may develop rapidly and be more generalized in distribution. Persists for months to years. Most drug-induced purpuras resolve more quickly after discontinuation of the drug. Usually asymptomatic but may be mildly pruritic.
- **Management:** Topical low- and middle-potency glucocorticoid preparations may inhibit new purpuric lesions. Systemic tetracycline or minocycline (50 mg twice daily) are effective. PUVA is effective in severe forms. *Supportive stockings required in all forms.*

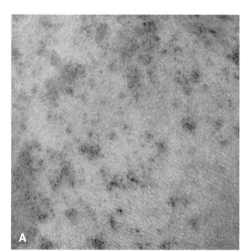
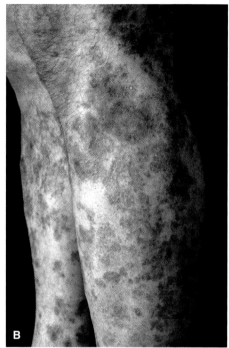

FIGURE 14-60 **Pigmented purpuric dermatosis: (A) Schamberg disease** Multiple discrete and confluent nonpalpable, nonblanching purpuric lesions on the leg. Acute microhemorrhages resolve with deposition of hemosiderin, creating a brown peppered stain. **(B) Majocchi disease** Multiple nonpalpable, nonblanching purpuric lesions arranged in annular configurations. Note disfiguring dark brown discoloration of old lesions.

KAWASAKI DISEASE ICD-10: M30.3

- Kawasaki disease (KD) is an acute febrile illness of infants and children.
- Characterized by cutaneous and mucosal erythema and edema with subsequent desquamation, and cervical lymphadenitis.
- Bilateral bulbar nonexudative conjunctival injection and inflammation of oropharynx.
- Complications: Coronary abnormalities, including aneurysms (30%), myocarditis, arthritis, urethritis, and aseptic meningitis.
- Immediate treatment with intravenous immunoglobulin and aspirin reduces coronary aneurysms.
- *Synonym*: Mucocutaneous lymph node syndrome.

EPIDEMIOLOGY AND ETIOLOGY

AGE OF ONSET Peak incidence at 1 year, mean 2.6 years, uncommon after 8 years. Most cases of KD in adults probably represent toxic shock syndrome.
SEX Male predominance, 1.5:1.
RACE In United States: Japanese > African Americans > Causcasions.
ETIOLOGY Unknown.

SEASON Winter and spring.
GEOGRAPHY First reported in Japan, 1961; United States, 1971. Epidemics.

PATHOGENESIS

Generalized vasculitis. Endarteritis of vasa vasorum involves adventitia/intima of proximal coronary arteries with ectasia, aneurysm formation, vessel obstruction, and distal embolization with subsequent myocardial infarction. Other vessels: Brachiocephalic, celiac, renal, and iliofemoral arteries. Increased activated helper T cells and monocytes, elevated serum IL-1, TNF-α, IL-6, adreno-medullin, as well as vascular endothelial growth factor, anti-endothelial antibodies, and increased cytokine-inducible activation anti-gens on the vascular endothelium occur in KD. T-cell response is driven by a superantigen.

CLINICAL MANIFESTATION/PHASES

PHASE I: ACUTE FEBRILE PERIOD Abrupt onset of fever, lasting approximately 12 days, followed (usually within 1 to 3 days) by most of the other principal features. Constitutional symptoms of diarrhea, arthritis, and photophobia.

PHASE II: SUBACUTE PHASE Lasts approximately until day 30 of illness; fever, thrombocytosis, desquamation, arthritis, arthralgia, and carditis; highest risk for sudden death.

PHASE III: CONVALESCENT PERIOD Begins within 8 to 10 weeks after onset of illness when all signs of illness have disappeared and ends when ESR

returns to normal; very low mortality rate during this period.

Skin Lesions

PHASE I Lesions appear 1 to 3 days after onset of fever. Duration, 12 days average. Nearly all mucocutaneous abnormalities occur during this phase.

Exanthem. Erythema usually first noted on the palms and soles, spreading to involve trunk and extremities within 2 days. First lesions: Erythematous macules; lesions enlarge and become more numerous. Type: Urticaria-like lesions (most common); morbilliform pattern (common); scarlatiniform and EM like in <5% of cases. Confluent macules to plaque-type erythema on perineum, which persist after other findings have resolved. Edema of hands/feet: Deeply erythematous to viola-ceous; brawny swelling with fusiform fingers (Fig. 14-61). Palpation: Lesions may be tender.

Mucous Membranes. Bulbar conjunctival injection; noted 2 days after onset of fever; duration, 1 to 3 weeks (throughout the febrile course). Lips: Red, dry, fissured (Fig. 14-61),

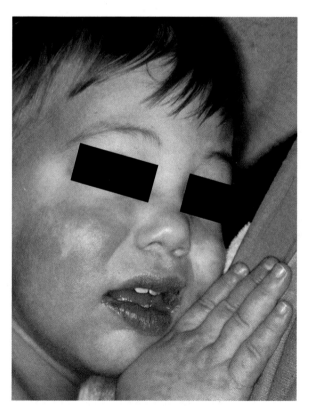

FIGURE 14-61 Kawasaki disease Cherry-red lips with hemorrhagic fissures, in a little boy with prolonged high fever. This child also had a generalized morbilliform eruption, injected conjunctivae, and "strawberry" tongue (not shown). Note erythema and edema of fingertips.

hemorrhagic crusts; duration, 1 to 3 weeks. Oropharynx: Diffuse erythema. Tongue: "Strawberry" tongue (erythema and protuberance of papillae of tongue).

Cervical Lymphnodes. Lymphadenopathy (Fig. 14-62) tender, firm, >1.5 cm.

PHASE II Desquamation highly characteristic; follows resolution of exanthem (Fig. 14-63). Begins on the tips of fingers and toes at the junction of nails and skin; desquamating sheets of palmar/plantar epidermis are progressively shed.

PHASE III Beau lines (transverse furrows on nail surface) may be seen (see Section 32). Possible telogen effluvium.

GENERAL FINDINGS Meningeal irritation. Pneumonia. Arthritis/arthralgias, knees, hips, elbows. Pericardial tamponade, dysrhythmias, rubs, congestive heart failure, and left ventricular dysfunction.

LABORATORY EXAMINATIONS

CHEMISTRY Abnormal liver function tests.

HEMATOLOGY Leukocytosis (>18,000/μL). Thrombocytosis after the 10th day of illness. Elevated ESR in phase II. ESR returns to normal in phase III.

URINALYSIS Pyuria.

DERMATOPATHOLOGY Arteritis involving small- and medium-sized vessels with swelling of endothelial cells in postcapillary venules, dilatation of small blood vessels, lymphocytic/monocytic perivascular infiltrate in arteries/arterioles of dermis.

ELECTROCARDIOGRAPHY Prolongation of PR and QT intervals; ST-segment and T-wave changes.

ECHOCARDIOGRAPHY AND ANGIOGRAPHY Coronary aneurysms in 20% of cases.

DIAGNOSIS AND DIFFERENTIAL DIAGNOSIS

DIAGNOSTIC CRITERIA Fever spiking to >39.4°C, lasting ≥5 days without other cause, associated with four of five criteria: (1) bilateral conjunctival injection; (2) at least one of the following mucous membrane changes—injected/fissured lips, injected pharynx, "strawberry" tongue; (3) at least one of the following extremity changes—erythema of palms/soles, edema of hands/feet, generalized/periungual desquamation; (4) diffuse scarlatiniform or deeply erythematous maculopapular rash, iris lesions;

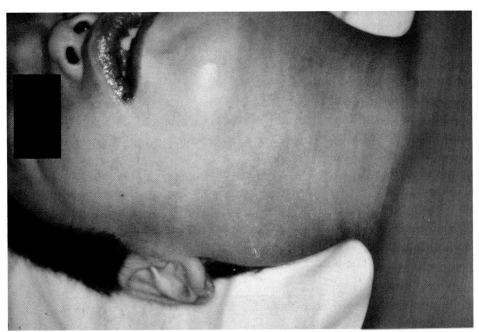

FIGURE 14-62 Kawasaki disease Lymphadenopathy. Visible cervical lymphadenopathy is seen in this child with Kawasaki disease. Note also cherry-red fissures lips and macular rash on neck. (Photo contributor: Tomisaku Kawasaki, MD. Reused with permission from *Knoop K, et al,* eds. *The Atlas of Emergency Medicine.* 3rd ed. New York, NY: McGraw-Hill; 2010.)

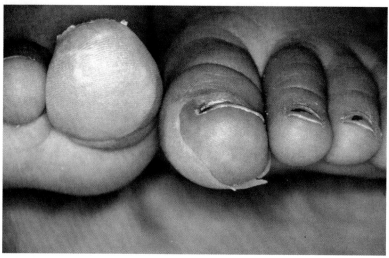

FIGURE 14-63 Kawasaki disease Periungual desquamation. This finding typically begins 2 to 3 weeks after the onset of Kawasaki disease, in contrast to perineal desquamation that occurs during the early course of the disease in infants. (Photo contributor: Tomisaku Kawasaki, MD. Reused with permission from *Knoop K, et al*, eds. *The Atlas of Emergency Medicine*. 3rd ed. New York, NY: McGraw-Hill; 2010.)

and (5) cervical lymphadenopathy (at least one lymph node ≥1.5 cm in diameter).

DIFFERENTIAL DIAGNOSIS Adverse cutaneous drug eruption, juvenile rheumatoid arthritis, infectious mononucleosis, viral exanthems, leptospirosis, Rocky Mountain spotted fever, toxic shock syndrome, staphylococcal scalded-skin syndrome, EM, serum sickness, SLE, and reactive arthritis syndrome.

COURSE AND PROGNOSIS

Clinical course triphasic. Uneventful recovery occurs in majority of patients. Cardiovascular system complications occur in 20%. Coronary artery aneurysms occur within 2 to 8 weeks, associated with myocarditis, myocardial ischemia/infarction, pericarditis, peripheral vascular occlusion, small-bowel obstruction, and stroke. Case fatality rate, 0.5 to 2.8% of cases, and is associated with coronary artery aneurysms.

MANAGEMENT

Diagnosis should be made early and attention directed at prevention of the cardiovascular complications.

HOSPITALIZATION Recommended during the phase I illness, monitoring for cardiac and vascular complications.

SYSTEMIC THERAPY **Intravenous Immunoglobulin.** 2 g/kg as a single infusion over 10 h together with aspirin as soon as possible. **Aspirin.** 100 mg/kg per day until fever resolves or until day 14 of illness, followed by 5 to 10 mg/kg per day until ESR and platelet count have returned to normal.

Glucocorticoids are Contraindicated. Associated with a higher rate of coronary aneurysms.

REACTIVE ARTHRITIS (formerly Reiter Syndrome) ICD-10: M02.3

- Reactive arthritis (RA) is defined by an episode of peripheral arthritis of >1 month's duration occurring in association with urethritis and/or cervicitis.
- Initiation by infection, usually in the genitourinary and gastrointestinal tract.
- *Salmonella, Campylobacter, Shigella, Yersinia*, and *Chlamydia* trigger RA but other infections can also be initiators.
- Frequently accompanied by keratoderma blennorrhagicum, circinate balanitis, conjunctivitis, and stomatitis.
- The classic triad is arthritis, urethritis, and conjunctivitis.

EPIDEMIOLOGY AND ETIOLOGY

AGE OF ONSET 22 years (median) in the type following sexually transmitted infection (STI).

SEX 90% of patients are males (postvenereal type).

RACE Most common in Caucasians from northern Europe; rare in Asians and African blacks.

GENETIC DIATHESIS HLA-B27 occurs in up to 75% of Caucasians with RA but in only 8% of healthy Caucasians. Patients who are HLA-B27 negative have a milder course, with significantly less sacroiliitis, uveitis, and carditis.

ASSOCIATED DISORDERS Incidence of RA may be increased in HIV-infected individuals.

ETIOLOGY Unknown.

PATHOGENESIS

RA appears linked to *genetic factors*, i.e., HLA-B27 and *enteric pathogens* such as *Salmonella enteritidis, S. typhimurium, S. heidelberg; Yersinia enterocolitica, Y. pseudotuberculosis; Campylobacter fetus; Shigella flexneri;* or genitourinary pathogens (such as *Chlamydia* or *Ureaplasma urealyticum*). Two patterns are observed: the *epidemic form*, which follows STI (most common type in the United States and the United Kingdom), and the *postdysenteric form* following GI infection (most common type in continental Europe and North Africa).

CLINICAL MANIFESTATION

Onset 1 to 4 weeks after infection: Enterocolitis, nongonococcal urethritis. Urethritis and/or conjunctivitis usually first to appear, followed by arthritis.

Symptoms consist of malaise, fever, dysuria, and urethral discharge. Eyes: Red, slightly sensitive, and seronegative arthritis.

SKIN LESIONS Resemble those of psoriasis, especially on the palms/soles, and glans penis. *Keratoderma blennorrhagicum:* Brownish-red papules or macules, sometimes topped by vesicles that enlarge; centers of lesions become pustular and/or hyperkeratotic, crusted (Fig. 14-64), mainly on palms and soles. Scaling erythematous, psoriasiform plaques on scalp, elbows, and buttocks. Erosive patches resembling pustular psoriasis may occur, especially on shaft of penis and scrotum. *Circinate balanitis* (Fig. 14-65): Shallow erosions with serpiginous, micropustular borders if uncircumcised; crusted and/or hyperkeratotic plaques if circumcised, i.e., psoriasiform.

NAILS Small subungual pustules → onycholysis and subungual hyperkeratosis.

MUCOUS MEMBRANES **Urethra.** Sterile serous or mucopurulent discharge. **Mouth.** Erosive lesions on tongue or hard palate, resembling migratory glossitis.

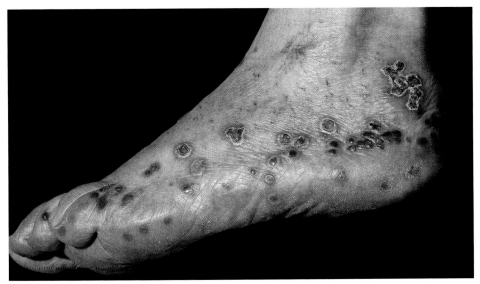

FIGURE 14-64 Reactive arthritis: keratoderma blennorrhagicum Red-to-brown papules, vesicles, and pustules with central erosion and characteristic crusting and peripheral scaling on the dorsolateral and plantar foot.

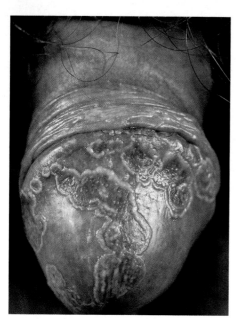

FIGURE 14-65 Reactive arthritis: balanitis circinata Moist, well-demarcated erosions with a slightly raised micropustular circinate border on the glans penis.

Eyes. Conjunctivitis, mild, evanescent, or bilateral; anterior uveitis.

SYSTEMIC FINDINGS Seronegative arthritis: Oligoarticular, asymmetric; most commonly knees, ankles, small joints of feet; diffuse swelling of fingers and toes, and enthesitis.

LABORATORY EXAMINATIONS

HEMATOLOGY Anemia, leukocytosis, thrombocytosis, and elevated ESR.

CULTURE Urethral culture negative for gonococcus, may be positive for *Chlamydia* or

Ureaplasma. Stool culture: May be positive for *Shigella, Yersinia,* and others.

DERMATOPATHOLOGY Spongiosis, vesiculation; later, psoriasiform epidermal hyperplasia, spongiform pustules, and parakeratosis. Perivascular neutrophilic infiltrate in superficial dermis; edema.

DIAGNOSIS AND DIFFERENTIAL DIAGNOSIS

Rule out skin lesions with other spondylo- and reactive arthropathies: psoriasis vulgaris with psoriatic arthritis, disseminated gonococcal infection, SLE, ankylosing spondylitis, rheumatoid arthritis, gout, and Behçet disease.

COURSE AND PROGNOSIS

Only 30% develop complete triad of arthritis, urethritis, conjunctivitis; 40% have only one manifestation. Majority have self-limited course, with resolution in 3 to 12 months. RA may relapse over many years in 30%. Chronic deforming arthritis in 10 to 20%.

MANAGEMENT

PRIOR INFECTION Role of antibiotic therapy unproven in altering course of postvenereal RA.

CUTANEOUS MANIFESTATIONS Similar to management of psoriasis (see Section 3). Balanitis: low-potency glucocorticoids. Palmar/plantar: Potent glucocorticoid preparations, which are more effective under plastic occlusion. Extensive or refractory disease: systemic retinoids (acitretin, 0.5 to 1 mg/kg body weight), phototherapy, and PUVA. Anti-TNF agents.

PREVENTION OF ARTICULAR INFLAMMATION/ JOINT DEFORMITY Rest, nonsteroidal antiinflammatory agents. Methotrexate, acitretin. In HIV/AIDS, antiretroviral therapy may ameliorate RA.

SARCOIDOSIS ICD-10: D86

- A systemic granulomatous disease of unknown cause.
- Primarily affecting the lungs (bilateral lymphadenopathy and pulmonary infiltration).
- Skin: Papules, translucent yellow-red with apple jelly appearance on diascopy; nodules and bluish-red plaques.
- Often localizes in scars.
- Histologically, noncaseating, and "naked" granulomas.
- Erythema nodosum is the most common nonspecific lesion in the skin in early sarcoidosis; it suggests a good prognosis.

EPIDEMIOLOGY

AGE OF ONSET Under 40 years (range 12 to 70 years).

SEX Equal incidence in males and females.

RACE The disease occurs worldwide, frequently in Scandinavia. All races. In the United States and South Africa, much more frequent in dark skinned ethnicities.

OTHER FACTORS Etiology unknown. The disease can occur in families.

CLINICAL MANIFESTATION

Onset of lesions: Days (presenting as acute erythema nodosum) or months (presenting as asymptomatic sarcoidal papules or plaques on the skin or pulmonary infiltrate discovered on routine chest radiography). Constitutional symptoms such as fever, fatigue, weight loss, and arrhythmia.

SKIN LESIONS Earliest lesions are skin-colored or brownish papules, occurring periorifically on the face (Fig. 14-66). Brownish or purple infiltrated plaques that may be annular, polycyclic, serpiginous, and occur mainly on the extremities, buttocks, and trunk (Fig. 14-67). Central clearing with slight atrophy may occur. Occasionally, nodules, firm, purple or brown, may arise on the face, trunk, or extremities, particularly the hands. *Lupus pernio*: Diffuse, violaceous, soft doughy infiltrations on the nose, cheeks (Fig. 14-68), or earlobes. Swelling of individual digits because of osteitis cystica (Fig. 14-69). Sarcoidosis tends to infiltrate old scars, which then exhibit translucent purple-red or yellowish papules or nodules (Fig. 14-70). *Note*: On blanching with glass slide, all cutaneous lesions of sarcoidosis reveal "apple jelly" semitranslucent yellowish brown color. On the scalp, sarcoidosis may cause scarring alopecia (see Section 31).

SYSTEMS REVIEW Enlarged parotids, pulmonary infiltrates, cardiac dyspnea, neuropathy, uveitis, kidney stones. *Löfgren syndrome*: erythema nodosum, fever, arthralgias, acute bilateral hilar adenopathy. *Hereford (-Waldenström) syndrome*: fever, parotitis, uveitis, facial palsy.

LABORATORY EXAMINATIONS

DERMATOPATHOLOGY Large islands of epithelioid cells with a few giant cells and lymphocytes (so-called naked tubercles). Asteroid bodies in large histiocytes; occasionally fibrinoid necrosis.

SKIN TESTS Intracutaneous tests for recall antigens usually but not always negative.

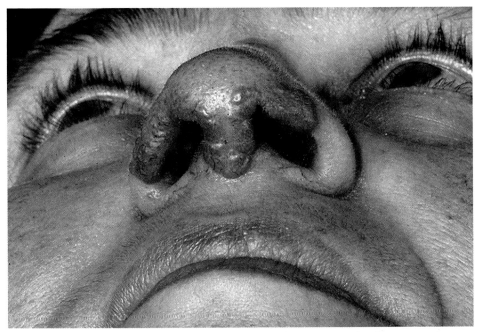

FIGURE 14-66 Sarcoidosis Brownish-to-purple papules coalescing to irregular plaques, occurring on the nose of this woman who also had massive pulmonary involvement. Blanching with a glass slide reveals "apple-jelly" color in the lesions.

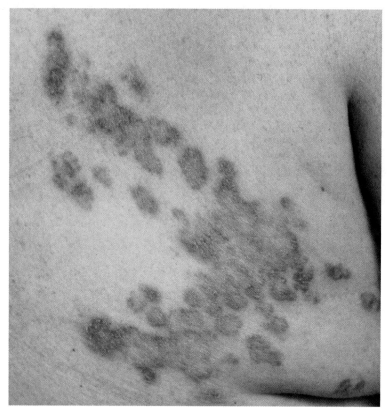

FIGURE 14-67 Sarcoidosis: granulomatous lesions Multiple, circinate, confluent, firm, brownish-red, infiltrated plaques that show a tendency to resolve in the
center. Thus, the annular and multicentric appearance. The lesions are diascopy positive, i.e., an "apple-jelly" tan-pink color remains in lesions after compression with glass.

IMAGING Systemic involvement is verified radio-
logically by gallium scan and transbronchial, liver,
or lymph node biopsy. In 90% of patients: Hilar
lymphadenopathy, pulmonary infiltrate. Cystic
lesions in phalangeal bones (osteitis cystica).
BLOOD CHEMISTRY Increased level of serum
angiotensin-converting enzyme, hypergammaglobulinemia, and hypercalcemia.

DIAGNOSIS

Lesional biopsy of skin or lymph nodes is the
best criterion for diagnosis of sarcoidosis.

MANAGEMENT

SYSTEMIC SARCOIDOSIS Systemic glucocorticoids
for active ocular disease, active pulmonary

disease, cardiac arrhythmia, CNS involvement,
or hypercalcemia.
CUTANEOUS SARCOIDOSIS **Glucocorticoids.**
Local: Intralesional triamcinolone, 3 mg/mL,
effective for small lesions. *Systemic*: Glucocorticoids for widespread or disfiguring involvement.
Hydroxychloroquine. 100 mg twice daily for
widespread or disfiguring lesions refractory to
intralesional triamcinolone. Only sometimes
effective.
Methotrexate. Low-dose for widespread skin
and systemic involvement, although not always
effective. Cyclophosphamide is used only for
potentially life-threatening disease.
Anti-TNF-α Agents, including thalidomide
(monitor for tuberculosis).

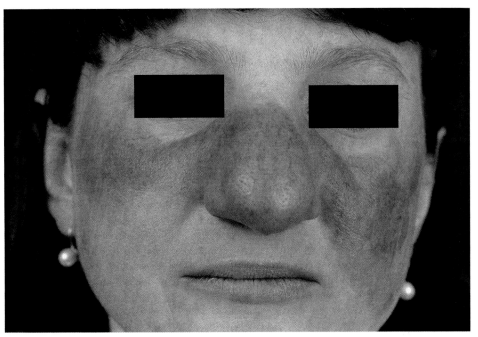

FIGURE 14-68 Sarcoidosis This is the classic appearance of "lupus pernio" with violaceous, soft, doughy infiltrations on cheeks and nose, which is grossly enlarged.

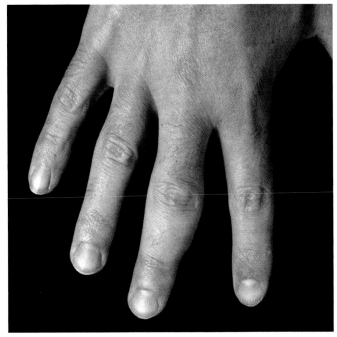

FIGURE 14-69 Sarcoidosis Firm swelling of the third digit resulting from osteitis cystica in a 52-year-old man with pulmonary involvement.

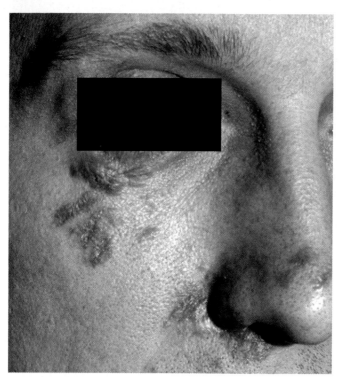

FIGURE 14-70 Sarcoidosis in scars Bizarre scars are almost replaced by brownish-red sarcoidal infiltrates. Years previously this man had a motorcycle accident suffering facial lesions when he skidded on a dirt road.

GRANULOMA ANNULARE (GA) ICD-10: L92.0

- A common self-limited, asymptomatic, chronic dermatosis of the dermis.
- Usually occurs in children and young adults. Female: male ratio: 2:1.
- Etiology and pathogenesis unknown but may be associated with diabetes.
- Consists of skin-colored or brownish-red, shiny beaded papules in an annular arrangement, commonly arising on the dorsa of the hands and feet, elbows, and knees (Fig. 14-71A).
- Sometimes becomes generalized in distribution with multiple lesions on the extremities and trunk. May annular (Fig. 14-71B) or micropapular (Fig. 14-71C).
- **Variants:** *Subcutaneous GA:* Painless, single or multiple nodules on fingers and toes (Fig. 14-71D). *Perforating* lesions are very rare and mostly on the hands; central umbilication followed by crusting and ulceration. May rarely involve fascia and tendons, causing sclerosis. Generalized GA: in this form, a search for diabetes mellitus should be made.
- **Dermatopathology.** Foci of chronic inflammatory and histiocytic infiltrations in superficial and mid-dermis, with necrobiosis of connective tissue surrounded by a wall of palisading histiocytes and multinucleated giant cells.
- The disease disappears in 75% of patients in 2 years. Recurrences are common (40%), but they also disappear.
- Management GA is a local skin disorder and not a marker for internal disease, and spontaneous remission is the rule. No treatment is an option if the lesions are not disfiguring. Lesions may resolve after biopsy. *Intralesional Triamcinolone.* **3 mg/mL into lesions is very effective.** *Cryospray.* **Superficial lesions respond to liquid nitrogen, but atrophy may occur.** *PUVA Photochemotherapy.* **Effective in generalized GA.** *Systemic Glucocorticoids.* Effective in generalized GA, but recurrences are common.

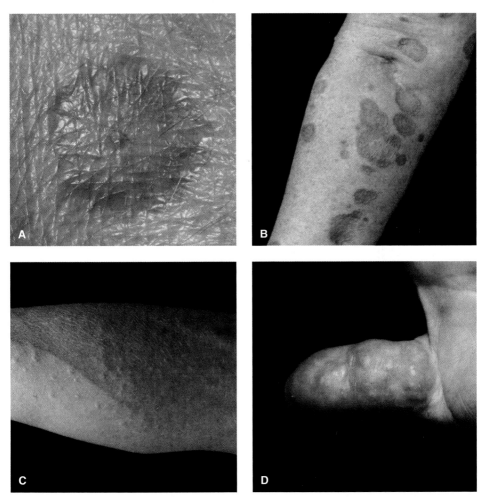

FIGURE 14-71 Granuloma annulare (A) Confluent, pearly papules forming a well-demarcated ring with central regression. **(B)** Multiple granulomata forming annular and semicircular plaques with central regression on the arm of a 60-year-old woman. **(C)** Disseminated granuloma annulare. Multiple, well-defined, pearly-white papules, some of which show a central depression. **(D)** Subcutaneous nodular GA on the thumb.

SYSTEMIC AL AMYLOIDOSIS ICD-10: E85.3

- Amyloidosis is an extracellular deposition in various tissues of amyloid fibril proteins and of a protein called *amyloid P component* (AP); the identical component of AP is present in the serum and is called *SAP*. These amyloid deposits can affect normal body function.
- AL amyloidosis is rare, occurs in many, but not all, patients with multiple myeloma and B cell dyscrasia.
- **Skin Lesions:** Smooth, waxy papules (Fig. 14-72), also nodules on the face, especially around the eyes (Fig. 14-73) and elsewhere. Purpura following trauma, "pinch" purpura in waxy papules (Fig. 14-73) sometimes also involving large surface areas without nodular involvement. Predilection sites are around the eyes, central face, extremities, body folds, axillae, umbilicus, and anogenital area. Nail changes: similar to lichen planus (see Section 32). Macroglossia: diffusely enlarged and firm, "woody" (Fig. 14-74).
- **Systemic Manifestations:** Fatigue, weakness, anorexia, weight loss, malaise, dyspnea; symptoms related to hepatic, renal, and GI involvement; paresthesia related to carpal tunnel syndrome, neuropathy.
- **General Examination:** Kidney—nephrosis; nervous system—peripheral neuropathy, carpal tunnel syndrome; cardiovascular—partial heart block, congestive heart failure; hepatic—hepatomegaly; GI—diarrhea, sometimes hemorrhagic, malabsorption; lymphadenopathy.
- **Laboratory:** May reveal thrombocytosis >500,000/μL. Proteinuria and increased serum creatinine; hypercalcemia. Increased IgG. Monoclonal protein in two-thirds of patients with primary or myeloma-associated amyloidosis. Bone marrow: myeloma.
- **Dermatopathology:** Accumulation of faintly eosinophilic masses of amyloid in the papillary body near the epidermis, in the papillary and reticular dermis, in sweat glands, around and within blood vessel walls. Immunohistochemistry to assess the proportion of kappa and lambda light chains.

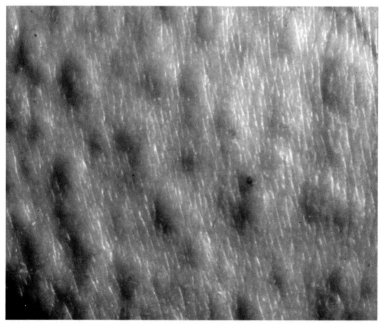

FIGURE 14-72 Systemic AL amyloidosis Waxy papules on the trunk of a 58-year-old male patient with myeloma.

FIGURE 14-73 Systemic AL amyloidosis: "pinch purpura" The topmost papule is yellowish and nonhemorrhagic; the lower portion is hemorrhagic. So-called pinch purpura of the upper eyelid can appear in amyloid nodules after pinching or rubbing the eyelid.

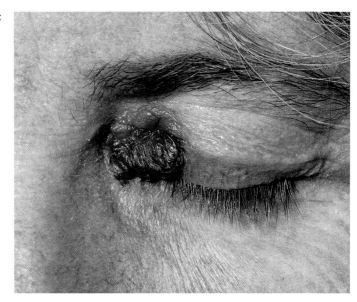

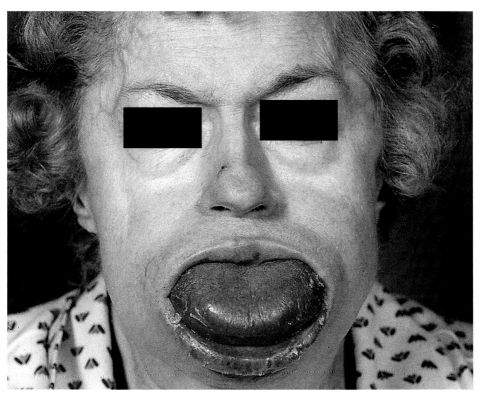

FIGURE 14-74 Systemic AL amyloidosis: macroglossia Massive infiltration of the tongue with amyloid has caused immense enlargement; the tongue cannot be retracted completely into the mouth because of its size. (Used with permission from Evan Calkins, MD.)

SYSTEMIC AA AMYLOIDOSIS ICD-10: E85.3

- A reactive type of amyloidosis.
- Occurs in any disorder associated with a sustained acute-phase response.
- 60% have inflammatory arthritis. The rest, other chronic inflammatory infective or neoplastic disorders.
- Amyloid fibrils are derived from cleavage fragments of the circulating acute-phase reactant serum amyloid A protein.
- Presents with proteinuria followed by progressive renal dysfunction; nephrotic syndrome.
- There are no characteristic skin lesions in AA amyloidosis.

LOCALIZED CUTANEOUS AMYLOIDOSIS ICD-10: E85.91

- Three varieties of localized amyloidosis that are unrelated to the systemic amyloidoses.
- *Nodular amyloidosis*: Single or multiple, smooth, nodular lesions with or without purpura on the limbs, face, or trunk (Fig. 14-75A).
- *Lichenoid amyloidosis:* Discrete, very pruritic, brownish-red papules on the legs (Fig. 14-75B).
- *Macular amyloidosis*: pruritic, gray-brown, reticulated macular lesions occurring principally on the upper back (Fig. 14-76); the lesions often have a distinctive "ripple" pattern.
- In lichenoid and macular amyloidosis, the amyloid fibrils in skin are keratin derived. Although these three localized forms of amyloidosis are confined to the skin and unrelated to systemic disease, the skin lesions of nodular amyloidosis are identical to those that occur in AL, in which amyloid fibrils derive from immunoglobulin light chain fragments.

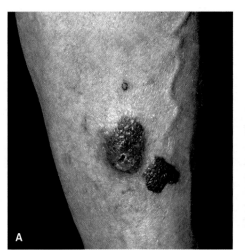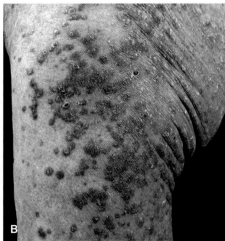

FIGURE 14-75 Localized cutaneous amyloidosis (A) Nodular. Two plaque-like nodules, waxy, yellowish-orange with hemorrhage. **(B)** Lichenoid amyloidosis. Grouped confluent scaly papules of livid, violaceous color. This is a purely cutaneous disease.

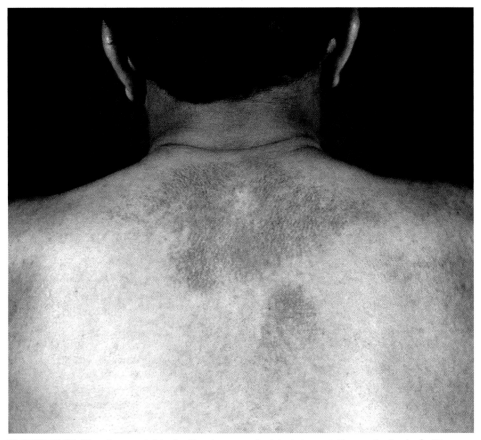

FIGURE 14-76 Macular amyloidosis Gray-brown, reticulated pigmentation on the back of a 56-year-old Arab.

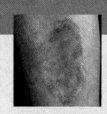

ENDOCRINE, METABOLIC, AND NUTRITIONAL DISEASES

SKIN DISEASES ASSOCIATED WITH DIABETES MELLITUS

- Acanthosis nigricans (see Section 5) and lipodystrophy.
  Associated with insulin resistance in diabetes mellitus. Insulin-like epidermal growth factors may cause epidermal hyperplasia.
- Adverse cutaneous drug reactions in diabetes (see Section 23).
  Insulin: Local reactions—lipodystrophy with decreased adipose tissue at the sites of subcutaneous injection; Arthus-like reaction with urticarial lesion at site of injection.
  Systemic insulin allergy: Urticaria, serum sickness–like reactions.
  Oral hypoglycemic agents: Exanthematous eruptions, urticaria, erythema multiforme, and photosensitivity.
- Calciphylaxis (see Section 18).
- Cutaneous perforating disorders.
  Rare conditions in which horny plugs perforate into the dermis or dermal debris is eliminated through the epidermis. Not always associated with diabetes (see Section 18).
- Diabetic bullae (bullosis diabeticorum) (p. 379).
- Diabetic dermopathy (p. 381).
- Eruptive xanthomas (p. 391).
- Granuloma annulare (see Section 14).
- Infections (see Sections 25 and 26).
  Poorly controlled diabetes associated with increased incidence of primary and secondary *Staphylococcus aureus* infections, cellulitis (*S. aureus*, group A streptococcus), erythrasma, dermatophytoses, candidiasis, and mucormycosis with necrotizing nasopharyngeal infections.
- Necrobiosis lipoidica (p. 382).
- Peripheral neuropathy (diabetic foot) (p. 380).
- Peripheral vascular disease (see Section 17).
  Small-vessel vasculopathy (microangiopathy): Involves arterioles, venules, and capillaries. Characterized by basement membrane thickening and endothelial cell proliferation. Presents clinically as acral erysipelas-like erythema, and ± ulceration.
  Large-vessel vasculopathy: Incidence greatly increased in diabetes. Ischemia is most often symptomatic on lower legs and feet with gangrene and ulceration. Predisposes to infections.
- Scleredema diabeticorum.
  Synonym: Scleredema adultorum of Buschke. Need not be associated with diabetes. Onset correlates with duration of diabetes and with the presence of microangiopathy. Skin findings: Poorly demarcated scleroderma-like induration of the skin and subcutaneous tissue of the upper back, neck, and proximal extremities. Rapid onset and progression.
- Scleroderma-like syndrome. Scleroderma-like thickening of skin and limited joint mobility ("prayer sign").

DIABETIC BULLAE ICD-10: E14.650

- Large, intact bullae arise spontaneously on the lower legs, feet, dorsa of the hands, and fingers on noninflamed bases (**Fig. 15-1**).
- When ruptured, oozing bright red erosions result but heal after several weeks.
- Localization on dorsa of hand and fingers suggests porphyria cutanea tarda, but abnormalities of porphyrin metabolism are not found.
- Neither trauma nor an immunologic mechanism has been implicated. Histologically, bullae show intra- or subepidermal clefting without acantholysis.

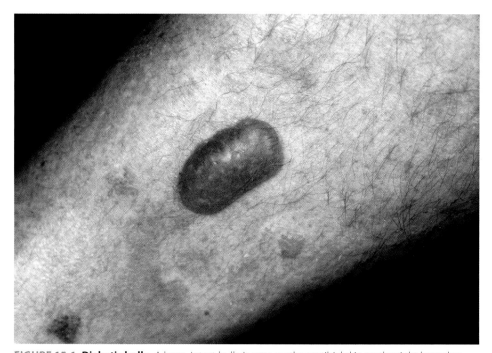

FIGURE 15-1 Diabetic bulla A large, intact bulla is seen on the pretibial skin on the right lower leg. The patient had many of the vascular complications of diabetes mellitus, i.e., renal failure, retinopathy, and atherosclerosis obliterans resulting in amputation of the left big toe.

"DIABETIC FOOT" AND DIABETIC NEUROPATHY ICD-10: E14.540

- Peripheral neuropathy is responsible for the "diabetic foot."
- Other factors are angiopathy, atherosclerosis, and infection; most often they are combined.
- Diabetic neuropathy is combined motor and sensory. Motor neuropathy leads to weakness and muscle wasting distally.
- Autonomic neuropathy accompanies sensory neuropathy and leads to anhidrosis, which may not be confined to the distal extremities.
- Sensory neuropathy predisposes to neurotropic ulcers over bony prominences of feet, usually on the great toe and sole (Fig. 15-2).
- Ulcers are surrounded by a ring of callus and may extend to interlying joint and bone, leading to osteomyelitis.

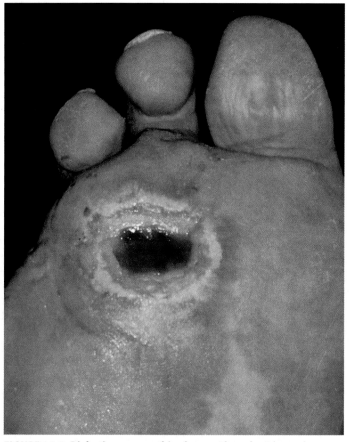

FIGURE 15-2 Diabetic, neuropathic ulcer on the sole A large ulcer overlying the second left metacarpophalangeal joint. The patient, a 60-year-old male with diabetes mellitus of 25 years' duration, has significant sensory neuropathy of the feet and lower legs as well as peripheral vascular disease, which resulted in the amputation of the fourth and fifth toes.

DIABETIC DERMOPATHY ICD-10: E14:560

- Circumscribed, atrophic, slightly depressed lesions on the anterior lower legs that are asymptomatic (Fig. 15-3).
- They arise in crops and gradually resolve, but new lesions appear and occasionally may ulcerate.
- The pathogenic significance of diabetic dermopathy remains to be established, but it is often accompanied by microangiopathy.

FIGURE 15-3 Diabetic dermopathy
A crusted erosion at the site of traumatic injury and many old pink depressed areas and scars are seen on the anterior leg of a 56-year-old male with diabetes mellitus. Identical findings were on the other leg.

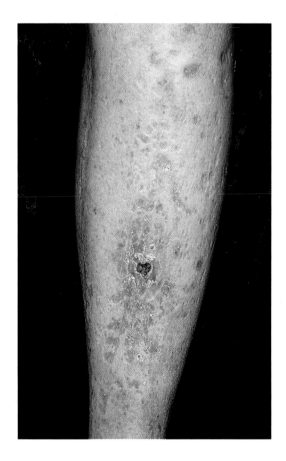

NECROBIOSIS LIPOIDICA ICD-10: E14.640

- Necrobiosis lipoidica (NL) is a cutaneous disorder often, but not always, associated with diabetes mellitus.
- Young adults, early middle age, but not uncommon in juvenile diabetics. Female:male ratio: 3:1.
- Incidence: From 0.3% to 3% of diabetic individuals. One-third of patients have clinical diabetes, one-third have abnormal glucose tolerance only, and one-third have normal glucose tolerance.
- The severity of NL is not related to the severity of diabetes. Control of the diabetes has no effect on the course of NL.
- Lesion starts as brownish-red or skin-colored papule that slowly evolves into a well-demarcated waxy plaque of variable size (Fig. 15-4). The sharply defined and slightly elevated border retains a brownish-red color, whereas the center becomes depressed and acquires a yellow-orange hue. Multiple telangiectasias of variable size. Larger lesions formed by centrifugal enlargement or merging of smaller lesions acquiring a serpiginous or polycyclic configuration. Ulceration may occur and healed ulcers result in depressed scars. Burned-out lesions are tan with telangiectasia.
- Usually one to three lesions; >80% occur on the shin; at times symmetric. Less commonly on feet, arms, trunk, or face and scalp; rarely may be generalized.
- Dermatopathology: Sclerosis, obliteration of the bundle pattern of collagen → necrobiosis, surrounded by concomitant granulomatous infiltration in lower dermis. Microangiopathy.
- Biopsy confirmation is usually not necessary; however, biopsy may be required in early stages to rule out granuloma annulare (which frequently coexists with NL), sarcoidosis, or xanthoma.
- Glucocorticoids. *Topical:* Under occlusion is helpful; however, ulcerations may occur when NL is occluded. *Intralesional:* triamcinolone, 5 mg/mL, into active lesions or lesion margins usually arrests extension of plaques of NL. Ulceration: Most ulcerations within NL lesions heal with local wound care; if not, excision of the entire lesion with grafting may be required.

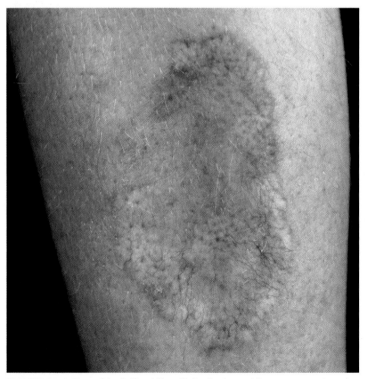

FIGURE 15-4 Necrobiosis lipoidica diabeticorum A large, symmetric plaque with active tan-pink, yellow, well-demarcated, raised, firm border and a yellow center in the pretibial region of a 28-year-old diabetic female. The central parts of the lesion are depressed with atrophic changes of epidermal thinning and telangiectasia against a yellow background.

CUSHING SYNDROME AND HYPERCORTICISM ICD-10: E24.900

- *Cushing syndrome* (CS) is characterized by truncal obesity, moon face, abdominal striae, hypertension, decreased carbohydrate tolerance, protein catabolism, psychiatric disturbances, and amenorrhea and hirsutism in females. It is associated with excess adrenocorticosteroids of endogenous or exogenous source.
- *Cushing disease* refers to CS associated with pituitary adrenocorticotropic hormone (ACTH)-producing adenoma.
- *CS medicamentosum* refers to CS caused by exogenous administration of glucocorticoids.
- Skin lesions: A plethoric obese person with a "classic" habitus that results from the redistribution of fat: moon facies (Fig. 15-5), "buffalo" hump, truncal obesity, and thin arms and legs. Purple striae, mostly on the abdomen and trunk; atrophic skin with easy bruising and telangiectasia. Facial hypertrichosis with pigmented hairs and often increased lanugo hairs on the face and arms; androgenetic alopecia in females. Acne of recent onset (without comedones) or flaring of existing acne.
- General symptoms: Fatigue and muscle weakness, hypertension, personality changes, amenorrhea in females, polyuria, and polydipsia.
- Workup includes determination of blood glucose, serum potassium, and free cortisol in 24-h urine. Abnormal dexamethasone suppression test with failure to suppress endogenous cortisol secretion when dexamethasone is administered. Elevated ACTH. CT scan of the abdomen and the pituitary. Assessment of osteoporosis.
- Management consists of elimination of exogenous glucocorticoids or the detection and correction of underlying endogenous cause.

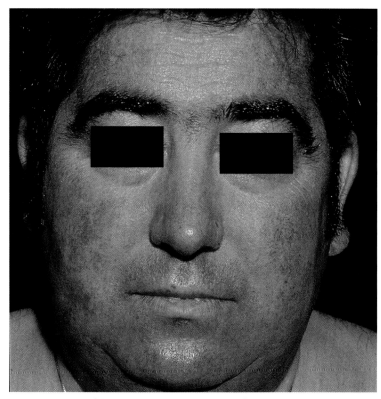

FIGURE 15-5 Cushing syndrome Plethoric moon facies with erythema and telangiectases of cheeks and forehead; the face and neck and supraclavicular areas (not depicted here) show increased deposition of fat.

GRAVES DISEASE AND HYPERTHYROIDISM ICD-10: E05.900

- Graves disease (GD) is a disorder with three major manifestations: Hyperthyroidism with diffuse goiter, ophthalmopathy, and dermopathy. These often do not occur together, may not occur at all, and run courses that are independent of each other.
- *Ophthalmopathy*: GD ophthalmopathy has two components, spastic (stare, lid lag, lid retraction) and mechanical [proptosis (Fig. 15-6A), ophthalmoplegia, congestive oculopathy, chemosis, conjunctivitis, periorbital swelling, and potential complications of corneal ulceration, optic neuritis, optic atrophy]. Exophthalmic ophthalmoplegia: Ocular muscle weakness with inward gaze, convergence, strabismus, and diplopia.
- *Acropachy*, which represents diaphyseal proliferation of the periosteum and clubbing of fingers (Fig. 15-6B).
- *Dermopathy (pretibial myxedema)*: Early lesions—bilateral, asymmetric, firm, nonpitting nodules and plaques that are pink, skin-colored, or purple (Fig. 15-6C). Late lesions—confluence of early lesions, which symmetrically involve the pretibial regions and may, in extreme cases, result in grotesque involvement of entire lower legs and dorsa of feet; smooth surface with orange peel–like appearance, later becomes verrucous.
  Note: Dermopathy may also occur *after* treatment of hyperthyroidism.
- *Thyroid:* Diffuse toxic goiter, asymmetric, and lobular. Asymmetric and lobular thyroid enlargement, often with the presence of a bruit.
- Management: *Thyrotoxicosis*—Antithyroid agents. Ablation of thyroid tissue, surgically or by radioactive iodine. *Ophthalmopathy*—Symptomatic treatment in mild cases. Severe cases: prednisone 100 to 120 mg/d initially, tapering to 5 mg/d. Orbital radiation. Orbital decompression. *Dermopathy*—Topical glucocorticoid under plastic occlusion. Low-dose oral glucocorticoids (prednisone, 5 mg/d). Intralesional triamcinolone 3 to 5 mg/mL for smaller lesions.

HYPOTHYROIDISM AND MYXEDEMA ICD-10: E03.9

- Myxedema results from insufficient production of thyroid hormones and can be caused by multiple disturbances.
- Hypothyroidism may be *thyroprivic* (e.g., congenital, primary idiopathic, postablative); *goitrous* (e.g., heritable biosynthetic defects, maternally transmitted, iodine deficiency, drug-induced, or chronic thyroiditis); *trophoprivic* (e.g., pituitary); or *hypothalamic* [e.g., infection (encephalitis), neoplasm].
- Early symptoms of *myxedema* are fatigue, lethargy, cold intolerance, constipation, stiffness and cramping of muscles, carpal tunnel syndrome, menorrhagia, slowing of intellectual and motor activity, decline in appetite, increase in weight, and deepening of voice.
- There is a dull, expressionless facies (Fig. 15-7), with puffiness of eyelids. Skin appears swollen, cool, waxy, dry, coarse, and pale with increased skin creases.
- The hair is dry, coarse, and brittle. Thinning of the scalp, beard (Fig. 15-7), and sexual areas. Eyebrows: Alopecia of the lateral one-third. Nails brittle and slow growing.
- Large, smooth, red, and clumsy tongue.
- Workup includes thyroid function tests, thyroid-stimulating hormone, scintigraphic imaging, and serum cholesterol (↑).
- Management is by replacement therapy.

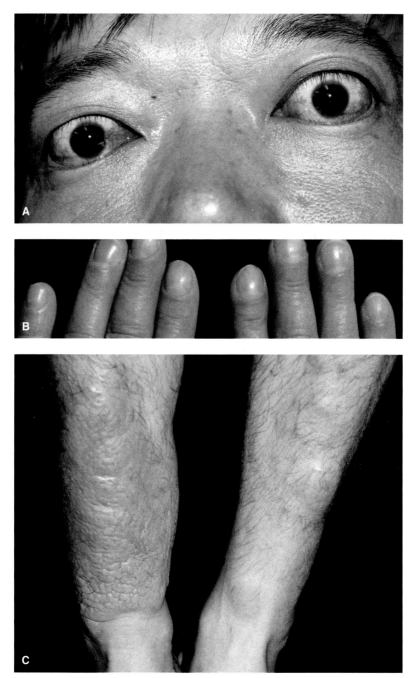

FIGURE 15-6 Graves disease (A) Proptosis, lid retraction, and telangiectasia and hemorrhage in the bulbar conjunctiva. **(B)** Thyroid acropachy (osteoarthropathy) with clubbing of fingers. **(C)** The pink- and skin colored papules, nodules, and plaques in the pretibial region are called dermopathy (formerly pretibial myxedema).

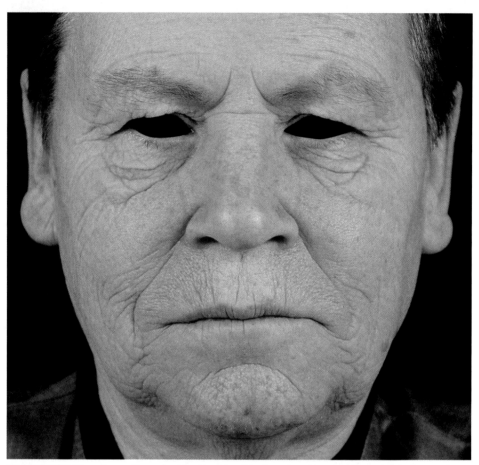

FIGURE 15-7 Myxedema Dry, pale skin; thinning of the lateral eyebrows; puffiness of the face and eye-lids; increased number of skin creases; dull, expressionless, beardless facies.

ADDISON DISEASE ICD-10: E27.1

- Addison disease is a syndrome resulting from adrenocortical insufficiency.
- It is insidious and is characterized by progressive generalized brown hyperpigmentation, slowly pro-gressive weakness, fatigue, anorexia, nausea, and, frequently, GI symptoms (vomiting and diarrhea).
- Suggestive laboratory changes include low serum sodium, high serum potassium, and elevation of the blood urea nitrogen. The diagnosis is confirmed by specific tests of adrenal insufficiency.
- Skin: The patient may appear completely normal except for a generalized brown hyperpigmentation: (1) In areas where pigmentation normally occurs either habitually or UV induced such as around the eyes, face, and dorsa of the hands (**Fig. 15-8A**), nipples, in the linea nigra (abdomen), axillae, and anogenital areas in males and females. (2) In new areas: Gingival or buccal mucosa, creases of palms (**Fig. 15-8B**), and bony prominences. Also in new scars following surgery.
- This disease should be managed by an endocrinologist.

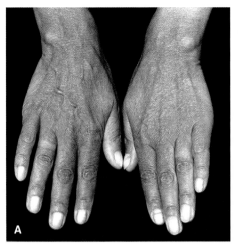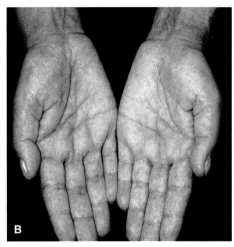

FIGURE 15-8 Addison disease (A) Hyperpigmentation representing an accentuation of normal pigmentation of the hands of a patient with Addison disease. **(B)** Note accentuated pigmentation in the palmar creases.

METABOLIC AND NUTRITIONAL CONDITIONS

XANTHOMAS ICD-10: E78.280

- Cutaneous xanthomas are yellow-brown, pinkish, or orange macules, papules, plaques, nodules, or infiltrations in tendons.
- Histologically, there are accumulations of xanthoma cells—macrophages containing droplets of lipids.
- Xanthomas may be symptoms of a general metabolic disease, a generalized histiocytosis, or a local fat phagocytosing storage process.
- The classification of metabolic xanthomas is based on this principle: (1) xanthomas caused by hyperlipidemia and (2) normolipidemic xanthomas.
- The cause of xanthomas in the first group may be a primary hyperlipidemia, mostly genetically determined (Table 15-1), or secondary hyperlipidemia, associated with certain internal diseases such as biliary cirrhosis, diabetes mellitus, chronic renal failure, alcoholism, hyperthyroidism, and monoclonal gammopathy, or with intake of certain drugs such as beta-blockers and estrogens.
- Some of the xanthomas are associated with high plasma low-density lipoprotein (LDL)-cholesterol levels, and therefore with a serious risk of atheromatosis and myocardial infarction. For this reason, laboratory investigation of plasma lipid levels is always necessary. In some cases, an apoprotein deficiency is present.
- Table 15-2 shows correlations of clinical xanthoma type and lipoprotein disturbances.

TABLE 15-1 Classification of Genetic Hyperlipidemias

Frederickson Type	Classification	Lipid Profile
I	Familial lipoprotein lipase deficiency (hyperchylomicronemia, hypertriglyceridemia)	TG++, C normal, CM++, HDL−/normal
IIa	Familial hypercholesterolemia	TG normal, C+, LDL+
IIb	Familial combined hyperlipidemia	TG+, C+, LDL+, VLDL+
III	Familial dysbetalipidemia (remnant particle disease)	TG+, C+, IDL+, CM remnants+
IV	Familial hypertriglyceridemia	TG+, C normal/+, LDL++, VLDL++
V	Familial combined hypertriglyceridemia	TG+, C+, VLDL++, CM++

TG, triglycerides; C, cholesterol; CM, chylomicrons; HDL, high-density lipoproteins; LDL, low-density lipoproteins; VLDL, very low density lipoproteins; IDL, intermediate-density lipoproteins; +, raised; −, lowered.

TABLE 15-2 Clinical Presentations of Xanthomas

Type of Xanthoma	Genetic Disorders	Secondary Disorders
Eruptive	Familial lipoprotein lipase deficiency Apo-C2 deficiency Apo-AI and apo-AI/CIII deficiency Familial hypertriglyceridemia Familial hypertriglyceridemia with chylomicronemia	Obesity Cholestasis Diabetes Medications: retinoids, estrogen therapy, protease inhibitors
Tuberous	Familial hypercholesterolemia Familial dysbetalipoproteinemia Phytosterolemia	Monoclonal gammopathies Multiple myeloma Leukemia
Tendinous	Familial hypercholesterolemia Familial defective apo-B Familial dysbetalipoproteinemia Phytosterolemia Cerebrotendinous xanthomatosis	
Planar		
Palmar	Familial dysbetalipoproteinemia Homozygous apo-AI deficiency	
Intertriginous	Familial homozygous hypercholesterolemia	Cholestasis
Diffuse		Monoclonal gammopathies, cholestasis
Xanthelasma	Familial hypercholesterolemia Familial dysbetalipoproteinemia	Monoclonal gammopathies
Other		
Corneal arcus	Familial hypercholesterolemia	
Tonsillar	Tangier disease	

Apo, apolipoprotein.

Source: Reproduced with permission from Schaefer EJ, Santos RD. Xanthomas and lipoprotein disorders. In: Goldsmith LA, Katz SI, Gilchrest BA, et al, eds. *Fitzpatrick's Dermatology in General Medicine*. 8th ed. New York, NY: McGraw-Hill; 2012, p. 1601.

XANTHELASMA ICD-10: H02.6

- Most common of all xanthomas. In most cases, an isolated finding unrelated to hyperlipidemia.
- Occurs in individuals >50 years; however, when in children or young adults, it is associated with familial hypercholesterolemia (FH) or familial dysbetalipoproteinemia (FD).
- Skin lesions are asymptomatic. Soft, polygonal yellow-orange papules and plaques localized to upper and lower eyelids (Fig. 15-9) and around inner canthus. Slow enlargement from tiny spots over months to years.
- Cholesterol should be estimated in plasma; if enhanced, screening for type of hyperlipidemia (FH or FD). If resulting from hyperlipidemia, complication with atherosclerotic cardiovascular disease may be expected.
- Laser, excision, electrodesiccation, or topical application of trichloroacetic acid. Recurrences are not uncommon.
- *Synonyms*: Xanthelasma palpebrarum, periocular xanthoma.

XANTHOMA TENDINEUM ICD-10: E75.510

- These subcutaneous tumors are yellow or skin colored and move with the extensor tendons (Fig. 15-10).
- They are a symptom of FH that presents as type IIa hyperlipidemia.
- This condition is autosomal recessive with a different phenotype in the heterozygote and homozygote.
- In the homozygote, the xanthomata appear in early childhood and the cardiovascular complications in early adolescence; the elevation of the LDL content of the plasma is extreme. These patients rarely attain ages above 20 years.
- *Management*: A diet low in cholesterol and saturated fats, supplemented by cholestyramine or statins. In extreme cases, measures such as portacaval shunt or liver transplantation have to be considered.
- *Synonym*: Tendinous xanthoma.

XANTHOMA TUBEROSUM ICD-10: E78.230

- This condition comprises yellowish nodules (Fig. 15-11) located especially on the elbows and knees by confluence of concomitant eruptive xanthomas.
- They are to be found in patients with FD, familial hypertriglyceridemia with chylomicronemia (type V) and FH (Table 15-2).
- In homozygous patients with FH, the tuberous xanthomas are flatter and skin colored. They are not accompanied by eruptive xanthomas (see the following discussion).
- *Management*: Treatment of the underlying condition.
- *Synonym*: Tuberous xanthoma.

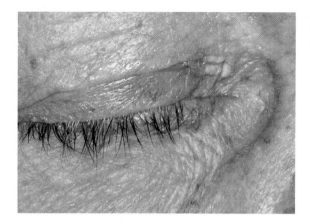

FIGURE 15-9 Xanthelasma Multiple creamy-orange, slightly elevated dermal papules on the eyelids of a normolipemic individual.

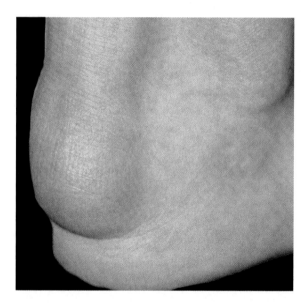

FIGURE 15-10 Tendinous xanthoma Large subcutaneous tumor adherent to the Achilles tendon.

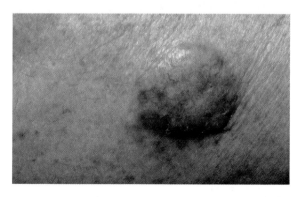

FIGURE 15-11 Tuberous xanthoma Flat-topped, yellow, firm nodule.

ERUPTIVE XANTHOMA ICD-10: E78.220

- These discrete inflammatory-type papules "erupt" suddenly and in showers, appearing typically on the buttocks, elbows, lower arms (**Fig. 15-12**), and knees.
- A sign of FHT, FD, the very rare familial lipoprotein lipase deficiency (**Table 15-2**), and out of control diabetes.
- Papules are dome shaped, discrete, initially red, then yellow center with red halo (**Fig. 15-12**).
- Lesions may be scattered, discrete, in a localized region [e.g., elbows, knees (**Fig. 15-12**), and buttocks] or appear as "tight" clusters that become confluent to form nodular "tuberoeruptive" xanthomas.
- *Management*: React very favorably to a low-calorie and low-fat diet.

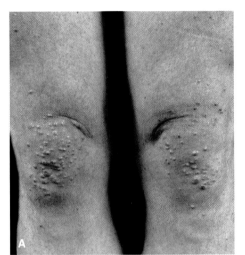 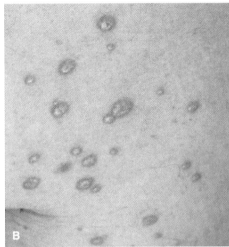

FIGURE 15-12 Papular eruptive xanthomas (A) Multiple, discrete, red-to-yellow papules becoming confluent on the knees of an individual with uncontrolled diabetes mellitus; lesions were also present on both elbows and buttocks. **(B)** Higher magnification of xanthomas on the trunk of another patient.

XANTHOMA STRIATUM PALMARE ICD-10: E78.260

- This condition is characterized by yellow-orange, flat or elevated infiltrations of the volar *creases* of palms and fingers (Fig. 15-13).
- Pathognomonic for FD (type III) (Table 15-2). Next to xanthoma striatum palmare, FD also presents with tuberous xanthoma (Fig. 15-11) and xanthelasma palpebrarum (Fig. 15-9).
- Patients with FD are prone to atherosclerotic cardiovascular disease, especially ischemia of the legs and coronary vessels.
- *Management*: Patients with FD react very favorably to a diet low in fats and carbohydrates. If necessary, this may be supplemented with statins, fibrates, or nicotinic acid.

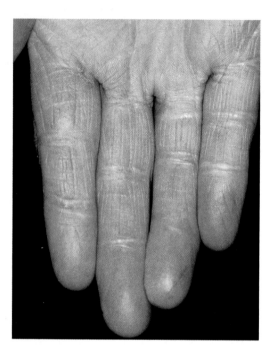

FIGURE 15-13 Xanthoma striatum palmare The palmar creases particularly over the interphalangeal joints, are yellow, often a very subtle lesion noticeable only upon close examination.

NORMOLIPEMIC PLANE XANTHOMA

- Xanthoma planum is a normolipemic xanthoma that consists of diffuse orange-yellow color and slight elevations of the skin (Fig. 15-14). There is a recognizable border.
- These lesions can be idiopathic or secondary to leukemia, but the most common association is with multiple myeloma.
- The lesions may precede the onset of multiple myeloma by many years.

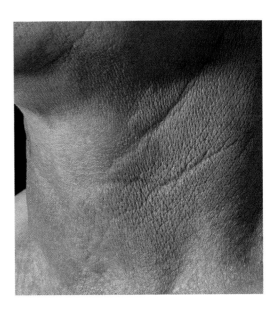

FIGURE 15-14 Plane xanthoma Yellowish-red, slightly elevated plaques on the neck, noticeable mainly because of the accentuation of the skin texture in a normolipemic patient with lymphoma. Plane xanthomas occur most commonly on the upper trunk and neck and most commonly occur in individuals with myeloma.

SCURVY ICD-10: E54.X00

- Scurvy is an acute or chronic disease caused by dietary deficiency of ascorbic acid (vitamin C).
- Scurvy occurs in infants or children on a diet consisting of only processed milk or in edentulous adult persons who do not eat salads and uncooked vegetables.
- *Precipitating factors*: Pregnancy, lactation, and thyrotoxicosis; most common in alcoholism.
- Symptoms of scurvy occur after 1–3 months cessation of vitamin C uptake. Lassitude, weakness, arthralgia, and myalgia.
- *Skin lesions*: Petechiae, follicular hyperkeratosis with perifollicular hemorrhage, especially on the lower legs (Fig. 15-15A). Hair becomes fragmented and buried in these perifolliculár hyperkeratotic papules (corkscrew hairs, Fig. 15-15B); also, extensive ecchymoses (Fig. 15-15C), which can be generalized. Nails: splinter hemorrhages.
- Gingiva: Swollen, purple, spongy, and bleeds easily. Loosening and loss of teeth.
- Hemorrhage occurring into periosteum of long bones and into joints → painful swellings and, in children, epiphyseal separation. Sternum sinks inward: Scorbutic rosary (elevation at rib margins). Retrobulbar, subarachnoid, and intracerebral hemorrhage can cause death.
- *Laboratory*: Normocytic, normochromic anemia. Folate deficiency, resulting in macrocytic anemia. Positive capillary fragility test. Serum ascorbic acid level zero. X-ray findings are diagnostic.
- Unless treated, scurvy is fatal. On treatment, spontaneous bleeding ceases within 24 h, muscle and bone pain fade quickly, bleeding from gums stops in 2 to 3 days.
- *Management*: Ascorbic acid 100 mg three to five times daily until 4 g is given; then 100 mg/d is curative in days to weeks.

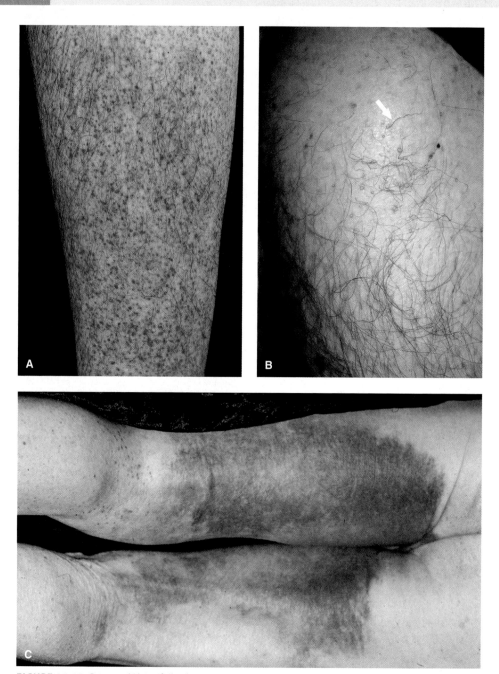

FIGURE 15-15 Scurvy (A) Perifollicular purpura on the leg. The follicles are often plugged by keratin (perifollicular hyperkeratosis). This eruption occurred in a 46-year-old alcoholic, homeless male, who also had bleeding gums and loose teeth. **(B) Perifollicular hyperkeratosis** often lead to corkscrew hairs (*arrow*) (Used with permission from Adam Lipworth, MD.). **(C)** These extensive ecchymoses occurred in an edentulous 65-year-old male who lived alone and whose food intake consisted mainly of biscuits soaked in water.

ACQUIRED ZINC DEFICIENCY AND ACRODERMATITIS ENTEROPATHICA ICD-10: E60.X10, E83.210

- Acquired zinc deficiency (AZD) occurs in older individuals caused by dietary deficiency or failure of intestinal absorption of zinc (malabsorption, alcoholism, or prolonged parenteral nutrition).
- Acrodermatitis enteropathica is a genetic disorder of zinc absorption. Autosomal recessive trait. It occurs in infants, bottle-fed with bovine milk, days to few weeks or in breast-fed infants, soon after weaning.
- *Skin Findings*: Identical in AZD and AE. Patches and plaques of dry, scaly, sharply marginated and brightly red, eczematous dermatitis evolving into vesiculobullous, pustular, erosive, and crusted lesions (**Figs. 15-16** and **15-17A**). Initially in the perioral and anogenital areas; later, scalp, hands and feet, flexural regions, and trunk. Fingertips glistening, erythematous, with fissures and secondary paronychia. Perlèche. Lesions become secondarily infected with *Candida albicans, S. aureus*. Impaired wound healing.
- Diffuse alopecia, graying of hair. Paronychia, nail ridging, and loss of nails.
- Red, glossy tongue; superficial aphthous-like erosions; secondary oral candidiasis.
- Photophobia; irritable, depressed mood. Children with AE whine and cry constantly. Failure of growth.
- Anemia, low serum/plasma zinc levels; reduced urinary zinc excretion.
- After zinc replacement, severely infected and erosive skin lesions heal within 1 to 2 weeks (**Fig. 15-17B**), diarrhea ceases, and irritability and depression of mood improve within 24 h.
- *Management*: Dietary or IV supplementation with zinc salts in two to three times the required daily amount restores normal zinc status in days to weeks.

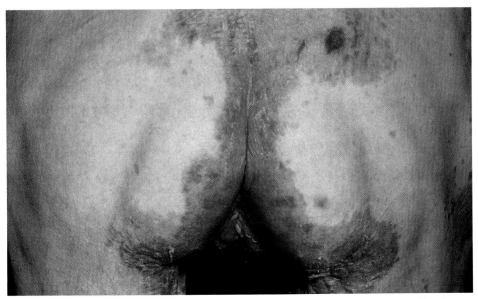

FIGURE 15-16 Acquired zinc deficiency Well-demarcated, psoriasiform and eczematous-like plaques with scaling and erosions overlying the sacrum, intergluteal cleft, buttocks, and hip in a 60-year-old alcoholic female whose diet had consisted of pickles and cheap wine. She also had a similar eruption around the mouth, perlèche, atrophic glossitis, and had glistening, shiny, oozing fingertips.

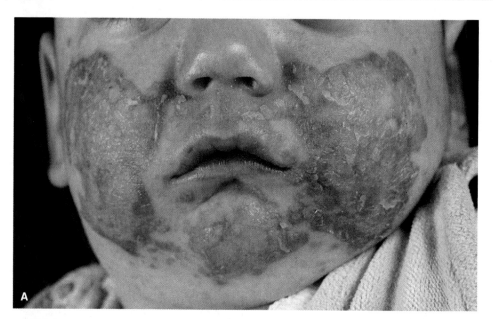

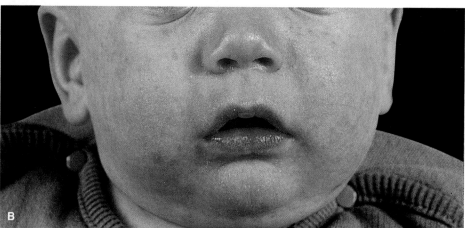

FIGURE 15-17 Acrodermatitis enteropathica (A) Sharply demarcated, symmetric, partially erosive, scaly, and crusted plaques on the face of an infant after weaning. Similar lesions were also found in the perigenital and perianal regions and on the fingertips. The child was highly irritable, whining, and crying and had diarrhea. **(B)** Within 24 h after zinc replacement, the irritability and diarrhea ceased and the infant's mood improved; and after 10 days (shown here), the perioral and perigenital lesions had healed.

PELLAGRA ICD-10: E52

- Pellagra arises from a diet deficient in niacin or tryptophan, or both. Tryptophan is converted in the body to niacin. A predominantly maize-based diet is usually implicated.
- Pellagra is characterized by the three Ds: *d*ermatitis, *d*iarrhea, and *d*ementia. Skin changes are determined by exposure to sunlight and pressure.
- The disorder begins with a symmetric itching and smarting erythema on the dorsa of the hands, neck, and face. Vesicles and bullae may erupt and break, so that crusting occurs and lesions become scaly (Fig. 15-18A). Later, skin becomes indurated, lichenified, rough, covered by dark scales and crusts; there are cracks and fissures and a sharp demarcation from normal skin (Fig. 15-18B).
- Distribution: dorsa of hands and fingers ("gauntlet") (Fig. 15-18B), band-like around the neck ("Casal necklace") (Fig. 15-18A), dorsa of feet up to malleoli with sparing of the heel, and butterfly region of the face.
- Diagnosis is verified by detection of decreased levels of urinary metabolites.
- 100 to 300 mg niacinamide orally plus other B vitamins lead to complete resolution.

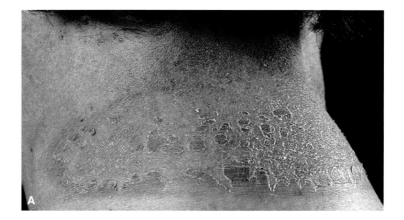

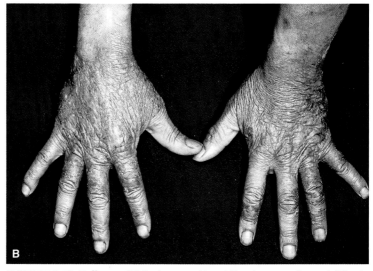

FIGURE 15-18 Pellagra (A) Scaly crusted band-like plaque on the neck ("Casal necklace"). **(B)** "Gauntlet" of pellagra; indurated, lichenified, pigmented, and scaly skin on the dorsa of the hands. Note sharp demarcation to lower arm.

GOUT ICD-10: M10

- A clinical syndrome occurring in a group of diseases characterized by the deposition of monosodium urate crystals in synovial fluid and joints.
- Acute gouty arthritis usually occurs in middle age and usually affects a single joint in the lower extremities, usually the first metatarsophalangeal joint. It can also affect fingers (Fig. 15-19A).
- Intercritical gout describes the interval between attacks of gout. With time, attacks tend to be polyarticular.
- In chronic tophaceous gout, patients rarely have asymptomatic periods. Urate crystals are found in soft tissues, cartilage (Fig. 15-19B), and tendons.
- Gout may occur with and without hyperuricemia, renal disease, and nephrolithiasis.

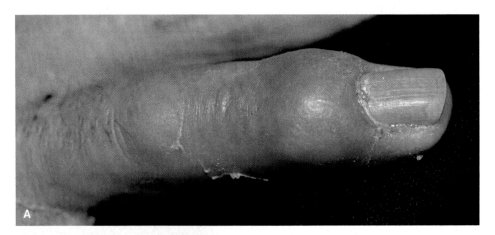

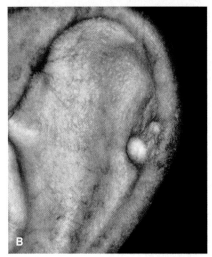

FIGURE 15-19 Acute gouty arthritis (A) Affecting the distal interphalangeal joint of the fifth digit. **(B)** Gouty tophi on helix.

SKIN DISEASES IN PREGNANCY

■ Normal skin changes associated with pregnancy are darkening of linea alba (linea nigra), melasma (see Section 13), and striae distensae (**Fig. 15-20**).

■ Pruritus occurring in pregnancy may result from a flare of preexisting dermatosis or a pregnancy-specific dermatosis.

■ Pregnancy-specific dermatoses associated with fetal risk are cholestasis in pregnancy, pustular psoriasis of pregnancy (impetigo herpetiformis), and pemphigoid gestationis.

■ Pregnancy-specific dermatoses not associated with fetal risk are polymorphic eruption of pregnancy and prurigo gestationis.

■ An algorithm of an approach to a pregnant patient with a pruritus is shown in **Fig. 15-21**.

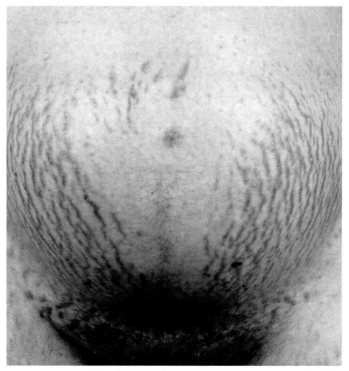

FIGURE 15-20 Striae distensae in a pregnant woman (36 weeks of gestation).

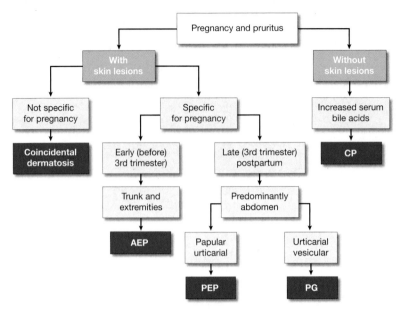

FIGURE 15-21 Algorithm of approach to a pregnant patient with pruritus
AEP, atopic eruption of pregnancy; PEP, polymorphic eruption of pregnancy;
PG, pemphigoid gestationis; CP, cholestasis of pregnancy.

CHOLESTASIS OF PREGNANCY (CP) ICD-10: O99.710

- Occurs in the third trimester.
- Leading symptoms: Pruritus, either localized (palms) or generalized. Most severe during the night.
- Cutaneous lesions invariably absent, but excoriations in severe cases.
- Elevation of serum bile acids.
- Fetal risks include prematurity, intrapartal distress, and fetal death.
- Treatment: Ursodeoxycholic acid, plasmapheresis.

PEMPHIGOID GESTATIONIS (PeG) ICD-10: O26.400

- Pemphigoid gestationis is a pruritic polymorphic inflammatory dermatosis of pregnancy and the postpartum period. It is an autoimmune process with circulating complement-fixing IgG antibodies in the serum. The condition is described in Section 6.

POLYMORPHIC ERUPTION OF PREGNANCY (PEP) ICD-10: 99.740

- PEP is a distinct pruritic eruption of pregnancy that usually begins in the third trimester, most often in primigravidae (76%). Common, estimated to be 1 in 120 to 240 pregnancies.
- There is no increased risk of fetal morbidity or mortality.
- The etiology and pathogenesis are not understood.
- Average time of onset is 36 weeks of gestation, usually 1 to 2 weeks before delivery. However, *symptoms and signs can start in the postpartum period.*
- Severe pruritus develops on the abdomen, often in the striae distensae. *Skin lesions* consist of erythematous papules, 1 to 3 mm, quickly coalescing into urticarial plaques (**Fig. 15-22**) with polycyclic shape and arrangement; blanched halos around the periphery of lesions. Target lesions. Tiny vesicles, 2 mm, but bullae are absent. Although pruritus is the chief symptom, excoriations are infrequent. Affected are the abdomen, buttocks, thighs (**Fig. 15-22**), upper inner arms, and lower back.
- The face, breasts, palms, and soles are rarely involved. The periumbilical area is usually spared. There are no mucous membrane lesions.
- Differential diagnosis includes all pruritic abdominal rashes in pregnancy (**Fig. 15-21**), drug reaction, allergic contact dermatitis, and metabolic pruritus.
- *Laboratory findings,* including histopathology and immunohistopathology, are noncontributory.
- The majority of women do not have a recurrence in the postpartum period, with subsequent pregnancies, or with the use of oral contraceptives. If a recurrence occurs, it is usually much milder.
- Management: High-potency topical steroids that often can be tapered off, oral prednisone in doses of 10 to 40 mg/d relieves symptoms in 24 h. Oral antihistamines are ineffective.
- *Synon*yms: PEP, toxemic rash of pregnancy, late-onset prurigo of pregnancy.

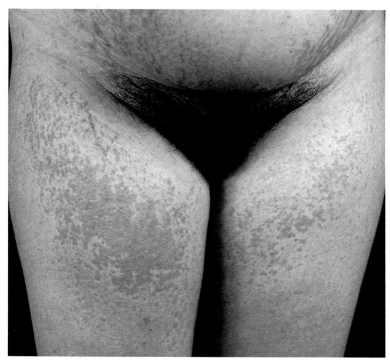

FIGURE 15-22 Polymorphic eruption of pregnancy [previously called pruritic urticarial papules and plaques of pregnancy (PUPPP)] Urticarial papules are present on both thighs where they coalesce to urticarial plaques. Similar papules and urticarial lesions are present within striae distensae on the abdomen of this pregnant woman at 35 weeks of gestation. Lesions were extremely pruritic, causing sleepless nights and great stress, yet there are no excoriations.

PRURIGO OF PREGNANCY AND ATOPIC ERUPTION OF PREGNANCY (AEP) ICD-10: L.20.900

- Prurigo of pregnancy is now reclassified as part of the AEP spectrum.
- Very common.
- AEP consists of flares of atopic dermatitis (also in patients who previously did not have AD); present either with eczematous or prurigo lesions (see Section 2).
- The cardinal symptom is pruritus.

PUSTULAR PSORIASIS IN PREGNANCY ICD-10: L40.120

- Previously called *impetigo herpetiformis.*
- Clinically and histopathologically indistinguishable from pustular psoriasis of von Zumbusch.
- Burning, smarting, not itching.
- May have hypocalcemia and decreased vitamin D levels.
- See "Pustular Psoriasis" in Section 3.

SKIN MANIFESTATIONS OF OBESITY

- Obesity is widely recognized as an epidemic in the Western world.
- Obesity is responsible for changes in skin barrier function, sebaceous glands and sebum production, sweat glands, lymphatics, collagen structure and function, wound healing, micro- and macrocirculation, and subcutaneous fat.
- Obesity is implicated in a wide spectrum of dermatologic diseases, including *acanthosis nigricans* (Section 5), acrochordons, keratosis pilaris (Section 4), *hyperandrogenism and hirsutism* (Section 31), *striae distensae, adipositas dolorosa* and fat redistribution, lymphedema, *chronic venous insufficiency,* (Section 17) and *plantar hyperkeratosis* (Section 4).
- *Cellulitis, skin infections* (Section 25), *hidradenitis suppurativa* (Section 1), *psoriasis* (Section 3), *insulin resistance syndrome,* and *tophaceous gout* (p. 398).

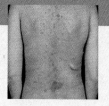

GENETIC DISEASES

PSEUDOXANTHOMA ELASTICUM ICD-10: Q82.810

- Pseudoxanthoma elasticum (PXE) is a serious hereditary disorder of connective tissue that involves the elastic tissue in the skin, blood vessels, and eyes. Autosomal recessive (most common) and autosomal dominant. *Incidence:* 1:40,000 to 1:100,000.
- *Etiology and Pathogenesis*: Pathogenic mutation in the *ABCC6* gene, which encodes MRP6, a member of the ATPase-dependent transmembrane transporter family of proteins. MRP6 can serve as an efflux pump transporting small-molecular-weight glutathione conjugates, which may facilitate calcification of elastic fibers. MRP6 is also thought to play a role in cellular detoxification.
- The principal skin manifestations are a distinctive *peau d' orange* surface pattern resulting from closely grouped clusters of yellow papules (cobblestoning) in a reticular pattern on the neck, axillae, and other body folds (Fig. 16-1).
- The effects on the vascular system include GI hemorrhage, hypertension occurring in young persons and resulting from involvement of renal arteries and claudication.
- Ocular manifestations ("angioid" streaks and retinal hemorrhages) can lead to blindness.
- *Dermatopathology*: Biopsy of a scar can detect characteristic changes of PXE *before typical skin changes are apparent*. Swelling and irregular clumping and basophilic staining of elastic fibers, which appear curled and "chopped up," with calcium deposition.
- The course is inexorably progressive. Gastric artery hemorrhage → hematemesis. Peripheral vascular disease → cerebrovascular accidents, atherosclerosis obliterans, or bowel angina. Pregnancies are complicated by miscarriage and cardiovascular complications. Blindness. Life span is often shortened resulting from myocardial infarction or massive GI hemorrhage.
- *Management*: Genetic counseling. Evaluate family members for PXE. Regular reevaluation by primary care physician and ophthalmologist is mandatory.
- *Support organization*: PXE International, *www.pxe.org*.

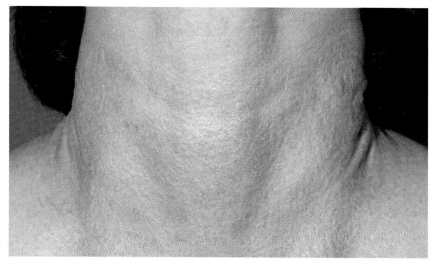

FIGURE 16-1 Pseudoxanthoma elasticum Multiple, confluent, yellow papules (pseudoxanthomatous) create a large, circumferential, pebbled plaque on the neck of a 32-year-old woman. Changes in the connective tissue in this condition lead to excessive folds on the lateral neck.

TUBEROUS SCLEROSIS (TS) ICD-10: Q85.1

- Tuberous sclerosis is an autosomal-dominant disease arising from a genetically programmed hyperplasia of ectodermal and mesodermal cells and manifested by a variety of lesions in the skin, CNS (hamartomas), heart, kidney, and other organs.
- The principal early manifestations are the triad of seizures, mental retardation, and congenital white spots.
- Facial angiofibromata are pathognomonic but do not appear until the 3rd or 4th year.

EPIDEMIOLOGY

INCIDENCE In mental institutions, 1:100 to 1:300; in general population, 1:20,000 to 1:100,000.

AGE OF ONSET Infancy.

SEX Equal incidence.

RACE All races.

HEREDITY Autosomal dominant. TS is caused by mutations in a tumor-suppressor gene, either *TSCS1* or *TSCS2*. *TSCS1* maps to chromosome 9q34. *TSCS2* maps to 16p13.3.

CLINICAL MANIFESTATION

White macules are present at birth or appear in infancy (>80% occur by 1 year of age, 100% appear by 2 years); >20% of angiofibromata are present at 1 year of age, 50% occur by 3 years. Seizures (infantile spasms) occur in 86%; the earlier the onset of seizures, the worse the mental retardation. Mental retardation (49%).

SKIN LESIONS (96% incidence).

Hypomelanotic Macules. "Off-white"; one or many, usually more than three. Polygonal or "thumbprint," 0.5 to 2 cm; lance ovate or "ashleaf" spots (Fig. 16-2), 3 to 4 cm (up to 12 cm); tiny white "confetti" macules, 1 to 2 mm (Fig. 16-3). White macules occur on trunk (>), lower extremities (>), upper extremities (7%), head and neck (5%). White macules shine up with Wood light (Fig. 16-2B)

Angiofibromas. 0.1 to 0.5 cm, dome-shaped and smooth, exhibiting red or skin color (Fig. 16-4). Occur in the center of the face. They are firm and disseminated but may coalesce; termed *adenoma sebaceum* but represent angiofibromas (present in 70%).

Plaques. Represent connective tissue nevi ("shagreen" patch), present in 40%; skin colored; occur on the back and buttocks (Fig. 16-5B).

Periungual Papules or Nodules. Ungual fibromas (Koenen tumors) present in 22%, arise late in childhood, and have the same pathology (angiofibroma) as facial papules (Fig. 16-5A).

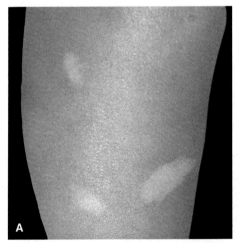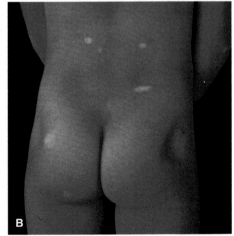

FIGURE 16-2 Tuberous sclerosis: ash-leaflet hypopigmented macules (A) Three well-demarcated, elongated (ash-leaflet shaped), hypomelanotic macules on the lower leg of a child with tan skin. **(B)** Ashleaflet hypomelanotic macules in pale skin are better visualized under Wood light where they light up.

FIGURE 16-3 Tuberous sclerosis: "confetti" macules Multiple, discrete, small, confetti-like, hypopigmented macules of variable size on the leg. These lesions are pathognomonic.

ASSOCIATED SYSTEMS

CNS (tumors producing seizures), eye (gray or yellow retinal plaques, 50%), heart (benign rhabdomyomas), and hamartomas of mixed cell type (kidney, liver, thyroid, testes, and GI system).

LABORATORY EXAMINATIONS

DERMATOPATHOLOGY **White Macules.**
Decreased number of melanocytes, decreased melanosome size, decreased melanin in melanocytes and keratinocytes.
Angiofibromata. Proliferation of fibroblasts, increased collagen, angioneogenesis, capillary dilatation, and absence of elastic tissue.
BRAIN PATHOLOGY "Tubers" are gliomas.

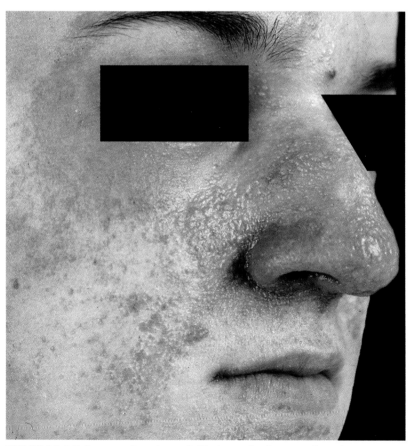

FIGURE 16-4 Tuberous sclerosis: angiofibromas Confluent, small, angiomatous (erythematous, glistening) papules on the cheek and nose. These lesions were not present during the first few years of life; appeared only after the age of 4 years.

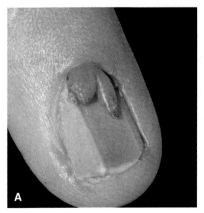
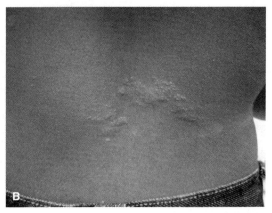

FIGURE 16-5 Tuberous sclerosis (A) Periungual fibroma (Koenen tumor). **(B)** Shagreen patch, slightly elevated, skin colored. This represents a connective tissue nevus. (Used with permission from Jennifer Tan, MD).

IMAGING **Skull X-Ray.** Multiple calcific densities.
CT Scan. Ventricular deformity and tumor deposits along the striothalamic borders.
MRI. Subependymal nodules.
Electroencephalography. Abnormal.
Renal Ultrasound. Reveals renal hamartoma.

DIAGNOSIS

More than five ash leaf macules (Fig. 16-2) in an infant are highly suggestive. Confetti spots (Fig. 16-2) are virtually pathognomonic. Evaluate the patient with a study of the family members and by obtaining various types of imaging as well as electroencephalography. Mental retardation and seizures may be absent.

DIFFERENTIAL DIAGNOSIS

WHITE SPOTS Focal vitiligo, nevus anemicus, tinea versicolor, nevus depigmentosus, pityriasis alba, and postinflammatory hypomelanosis.

ANGIOFIBROMAS Tricholemmona, syringoma, skin-colored papules on the face, and dermal nevi. *Note*: Angiofibromata of the face (Fig. 16-4) have been mistaken for and treated as acne vulgaris or rosacea.
PERIUNGUAL FIBROMAS Verruca vulgaris.

COURSE AND PROGNOSIS

Tuberous sclerosis is a serious autosomal disorder that causes major problems in behavior, caused by mental retardation, and in therapy, the aim is to control the seizures.

In severe cases, 30% die before the fifth year of life, and 50 to 75% die before reaching adult age. Malignant gliomas are not uncommon. Genetic counseling is imperative.

MANAGEMENT

PREVENTION Counseling.
TREATMENT Laser surgery for angiofibromas.
Support Organization: *http://www.support-group.com.*

NEUROFIBROMATOSIS (NF) ICD-10: Q85.0

- NF is an autosomal-dominant trait manifested by changes in the skin, nervous system, bones, and endocrine glands. These changes include a variety of congenital abnormalities, tumors, and hamartomas.
- Two major forms of NF are recognized: (1) classic von Recklinghausen NF, termed *NF1*, and (2) central or acoustic NF, termed *NF2*. *Several less common variants have also been reported (variants NF3- NF7).*
- Both common types have café-au-lait macules and neurofibromas, but only NF2 has *bilateral* acoustic neuromas (unilateral acoustic neuromas are a variable feature of NF1).
- An important diagnostic sign present only in NF1 is pigmented hamartomas of the iris (Lisch nodules).
- *Synonym*: von Recklinghausen disease.

EPIDEMIOLOGY

INCIDENCE *NF1*: 1:4000; *NF2*: 1:50,000.
RACE All races.
SEX Males slightly more than females.
HEREDITY Autosomal dominant; the gene for NF1 is on chromosome 17 (q1.2) and the gene codes for a protein named neurofibromin. The gene for NF2 is on chromosome 22 and codes for a protein called merlin.

CLINICAL MANIFESTATION

Café-au-lait (CAL) macules are not usually present at birth but appear during the first 3 years; neurofibromata appear during late adolescence. Clinical manifestations in various organs are related to pathology such as hypertensive headaches (pheochromocytomas), pathologic fractures (bone cysts), mental retardation, brain tumor (astrocytoma), short stature, and precocious puberty (early menses or clitoral hypertrophy).

SKIN LESIONS **CAL Macules.** Light or dark brown *uniform* melanin pigmentation with sharp margination. Lesions vary in size from multiple "freckle-like" tiny macules <2 mm (Fig. 16-6, "axillary freckling" is pathognomonic) to large brown macules >20 cm (Fig. 16-7). CAL macules also vary in number, from a few to hundreds.

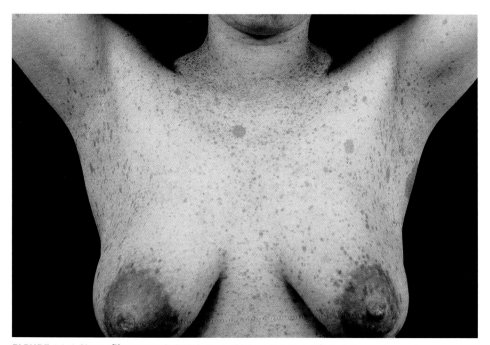

FIGURE 16-6 Neurofibromatosis (NF1) Several larger (>1 cm) café-au-lait macules on the upper chest and multiple small macules on the axillae (axillary "freckling") in a brown-skinned female. Myriads of early, small, pink-tan neurofibromas on the chest, breasts, and neck.

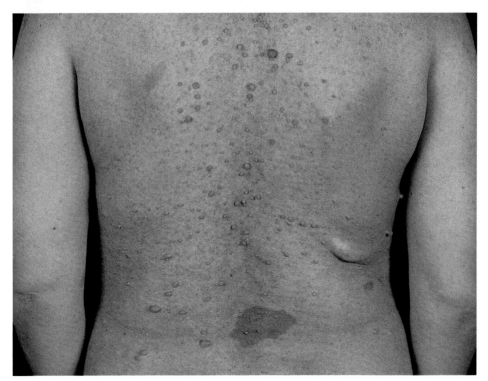

FIGURE 16-7 Neurofibromatosis (NF1) Skin-colored and pink-tan, soft papules and nodules on the back are neurofibromas. The lesions first appeared during late childhood. One large café-au-lait macule on the back. The large, soft, ill-defined, subcutaneous nodule on the right lower back and on the right posterior axillary line are plexiform neuromas.

Papules/Nodules (Neurofibromas). Skin-colored, pink, or brown (Fig. 16-7); flat, dome shaped or pedunculated (Fig. 16-8); soft or firm, sometimes tender; "buttonhole sign"—invagination with the tip of the index finger is pathognomonic.

Plexiform Neuromas. Drooping, soft (Figs. 16-7 and 16-9), doughy; may be massive, involving entire extremity, the head, or a portion of the trunk.

Distribution. Randomly distributed but may be localized to one region (segmental NF1). The segmental type may be heritable or a sporadic hamartoma.

OTHER PHYSICAL FINDINGS *Eyes.* Pigmented hamartomas of the iris (Lisch nodules) begin to appear at the age of 5 and are present in 20% of children with NF before age 6 but can be found in 95% of patients with NF1 in adolescence (Fig. 6-10). They do not correlate with the severity of the disease. They are not present in NF2.

Adrenal Pheochromocytoma. Elevated blood pressure and episodic flushing.

Peripheral Nervous System. Elephantiasis neuromatosa (gross disfigurement from NF of the nerve trunks).

Central Nervous System. Optic glioma, acoustic neuroma (rare in NF1 and unilateral, but common and bilateral in NF2), astrocytoma, meningioma, and neurofibroma.

Hematologic: Juvenile chornic myelogenous leukemia may be overrepresented.

LABORATORY EXAMINATIONS

WOOD LAMP EXAMINATION In white persons with pale skin, the CAL macules are more easily visualized with Wood lamp examination.

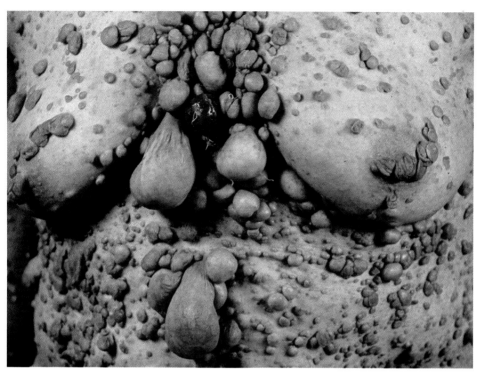

FIGURE 16-8 Neurofibromatosis (NF1) An excessively large number of small and large, pedunculated neurofibromas on the chest of a 56-year-old woman who also had a severely distorted face caused by multiple neurofibromas and plexiform neuromas.

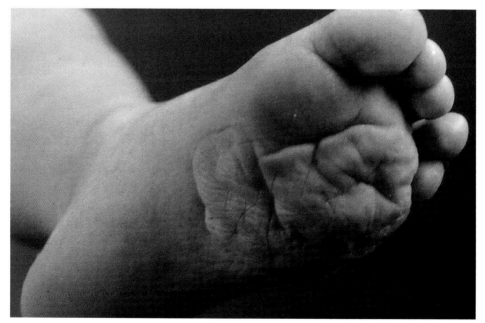

FIGURE 16-9 Neurofibromatosis (NF1) Plexiform neuroma on the sole of the foot of a child. This ill-defined subcutaneous mass is soft and asymptomatic. The patient has café-au-lait macules and multiple neurofibromas.

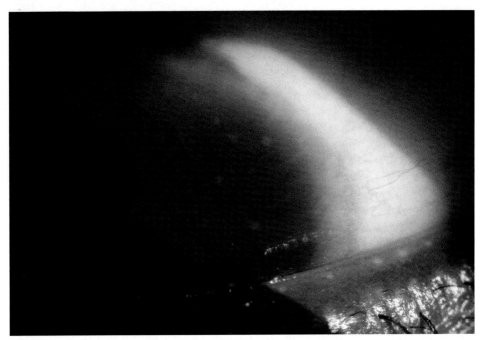

FIGURE 16-10 Lisch nodules are visible only by slit-lamp examination and appear as "glossy" transient dome-shaped yellow to brown papules of up to 2 mm.

DIAGNOSIS AND DIFFERENTIAL DIAGNOSIS

Two of the following criteria:

- Multiple CAL macules—more than six lesions with a diameter of 1.5 cm in adults and more than five lesions with a diameter of 0.5 cm or more in children younger than 5 years.
- Multiple freckles in the axillary and inguinal regions.
- Based on clinical and histologic grounds, two or more neurofibromas of any type, or one plexiform neurofibroma.
- Sphenoid wing dysplasia or congenital bowing or thinning of long bone cortex, with or without pseudoarthrosis.
- Bilateral optic nerve gliomas.
- Two or more Lisch nodules on slit-lamp examination.
- First-degree relative (parent, sibling, or child) with NF1 by the preceding criteria.

DIFFERENTIAL DIAGNOSIS Brown CAL-type macules: Albright syndrome (polyostotic fibroma, dysplasia, and precocious puberty); note: a few CAL macules (three or less) may be present in 10 to 20% of normal population.

COURSE AND PROGNOSIS

There is variable involvement of the organs affected over time, from only a few pigmented macules to marked disfigurement with thousands of nodules, segmental hypertrophy, and plexiform neuromas. The mortality rate is higher than in the normal population, principally because of the development of neurofibrosarcoma during adult life. Other serious complications are relatively infrequent.

MANAGEMENT

COSMETIC COUNSELING NF support groups help with social adjustment in severely affected persons.

An orthopedic physician should manage the two major bone problems: kyphoscoliosis and tibial bowing. A plastic surgeon is involved in reconstructive surgery for facial asymmetry. The language disorders and learning disabilities should be evaluated by a psychologist. Close follow-up annually should be mandatory to detect sarcomas that may arise within plexiform neuromas.

Support Group: http://www.support-group. com

HEREDITARY HEMORRHAGIC TELANGIECTASIA ICD-10: I78.0

- Hereditary hemorrhagic telangiectasia is an autosomal-dominant condition affecting blood vessels, especially in the mucous membranes of the mouth and the GI tract. It is caused by variants in genes involved in the TFG-β/BMP signaling cascade: *ENG* (codes for endoglin), *ACVRL1* (cell surface receptor); *SMAD4* (intracellular signaling molecule); *GDF2* (growth factor).
- The disease is frequently heralded by recurrent epistaxis that appears often in childhood.
- The diagnostic lesions are small, pulsating, macular and papular, usually punctate, telangiectases (Figs. 16-11A and B) on the lips, tongue, face, palms/soles, fingers/toes, nail beds, tongue, conjunctivae, nasopharynx, and throughout the GI and genitourinary tracts. In the 18-year-old male, shown in Figure 16-11A, there had been repeated epistaxis, but the telangiectasias had gone unnoticed until the patient was evaluated for anemia. Careful history revealed that the patient's father had a minor form of the same condition.
- Pulmonary arteriovenous fistulas may occur.
- Chronic blood loss results in anemia.
- Electrocautery and pulse dye laser are used to destroy cutaneous and accessible mucosal lesions. Estrogens have been used to treat recalcitrant bleeding.
- *Synonym*: Osler–Weber–Rendu syndrome.

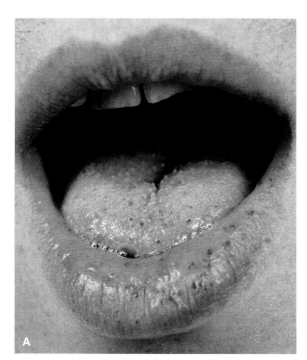 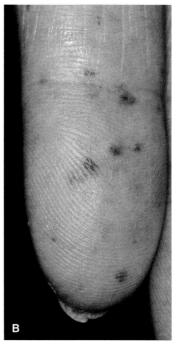

FIGURE 16-11 Hereditary hemorrhagic telangiectasia (A) Multiple 1 to 2 mm, discrete, red macular and papular telangiectases on the lower lip and tongue. **(B)** Multiple pinpoint telangiectases on the index finger of another patient. Using dermatoscopy or a glass slide, the lesions can be shown to pulsate.

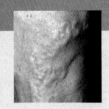

SKIN SIGNS OF VASCULAR INSUFFICIENCY

ATHEROSCLEROSIS, ARTERIAL INSUFFICIENCY, AND ATHEROEMBOLIZATION ICD-10: I70

- Atherosclerosis obliterans (ASO) is associated with spectrum of cutaneous findings of slowly progressive ischemic changes, especially when occurring on the lower extremities.
- Symptoms range from acute ischemia to intermittent claudication with exertional muscle pain and fatigue to limb ischemia with rest pain and tissue damage.
- Cutaneous findings range from dry skin, hair loss, onychodystrophy, gangrene, and ulceration.
- Atheroembolism is the phenomenon of dislodgment of atheromatous debris from a proximal affected artery or aneurysm with centrifugal microembolization and resultant acute ischemic and infarctive cutaneous lesions.
- More common with advanced age and invasive procedures.
- Manifestations are blue or discolored toes ("blue toe"), livedo reticularis, and gangrene.

EPIDEMIOLOGY

AGE OF ONSET Middle aged to elderly. Males > females.

INCIDENCE Atherosclerosis is the cause of 90% of arterial disease in developed countries.

RISK FACTORS FOR ATHEROSCLEROSIS Cigarette smoking, hyperlipidemia, low high-density lipoprotein, high low-density lipoprotein (LDL), high cholesterol, hypertension, diabetes mellitus, hyperinsulinemia, abdominal obesity, family history of premature ischemic heart disease, and personal history of cerebrovascular disease or occlusive peripheral vascular disease.

PATHOGENESIS

Atherosclerosis is the most common cause of arterial insufficiency and may be generalized or localized to the coronary arteries, aortic arch vessels to the head and neck, or those supplying the lower extremities, i.e., femoral, popliteal, anterior, and posterior tibial arteries. In addition to large-vessel arterial obstruction, individuals with diabetes mellitus often have microvasculopathy (see Section 15, Endocrine, Metabolic and Nutritional Diseases).

ATHEROEMBOLISM Multiple small deposits of fibrin, platelet, and cholesterol debris embolize from proximal atherosclerotic lesions or aneurysmal sites. Occurs spontaneously or after intravascular surgery or procedures such as arteriography, fibrinolysis, or anticoagulation.

CLINICAL MANIFESTATION

Atherosclerosis/Arterial Insufficiency of Lower Extremity Arteries

SYMPTOMS Pain on exercise, i.e., *intermittent claudication*. With progressive arterial insufficiency, pain and/or paresthesias at rest occur in the leg and/or foot, especially at night. Pallor, cyanosis, livedoid vascular pattern (Fig. 17-1), and loss of hair on affected limb. Earliest infarctive changes include well-demarcated maplike areas of epidermal necrosis. Later, dry black gangrene may occur over the infarcted skin (purple cyanosis → white pallor → black gangrene) (Fig. 17-2). Shedding of slough leads to well-demarcated ulcers in which underlying structures such as tendons can be seen.

GENERAL EXAMINATION **Pulses.** Pulse of large vessels usually diminished or absent. In diabetic patients with mainly microangiopathy, gangrene may occur in the setting of adequate pulses.

Bürger Sign. With significant reduction in arterial blood flow, limb elevation causes pallor (best noted on plantar foot); dependency causes delayed and exaggerated hyperemia.

Pain. Ischemic ulcers are painful; in diabetic patients with neuropathy and ischemic ulcers, pain may be minimal or absent.

Distribution. Ischemic ulcers may first appear between the toes at sites of pressure and begin as fissures on the plantar heel. Dry gangrene of feet, starting at the toes or at pressure sites, or of finger (Fig. 17-2B).

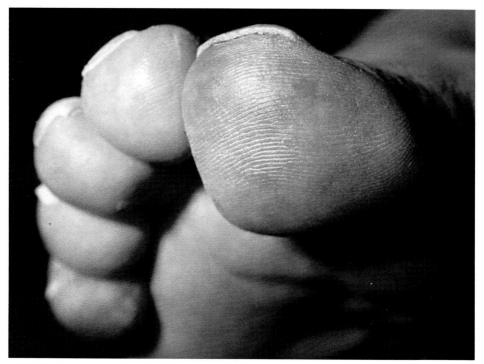

FIGURE 17-1 **Atherosclerosis obliterans, early** The great toe shows pallor and there is mottled, livedoid erythema on the tip of the toe. In this 68-year-old diabetic man, the iliac artery was occluded.

Atheroembolization

Symptoms. Acute pain and tenderness at site of embolization.

SKIN LESIONS Violaceous livedo reticularis on legs and feet, but also as high up as the buttocks. Ischemic changes with poor return of color after compression of skin. "Blue toe" (Fig. 17-3): Indurated, painful plaques often following livedo reticularis on the calves and thighs that may undergo necrosis (Fig. 17-4), become black and crusted, or ulcerate.

GENERAL EXAMINATION **Pulses.** Distal pulses may remain intact.

LABORATORY EXAMINATIONS

HEMATOLOGY Rule out anemia, polycythemia.
LIPID STUDIES Hypercholesterolemia (>240 mg/dL), often associated with a rise in LDL. Hypertriglyceridemia (250 mg/dL) is often associated with a rise in very low-density lipoproteins.
DERMATOPATHOLOGY OF ATHEROEMBOLISM Deep skin and muscle biopsy specimen shows arterioles occluded by fibrosis with multinucleated giant cells surrounding biconvex, -needle-shaped clefts corresponding to cholesterol crystal microemboli.

DOPPLER STUDIES Show reduced or interrupted blood flow.
ARTERIOGRAPHY Atherosclerosis is best visualized by angiography. Ulceration of atheromatous plaques seen in abdominal aorta or more distally.

DIAGNOSIS AND DIFFERENTIAL DIAGNOSIS

DIFFERENTIAL DIAGNOSIS **Intermittent Claudication.** Pseudoxanthoma elasticum, Bürger disease (thromboangiitis obliterans), arthritis, and gout.
Painful Foot. Gout, interdigital neuroma, flat feet, calcanean bursitis, plantar fasciitis, and rupture of the plantar muscle.
Ischemic and Infarctive Lesions of Leg/Foot. Vasculitis, Raynaud phenomenon (vasospasm), disseminated intravascular coagulation, cryoglobulinemia, hyperviscosity syndrome (macroglobulinemia), septic embolization (infective endocarditis), nonseptic

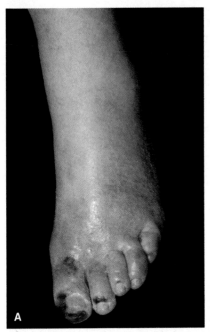
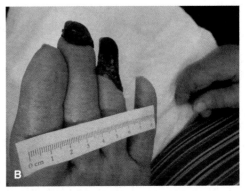

FIGURE 17-2 Atherosclerosis obliterans (A) There is pallor of the forefoot and mottled erythema distally with incipient gangrene on the great toe and the second digit. This is a female diabetic with partial occlusion of the femoral artery. The patient was a smoker. **(B)** More advanced gangrene of the distal digits. The patient had longstanding arterial insufficiency and subacutely noticed discoloration with eventual loss of sensation in spite of attempts for revascularization and restoring of blood flow. (Used with permission from Virginia Capasso, PhD, APRN.)

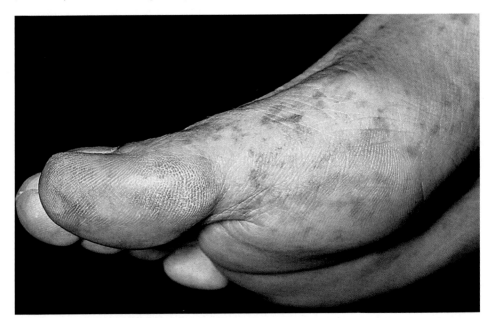

FIGURE 17-3 Atheroembolism after angiography A mottled ("blue toe"), violaceous, vascular pattern on the forefoot and great toe. The findings were noted after intravascular catheterization and angiography in an individual with ASO.

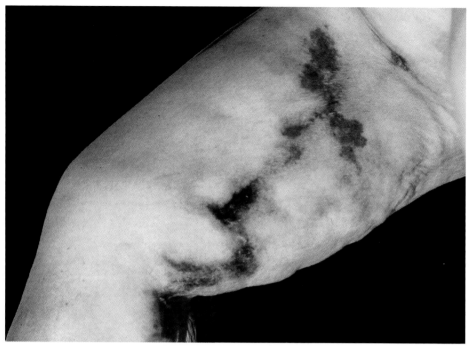

FIGURE 17-4 Atheroembolism with cutaneous infarction Violaceous discoloration and cutaneous infarctions with a linear arrangement on the medial thigh of a 73-year-old woman with atherosclerosis, heart failure, and diabetes.

embolization, drug-induced necrosis (warfarin and heparin), ergot poisoning, intra-arterial injection, livedo reticularis syndromes, and external compression (popliteal entrapment).

COURSE AND PROGNOSIS

Arterial insufficiency is a slowly progressive disease. Atherosclerosis of coronary and carotid arteries usually determines survival of the patient. Amputation rates have been lowered from 80% to <40% by aggressive vascular surgery. *Atheroembolism* may be a single episode if atheroembolization follows the intra-arterial procedure. May be recurrent if spontaneous and associated with significant tissue necrosis.

MANAGEMENT

PREVENTION Goal of management is the prevention of atherosclerosis.
Medical Management *of primary hyperlipidemia*: By statins, diet, and exercise. Reduce elevated blood pressure. *Discontinue cigarette smoking.* Encourage walking to create new collateral vessels. Position the ischemic foot as low as possible without edema. Heparin and warfarin. IV prostacyclins. Analgesics.
SURGICAL MANAGEMENT Endarterectomy or bypass for iliac occlusions. Debridement of necrotic tissue locally. Amputation of leg/foot is indicated when medical and surgical management has failed.

THROMBOANGIITIS OBLITERANS (TO) ICD-10: I73.1

- A rare inflammatory occlusive disease of medium-sized and small arteries and veins.
- Predominantly in males, 20 to 40 years of age.
- Very strong association with smoking.
- An angiitis clinically indistinguishable from TO occurs in persons consuming cannabis.
- Clinical manifestations are cold sensitivity; ischemia: claudication of the leg, foot, arm, or hand.
- Peripheral cyanosis, ischemic ulcers, gangrene (**Fig. 17-5**), and superficial thrombophlebitis.
- Therapy: Smoking cessation, analgesics, wound care; antiplatelet agents, prostacyclins, pentoxifylline, angioplasty, sympathectomy, and amputation.
- *Synonym*: Bürger disease.

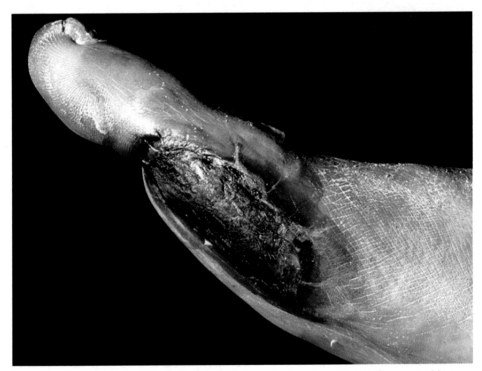

FIGURE 17-5 Thromboangiitis obliterans Infarctive necrosis on the great toe of a 28-year-old man. The lesion is exquisitely painful. (The yellowish-brownish color is from iodine disinfection.)

THROMBOPHLEBITIS AND DEEP VENOUS THROMBOSIS
ICD-10: I 80 ICD-9: 433.40 ∘ ICD-10: I 80.2

- Superficial phlebitis (SP) is an inflammatory thrombosis of a superficial *normal* vein, usually due to infection or trauma from needles and catheters.
- Inflammatory thrombosis of *varicose* veins usually in the context of the chronic venous insufficiency (CVI) syndrome.
- Deep venous thrombosis (DVT) is due to thrombotic obstruction of a vein with or without an inflammatory response.
- Occurs due to slow blood flow, hypercoagulability, or changes in the venous walls.

Predisposing Factors and causes of Deep Venous Thrombosis

Common Factors
- Major surgery
- Fractures
- Congestive heart failure
- Acute myocardial infarction
- Stroke
- Pregnancy and postpartum
- Spinal cord injuries
- Shock

Less Common Factors
- Sickle cell anemia
- Homocystinuria
- Protein C or S deficiency
- Oral contraceptives
- Malignancies
- Venous varicosities
- Previous history of venous thrombosis
- Leiden factor V mutation
- Severe pulmonary insufficiency
- Prolonged immobilization
- Antithrombin III deficiency
- Antiphospholipid antibodies
- Ulcerative colitis

ETIOLOGY AND PATHOGENESIS

The thrombus originates in an area of low venous flow. An inflammatory response to the thrombus causes pain and tenderness. Organization of the thrombus in the vein destroys the venous walls, which leads to postthrombotic syndrome.

CLINICAL MANIFESTATION

Patients complain of pain or aching in the involved limb or notice limb swelling. Some patients may have no symptoms. Pulmonary embolus may be the first indication of DVT.

Superficial thrombophlebitis is diagnosed by the characteristic induration of a superficial vein with redness, tenderness, and increased heat (Fig. 17-6A). DVT presents with a swollen, warm, and tender limb (Fig. 17-6B) with prominent distended collateral veins. Two types of exam complexes are recognized: The limb may be very pale and painful (*phlegmasia alba dolens*) (Fig. 17-6B) or may be cyanotic and painful with cold digits if the arterial inflow is also compromised (*phlegmasia coerulea dolens*).

Migratory phlebitis describes an inflammatory induration of superficial veins that migrates within a defined region of the body; it may be associated with thromboangiitis obliterans and malignancies. *Mondor disease* (sclerosing phlebitis) is an indurated, subcutaneous vein from the breast to the axillary region that during healing leads to a shortening of the venous cord, which puckers the skin.

LABORATORY EXAMINATIONS

Venous imaging by color-coded duplex ultrasound and Doppler examination reveals an absence of flow or of the normal respiratory venous flow variations in proximal venous occlusions.

DIFFERENTIAL DIAGNOSIS

Lymphedema, cellulitis, erysipelas, superficial phlebitis, and lymphangitis. An uncommon differential diagnosis is rupture of the plantar muscle, which produces pain, swelling, and ecchymotic areas in the dependent ankle area.

MANAGEMENT

The treatment of SP is compression, antiplatelet drugs, and nonsteroidal anti-inflammatory agents.

The treatment of DVT is anticoagulation. IV heparin and low molecular weight heparins. Warfarin can be started orally at the same time. Newer anticoagulant agents including fondaparinux, rivaroxaban, dabigatran, apixaban, and edoxaban have recently been approved by the FDA for treatment of DVT and PE in specific circumstances.

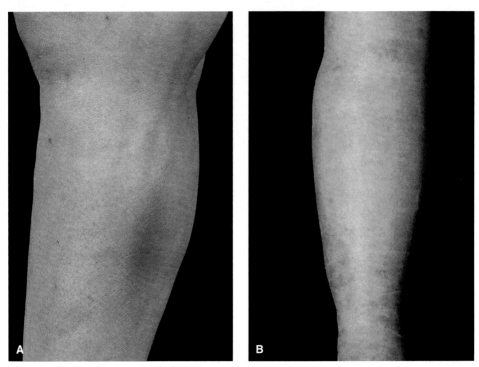

FIGURE 17-6 Superficial phlebitis and deep venous thrombosis (A) A linear painful erythematous cord extending from the popliteal fossa to the mid-calf in a 35-year-old man who had moderate varicosities. Phlebitis occurred after a 15-h flight. **(B)** The leg is swollen, pale, with a bloody cyanotic discoloration and is painful. The episode occurred after abdominal surgery (the circular marks are from a compression bandage).

CHRONIC VENOUS INSUFFICIENCY (CVI) ICD-10: I87.2

- Chronic venous insufficiency results from failure of centripetal return of venous blood and increased capillary pressure.
- The resultant changes include edema, stasis dermatitis, hyperpigmentation, fibrosis of the skin and subcutaneous tissue (lipodermatosclerosis) of the leg, and ulceration.
- Venous ulcers are the most common chronic wounds in humans.

EPIDEMIOLOGY AND ETIOLOGY

Varicose veins: Peak incidence of onset 30 to 40 years. Varicose veins are three times more common in women than in men.

ETIOLOGY CVI is most commonly associated with varicose veins and the postphlebitic syndrome. Varicose veins are an inherited characteristic.

AGGRAVATING FACTORS Pregnancy, increased blood volume, increased cardiac output, increased venocaval pressure, and progesterone.

PATHOGENESIS

The damaged valves of the deep veins of the calf are incompetent at restricting backflow of blood. Fibrin is deposited in the extravascular space, resulting in sclerosis and obliteration of lymphatics and microvasculature.

This cycle repeats itself: initial event → aggravation of venous stasis and varicose vein dilatation → thrombosis → lipodermatosclerosis → stasis dermatitis → ulceration.

CLINICAL MANIFESTATION

CVI is commonly associated with heaviness or aching of the leg, which is aggravated by standing (dependency) and relieved by walking. Lipodermatosclerosis may limit movement of the ankle and cause pain and limitation of movement, which in turn increases stasis.

Skin Lesions

VARICOSE VEINS Superficial leg veins are enlarged, tortuous, with incompetent valves; best evaluated with the patient standing (Fig. 17-7A). "Blow-out" at sites of incompetent communicating veins. Varicose veins may or may not be associated with starburst phlebectasia usually overlying the area of an incompetent communicating vein (Fig. 17-7B).

EDEMA Dependent; improved or resolved in the morning after a night in the horizontal position. Dorsa of feet, ankles, and lower legs.
ECZEMATOUS (STASIS) DERMATITIS Occurs in setting of CVI around the lower legs and ankles (Fig. 17-8). It is a classic eczematous dermatitis with inflammatory papules, scaly and crusted erosions; in addition, there is pigmentation, stippled with recent and old hemorrhages; dermal sclerosis; and excoriations due to scratching. If eczematous stasis dermatitis is extensive, it may be associated with generalized eczematous dermatitis, i.e., "id" reaction or autosensitization (see Section 2).
ATROPHIE BLANCHE Small ivory-white depressed patches (Fig. 17-9) on the ankle and/or foot; stellate and irregular, coalescing; stippled pigmentation; hemosiderin-pigmented border, usually within stasis dermatitis. Often following trauma.

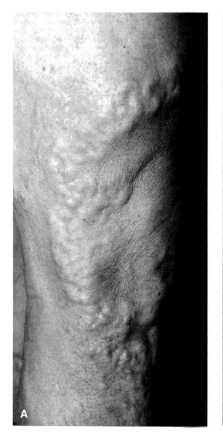
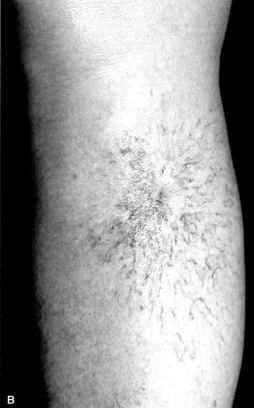

FIGURE 17-7 **Varicose veins (A)** There are meandering and convoluted irregular varicose veins and the thigh and below the knee of a 70-year-old man who also had lipodermatosclerosis and stasis dermatitis on the lower legs. **(B)** *Starburst venectasias on the calf.* This is an area overlying an insufficient communicating vein.

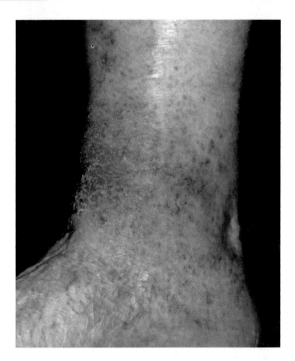

FIGURE 17-8 Stasis dermatitis in CVI
A patch of eczematous dermatitis overlying venous varicosities on the medial ankle in a 59-year-old woman. The lesion is papular, scaly and pruritic.

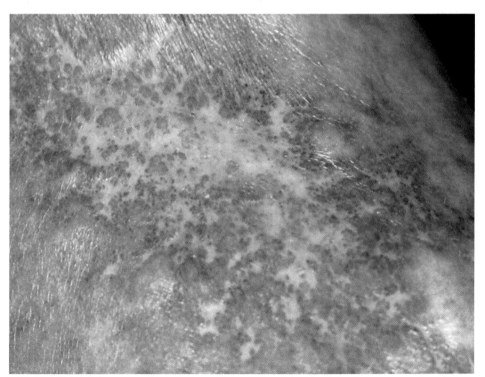

FIGURE 17-9 Chronic venous insufficiency. Atrophie blanche An area of diffuse and mottled pigmentation due to hemosiderin and ivory-white patches of atrophie blanche. Such lesions are both itchy and painful.

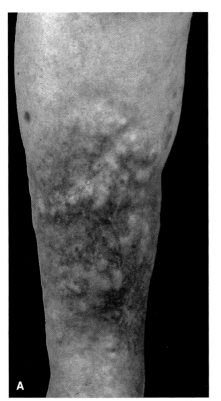
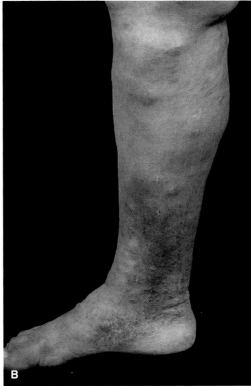

FIGURE 17-10 Chronic venous insufficiency and lipodermatosclerosis (A) The ankle is relatively thin and the upper calf edematous, creating a "champagne bottle" or "piano-leg" appearance. **(B)** Varicose veins are less visible here but can be easily palpated in the sclerotic plaque encasing the entire calf ("groove" sign). There is also pigmentation and minor papular stasis dermatitis.

LIPODERMATOSCLEROSIS Inflammation, induration, pigmentation of the lower third of the leg creating a "champagne bottle" or "piano leg" appearance with edema above and below the sclerotic region (Fig. 17-10A). "Groove sign" created by varicose veins meandering through the sclerotic tissue. A verrucous epidermal change can occur overlying the sclerosis and can be combined with chronic lymphedema.
ULCERATION Occurs in 30% of cases; very painful "hyperalgesic microulcer" in area of atrophie blanche; necrotic base surrounded by atrophie blanche, stasis dermatitis, and lipodermatosclerosis (Figs. 17-10B and 17-11). Venous ulcers usually occur medially and above the ankles (Fig. 17-11).

LABORATORY EXAMINATIONS

DOPPLER AND COLOR-CODED DUPLEX SONOGRAPHY These detect incompetent veins and venous occlusion due to thrombus.
DERMATOPATHOLOGY *Early*: Dilated small venules and lymphatics; edema of extracellular space. *Later*: Capillaries dilated, congested with tuft formation and tortuosity of venules; deposition of fibrin. *Endothelial cell hypertrophy;* venous thrombosis; angioendotheliomatous proliferation mimicking Kaposi sarcoma. In all stages, extravasation of red blood cells that break down forming hemosiderin, which is taken up by macrophages. Lymphatic vessels become encased in a fibrotic stroma, i.e., lipodermatosclerosis.

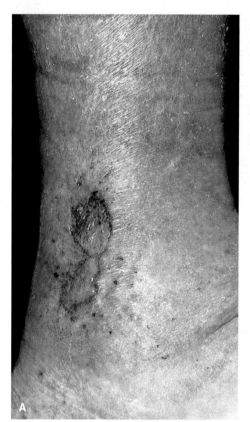 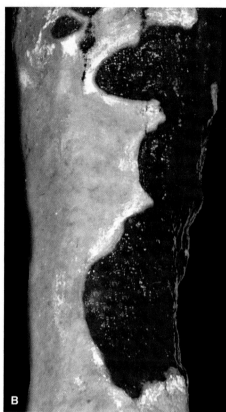

FIGURE 17-11 Venous insufficiency (A) Two coalescing ulcers with a necrotic base in an area of atrophie blanche, lipodermatosclerosis, and stasis dermatitis. Scratch marks indicate itchiness of surrounding skin, while the ulcers are painful. **(B)** A giant ulcer, well-defined with scalloped borders and a beefy red base in a leg with lipodermatosclerosis.

DIAGNOSIS

Usually made on history, clinical findings, and Doppler and color-coded Duplex sonography.

MANAGEMENT

PREREQUISITE Compression dressings or stockings; Unna boot.

ATROPHIE BLANCHE Avoid trauma to the area involved. Intralesional triamcinolone into painful lesions.

STASIS DERMATITIS Topical glucocorticoids (short term). Topical antibiotic treatments (e.g., mupirocin) when secondarily infected. Culture for methicillin-resistant *Staphylococcus aureus*.

VARICOSE VEINS **Injection Sclerotherapy.** A sclerosing agent is injected into varicosities, followed by prolonged compression.

Vascular Surgery. Incompetent perforating veins are identified, ligated, and cut, followed by stripping long and/or short saphenous veins out of the main trunk.

Endovascular Techniques. These new technologies encompass endoscopic subfascial dissection of perforating veins (employed primarily in the elimination of insufficient perforating veins in CVI) and endoscopic endovenous diode laser or radio frequency thermal heating, which leads to occlusion of the varicose vein.

MOST COMMON LEG/FOOT ULCERS ICD-10: I83.0

- Leg ulcers occur commonly in late middle and old age.
- They arise in association with CVI, chronic arterial insufficiency, or peripheral sensory neuropathy.
- Particularly in diabetes, leg ulcers are common.
- Leg ulcers are associated with significant long-term morbidity and often do not heal unless the underlying problem(s) is (are) corrected.
- Rarely squamous cell carcinoma (SCC) can arise in chronic venous ulcers.

VENOUS ULCERS The prevalence of venous ulcers is estimated to be approximately 1%. It rises with patient age, obesity, previous leg injury (fractures), DVT, and phlebitis. Venous ulcers are associated with at least one or all of the symptoms of CVI (Fig. 17-11); single or multiple; they are usually on the medial lower calf, especially over the malleolus (medial > lateral), in the area supplied by incompetent perforating veins (Fig. 17-11). They can involve the circumference of the entire lower leg (Fig. 17-11B). They are sharply defined, irregularly shaped, relatively shallow with a sloping border, and are usually painful. The base is usually covered by fibrin and necrotic material (Fig. 17-11A), and there is always secondary bacterial colonization. SCC can arise in a long-standing venous ulcer (Fig. 17-12) of the leg.

ARTERIAL ULCERS Arterial ulcers are associated with peripheral arterial disease (atherosclerosis obliterans, see p. 408). Characteristically painful at night. Occur on the pretibial, supramalleolar (usually lateral), and at distant points, such as the toes. Punched out, with sharply demarcated borders (Fig. 17-13).

A special type of arterial ulcer is the *Martorell ulcer*, which is associated with labile hypertension and lacks clinical signs of ASO. The ulcer(s) start with a black eschar surrounded by erythema and after sloughing of necrotic tissue are punched out with sharply demarcated borders, with surrounding erythema; very painful on the anterior lateral lower leg.

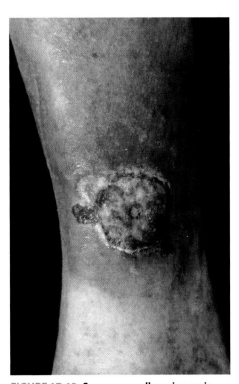

FIGURE 17-12 Squamous cell carcinoma in chronic venous ulcer A venous ulcer had been present >10 years in an area of lipodermatosclerosis and stasis dermatitis. Eventually, the base of the ulcer became elevated, hard, and less painful. Deep biopsy (circular mark in the center) revealed necrosis and at the base invasive squamous cell carcinoma.

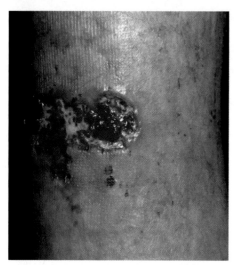

FIGURE 17-13 Chronic arterial insufficiency with a sharply defined, "punched out" ulcer with irregular outlines The extremity was pulseless, and there was massive ischemia on the toes.

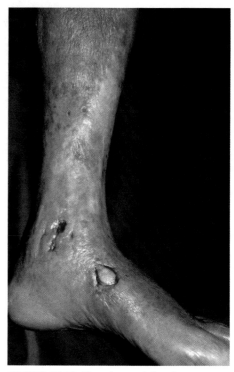

FIGURE 17-14 Chronic arterial and venous insufficiency, "combined" arterial and venous ulcers Note pronounced lipodermatosclerosis and ulceration on the supramalleolar lower leg (venous component) and purple discoloration of forefoot and toes with punched-out ulcer revealing tendon over metatarsal site (arterial component).

TABLE 17-1 Differential Diagnosis of Three Major Types of Leg Ulcers

	Lesion	Site	Surrounding Skin	General Examination
Venous	Irregular	Malleolar and supramalleolar (medial)	Lipodermatosclerosis	Varicose veins
	Sloped borders		Stasis dermatitis	Pain, worse in dependent state
	Necrotic base Fibrin		Atrophie blanche Pigmentation Lymphedema	
Arterial	Punched out	Pressure sites: distal (toes), pretibial, supramalleolar (lateral)	Atrophic, shiny	Weak/absent pulses
	Necrotic base		Hair loss	Pallor on elevation of leg
			Pallor or reactive hyperemia	Pain worse on elevation of leg
Neuropathic	Punched out	Pressure sites	Callus before ulceration and surrounding ulcer	Peripheral neuropathy
		Plantar		Decreased sensation No pain

COMBINED ARTERIAL AND VENOUS ULCERS These ulcers arise in patients who have both CVI and ASO (Fig. 17-14).

NEUROPATHIC ULCERS Soles, toes, and heels. Most commonly associated with diabetes of many years' duration (see Diabetic Foot, Section 15).

DIFFERENTIAL DIAGNOSIS

A differential diagnosis of the three main types of leg/foot ulcers is shown in Table 17-1. Other differential diagnostic considerations include ulcerated SCC, basal cell carcinoma, injection drug use (skin popping), and pressure ulcer (ski boot). Ulcerations also occur in vasculitis (particularly polyarteritis nodosa), erythema induratum, calciphylaxis, and various infections [ecthyma, Buruli ulcer, *Mycobacterium marinum* infection, gumma, leprosy, invasive fungal infection, and chronic herpes simplex virus (HSV) ulcer] and in sickle cell anemia, polycythemia vera, pyoderma gangrenosum, necrobiosis lipoidica with ulceration, and factitia.

COURSE AND PROGNOSIS

Course and prognosis are dependent on the underlying disease.

MANAGEMENT

GENERAL MANAGEMENT In general, factors such as anemia and malnutrition should be corrected to facilitate healing. Control hypertension, weight reduction in the obese, exercise; mobilize patient; correct edema caused by cardial, renal, or hepatic dysfunction. Of utmost importance is treatment of the underlying disease. In neuropathic ulcers, correct underlying diabetes, rule out underlying osteomyelitis, distribute weight of pressure points with special shoes in neuropathic ulcers. *Note:* Diabetic patients are particularly predisposed to ulcers and frequently have several etiologic factors in play, i.e., peripheral vascular disease, neuropathy, infection, and impaired healing.

LOCAL TREATMENT OF ULCER AND SURROUNDING SKIN Treat stasis dermatitis in CVI with wet dressings and moderate to potent glucocorticoid ointment. Debridement of necrotic material mechanically (surgically) or by enzymatic debriding agents; antiseptics and antibiotics to counteract infection. Hydrocolloid dressings. For cleaned ulcers that heal slowly surgical procedures either by pinch grafts, split-thickness skin grafts, epidermal grafts, cultured keratinocyte allografts, or composite grafts.

LIVEDOID VASCULITIS (LV) ICD-10: L95.0

- LV is a thrombotic vasculopathy of dermal vessels confined to the lower extremities and starting mostly in the ankle region.
- A triad of livedo reticularis, atrophie blanche, and very painful, small punched-out ulcers that have a very poor tendency for healing (Fig. 17-15).
- Atrophie blanche in LV is clinically indistinguishable from that seen in CVI, except for varicose veins (compare Figs. 17-15 and 17-9). LV is a reaction pattern of the skin that often recurs in winter or summer ("livedo reticularis with winter and summer ulcerations").
- Histologically, there are fibrin thrombi in small and medium-sized dermal veins and arteries with wedge-shaped necrosis and hyalinization of the vessel walls (segmental hyalinizing vasculitis).
- LV may be idiopathic or may be associated with Sneddon syndrome (see Fig. 14-42), antiphospholipid antibody syndrome, or conditions of hypercoagulability or hyperviscosity.
- Treatment: Bed rest, analgesics, low-dose heparin, and platelet aggregation inhibitors. Pain can be relieved and healing accelerated by systemic glucocorticoids. Anabolic agents such as danazol and stanozolol have been anecdotally reported to be effective.
- Larger ulcers will have to be excised and grafted.

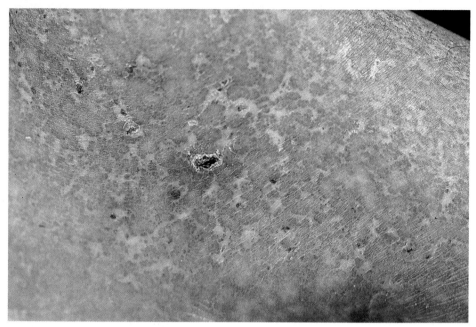

FIGURE 17-15 Livedoid vasculitis This is characterized by the triad of livedo reticularis, atrophie blanche, and small, painful, and crusted ulcers. This is clinically indistinguishable from atrophie blanche seen in CVI except for the absence of varicose veins.

CHRONIC LYMPHATIC INSUFFICIENCY ICD-10: I87.2

- Lymphedema in childhood and early adult life are genetic and are often caused by defects in vascular endothelial growth factor receptor 3 and FoxC2, a transcription factor.
- Acquired lymphedema of adults may be related to chronic venous insufficiency; chronic, recurring soft-tissue infections (erysipelas and cellulitis, see Section 25); node dissection and radiation after cancer; and in some geographic regions by filariasis.
- Clinical manifestations: swelling of extremities, pitting edema initially slowly evolving into nonpitting woody induration.
- Prolonged lymphedema may lead to grotesque enlargement of extremity; epidermal hyperplasia with verrucosis (**Fig. 17-16**).
- Secondary, soft-tissue infection (erysipelas and cellulitis) is common, recurrent, and leads to worsening of the condition.
- Treatment is mainly compression (as in CVI) and manual lymphatic drainage; antibiotics in secondary infection.
- Lymphangiosarcoma (in postmastectomy lymphedema) is a rare complication: Stewart-Treves syndrome.

FIGURE 17-16 **Chronic lymphatic insuffi-**
ciency: lymphedema Lower legs are thickened of
woody consistency and three is massive hyperkeratosis and pebbly and papillomatous overgrowths.
The 60-year-old patient had innumerable episodes
of erysipelas and cellulitis. There is also diabetes
and atherosclerosis.

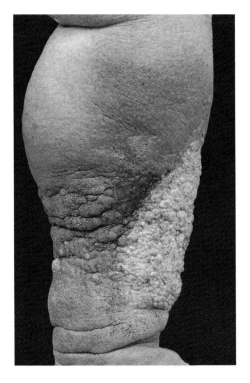

PRESSURE ULCERS ICD-10: L89

- Pressure ulcers develop at body-support interfaces over bony prominences as a result of external compression of the skin, shear forces, and friction, which produce ischemic tissue necrosis.
- Occurs in patients who are obtunded mentally or have diminished sensation (as in spinal cord disease) in the affected region. Secondary infection results in localized cellulitis, which can extend locally into bone or muscle or into the bloodstream.

EPIDEMIOLOGY

AGE OF ONSET Any age, but the greatest prevalence of pressure ulcers is in elderly, chronically
bedridden patients.
SEX Equally prevalent in both sexes.

PATHOGENESIS

Risk factors: Inadequate nursing care, diminished sensation/immobility (obtunded mental
status, spinal cord disease), hypotension, fecal or
urinary incontinence, the presence of fracture,
hypoalbuminemia, and poor nutritional status.
Infection also impairs or prevents healing.

CLINICAL MANIFESTATION

SKIN LESIONS **Clinical Categories of Pressure**
Ulcers. Early change: Localized erythema that
blanches on pressure.
 Stage I: Nonblanching erythema of intact
skin.
 Stage II: Necrosis, superficial or partial
thickness involving the epidermis and/or
dermis. Bullae → necrosis of dermis (black) →
shallow ulcer.
 Stage III: Deep necrosis, crateriform ulceration with full-thickness skin loss (Fig. 17-17);
damage or necrosis can extend down to, but
not through, fascia.

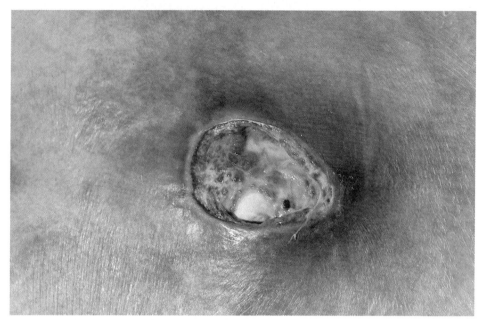

FIGURE 17-17 Pressure ulcer, stage III Well-demarcated crateriform ulcer with full-thickness skin loss extending down to fascia over greater trochanteric region.

Stage IV: Full-thickness necrosis (→ ulceration) with involvement of supporting structures such as muscle and bone (Fig. 17-18). May enlarge to many centimeters. May or may not be tender. Borders of ulcers may be undetermined.

Well-established pressure ulcers with devitalized tissue at the base (eschar) have a higher chance of secondary infection.

Distribution. Occur over bony prominences: sacrum (60%) > ischial tuberosities, greater trochanter (Fig. 17-17), heel (Fig. 17-18) > elbow, knee, ankle, and occiput.

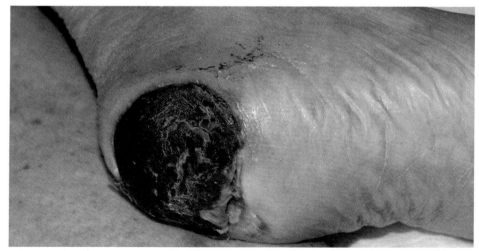

FIGURE 17-18 Pressure ulcer, stage IV on the heel The black necrosis seen here extended into the calcaneal bone which also had to be debrided.

LABORATORY EXAMINATIONS

Hematologic Studies

WOUND CULTURE For aerobic and anaerobic bacteria.

BLOOD CULTURE Bacteremia often follows manipulation of ulcer.

PATHOLOGY **Skin Biopsy.** Epidermal necrosis with eccrine duct and gland necrosis. Deep ulcers show wedge-shaped infarcts of the subcutaneous tissue.

Bone Biopsy. Essential for diagnosing continuous osteomyelitis.

DIAGNOSIS AND DIFFERENTIAL DIAGNOSIS

Usually made clinically. Differential diagnosis includes infectious ulcer (actinomycotic infection, deep fungal infection, chronic herpetic ulcer), thermal burn, malignant ulcer, pyoderma gangrenosum, and rectocutaneous fistula.

COURSE AND PROGNOSIS

If pressure is relieved, some changes are reversible. Osteomyelitis occurs in nonhealing pressure ulcers (32 to 81%). Septicemia is associated with a high mortality rate. With proper treatment, stages I and II ulcers heal in 1 to 4 weeks and stages III and IV ulcers heal in 6 to >12 weeks.

MANAGEMENT

PROPHYLAXIS IN AT-RISK PATIENTS Reposition patient every 2 h (more often if possible); inspect for areas of skin breakdown over pressure points; minimize friction and shear forces.

- Use interface air mattress to reduce compression.
- Minimize skin exposure to excessive moisture from incontinence, perspiration, or wound drainage.
- Evaluate and correct nutritional status; consider supplements of vitamin C and zinc.

STAGES I AND II ULCERS Topical antibiotics (not neomycin) under moist sterile gauze may be sufficient for early erosions. Hydrogels or hydrocolloid dressings.

STAGES III AND IV ULCERS Surgical management: Debridement of necrotic tissue, bony prominence removal, flaps, and skin grafts.

INFECTIOUS COMPLICATIONS Prolonged course of antimicrobial agent depending on sensitivities and with surgical debridement of necrotic bone in osteomyelitis.

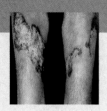

SECTION 18

SKIN SIGNS OF RENAL INSUFFICIENCY

CLASSIFICATION OF SKIN CHANGES

- Acute renal failure
  - Edema
  - Uremic frost (deposition of urea crystals on the skin's surface in severe uremia)
- Chronic renal failure
  - Edema
  - Uremic frost
  - Calciphylaxis
  - Bullous disease of hemodialysis (pseudoporphyria, see Section 23)
  - Nephrogenic fibrosing dermopathy
  - Acquired perforating dermatosis

CALCIPHYLAXIS ICD-10: E83.59

- Calciphylaxis is characterized by progressive cutaneous necrosis associated with small- and medium-sized vessel vasculitis, calcification, and thrombosis.
- It occurs in the setting of end-stage renal disease, diabetes mellitus, and secondary hyperparathyroidism. Most often follows initiation of hemo or peritoneal dialysis.
- Precipitating factors: glucocorticosteroids, albumin infusions, IM tobramycin, iron dextran complex, calcium heparinate, and vitamin D.
- Preinfarctive lesions show mottling or a livedo reticularis pattern, dusky red (**Fig. 18-1A**).
- Turn into black, leathery eschar (**Fig. 18-1B**) and ulcer with tightly adherent black or leathery slough. Ulcers enlarge over weeks to months; when debrided reach down to fascia and beyond; areas of plate-like induration can be palpated surrounding infarcted or ulcerated lesions (**Fig. 18-2**).
- Extremely painful.
- Lower extremities, abdomen, buttocks, and penis.
- Azotemia. Calcium X phosphate ion product usually elevated. Parathormone levels usually but not always elevated. Dermatopathology: Calcification of media of small- and medium-sized blood vessels in dermis and subcutaneous tissues.
- Slowly progressive, despite therapy. Ulcers become secondarily infected.
- Management: Treatment of renal failure, partial parathyroidectomy when indicated, and debridement of necrotic tissue.

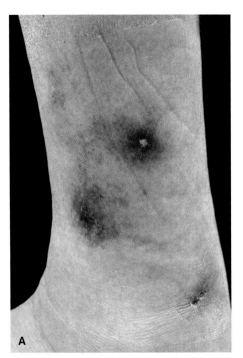
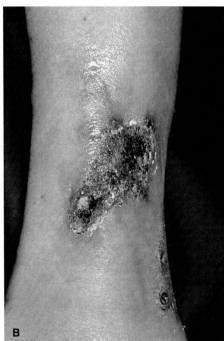

FIGURE 18-1 Calciphylaxis (A) Early stage. An area of mottled erythema, starburst-like, and reminiscent of livedo reticularis with two small ulcerations. Patient has chronic renal failure and is on hemodialysis. Even at this early stage, lesions are extremely painful. **(B)** Calciphylaxis, more advanced lesion. An area of jagged necrosis on the lower leg in a patient with diabetes and chronic renal failure who is on hemodialysis. The surrounding skin is indurated and represents a plate-like subcutaneous mass that is appreciated only upon palpation.

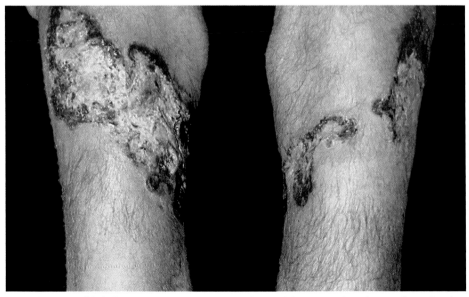

FIGURE 18-2 Calciphylaxis, extensive Lesions are ulcerated; the surrounding skin is indurated and best seen on left thigh where skin is hairless. Similar lesions are also found on the abdomen.

NEPHROGENIC FIBROSING DERMOPATHY (NFD) ICD-10: L90.8

- NFD is a fibrosing disorder in patients with acute or chronic renal failure.
- Most patients receive hemodialysis or peritoneal dialysis; in acute renal failure, NFD occurs without dialysis.
- It is part of a wider spectrum of *nephrogenic systemic fibrosis* involving the heart, lungs, diaphragm, skeletal muscle, liver, genitourinary tract, and central nervous system.
- Etiology unknown but exposure to gadodiamide containing contrast media for MR angiography is a strong association. Gadodiamide is found only in lesions and not in normal tissue.
- NFD is characterized by acute onset, brawny indurations, plaque-like or nodular, bound down upon palpation (**Fig. 18-3**); up to 20 cm and more in diameter, with an uneven rippled surface.
- Mostly on lower extremities, less often on upper extremities and torso but not the face.
- Tingling, tender, and often painful.
- Differential diagnosis: Morphea, pretibial myxedema, lipodermatosclerosis, and panniculitis.
- Course is chronic and unremitting; prognosis guarded.
- Therapy unknown. Imatinib may be beneficial. Sodium thiosulfate may be given during dialysis but this can be complicated by metabolic acidosis. Intralesional sodium thiosulfate has been used with some success.

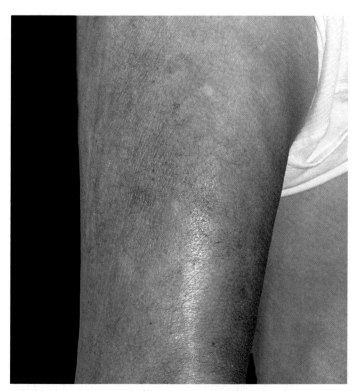

FIGURE 18-3 Nephrogenic fibrosing dermopathy A brawny plate-like induration bound down upon palpation, with an uneven surface on the legs. This patient had end-stage chronic renal failure and was on hemodialysis.

ACQUIRED PERFORATING DERMATOSES ICD-10: L87.0

- Occurs in chronic renal failure and diabetes mellitus; in up to 10% of patients undergoing hemodialysis.
- Chronic pruritic condition triggered by trauma.
- Umbilicated papules with central hyperkeratotic crust (**Fig. 18-4**).
- Transepidermal elimination of collagen.
- Relationship with other perforating disorders not clear.

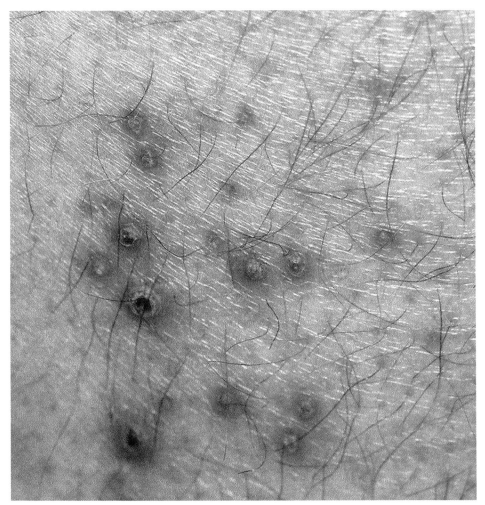

FIGURE 18-4 Acquired perforating dermatosis in a patient undergoing hemodialysis There are purpuric umbilicated papules with a central hyperkeratotic crust.

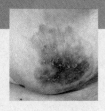

SKIN SIGNS OF SYSTEMIC CANCERS

MUCOCUTANEOUS SIGNS OF SYSTEMIC CANCERS ICD-10: M8000/6

- Mucocutaneous findings may suggest systemic cancers in several ways:
  - Associations of heritable mucocutaneous disorders with systemic cancers.
  - By action at a distance, i.e., paraneoplastic syndromes.
- Or spread of cancer to the skin or mucosal sites by direct, lymphatic, or hematogenous extension (cutaneous metastasis).

CLASSIFICATION OF SKIN SIGNS OF SYSTEMIC CANCER[1]

METASTATIC CANCERS

PERSISTENT TUMOR Lymphatic extension and hematogenous spread.
DIRECT EXTENSION Paget disease and extramammary Paget disease.
  Lymphomas with secondary skin involvement (Section 21).

HERITABLE DISORDERS

Cowden Syndrome

Peutz–Jeghers Syndrome

Neurofibromatosis (see Section 16).
Tuberous sclerosis (see Section 16).
Multiple endocrine neoplasia (types 1 and 2b).

PARANEOPLASTIC SYNDROMES

Acanthosis nigricans, malignant, tripe palms
- Acquired ichthyosis
- Bazex syndrome
- Carcinoid syndrome
- *Dermatomyositis* (see Section 14)
- Ectopic ACTH syndrome
- Erythema gyratum repens
- Gardner syndrome

Glucagonoma syndrome
- Hypertrichosis lanuginosa
- Muir–Torre syndrome
- Palmar keratoses

Paraneoplastic pemphigus (paraneoplastic autoimmune multiorgan syndrome)
- *Pruritus*
- *Pyoderma gangrenosum* (see Section 7)
- *Sweet syndrome* (see Section 7)
- *Vasculitis* (see Section 14)

---

[1]Conditions covered in this section are printed in **bold**, conditions dealt with in other sections are in *italics*. Numbers in parentheses indicate page numbers. Rare conditions not discussed in this book are described in CA deWitt et al, in K Wolff et al (eds): *Fitzpatrick's Dermatology in General Medicine* 7th ed. New York, McGraw-Hill, 2008, pp. 1493–1507.

METASTATIC CANCER TO THE SKIN* ICD-10: M8000/6

- Metastatic cancer to the skin is characterized by solitary or multiple dermal or subcutaneous nodules, occurring as metastatic cells from a distant noncontiguous primary malignant neoplasm.
- They are transported to and deposited in the skin or subcutaneous tissue by one of the following routes:
  - Lymphatic routes.
  - Hematogenous spread.
  - Contiguous spread across the peritoneal cavity or other tissues.
- *Skin lesions* nodule (**Figs. 19-1** and **19-2**), raised plaque, thickened fibrotic area. First detected when <5 mm. The fibrotic area may resemble morphea; occurring on scalp, may produce alopecia. Initially, epidermis is intact and stretched over nodule; in time, the surface may become ulcerated (**Fig. 19-3**) or hyperkeratotic. It may appear inflammatory, i.e., pink to red or hemorrhagic. Firm to indurated. May be solitary, few, or multiple. May acquire considerable size and may be mistaken for a primary skin cancer (**Fig. 19-3**).

*For metastatic nonmelanoma skin cancers and melanoma, see Sections 11 and 12.

SPECIAL PATTERNS OF CUTANEOUS INVOLVEMENT

Breast

Inflammatory metastatic carcinoma (carcinoma erysipelatodes): Erythematous patch or plaque with an active spreading border (Fig. 19-4). Most often with breast cancer that may spread within lymphatics to the skin of involved breast, resulting in inflammatory plaques resembling erysipelas (hence, the designation *carcinoma erysipelatodes*). Occurs with other cancers as well [pancreas, parotid, tonsils, colon, stomach, rectum, melanoma, pelvic organs, ovary (Fig. 19-5), uterus, prostate, lung, and mesothelioma (Fig. 19-6)].

Telangiectatic metastatic carcinoma (*carcinoma telangiectaticum*): Breast cancer appearing as pinpoint telangiectases with dilated capillaries within carcinoma erysipelatodes. Violaceous papules or papulovesicles resembling lymphangioma circumscriptum.

En cuirasse metastatic carcinoma: Diffuse morphea-like induration of skin (Fig. 19-7). Usually local extension of breast cancer occurring in breast and presternal region. Sclerodermoid plaque may encase the chest and resembles a metal breastplate of a cuirassier. Also occurs with primary of lung, GI tract, and kidney.

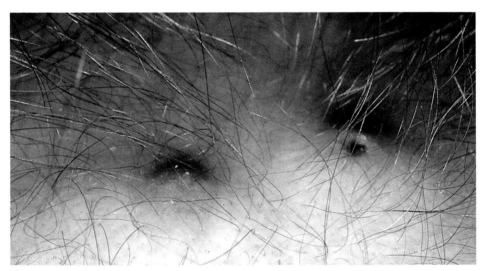

FIGURE 19-1 Metastatic cancer to the skin: bronchogenic cancer Dermal nodules on the scalp of a patient undergoing chemotherapy for metastatic lung cancer; the nodules were only apparent following loss of hair during chemotherapy. The nodule on the left is asymptomatic, erythematous, but noninflamed. The nodule on the right has a central depression marking a punch biopsy site.

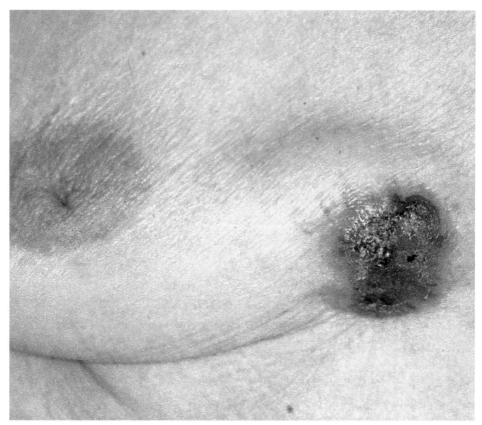

FIGURE 19-2 Metastatic cancer to the skin *Breast cancer.* Large nodule on breast in a 40-year-old woman with breast cancer, present for 4 months.

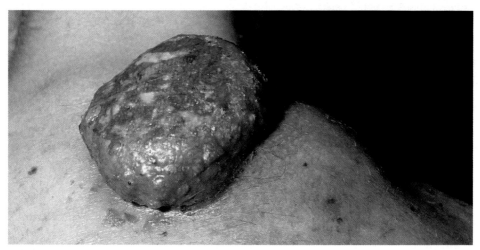

FIGURE 19-3 Metastatic cancer to the skin Adenocarcinoma of the GI tract. This fungating mass was just the tip of the iceberg: a much larger mass was in the subcutis.

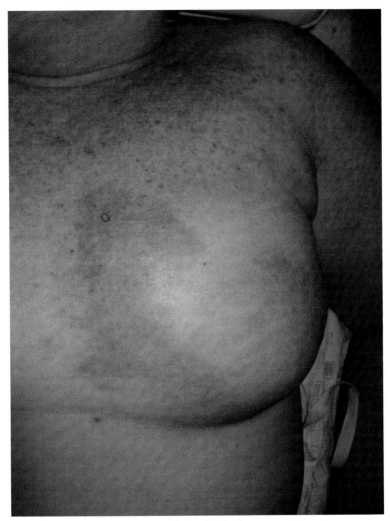

FIGURE 19-4 Metastatic cancer of the skin: inflammatory breast cancer (carcinoma erysipelatodes) A large erythematous and only minimally indurated lesion covering the entire breast and presternal region; the lesion is red and sharply defined and thus looks like erysipelas. There was a 2 × 2 cm lump in the breast upon palpation.

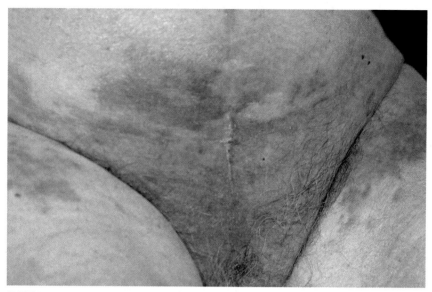

FIGURE 19-5 Metastatic ovarian cancer Manifesting as carcinoma erysipelatodes on the lower abdomen and inguinal region. Workup disclosed ovarian cancer with peritoneal carcinomatosis.

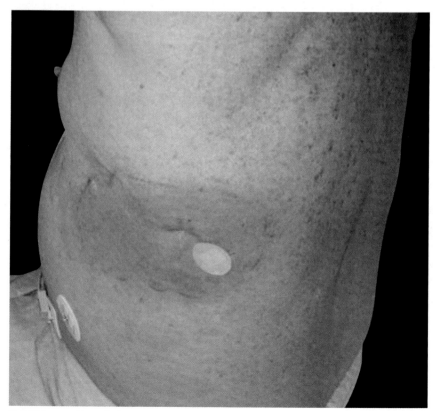

FIGURE 19-6 Mesothelioma An indurated erythematous patch on the lateral chest represents carcinoma erysipleatodes from mesothelioma.

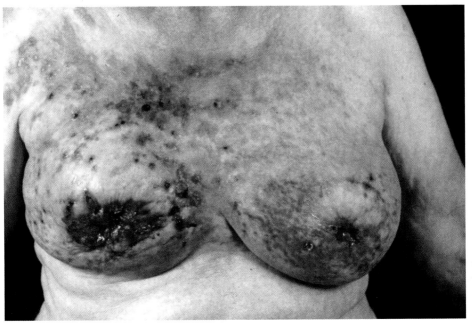

FIGURE 19-7 Metastatic breast cancer: cancer en cuirasse Both breasts are hard upon palpation, like an armor plate. There are multiple small and large, ulcerated nodules and there is a background of erysipelas-like erythema (carcinoma erysipelatodes).

Paget disease: See below.

Multiple smooth nodules on scalp: Prostate adenocarcinoma, lung cancer, and breast cancer (Fig. 19-1).

Alopecia neoplastica: On scalp, areas of hair loss resembling alopecia areata; well-demarcated, red-pink, smooth surface, and flat.

Large Intestine. Often presents on skin of abdomen or perineal regions; also, on the scalp or face. Most originate in rectum. May present with metastatic inflammatory carcinoma (like carcinoma erysipelatodes) of inguinal region, supraclavicular area, or face and neck. Less commonly, sessile or pedunculated nodules on buttocks, grouped vascular nodules of groin or scrotum, or facial tumor. Rarely, cutaneous fistula after appendectomy or resembling hidradenitis suppurativa.

Lung Carcinoma. May produce a large number of metastatic nodules in a short period.

Most commonly, reddish nodule(s) on scalp (Fig. 19-1). Trunk: Symmetric; along direction of intercostal vessels, may be zosteriform; in scar (thoracotomy site or needle aspiration tract).

Hypernephroma. Can produce solitary lesion; also widespread. Usually appear vascular, ± pulsatile and ± pedunculated; can resemble pyogenic granuloma. Most common on the head (scalp) and neck; also trunk and extremities.

Carcinoma of Bladder, Ovary. Can spread contiguously to abdominal and inguinal skin similarly to breast cancer, as previously described, and look like erysipelas (Fig. 19-5).

MISCELLANEOUS PATTERNS With dilation of lymphatics and superficial hemorrhage, may resemble lymphangioma. With lymph stasis and dermal edema, resembles pigskin or orange peel.

MAMMARY PAGET DISEASE ICD-10: C50.01

- Mammary Paget disease (MPD) is a malignant neoplasm that unilaterally involves the nipple or areola and simulates a chronic eczematous dermatitis.
- It represents contiguous spread of underlying intraductal carcinoma of the breast (1 to 4% of breast cancers).
- Usually occurring in females (>50 years); there are rare examples in males.
- Onset is insidious over several months or years. May be asymptomatic or there may be pruritus, pain, burning, discharge, bleeding, ulceration, and nipple invagination.
- Skin lesion presents as red, scaling plaque, rather sharply marginated, oval with irregular borders. When scale is removed, the surface is moist and oozing (**Fig. 19-8**). Lesions range in size from 0.3 to 15 cm (**Fig. 19-9**). In early stages, there is no induration of the plaque; later, induration and infiltration develop and nodules may be palpated in breast. At initial, there is flattening or retraction of the nipple, an underlying breast mass is palpable in fewer than one-half of patients. May be bilateral. Lymph node metastases occur more often when MPD is associated with an underlying palpable mass.
- Differential diagnosis includes eczematous dermatitis, psoriasis, benign ductal papilloma, nipple-areola retention hyperkeratosis, impetigo, SCC in situ, and familial pemphigus.
- *Eczematous dermatitis of the nipples* is usually bilateral; it is without any induration and responds rapidly to topical glucocorticoids. Nevertheless, be suspicious of Paget disease if "eczema" persists for >3 weeks. Diagnosis verified by biopsy showing neoplastic cells in epidermis following a pathognomonic pattern of spread. Define underlying intraductal carcinoma by mammography.
- Management consists of surgery, radiotherapy, and/or chemotherapy as in any other breast carcinomas. Lymph node dissection is suggested if regional nodes are palpable. Prognosis varies. When breast mass is not palpable, 92% of patients survive 5 years after excision; 82% survive 10 years. When breast mass is palpable, 38% survive 5 years; 22% survive 10 years. Prognosis is worse when there is lymphadenopathy.

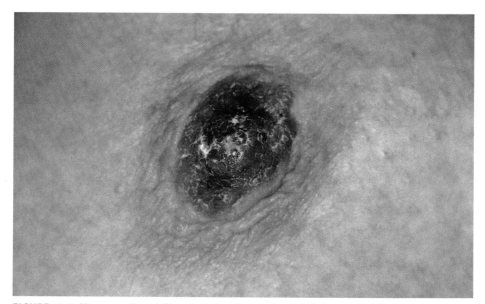

FIGURE 19-8 Mammary Paget disease A sharply demarcated red plaque mimicking eczema or psoriasis on the nipple. The plaque is slightly indurated and there is slight scaling; any red, eczema-like lesion on the nipple and areola that does not respond to topical glucocorticoids should be biopsied.

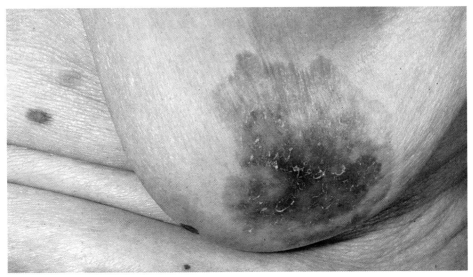

FIGURE 19-9 Mammary Paget disease A sharply defined psoriasiform plaque that has obliterated the areola and nipple. There was a lump in the breast and a small axillary mass.

EXTRAMAMMARY PAGET DISEASE ICD-10: L87.9

- Extramammary Paget disease (EPD) is a neoplasm of the anogenital and axillary skin, histologically identical, and clinically similar to Paget disease of the breast.
- Often representing an intraepidermal extension of a primary adenocarcinoma of underlying apocrine glands or of the lower gastrointestinal, urinary, or female genital tracts.
- Often, however, it is unassociated with underlying cancer.
- The histogenesis of EPD is not uniform. Occurs as an in situ upward extension of an in situ adenocarcinoma in deeper glands (25%). Alternatively, EPD may have a multifocal primary origin in the epidermis and its appendages. Primary tumors in the anorectum can arise within the rectal mucosa or intramural glands.
- Insidious onset, slow spread, plus itching. The lesion presents as erythematous plaque, plus scaling, plus erosion (Fig. 19-10), plus crusting, plus exudation; eczematous-appearing lesions, but borders are sharply defined (Fig. 19-10), geographic configuration. Lesions should always be biopsied.
- Histopathologically, paget cells are dispersed between keratinocytes, occur in clusters, and extend down into adnexal structures (hair follicles and eccrine ducts). Adnexal adenocarcinoma is often found when carefully searched for.
- In perineal/perianal EPD, underlying carcinoma should be searched for by *rectal examination, proctoscopy, sigmoidoscopy,* and *barium enema.* In genital EPD, search for underlying carcinoma by *cystoscopy, intravenous pyelogram;* in vulvar EPD, by *pelvic examination.*
- Differential diagnosis includes all red plaques: eczematous dermatitis, lichen simplex chronicus, lichen sclerosus et atrophicus, lichen planus, intertriginous psoriasis, *Candida* intertrigo, SCC in situ (erythroplasia of Queyrat), human papilloma virus–induced SCC in situ, and amelanotic superficial spreading melanoma.
- EPD is usually much larger than is apparent clinically. Surgical excision must be controlled histologically (Mohs micrographic surgery). If Paget cells are in dermis and regional lymph nodes are palpable, lymph node dissection may improve prognosis, which is related to underlying adenocarcinoma. EPD remains in situ in the epidermis and adnexal epithelium in >65% of cases. When no underlying neoplasm is present, there is nonetheless a high recurrence rate, even after apparently adequate excision; this is due to the multifocal origin in the epidermis and adnexal structures.

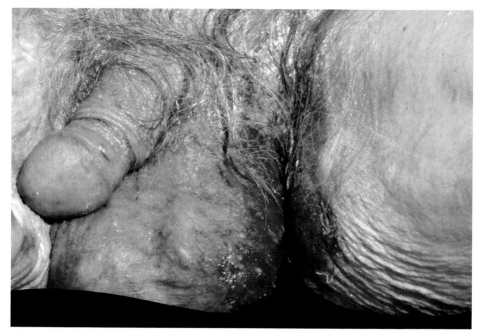

FIGURE 19-10 Extramammary Paget disease Moist, well-demarcated, eroded, oozing, erythematous plaque on the scrotum and inguinal fold in an older male. The lesion is commonly mistaken for *Candida* intertrigo and unsuccessfully treated as such.

COWDEN SYNDROME (MULTIPLE HAMARTOMA SYNDROME)
ICD-10: Q85.9

- Cowden syndrome (named after the propositus) is a rare, autosomal-dominant heritable cancer syndrome with variable expressivity in a number of systems in the form of multiple hamartomatous neoplasms of ectodermal, mesodermal, and endodermal origin.
- Germ-line mutations in the tumor-suppressor gene *PTEN* are located on chromosome 10q22–23 in most cases.
- There is a special susceptibility for breast and thyroid cancers, and the skin lesions are important markers.
- Skin lesions may appear first in childhood and develop over time. They consist of trichilemmomas, skin-colored, pink (**Fig. 19-11B**), or brown papules and have the appearance of flat warts on the central area of the face, lips, and the ears; *translucent punctate keratoses* of the palms and soles; and *hyperkeratotic, flat-topped papules* on the dorsa of the hands and forearms. Mucous membranes: *papules* of the gingival, labial (**Fig. 19-11A**), and palatal surfaces that coalesce, giving a "cobblestone" appearance. *Papillomas* of the buccal mucosa and the tongue.
- In addition to breast cancer (20%), which is often bilateral, and thyroid cancer (8%), there are various internal hamartomas:
  - *Breast:* Fibrocystic disease, fibroadenomas, adenocarcinoma, and gynecomastia in males.
  - *Thyroid:* Goiter, adenomas, thyroglossal duct cysts, and follicular adenocarcinoma.
  - *GI tract:* Hamartomatous polyps throughout tract but increased in large bowel; adenocarcinoma arising in polyp.
  - *Female genital tract:* Ovarian cysts and menstrual abnormalities.
  - *Musculoskeletal:* Craniomegaly, kyphoscoliosis, "adenoid" facies, and high-arched palate.
  - *CNS:* Mental retardation, seizures, neuromas, ganglioneuromas, and meningiomas of the ear canal.
- It is important to establish the diagnosis of Cowden syndrome so that these patients can be followed carefully to detect breast and thyroid cancers early.

FIGURE 19-11 Cowden syndrome
(A) Multiple reddish, confluent papules on the oral mucosa giving a cobblestone appearance. **(B)** Multiple skin-colored warty papules on the face, which represent trichilemmomas.

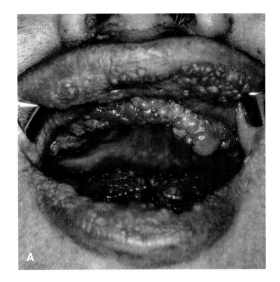

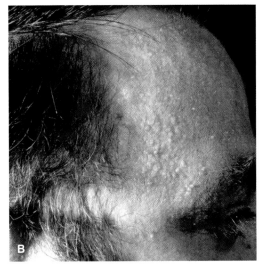

PEUTZ–JEGHERS SYNDROME ICD-10: Q85.8

- Peutz–Jeghers syndrome is a familial (autosomal dominant, spontaneous mutation in 40%) polyposis characterized by many small, pigmented brown macules (lentigines) on the lips, oral mucous membranes (brown to bluish black), and on the bridge of the nose, palms, and soles.
- The gene has been mapped to 19p13.3.
- Macules on the lips may disappear over time, but not the pigmentation of the mouth; therefore, the mouth pigmentation is the sine qua non for the diagnosis (Fig. 19-12).
- There are usually, but not always, multiple hamartomatous polyps in the small bowel, as well as in the large bowel and stomach, that cause abdominal symptoms such as pain, GI bleeding, and anemia.
- Although pigmented macules are congenital or develop in infancy and early childhood, polyps appear in late childhood or before the age of 30 years.
- Adenocarcinoma may develop in polyps, and there is an increased incidence of breast, ovarian, and pancreatic cancer.
- There is a normal life expectancy unless carcinoma develops in the GI tract. Malignant neoplasms may be more frequent in Japanese patients with this syndrome. Prophylactic colectomy has been recommended for these patients.

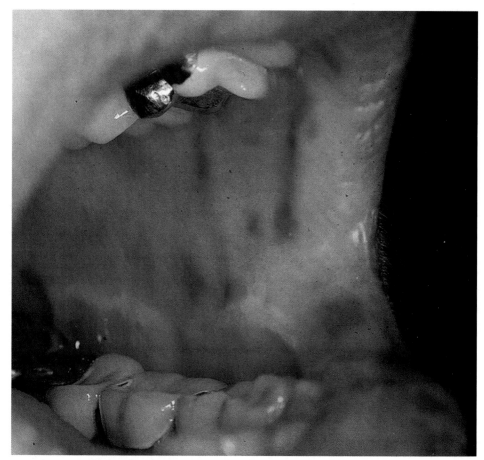

FIGURE 19-12 **Peutz–Jeghers syndrome** Multiple, dark-brown lentigines on the vermilion border of the lip and the buccal mucosa. This patient had GI bleeding due to hamartomatous polyps in the small bowel.

GLUCAGONOMA SYNDROME ICD-10: M8152/0

- Glucagonoma syndrome is a rare but well-described clinical entity caused by excessive production of glucagon in an α-cell tumor of the pancreas.
- Characterized by superficial migratory necrolytic erythema (MNE) with erosions that crust and heal with hyperpigmentation.
- Inflammatory patches and red plaques (**Figs. 19-13** and **19-14**) of gyrate, circinate, arcuate, or annular shape that enlarge with central clearing, resulting in geographic areas that become confluent (**Fig. 19-14**). Borders show vesiculation to bulla formation, crusting, and scaling.
- Lesions involve perioral and perigenital regions and flexures and intertriginal areas.
- Fingertips are red, shining, and erosive (**Fig. 19-15**).
- There is glossitis, angular cheilitis (**Fig. 19-13**), and blepharitis.
- General examination reveals wasting and malnutrition.
- Most cases are associated with glucagonoma, but the pathogenesis of MNE is not known. There exists MNE without glucagonoma.
- *Differential diagnosis*: Includes all moist red plaque(s): Acrodermatitis enteropathica, zinc deficiency, pustular psoriasis, mucocutaneous candidiasis, Hailey–Hailey disease (familial pemphigus).
- *Laboratory*: Fasting plasma glucagon level increased to >1000 ng/L (normal 50 to 250 ng/L) and makes the diagnosis. There is also hyperglycemia, reduced glucose tolerance, severe malabsorption, gross hypoaminoacidemia, and low serum zinc. CT scan angiography will locate tumors within pancreas and metastases in the liver.
- Dermatopathology of early skin lesions shows band-like upper epidermal necrosis with retention of pyknotic nuclei and pale keratinocyte cytoplasm.
- Prognosis depends on the aggressiveness of the glucagonoma. Hepatic metastases have occurred in 75% of patients at the time of diagnosis. If these are slow growing, patients may have prolonged survival, even with metastatic disease.
- MNE responds poorly to all types of therapy. Some cases have responded partially to zinc replacement. MNE resolves after tumor excision. However, surgical excision of glucagonoma achieves a cure in only 30% of cases because of persistent metastases (usually liver). There is poor response to chemotherapy.

FIGURE 19-13 Glucagonoma syndrome: migratory necrolytic erythema Inflammatory dermatosis with angular cheilitis, inflammatory, scaly, erosive, and crusted plaques and fissures around the nose and mouth.

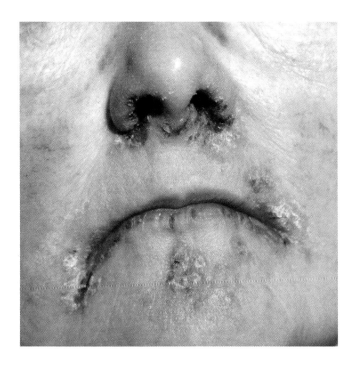

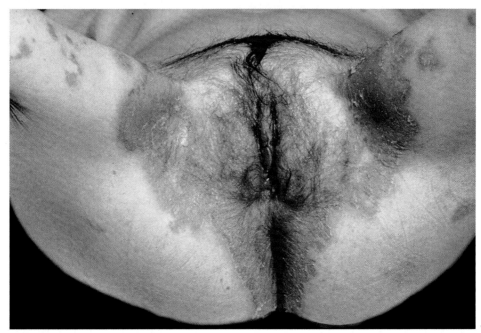

FIGURE 19-14 Glucagonoma syndrome: migratory necrolytic erythema Polycyclic erosions in the anogenital gluteal and sacral regions. Sharply defined with necrotic flaccid epidermis still covering part of these erosions.

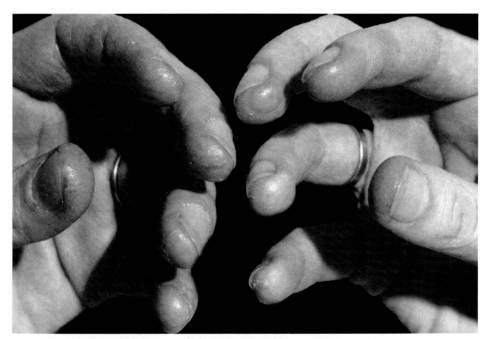

FIGURE 19-15 Glucagonoma syndrome Fingertips are red, glistening, and partially erosive.

MALIGNANT ACANTHOSIS NIGRICANS ICD-10: L83

- Like other forms of acanthosis nigricans (AN) (see Section 5), malignant AN starts as a diffuse, velvety thickening and hyperpigmentation chiefly on the neck, axillae, and other body folds, as well as on the perioral and periorbital, umbilical, mamillary, and genital areas, giving the skin a dirty appearance (see **Fig. 5-1**).
- Malignant AN differs from other forms of AN primarily because of (1) the more pronounced velvety hyperkeratosis and hyperpigmentation, (2) the pronounced mucosal involvement and involvement of the mucocutaneous junction, (3) tripe hands, and (4) weight loss and wasting due to the underlying malignancy.
- AN may precede by 5 years other symptoms of a malignancy, usually adenocarcinoma of the GI or GU tract, bronchial carcinoma, or, less commonly, lymphoma. Malignant AN is a truly paraneoplastic disease, and a search for underlying malignancies is imperative. Removal of malignancy is followed by regression of AN.
- See "Acanthosis Nigricans" in Section 5.

PARANEOPLASTIC PEMPHIGUS (PNP) (PARANEOPLASTIC AUTOIMMUNE MULTIORGAN SYNDROME) ICD-10: L10.82

- Mucous membranes are primarily and most severely involved.
- Lesions combine features of pemphigus vulgaris (Section 6) and erythema multiforme (Section 14), clinically, histologically, and immunopathologically.
- Most prominent clinical findings consist of severe oral (**Fig. 19-16**) and conjunctival erosions in a patient with an underlying neoplasm.
- These neoplasms are in order of frequency: Non-Hodgkin lymphomas, chronic lymphatic leukemia, Castleman disease, thymoma, sarcoma, and Waldenström macroglobulinemia.
- Patients with PNP may also have clinical and serologic evidence of myasthenia gravis and autoimmune cytopenia.
- PNP sera contain autoantibodies to plakin antigens (in the intercellular plaque of desmosomes), envoplakin and periplakin, and to desmoplakin I and II. Less commonly patient sera may contain autoantibodies that recognize bullous pemphigoid antigen (230 kDa), plectin, and plakoglobin.
- Autoantibodies of PNP cause blistering in neonatal mice and are detected by indirect immunofluorescence on rodent urinary bladder epithelium.
- Treatment is directed toward elimination or suppression of malignancy but may also require systemic glucocorticoids.

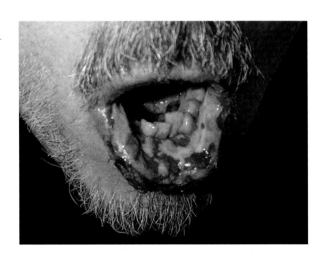

FIGURE 19-16 Paraneoplastic pemphigus Severe erosions covering practically the entire mucosa of the oral cavity partially covered by fibrin. Lesions are extremely painful, interfering with adequate food intake.

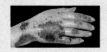

SKIN SIGNS OF HEMATOLOGIC DISEASE

THROMBOCYTOPENIC PURPURA   ICD-10: D69.3

- Thrombocytopenic purpura (TP) is characterized by cutaneous hemorrhages occurring in association with a reduced platelet count.
- Occur at sites of minor trauma/pressure (platelet count <40,000/μL) or spontaneously (platelet count <10,000/μL).
- Due to decreased platelet production, splenic sequestration, or increased platelet destruction.
- *Decreased platelet production.* Direct injury to bone marrow, drugs (cytosine arabinoside, daunorubicin, cyclophosphamide, busulfan, methotrexate, 6-mercaptopurine, vinca alkaloids, thiazide diuretics, ethanol, estrogens), replacement of bone marrow, aplastic anemia, vitamin deficiencies, and Wiskott–Aldrich syndrome.
- *Splenic sequestration.* Splenomegaly and hypothermia.
- *Increased platelet destruction. Immunologic*: Autoimmune TP, drug hypersensitivity (sulfonamides, quinine, quinidine, carbamazepine, digitoxin, or methyldopa), after transfusion. *Nonimmunologic*: Infection, prosthetic heart valves, disseminated intravascular coagulation, and thrombotic TP (microangiopathic hemolytic anemia, thrombocytopenia, neurologic abnormalities, fever and renal disease).
- **Skin Lesions.** *Petechiae*—Small (pinpoint to pinhead), red, nonblanching macules that are not palpable and turn brown as they get older (**Fig. 20-1**); later acquiring a yellowish-green tinge. *Ecchymoses*—Black-and-blue spots; larger area of hemorrhage. *Vibices*—linear hemorrhages (**Fig. 20-1**), due to trauma or pressure. Most common on legs and upper trunk, but may occur anywhere.
- **Mucous Membranes.** *Petechiae*—Most often on palate (**Fig. 20-2**) and gingival bleeding.
- **General Examination.** Possible CNS and internal hemorrhage, anemia.
- **Laboratory Hematology.** Thrombocytopenia.
- **Serology.** Rule out HIV disease; antibodies against ADAMTS 13 (a protease).
- **Lesional Skin Biopsy** (bleeding usually can be controlled by suturing biopsied site) to rule out vasculitis.
- **Differential diagnosis.** Senile purpura, purpura of scurvy, progressive pigmentary purpura (Schamberg disease), purpura following severe Valsalva maneuver (coughing, vomiting/retching), traumatic purpura, factitial or iatrogenic purpura, and vasculitis.
- **Management.** Identify underlying cause and correct, if possible. Oral glucocorticoids, high-dose IV immunoglobulins, or platelet transfusion for chronic ITP (splenectomy may be indicated).

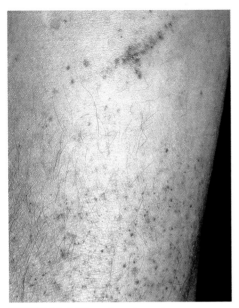

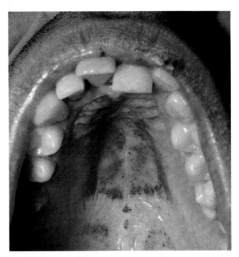

FIGURE 20-2 Thrombocytopenic purpura
Can first manifest on the oral mucosa or conjunctiva. Here, multiple petechial hemorrhages are seen on the palate.

FIGURE 20-1 Thrombocytopenic purpura
Multiple petechiae on the upper arm of an HIV-infected 25-year-old male were the presenting manifestation of his disease. The linear arrangement of petechiae at the site of minor trauma is called vibices.

DISSEMINATED INTRAVASCULAR COAGULATION ICD-10: D65

- Disseminated intravascular coagulation (DIC) is a widespread blood clotting disorder occurring within blood vessels.
- Associated with a wide range of clinical circumstances: Bacterial sepsis, obstetric complications, disseminated malignancy, and massive trauma.
- Manifested by purpura fulminans (cutaneous infarctions and/or acral gangrene) or bleeding from multiple sites.
- The spectrum of clinical symptoms associated with DIC ranges from relatively mild and subclinical to explosive and life threatening.
- *Synonyms*: Purpura fulminans, consumption coagulopathy, defibrination syndrome, and coagulation fibrinolytic syndrome.

EPIDEMIOLOGY

AGE OF ONSET All ages; occurs in children.

ETIOLOGY AND PATHOGENESIS

- *Events that initiate DIC:* Tumor products, crushing trauma, extensive surgery, severe intracranial damage; retained contraception products, placental abruption, amniotic fluid embolism; certain snake bites; hemolytic transfusion reaction; acute promyelocytic leukemia.
- *Extensive destruction of endothelial surfaces:* Vasculitis in Rocky Mountain spotted fever, meningococcemia, or occasionally gram-negative septicemia; group A streptococcal infection, heat stroke, malignant hyperthermia; extensive pump oxygenation (repair of aortic aneurysm); eclampsia, preeclampsia; tufted angioma and Kaposiform hemangioendothelioma; Kasabach–Merritt syndrome; immune complexes; postvaricella purpura gangrenosa.

■ *Events that complicate and propagate DIC:* Shock and complement pathway activation.

Uncontrolled activation of coagulation results in thrombosis and consumption of platelets/clotting factors II, V, and VIII. Secondary fibrinolysis. If the activation occurs slowly, excess activated products are produced, predisposing to vascular infarctions/venous thrombosis. If the onset is acute, hemorrhage surrounding wound sites and IV lines/catheters or bleeding into deep tissues.

CLINICAL MANIFESTATION

Hours to days; rapid evolution. Fever and chills associated with onset of hemorrhagic lesions.
SKIN LESIONS *Infarction (purpura fulminans)* (Figs. 20-3 to 20-5): Massive ecchymoses with sharp, irregular ("geographic") borders with deep purple to blue color (Fig. 20-5) and erythematous halo, ± evolution to hemorrhagic bullae (Fig. 20-3), and blue to black gangrene (Fig. 20-5); multiple lesions are often symmetric; distal extremities, areas of pressure; lips, ears, nose, and trunk; peripheral acrocyanosis followed by gangrene on the hands, feet, and tip of nose, with subsequent autoamputation if patient survives.

Hemorrhage from multiple cutaneous sites, i.e., surgical incisions, venipuncture, or catheter sites.
MUCOUS MEMBRANES Hemorrhage from gingiva.
GENERAL EXAMINATION High fever, tachycardia, ± shock. Multitude of findings depending on the associated medical/surgical problem.

LABORATORY EXAMINATIONS

DERMATOPATHOLOGY Occlusion of arterioles with fibrin thrombi. Dense neutrophilic infiltrate around infarct and massive hemorrhage.
HEMATOLOGIC STUDIES **CBC.** Schistocytes (fragmented RBCs), arising from RBC entrapment and damage within fibrin thrombi, seen on blood smear; platelet count low. Leukocytosis.
Coagulation Studies. Reduced plasma fibrinogen; elevated fibrin degradation products; prolonged prothrombin time, partial thromboplastin time and thrombin time.
BLOOD CULTURE For bacterial sepsis.

DIAGNOSIS AND DIFFERENTIAL DIAGNOSIS

Clinical suspicion confirmed by coagulation studies. Differential diagnosis of *large cutaneous infarctions*: Necrosis after initiation of warfarin therapy, heparin necrosis, and calciphylaxis, atheroembolization.

COURSE AND PROGNOSIS

Mortality rate is high. Surviving patients require skin grafts or amputation for gangrenous tissue. Common complications: Severe bleeding, thrombosis, tissue ischemia/necrosis, hemolysis, and organ failure.

MANAGEMENT

Vigorous antibiotic therapy for infections. Control bleeding or thrombosis: Heparin, pentoxifylline, protein C concentrate, intravenous immunoglobulin, and FFP.

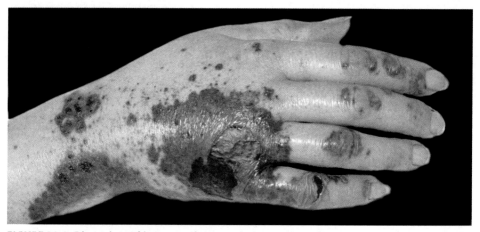

FIGURE 20-3 Disseminated intravascular coagulation: purpura fulminans Extensive geographic area of cutaneous infarction with hemorrhage involving the hand. Similar lesions were on the face, the other hand, and the feet.

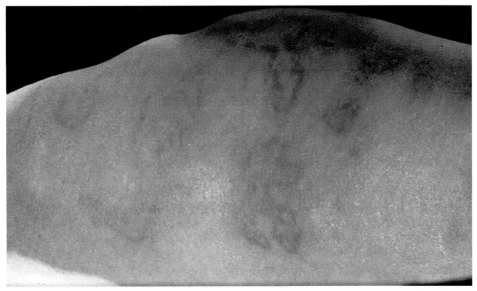

FIGURE 20-4 Extensive cutaneous infarction with hemorrhage involving the entire leg This catastrophic event followed sepsis after abdominal surgery.

FIGURE 20-5 Disseminated intravascular coagulation: purpura fulminans Geographic cutaneous infarctions on the chest; lesions were also present on the hands, elbows, thighs, and feet. The patient was a diabetic with *Staphylococcus aureus* sepsis.

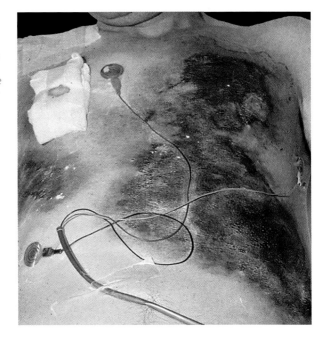

CRYOGLOBULINEMIA ICD-10: D89.1

- Cryoglobulinemia (CG) is the presence of serum immunoglobulin (precipitates at low temperature and redissolves at 37°C) complexed with other immunoglobulins or proteins.
- Associated clinical findings include purpura in cold-exposed sites, Raynaud phenomenon, cold urticaria, acral hemorrhagic necrosis, bleeding disorders, vasculitis, arthralgia, neurologic manifestations, hepatosplenomegaly, and glomerulonephritis.
- Precipitation of cryoglobulins (when present in large amounts) causes vessel occlusion, and is also associated with hyperviscosity.
- Platelet aggregation/consumption of clotting factors by cryoglobulins, causing coagulation disorder.
- Immune complex deposition followed by complement activation and vasculitis.

ETIOLOGY AND PATHOGENESIS

Type I Cryoglobulins: Monoclonal immunoglobulins (IgM, IgG, IgA, light chains). *Associated with* plasma cell dyscrasias such as multiple myeloma, Waldenström macroglobulinemia, lymphoproliferative disorders such as B cell lymphoma.

Type II Cryoglobulins: Mixed cryoglobulins: Two immunoglobulin components, one of which is monoclonal (usually IgG, less often IgM) and the other polyclonal. *Associated with* multiple myeloma, Waldenström macroglobulinemia, chronic lymphocytic leukemia; rheumatoid arthritis, systemic lupus erythematosus, and Sjögren syndrome.

Type III Cryoglobulins: Polyclonal immunoglobulins that form cryoprecipitate with polyclonal IgG or a nonimmunoglobulin serum component occasionally mixed with complement and lipoproteins. Represents immune complex disease. *Associated with* autoimmune diseases; connective tissue diseases; wide variety of infectious diseases, i.e., hepatitis B, hepatitis C, Epstein–Barr virus infection, cytomegalovirus infection, subacute bacterial endocarditis, leprosy, syphilis, and streptococcal infections.

CLINICAL MANIFESTATION

There is cold sensitivity in <50% of cases. Chills, fever, dyspnea, and diarrhea may occur following cold exposure. Purpura also may follow long periods of standing or sitting. Due to other organ system involvement, arthralgia, renal symptoms, neurologic symptoms, abdominal pain, and arterial thrombosis.

- *Noninflammatory purpura* (usually type I), occurring at cold-exposed sites, e.g., helix (Fig. 20-6) or the tip of the nose.

- *Acrocyanosis* and *Raynaud phenomenon*, with or without severe resultant gangrene of fingertips and toes or elsewhere on arms or legs (usually type I or II) (Fig. 20-7).
- *Palpable purpura* with bullae and necroses (usually types II and III) due to hypersensitivity vasculitis, occurring in crops on lower extremities with extension to thighs and abdomen; precipitated by standing up (Fig. 20-8), less commonly by cold.
- *Livedo reticularis* mostly on lower and upper extremities.
- *Urticaria* induced by cold, associated with purpura.
- *Systemic involvement*: Between 30% and 60% of individuals with essential mixed

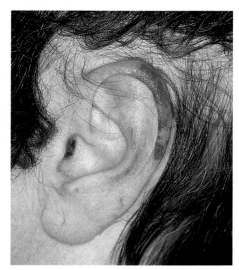

FIGURE 20-6 **Cryoglobulinemia: monoclonal (type I)** This noninflamed, purpuric lesion on the helix appeared on the first cold day in the fall.

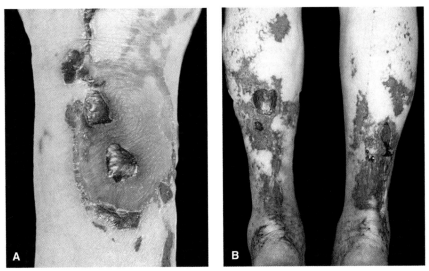

FIGURE 20-7 Cryoglobulinemia: mixed (type II) (A) Extensive necrosis and hemorrhage on the skin of the forearm. There was also digital gangrene on hands and feet. **(B)** Extensive hemorrhagic necrosis on both legs. There was also acral gangrene on four toes.

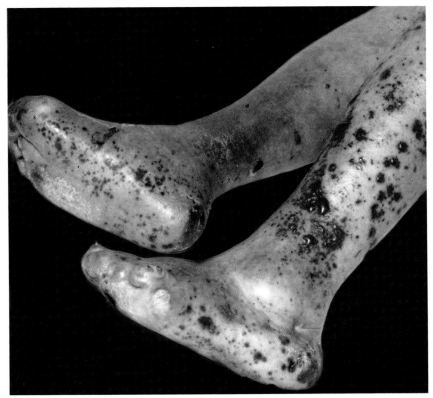

FIGURE 20-8 Cryoglobulinemia: polyclonal (type III) Palpable purpura with widespread hemorrhagic blisters and necrosis as in any other type of hypersensitivity vasculitis (compare with Fig. 14-57). Patient had diabetes and amputation of several toes.

CG (type II) develop renal disease with hypertension, edema, or renal failure. Neurologic involvement manifests as peripheral sensorimotor polyneuropathy, presenting as paresthesias or foot drop. Arthritis. Hepatosplenomegaly.

- *Diagnosis* is confirmed by determination of cryoglobulins (blood drawn into warmed syringe, RBC removed via warmed centrifuge; plasma refrigerated in a Wintrobe tube at 4°C for 24 to 72 h, then centrifuged and cryocrit determined) and diagnosis of underlying disease.
- The *course* is characterized by cyclic eruptions induced by cold or fluctuations of the activity of the underlying disease.
- *Treatment* is that of the underlying disease. Idiopathic disease can be treated with plasmapheresis, oral corticosteroids, and mycophenolate mofetil.

LEUKEMIA CUTIS ICD-10: C92.3

- Leukemia cutis (LC) is a localized or disseminated skin infiltration by leukemic cells. It is usually a sign of dissemination of systemic disease or relapse of existing leukemia. The term aleukemic leukemia cutis describes a rare disorder in which extracutaneous evidence of recurrent leukemia cannot be ascertained. Prognosis tends to be poor.
- Incidence varies from <5% to 50%, depending on the type of leukemia, both acute and chronic, including the leukemic phase of non-Hodgkin lymphoma and hairy cell leukemia.
- Most commonly occurs with acute monocytic leukemia M5 and acute myelomonocytic leukemia M4.
- Most common lesions are small (2 to 5 mm) papules (**Figs. 20-9** and **20-10**), nodules (**Figs. 20-11** and **20-12**), or plaques. LC lesions are usually somewhat more pink, violaceous, or darker than normal skin, always palpable, indurated, and firm.
- Localized or disseminated; usually on the trunk (**Fig. 20-9**), extremities (**Fig. 20-11**), and the face (**Fig. 20-10**) but may occur at any site. May be hemorrhagic when associated with thrombocytopenia or may ulcerate (**Fig. 20-12**). Erythroderma may (rarely) occur. Leukemic gingival infiltration (hypertrophy) occurs with acute monocytic leukemia.
- *Inflammatory disorders* occurring in patients with leukemia are modified by the participation of leukemic cells in the infiltrate, resulting in unusual presentations of such disorders, e.g., psoriasis with hemorrhage or erosions/ulcerations.
- Cutaneous inflammatory diseases that may be associated with leukemia are Sweet syndrome, bullous pyoderma gangrenosum, urticaria, and necrotizing vasculitis.
- Systemic symptoms are those associated with hematologic malignancy.
- The *diagnosis* is made by suspicion and verified by skin biopsy, immunophenotyping, and B- or T-cell receptor rearrangement studies. Hematologic studies with complete analysis of bone marrow aspirate and peripheral blood smear.
- The prognosis for LC is directly related to the prognosis for the systemic disease.
- *Therapy* is usually directed at the leukemia itself. However, systemic chemotherapy sufficient for bone marrow remission may not treat the cutaneous lesions effectively. Thus, a combination of systemic chemotherapy and local electron beam therapy or PUVA may be necessary for chemotherapy-resistant LC lesions. Intralesional chemotherapy has been used in management of localized, single, or a few lesions.

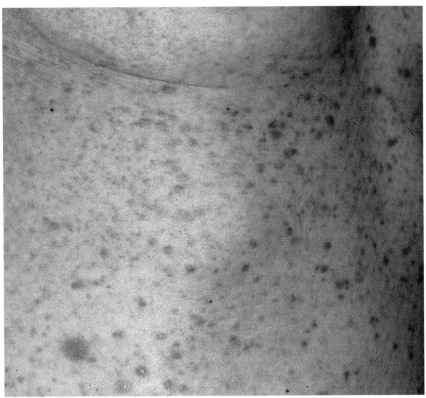

FIGURE 20-9 Leukemia cutis Hundreds of tan-pink papules and a nodule on the trunk of a female with acute myelogenous leukemia arose during a 1-week interval. These lesions are "nonspecific" and do not present a diagnosis, but when such an eruption is seen, one should perform a peripheral blood count and a biopsy.

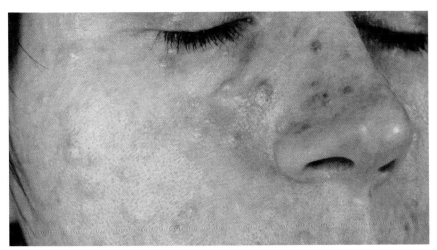

FIGURE 20-10 Leukemia cutis Multiple skin-colored and erythematous papules in a 38-year-old febrile woman that had erupted about 1 week before this picture was taken. The patient had acute myelogenous leukemia.

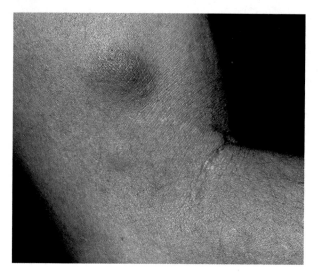

FIGURE 20-11 Leukemia cutis
A large, dark brown nodule on the upper arm of a male with acute myelogenous leukemia; six similar nodules were also present on the trunk.

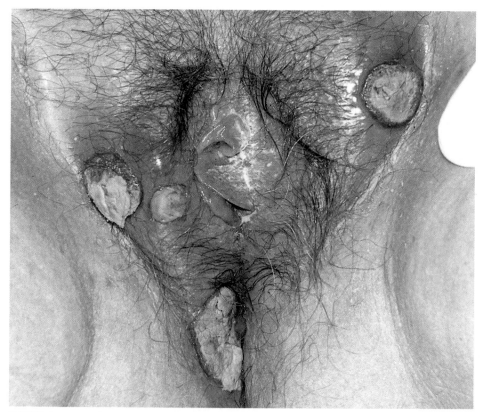

FIGURE 20-12 Leukemia cutis: chloroma Large, ulcerated, green-hued tumors (chloromas) in the inguinal and perineal regions of a female with acute myelogenous leukemia; similar lesions were also present in the axillae and on the tongue.

LANGERHANS CELL HISTIOCYTOSIS ICD-10: D76.0

- Langerhans cell histiocytosis (LCH) is an idiopathic group of disorders characterized histologically by proliferation and infiltration of tissue by Langerhans cell–type histiocytes that fuse into multinucleated giant cells and form granulomas with eosinophils.
- Etiology: A reactive versus neoplastic nature of LCH is debated.
- LCH is characterized clinically by cutaneous findings that range from soft-tissue swelling to seborrheic dermatitis–like changes to papular, pustular lesions, erosions, and ulcerations.
- Systemic lesions affect bones (lytic erosions), lungs, bone marrow, liver, spleen, and lymph nodes.
- The course is variable, ranging from localized self-healing forms to generalized and fatal cases.
- Therapy depends on the extent of the disease and systemic involvement.

CLASSIFICATION

The disorders of histiocytes are classified as LCH (LCH, formerly histiocytosis X), non-LCH,[1] and malignant histiocytosis. LCH is newly classified as shown in Table 20-1.

EPIDEMIOLOGY

AGE OF ONSET **Unifocal LCH.** Most commonly, childhood and early adulthood.
Multifocal unisystem LCH. Most commonly, childhood.
Multifocal multisystem LCH (previously Letterer-Siwe disease). Mostly seen in children under 2 years of age.
Pulmonary LCH. Mostly in cigarette smokers. The triad of diabetes insipidus, exophthalmos and lytic bone lesions was previously referred to as Hand-Schuller Christian disease.
SEX Males > females.
INCIDENCE Rare, estimated 0.5 per 100,000 children (estimate).

PATHOGENESIS

The stimulus for the proliferation of Langerhans cells is unknown. A reactive versus neoplastic nature is debated.

CLINICAL MANIFESTATION

UNIFOCAL LCH Systemic symptoms uncommon. Pain and/or swelling over underlying bony lesion. Disruption of teeth with mandibular disease, fracture, and otitis media due to mastoid involvement.
MULTIFOCAL LCH Erosive skin lesions are exudative, pruritic, or painful and may have an offensive odor. Otitis media caused by destruction of temporal and mastoid bones, proptosis due to orbital masses, loose teeth with infiltration of maxilla or mandible, pituitary dysfunction with involvement of sella turcica associated with growth retardation, and diabetes insipidus. Lung involvement associated with chronic cough or pneumothorax.

Skin Lesions

Unifocal LCH. (*Eosinophilic Granuloma*)

- Swelling over bony lesions (e.g., humerus, rib, or mastoid) and tender.

TABLE 20-1 Classification of LCH

Unifocal LCH	Most commonly manifested by a single osteolytic bony or skin or soft-tissue lesion
Multifocal LCH	Bony lesions are multiple and interfere with function of neighboring structures. Multifocal LCH also involves skin (second most frequently involved organ), soft tissue, lymph nodes, lungs, and pituitary glands. Rarely, thyroid gland may also be involved.
Clinical syndromes	
Eosinophilic granuloma	Unifocal skin, mucous membranes, or soft-tissue lesions
Hand–Schüller–Christian disease	The chronic, progressive multifocal form of LCH with skin and systemic involvement
Letterer–Siwe disease	The most aggressive multifocal LCH form, with skin and systemic involvement
Hashimoto–Pritzker syndrome	A benign, self-healing variant of LCH in childhood

[1]For the non-Langerhans cell histiocytoses, the reader is referred to Gelmeti C and Caputo R in Wolff K et al. (eds.), *Fitzpatrick's Dermatology in General Medicine*, 7th ed. New York, McGraw-Hill, 2008:1424–1434.

- Cutaneous/subcutaneous nodule, yellowish, may be tender and break down, occurring anywhere.
- Sharply marginated ulcer, usually in genital and perigenital regions or oral mucous membrane (gingival or hard palate). Necrotic base, draining, and tender (Fig. 20-13).

Multifocal LCH. As in unifocal LCH; in addition, regionally localized (head) or generalized (trunk) eruptions. Papulosquamous, seborrheic dermatitis–like (scaly, oily), eczematous dermatitis–like lesions (Fig. 20-14); sometimes vesicular or purpuric (Fig. 20-15). Turn necrotic and may become heavily crusted. Removal of crusts leaves small, shallow punched-out ulcers that heal with scars. Intertriginous lesions coalesce, may be erosive and exudative, become secondarily infected, and ulcerate. Mandibular and maxillary bone involvement may result in loss of teeth (Fig. 19-13). Ulceration of vulva and/or anus (Fig. 20-16).

GENERAL FINDINGS **Multifocal LCH.** Bony lesions occur in calvarium, sphenoid bone, sella turcica, mandible, long bones of upper extremities, and vertebrae. Associated findings of pituitary involvement.

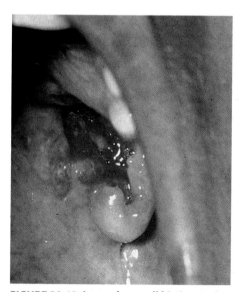

FIGURE 20-13 Langerhans cell histiocytosis: eosinophilic granuloma Solitary, ulcerated nodule with loss of teeth on the gingival ridge near the palate, associated with involvement of the maxillary bone. Lesion was asymptomatic and only when the molars were lost did the patient consult a physician.

Multifocal multisystem (HSCD). Lytic skull lesions, proptosis, diabetes mellitus, and skin lesions.

LSD. Hepatosplenomegaly, lymphadenopathy, involvement of lungs and other organs, and bone marrow; thrombocytopenia as well as widespread and ulcerating skin lesions (Figs. 20-15 and 20-16).

LABORATORY EXAMINATIONS

HISTOPATHOLOGY Proliferation of Langerhans cells with abundant pale eosinophilic cytoplasm and indistinct cell borders; a folded, indented, kidney-shaped nucleus with finely dispersed chromatin; epidermotropism. Langerhans cells in LCH have to be recognized by histochemical, and immunohistochemical markers [S-100 protein, CD1a, and CD207 (Langerin)]. In the past, morphologic, ultrastructural (Birbeck granules) were needed for diagnosis, but is now rarely done.

COURSE AND PROGNOSIS

UNIFOCAL LCH Benign course with excellent prognosis for spontaneous resolution but tissue destruction.

MULTIFOCAL LCH Spontaneous remissions possible. Prognosis poorer at extremes of age and with extrapulmonary involvement.

MANAGEMENT

UNIFOCAL LCH Curettage with or without bony chip packing. Low-dose (300 to 600 rad) radiotherapy. Intralesional corticosteroids. Extraosseous soft-tissue lesions: Surgical excision or low-dose radiotherapy.

MULTIFOCAL LCH Diabetes insipidus and growth retardation treated with vasopressin and human growth hormone. Low-dose radiotherapy to bony lesions. Systemic treatment with glucocorticoids and/or vinblastine, given as single agents or in combination and etoposide. Nonresponders: Polychemotherapy (vincristine and cytarabine and prednisone or vincristine and doxorubicin and prednisone), cladribine (2-chlorodeoxyadenosine). Bone marrow transplantation is an option.

CUTANEOUS LESIONS Glucocorticoids for discrete cutaneous lesions. Also topical tacrolimus, imiquimod. Extensive or generalized: Cutaneous lesions respond best to PUVA or topical nitrogen mustard but also to oral thalidomide. In rare cases, when the disease expresses CD30, brentuximab has been of clinical benefit.

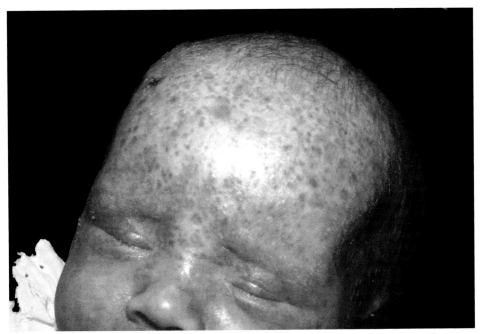

FIGURE 20-14 Langerhans cell histiocytosis Erythema and small, orange papules with a greasy scale on the face and scalp in this infant. These were the only lesions at first presentation and were mistaken for infantile seborrheic dermatitis. After lesions proved refractory to topical treatment and additional purpuric and crusted lesions appeared on the trunk, a biopsy was performed and the correct diagnosis was established.

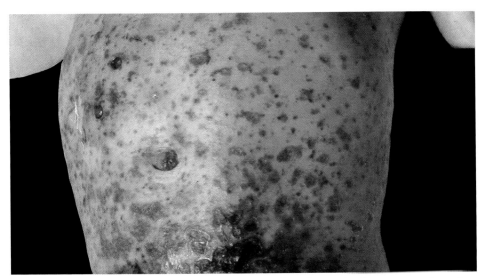

FIGURE 20-15 Langerhans cell histiocytosis: Letterer–Siwe disease Erythematous papules and vesicles with purpura and crusting, becoming confluent on the abdomen of an infant. Some lesions have ulcerated and are crusted.

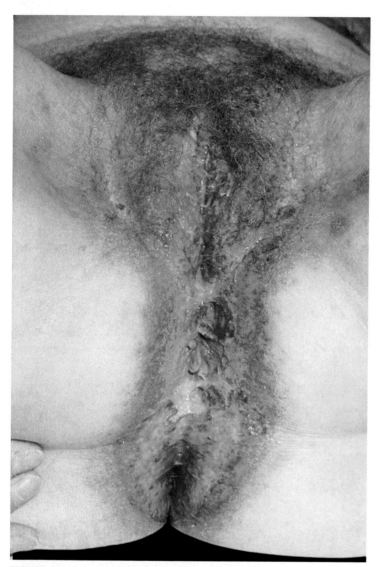

FIGURE 20-16 Langerhans cell histiocytosis: Letterer–Siwe disease in an adult Confluent erythematous plaques with necrosis and ulceration in the ano-genital and perineal region in a 65-year-old female.

MASTOCYTOSIS SYNDROMES ICD-10: Q82.2

- Mastocytosis is an abnormal accumulation of mast cells in the skin and at various organs.
- An abbreviated WHO classification of mastocytosis is shown in Table 20-2.
- The skin is the most commonly involved organ system.
- Skin lesions are localized nodular or generalized maculopapular (Table 20-3).
- Because of the release of pharmacologically active substances, cutaneous symptoms are urticarial swelling or blistering with pruritus; systemic symptoms are blushing, vomiting, diarrhea, headache, and syncope.
- Most patients with mastocytosis have only skin involvement, and most of these have no systemic symptoms. However, up to half of patients with systemic mastocytosis may not have any skin findings.

EPIDEMIOLOGY

AGE OF ONSET Between birth and 2 years of age (55%) (NCM, PPCM, UP), but mastocytosis can occur at any age; infancy-onset mastocytosis is rarely associated with systemic mastocytosis.
SEX Slight male preponderance.
PREVALENCE Unknown.

PATHOGENESIS

Human mast cell proliferation depends on the Kit ligand and the Kit is the receptor for the stem cell factor. c-*kit* mutations have been identified in the blood and tissues of patients with mastocytosis. Mast cells contain several pharmacologically active substances that are associated with the clinical findings in mastocytosis: Histamine (urticaria or GI symptoms), prostaglandin D_2 (flush, cardiovascular symptoms, bronchoconstriction, or GI symptoms), heparin (bleeding into tissue or osteoporosis), neutral protease/acid hydrolases (patchy hepatic fibrosis or bone lesions).

CLINICAL MANIFESTATION

Stroking lesion causes it to itch and to wheal (*Darier sign*) (see generalized mastocytosis, below: generalized. Various drugs are capable of causing mast cell degranulation and release of pharmacologically active substances that exacerbate skin lesions (whealing and itching) and cause flushing such as alcohol, dextran, polymyxin B, morphine, codeine, scopolamine, d-tubocurarine, and nonsteroidal anti-inflammatory drugs. Flushing episode can also be elicited by heat or cold and may be accompanied by headache, nausea, vomiting, diarrhea, dyspnea/wheezing, and syncope. Systemic involvement may lead to symptoms of malabsorption; portal hypertension. Bone pain. Neuropsychiatric symptoms (malaise and/or irritability).
SKIN LESIONS (CM) LOCALIZED **NCM.** Macular to papular to nodular lesions (mastocytoma) (Fig. 20-17), often solitary; may be multiple, but few. Yellow to tan-pink, which become erythematous and raised (urticate) when stroked due to degranulation of mast cells (Darier sign); in some patients, lesions become bullous.
GENERALIZED **PPCM.** Tan, occasionally yellowish plaques, up to 2 to 5 cm, sharply defined with irregular outlines. Darier sign positive (Fig. 20-18). No scaling, occasionally with bulla formation after rubbing. Occurs mostly in infants and children.

TABLE 20-2 Abbreviated WHO Classification of Mastocytosis

Cutaneous mastocytosis (CM)
Indolent systemic mastocytosis (ISM)
Systemic mastocytosis with an associated clonal hematologic nonmast cell lineage disease (SM-AHNMD)
Aggressive systemic mastocytosis (ASM)
Mast cell leukemia (MCL)
Mast cell sarcoma (MCS)
Extracutaneous mastocytoma

Source: Reproduced with permission from Jaffe ES, et al, eds. *WHO Classification of Tumours: Pathology and Genetics of Tumours of the Haematopoietic and Lymphoid Tissues.* Lyon: IARC Press; 2001.

TABLE 20-3 Classification of Cutaneous Mastocytosis (CM)

Localized	Nodular CM (mastocytoma, NCM)
Generalized	Maculopapular CM (MPCM)
	Papular plaque CM (PPCM)
	Urticaria pigmentosa (UP)
	Telangiectasia macularis eruptiva perstans (TMEP)
	Diffuse CM (DCM)

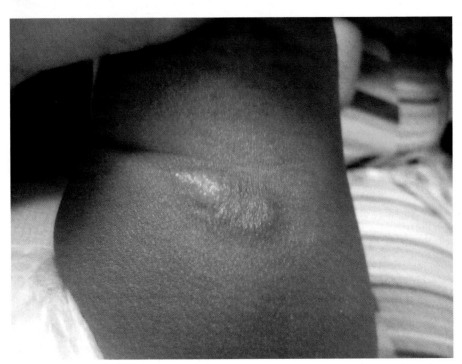

FIGURE 20-17 Mastocytosis: solitary mastocytoma (NCM) A single, tan plaque with poorly demarcated borders on the posterior calf of an infant. When stroked vigorously, the lesion became erythematous, raised, and a blister developed. (Used with permission from Jennifer Tan, MD.)

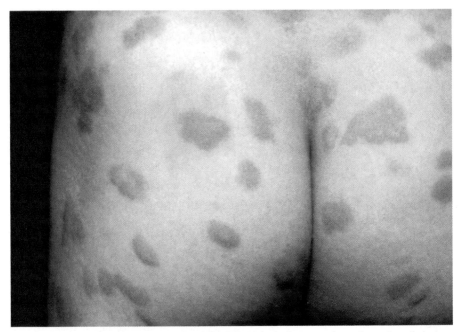

FIGURE 20-18 Mastocytosis: generalized (PPCM) Multiple, flat-topped papules and small plaques of brownish to yellowish color on the buttocks of a child. Lesions are asymptomatic. Rubbing one of the lesions on the left buttock has resulted in urtication and an axon flare, a positive Darier sign, and itching.

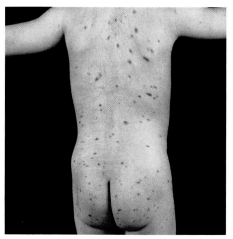

FIGURE 20-19 Mastocytosis: urticaria pigmentosa (UP) Multiple, generalized tan to brown papules in a child. The patient had occasional syncopes, diarrhea, and wheezing; workup revealed systemic mastocytosis.

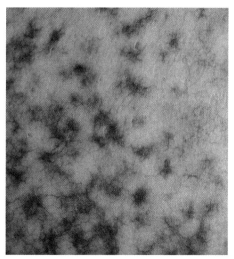

FIGURE 20-20 Mastocytosis: telangiectasia macularis eruptiva perstans (TMEP) Small, stellate erythematous macules and telangiectases on the back of a 45-year-old woman who had systemic (indolent) mastocytosis.

UP. Tan macules to slightly raised tan to brown papules (Fig. 20-19). Disseminated, few or >100 with widespread symmetric distribution. Darier sign (whealing) after rubbing; in infants, may become bullous. Occurs in infancy and/or de novo in adults. Bright red diffuse flushing occurring spontaneously, after rubbing of skin, or after ingestion of alcohol or mast cell-degranulating agents.

TMEP. Freckle-like, brownish to reddish macules (Fig. 20-20) with fine telangiectasia in long-standing lesions. Hundreds of lesions, on the trunk > extremities; lesions may be confluent. Urticate with gentle stroking. Dermatographism. Occur only in adults and very rare.

DCM. Yellowish, thickened appearance of large areas of skin; "doughy." Smooth with scattered elevation, resembling leather; "pseudoxanthomatous mastocytosis," skin folds exaggerated, especially in axilla/groin. Large bullae may occur after trauma or spontaneously. DCM may present as erythroderma (Fig. 20-21). Very rare, occurs at all ages.

LABORATORY EXAMINATIONS

DERMATOPATHOLOGY Accumulation of normal-looking mast cells in dermis. Mast cell infiltrates may be sparse (spindle-shaped) or densely aggregated (cuboidal shape) and have

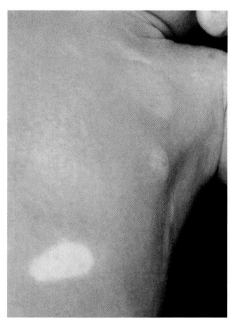

FIGURE 20-21 Mastocytosis: diffuse cutaneous mastocytosis (DCM) The skin of this infant is uniformly erythematous (erythroderma) secondary to infiltrating mast cells with several spared, white areas of normal skin. In this child, there were systemic symptoms associated with the flare of erythroderma: syncope, wheezing, and diarrhea.

a perivascular or nodular distribution. Various stains and immunoperoxidase methods can be used in difficult cases (metachromatic toluidine blue and Giemsa), such as tryptase and C-kit.

CBC Systemic mastocytosis: Anemia, leukocytosis, eosinophilia.

BLOOD Tryptase levels ↑, coagulation parameters.

URINE Patients with extensive cutaneous involvement may have increased 24-h urinary histamine excretion.

BONE SCAN AND IMAGING Define bone involvement (lytic bone lesions, osteoporosis, or osteosclerosis) and endoscopy for small-bowel involvement.

BONE MARROW Smear and/or biopsy for morphology and mast cell markers.

DIAGNOSIS

Clinical suspicion, positive Darier sign, confirmed by skin biopsy.

DIFFERENTIAL DIAGNOSIS

NCM Juvenile xanthogranuloma, Spitz nevus.

FLUSHING Carcinoid syndrome.

UP, PPCM, TMEP LCH, secondary syphilis, papular sarcoid, generalized eruptive histiocytoma, and non-LCH of childhood.

DCM Cutaneous T-cell lymphoma, pseudoxanthoma elasticum, and forms of erythroderma.

COURSE AND PROGNOSIS

Most cases of solitary mastocytosis and generalized UP and PPCM in children resolve spontaneously. They rarely have systemic involvement. Adults with onset of UP or TMEP with extensive cutaneous involvement have a higher risk for development of systemic mastocytosis (see Table 20-2). In young children, acute and extensive degranulation may be life threatening (shock).

MANAGEMENT

Avoidance of drugs that may cause mast cell degranulation and histamine release (see the preceding).

Antihistamines, both H_1 and H_2, either alone or with ketotifen. Disodium cromoglycate, 200 mg four times a day, may ameliorate pruritus, flushing, diarrhea, abdominal pain, and disorders of cognitive function but not skin lesions. Imatinib for patients with a KIT mutation at the F522C position but ineffective with other KIT mutations. PUVA treatment is effective for disseminated skin lesions, but recurrence is common. Vascular collapse is treated with epinephrine. NCM responds to potent glucocorticoid ointments under occlusion or to intralesional triamcinolone acetonide but may eventually recur.

CUTANEOUS LYMPHOMAS AND SARCOMA

■ Cutaneous lymphomas are clonal proliferations of neoplastic T or B cells, rarely natural killer cells, or plasmacytoid dendritic cells. Cutaneous lymphomas are the second most common group of extra-nodal lymphomas. The annual incidence is estimated to be 1 per 100,000.

ADULT T CELL LEUKEMIA/LYMPHOMA ICD-10: C83/E88

■ Adult T cell leukemia/lymphoma (ATLL) is a neoplasm of CD4+/CD25+ T cells, caused by human T cell lymphotrophic virus I (HTLV-I).

■ Manifested by skin infiltrates, hypercalcemia, visceral involvement, lytic bone lesions, and abnormal lymphocytes on peripheral smears.

■ HTLV-I is a human retrovirus. Infection by the virus does not usually cause disease, which suggests that other environmental factors are involved. Immortalization of some infected CD4+ T cells, increased mitotic activity, genetic instability, and impairment of cellular immunity can all occur after infection with HTLV-I.

■ ATLL occurs in southwestern Japan (Kyushu), Africa, the Caribbean Islands, and the southeastern United States. Transmission is by sexual intercourse, perinatally, or by exposure to blood or blood products (same as HIV).

■ There are four main categories. In the relatively indolent *smoldering* and *chronic* forms, the median survival is ≥2 years. In the *acute* and *lymphomatous* forms, it ranges from only 4 to 6 months.

■ Symptoms include fever, weight loss, abdominal pain, diarrhea, pleural effusion, ascites, cough, and sputum. Skin lesions occur in 50% of patients with ATLL. Single to multiple small, confluent erythematous, violaceous papules (Fig. 21-1), ±purpura; firm violaceous to brownish nodules (Fig. 21-2); papulosquamous lesions, large plaques, ±ulceration; trunk > face > extremities; generalized erythroderma; poikiloderma; diffuse alopecia. Lymphadenopathy (75%) sparing mediastinal lymph nodes. Hepatomegaly (50%) and splenomegaly (25%).

■ Patients are seropositive (ELISA, Western blot) to HTLV-I; in IV drug users, up to 30% have dual retroviral infection with both HTLV-I and HIV. WBC ranges from normal to 500,000/μL. Peripheral blood smears show polylobulated lymphocytic nuclei ("flower cells"). *Dermatopathology* reveals lymphomatous infiltrates composed of many large abnormal lymphocytes, ±giant cells, ±Pautrier microabscesses. There is hypercalcemia in 25% at time of diagnosis of ATLL and in >50% during clinical course; this is thought to be caused by osteoclastic bone resorption.

■ Management consists of various regimens of cytotoxic chemotherapy; the rates of complete response are <30% and responses lack durability, but good results have been obtained with the combination of oral zidovudine and subcutaneous interferon-α in acute and lymphoma-type ATLL patients. Allogeneic hematopoietic stem cell transplantation has shown some promise.

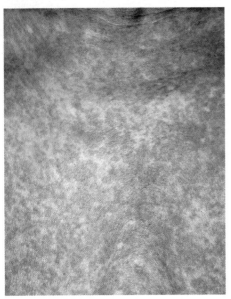

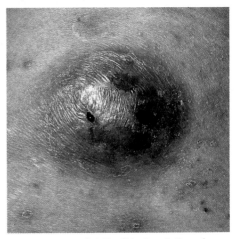

FIGURE 21-2 Adult T cell leukemia/lymphoma
Firm, violaceous to brownish nodules as shown here are another cutaneous manifestation of ATLL. These nodules may ulcerate.

FIGURE 21-1 Adult T cell leukemia/lymphoma
A generalized eruption of small, confluent violaceous papules with a predilection for the trunk. The patient had fever, weight loss, abdominal pain, massive leukocytosis with "flower cells" in smear, lymphadenopathy, hepatosplenomegaly, and hypercalcemia.

CUTANEOUS T CELL LYMPHOMA ICD-10: C84.0/C84.1

- Cutaneous T cell lymphoma (CTCL) is a term that applies to T cell lymphoma first manifested in the skin, but since the neoplastic process involves the entire lymphoreticular system, the lymph nodes and internal organs become involved in the course of the disease. CTCL is a malignancy of helper T cells (CD4+) but CD8 + predominant subtypes are also diagnosed.
- In the classic form of CTCL, called *mycosis fungoides* (MF), the malignant cells are cutaneous CD4+ cells, but the clinical entity of MF has now been expanded to the spectrum of CTCL including non-MF CTCLs.
- Whereas all MF is CTCL not all CTCLs are MF.
- Only the classic MF form is discussed here.

MYCOSIS FUNGOIDES (MF) ICD-10: C84.0/C84.1

- MF is the most common cutaneous lymphoma.
- Arising in mid-to-late adulthood with male predominance of 2:1.
- A clonal proliferation of skin-homing CTLA+ CD4+ T cells with an admixture of CD8+ T cells (antitumor response).
- Categorized as patch, plaque, or tumor stage.
- Related features are pruritus, alopecia, palmoplantar hyperkeratosis, and bacterial infections.
- Histologically, epidermotropism of T cells with hyperconvoluted nuclei. In the tumor stage, dermal nodular infiltrates.
- Prognosis related to stage.
- Treatment: Symptom-oriented and stage-adapted.

EPIDEMIOLOGY AND ETIOLOGY

AGE OF ONSET Median age at diagnosis 55 to 60 years.
SEX Male:female ratio 2:1.
INCIDENCE Uncommon but not rare.
ETIOLOGY Unknown. CTCL is a malignancy of skin-homing CTLA+ CD4+ T cells.

CLINICAL MANIFESTATIONS

For months to years, often preceded by various diagnoses such as psoriasis, nummular dermatitis, and "large plaque" parapsoriasis. Symptoms: Pruritus, often intractable, but may be none.
SKIN FINDINGS Skin lesions are classified into patches, plaques, and tumors. Patients may have simultaneously more than one type of lesion.
Patches. Randomly distributed, scaling or nonscaling patches in different shades of red (Fig. 21-3). Well- or ill-defined; at first superficial, much like eczema or psoriasis (Figs. 21-3 and 21-4) or mimicking dermatophytosis ("mycosis"), and later becoming thicker.
Plaques. Round, oval, but often also arciform, annular, and of bizarre configuration (Figs. 21-3 and 21-5). Lesions are randomly distributed but in early stages often spare exposed areas.
Tumors. Later lesions consist of nodules (Figs. 21-5 and 21-6) and tumors, with or without ulceration (Fig. 21-7). Extensive infiltration can cause leonine facies (Fig. 21-8). Confluence may lead to erythroderma (see Section 8). There is palmoplantar keratoderma and there may be hair loss. Poikiloderma may be present from the onset or develop later (Fig. 21-9).
GENERAL EXAMINATION Lymphadenopathy, usually after thick plaques and nodules have appeared.

LABORATORY EXAMINATIONS

DERMATOPATHOLOGY Bandlike and patchy infiltrate in upper dermis of atypical lymphocytes (mycosis cells) extending to epidermis and skin appendages. The classic finding is the epidermotropism of this T cell infiltrate, which will form microabscesses in the epidermis (Pautrier microabscesses). Fibroplasia of the upper dermis is often seen. Some cases fail to show significant lymphocytic atypia. In the plaque and tumor stage, the infiltrate extends deep into the dermis and beyond. Mycosis cells are T cells with hyperchromatic, irregularly shaped (cerebriform) nuclei. Mitoses vary from rare to frequent.

Mycosis cells are activated monoclonal CTLA+ CD4+ T cells. However, lesions of MF often have a CD8+ T cell component, and these cells are considered to reflect an antitumor response.
HEMATOLOGY Eosinophilia, 6 to 12%, can increase to 50%. Buffy coat: Abnormal circulating T cells (mycosis cell-type) and increased WBC (20,000/μL). Bone marrow examination

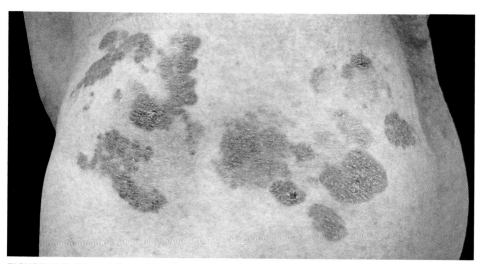

FIGURE 21-3 Mycosis fungoides In early stages, lesions consist of randomly distributed, well- and/or ill-defined patches and later plaques as shown here in a 37-year-old male. They may be scaly and appear in various shades of red. They mimic eczema, psoriasis, or dermatophytosis.

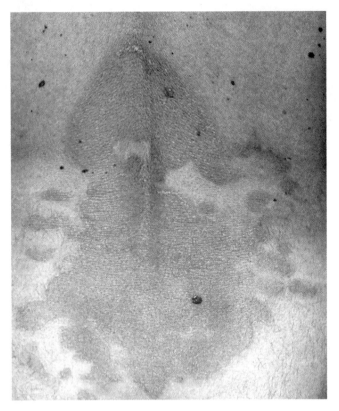

FIGURE 21-4 Mycosis fungoides: patches/plaque stage More advanced stages show confluence of patches and plaques with irregular configuration. This patient had been treated unsuccessfully for psoriasis for 2 years. Morphologically, he could also have extensive, confluent dermatophytosis (see Section 26), but a negative KOH preparation ruled out this diagnosis. Only after a biopsy had been done was the correct diagnosis of MF made.

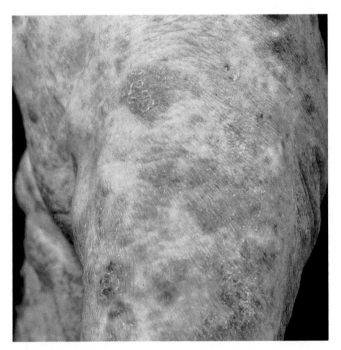

FIGURE 21-5 Mycosis fungoides Plaque and early nodular stage with reddish-brownish scaly, and crusted plaques and flat nodules.

FIGURE 21-6 Mycosis fungoides: tumor stage Scaly and crusted eczema-like plaques seen on the arm and chest have turned nodular on the shoulder. This patient had similar lesions elsewhere and was staged IIB (T_3 N_1 M_0).

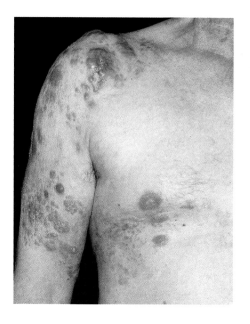

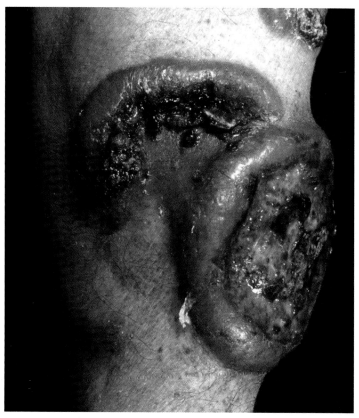

FIGURE 21-7 Mycosis fungoides: tumors Two large ulcerated tumors on the lower leg of a 58-year-old man. These lesions look like mushrooms.

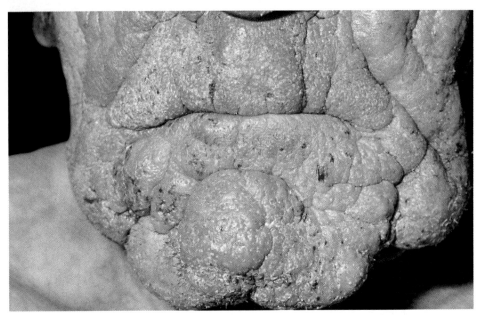

FIGURE 21-8 **Mycosis fungoides: leonine facies** In this 50-year-old patient, the disease had started with extremely pruritic, generalized eczema-like plaques on the trunk that had been treated as eczema over a course of 4 years. Massive nodular infiltration of the face occurred only recently leading to a leonine facies.

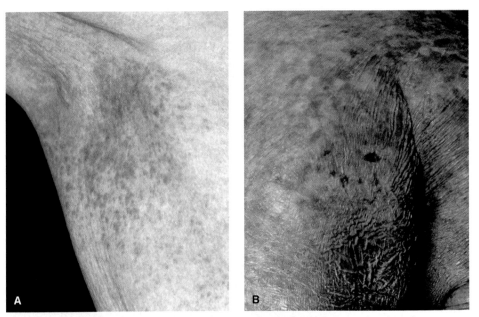

FIGURE 21-9 **Mycosis fungoides: poikilodermatous lesions** **(A)** Small reticulated, confluent papules mixed with superficial atrophy give the impression of poikiloderma. This patient had patches elsewhere on the body similar to those shown in **Fig. 20-3**. **(B)** Poikiloderma in MF can also result from treatment. This patient had been treated with electron beam.

is not helpful in early stages. Peripheral blood cytometry can also be helpful in detecting abnormal ratio of CD4+ cells. T cell receptor studies can be used to detect clonal expansion. IMAGING In stage I and stage II disease, diagnostic imaging (CT, gallium scintigraphy, liver–spleen scan, and lymphangiography) does not provide more information than biopsies of lymph nodes.

CT Scan. With more advanced disease, to search for retroperitoneal nodes in patients with extensive skin involvement, lymphadenopathy.

DIAGNOSIS AND DIFFERENTIAL DIAGNOSIS

In the early stages, the diagnosis of MF is a problem. Clinical lesions may be typical, but histologic confirmation may not be possible for years despite repeated biopsies. Immuno-phenotyping of infiltrating T cells by use of monoclonal antibodies and T cell receptor rearrangement studies. Lymphadenopathy and the detection of abnormal circulating T cells in the blood appear to correlate well with *internal* organ involvement.

DIFFERENTIAL DIAGNOSIS Mainly *scaling plaques.* High index of suspicion is needed in patients with atypical or refractory "psoriasis," "eczema," and poikiloderma. MF often mimics psoriasis in being a scaly plaque and disappearing with exposure to sunlight.

PATIENT EVALUATION IN MF AND STAGING This has to focus on an evaluation of tumor burden, the degree of atypia of malignant cells, and the state of immunocompetence of the patient. Table 21-1 shows a flow sheet of patient evalua-tion, and Table 21-2 shows the TNM classifica-tion and staging of MF.

TABLE 21-1 Patient Evaluation in MF

Skin
  Body surface area assessment
  Routine histology
  Immunophenotyping
  Polymerase chain reaction for T cell receptor
    rearrangement

Blood
  Complete blood count with smear examination
  Immunophenotyping

Lymph node
  Palpate all nodes
  Measure enlarged nodes by CT scan
  Biopsy enlarged nodes

COURSE AND PROGNOSIS

Unpredictable; MF (pre-MF) may be present for years. Course varies with tumor stage and the source of the patients studied. At the NIH,

---

TABLE 21-2 TNM Staging of Mycosis Fungoides

Classification	Definition
Stage	
T1	Patches, plaques, or both involving <10% body-surface area
T2	Patches, plaques, or both involving 10% of body-surface area
T3	One or more cutaneous tumors
T4	Erythroderma
N0	Lymph nodes clinically uninvolved
N1	Lymph nodes clinically palpable but histologically uninvolved
N2	Lymph nodes clinically nonpalpable but histologically involved
N3	Lymph nodes clinically enlarged and histologically involved
Nx	Abnormal lymph nodes, no histology available
M0	No visceral disease
M1	Visceral disease
B0	No circulating atypical cells (Sézary cells)
B1	Circulating atypical cells (Sézary cells)
B2	High tumor burden (>1000/μL Sézary cells)
Stage groups	
IA	T1N0M0
IB	T2N0M0
IIA	T1 or 2N1M0
IIB	T3N0–1M0
IIIA	T4N0M0
IIIB	T4N1M0
IVA	T1 to 4N2 to 3 M0
IVB	T1 to 4N0 to 3 M1

Source: Data from E Olsen et al: Revisions to the staging and classification of mycosis fungoides and Sezary syndrome: a proposal of the International Society for Cutaneous Lymphomas (ISCL) and the cutaneous lymphoma task force of the European Organization of Research and Treatment of Cancer (EORTC). Blood. 110:1713, 2007.

there was a median survival time of 5 years from the time of the histologic diagnosis, while in Europe a less malignant course is seen (survival time, up to 10 to 15 years). This, however, may result from patient selection. Prognosis is much worse when (1) tumors are present (mean survival, 2.5 years), (2) there is lymphadenopathy (mean survival, 3 years), (3) >10% of the skin surface is involved with pretumor-stage MF, and (4) there is a generalized erythroderma. Patients <50 years have twice the survival rate of patients >60 years.

MANAGEMENT

Therapy is symptom-oriented and extent of disease- and stage-adapted. In the pre-MF stage, in which the histologic diagnosis is only compatible, but not confirmed, PUVA photochemotherapy or narrowband UVB treatment is most effective. For histologically proven plaque-stage disease with no lymphadenopathy and no abnormal circulating T cells, PUVA photochemotherapy is also the method of choice, either alone or combined with oral isotretinoin or bexarotene or subcutaneous interferon-α. Also used at this stage are topical chemotherapy with nitrogen mustard in an ointment base (10 mg/dL), topical carmustine (BCNU) (for limited body surface area involvement), and total-body electron-beam therapy, singly or in combination. Isolated tumors are treated with local x-ray or electron-beam therapy. For extensive plaque stage with multiple tumors or in patients with lymphadenopathy or abnormal circulating T cells, electron-beam plus chemotherapy is probably the best combination for now; randomized, controlled studies of various combinations are in progress. Also, extracorporeal PUVA photochemotherapy is being evaluated in patients with Sézary syndrome, the leukemic form of the disease (see below).

MYCOSIS FUNGOIDES VARIANTS

- *Folliculotropic MF*: With preferential involvement of head and neck, with or without mucinosis, degeneration of hair follicles (previously "mucinosis follicularis," "alopecia mucinosa") (**Fig. 21-10**).
- *Hypopigmented MF*: Hypopigmented patches in patients with dark skin.
- *Pagetoid reticulosis (Woringer–Kolopp disease)* This is a special variant of MF consisting of *localized* patches and plaques (**Fig. 21-11**), with a proliferation of neoplastic T cells that expand intraepidermally following a pattern similar to Paget disease. Extracutaneous dissemination has not been observed, and there is an excellent prognosis.
- *Granulomatous slack skin*: Rare subtype of MF with folds of lax skin in the major skin folds (**Fig. 21-12**).
- *Sézary syndrome*: A leukemic variant, see page 470 and Section 8.

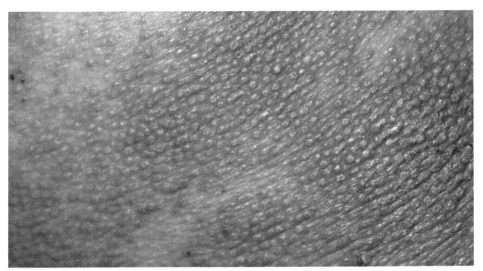

FIGURE 21-10 Folliculotropic MF Multiple small follicular papules. This is called "mucinosis follicularis."

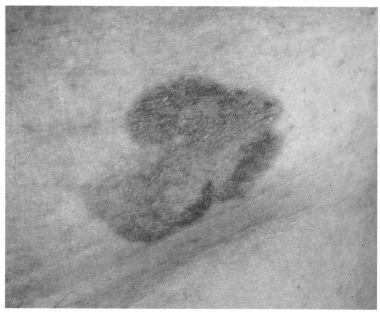

FIGURE 21-11 Pagetoid reticulosis This singular plaque in the groin of a 53-year-old woman looks like psoriasis with minimal scale. It was asymptomatic and had been present for 10 months. Histopathology revealed intraepidermal T cells in a pagetoid pattern.

FIGURE 21-12 Granulomatous slack skin Firm, platelike infiltrates on the neck and anterior chest and lax skin folds of the axillary and scapular region.

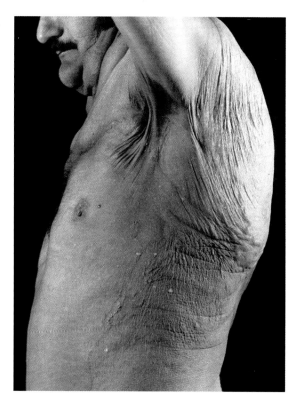

SÉZARY SYNDROME ICD-10: L84.1

- Sézary syndrome is a rare special variant of MF characterized by universal erythroderma, peripheral lymphadenopathy, and cellular infiltrates of atypical lymphocytes (Sézary cells) in the skin and in the blood.
- The disease may arise de novo or, less commonly, result from extension of a preexisting circumscribed MF. It usually occurs in patients >60 years and more commonly in males than in females.
- Patients appear sick, shivering, and scared and there is generalized scaling erythroderma with considerable thickening of the skin. Because of the bright red color, the syndrome has been called the "red man syndrome" (see Section 8 and **Fig. 8-3**). There is diffuse hyperkeratosis of the palms and soles, diffuse hair loss that can lead to baldness, and generalized lymphadenopathy.
- *Dermatopathology*: The same as MF but it may be much more subtle. The lymph nodes may contain nonspecific inflammatory cells (dermatopathic lymphadenopathy) or there can be a complete replacement of the nodal pattern by Sézary cells. The cell infiltrates in the viscera are the same as are present in the skin. *Immunophenotyping*: CD4+ T cells; T cell receptor rearrangement: monoclonal process. There may be a moderate leukocytosis or a normal WBC. The buffy coat contains from 15% to 30% atypical lymphocytes (Sézary cells).
- Diagnosis rests on three features: Erythroderma, generalized lymphadenopathy, and the presence of increased numbers of atypical lymphocytes in the buffy coat.
- Note that any exfoliative dermatitis can mimic Sèzary syndrome (see Section 8).
- Without treatment, the course is progressive and patients die from opportunistic infections. Management is as in MF, plus appropriate supportive measures required for erythroderma (see Section 8).

LYMPHOMATOID PAPULOSIS ICD-10: L41.2

- Lymphomatoid papulosis is an asymptomatic, chronic, self-healing, polymorphous eruption of unknown etiology.
- It is a low-grade, self-limited T cell lymphoma with a low but real risk of progression to more malignant forms of lymphoma.
- Incidence is 1.2 to 1.9 cases per million, occurring sporadically in both sexes from childhood to old age; average age 40 years.
- Characterized by recurrent crops of lesions that regress spontaneously, with histologic features of lymphocytic atypia.
- Pathogenesis unknown; considered to be a low-grade lymphoma perhaps induced by chronic antigenic stimulation and controlled by host mechanisms. It belongs in the spectrum of primary cutaneous CD30+ lymphoproliferative disorders.
- Close clinical resemblance to pityriasis lichenoides et varioliformis acuta (see **Fig. 3-23A and B**). Erythematous to red-brown papules (**Fig. 21-13**) and nodules, 2 to 5 mm in diameter, which are initially smooth and hemorrhagic, later hyperkeratotic, with central, black necrosis, crusting (**Fig. 21-13**), and ulceration. Few to hundreds of lesions, asymptomatic or pruritic, arranged at random and often grouped, recurrent, primarily on trunk and extremities; rarely, oral and genital mucosa. Individual lesions evolve over a 2- to 8-week period and resolve spontaneously. Atrophic hyper- or hypopigmented scarring following ulcerated lesions.
- Other organ systems are uninvolved.
- *Dermatopathology*: Superficial or deep, perivascular or interstitial mixed cell infiltrate, or wedge-shaped. Atypical cells may comprise 50% of infiltrate. *Type A*: Large CD30+, atypical histioid lymphocytes with abundant cytoplasm and convoluted nucleus. *Type B*: Smaller CD30–, atypical lymphocytes with cerebriform nuclei. *Type C*: Large CD30+ cells form sheets resembling cutaneous anaplastic large cell lymphoma (CACL, see p. 472).
- *Differential diagnosis*: Based on typical histology and immunohistochemistry, lack of systemic involvement by history and physical examination.
- *Course*: May remit in 3 weeks or continue for decades. In 10 to 20% of patients, lymphomatoid papulosis is preceded by, associated with, or followed by another type of lymphoma: MF, Hodgkin disease, or CD30+CALCL. May persist despite systemic chemotherapy for concurrent lymphoma.
- No treatments have proved consistently effective. Topical agents include glucocorticoids and carmustine (BCNU). Electron-beam irradiation, PUVA. Retinoids, methotrexate, chlorambucil, cyclophosphamide, cyclosporine; brentuximab, and interferon-α2b, none with lasting effect.

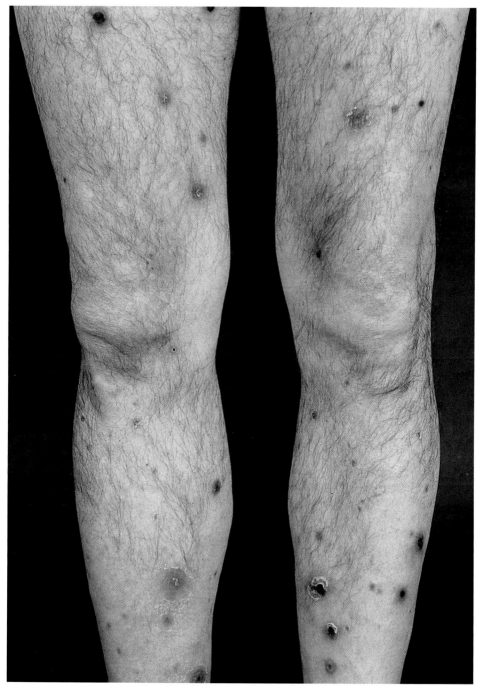

FIGURE 21-13 **Lymphomatoid papulosis** Crops of reddish-brown papules appear in waves involving the entire body. Lesions are asymptomatic, become hyperkeratotic, crusted, and necrotic in the center. Since lesions arise asynchronously, all stages in this evolution are present simultaneously.

CUTANEOUS ANAPLASTIC LARGE CELL LYMPHOMAS (CALCLS) ICD-10: 84.43

- CALCLs are cutaneous lymphomas consisting of large tumor cells that express CD30 antigen and have no evidence or history of lymphomatoid papulosis, MF, or other types of CTCL.
- They occur in adults and present as solitary, reddish to brownish nodules and tumors, which frequently tend to ulcerate (**Fig. 21-14**).
- The nodular infiltrates are nonepidermotropic, and neoplastic cells show an anaplastic morphology. At least 75% of the neoplastic cells are CD30+ and additionally express the CD4+ phenotype. Other markers have been used to determine whether the tumor is primary to skin or systemic, but follow up studies have shown that this approach is not reliable.
- CALCLs have a favorable prognosis with a disease-related 5-year survival rate of 90%.
- Treatment is radiotherapy, but successful treatment with PUVA in combination with interferon-α has been reported.

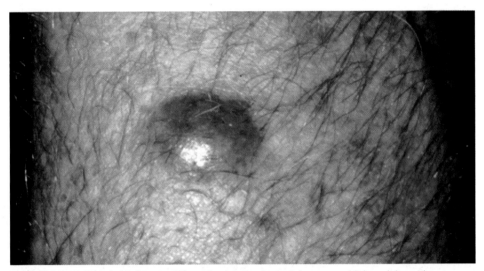

FIGURE 21-14 Anaplastic large cell lymphoma A solitary violaceous, reddish nodule on the forearm of a 46-year-old male patient. Histopathology revealed nonepidermotropic anaplastic mononuclear cells, most of which were of the CD4+, CD30+ phenotype. The lesion was excised and there was no recurrence.

CUTANEOUS B CELL LYMPHOMA ICD-10: C85.1

- A clonal proliferation of B lymphocytes can be confined to the skin or more often is associated with systemic B cell lymphoma. Rare. It comprises 20% of all cutaneous lymphomas.
- Occurs in individuals >50 years.
- Crops of asymptomatic nodules and plaques, red to plum color (Fig. 21-15) with a smooth surface, firm, nontender, cutaneous, or subcutaneous.
- Primary cutaneous follicle center cell lymphoma, primary cutaneous marginal zone lymphoma, primary cutaneous diffuse large B cell lymphoma (non-leg and leg types) and intravascular large B-cell lymphoma (not primarily cutaneous but affects skin: mantle cell lymphoma, lymphomatoid granulomatosis, chornic lymphocytic leukemia, and Nurkit lymphoma) are special defined entities.
- *Dermatopathology*: Dense nodular or diffuse monomorphous infiltrates of lymphocytes usually separated from the epidermis by a zone of normal collagen ("grenz zone"). B cell-specific monoclonal antibody studies facilitate differentiation of cutaneous B cell lymphoma from pseudolymphoma and CTCL and permit more accurate classification of the cell type. Most cases react with CD19, 20, 22, and 79A. Gene-typing studies confirm diagnosis with immunoglobulin gene rearrangement, usually IgH.
- Patients should be investigated thoroughly for nodal and extracutaneous disease; if found, bone marrow, lymph node, and peripheral blood studies will show morphologic, cytochemical, and immunologic features similar to those of the cutaneous infiltrates.
- *Management*: Consists of X-ray therapy to localized lesions and chemotherapy for systemic disease.

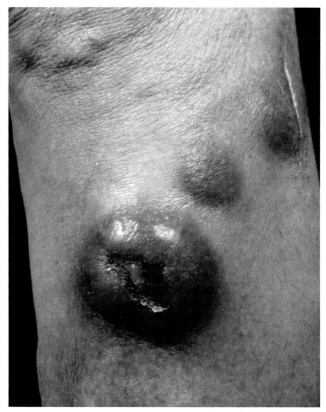

FIGURE 21-15 Cutaneous B cell lymphoma Smooth, cutaneous, and subcutaneous nodules on the lower leg. One is ulcerated. They were asymptomatic and firm and were the first signs of B cell lymphoma.

KAPOSI SARCOMA (KS) ICD-10: C46

- KS is a multifocal systemic tumor of endothelial cell origin.
- Invariably linked with human herpes virus type 8 (HHV-8) infection.
- Four clinical variants: Classic KS, endemic African KS, immunosuppressive therapy-related KS, and HIV/AIDS-related KS.
- Stage- and variant-dependent localized and/or generalized disease: patches, plaques, and nodules.
- Systemic involvement: Mainly GI tract and lung.
- Responds to radiation and chemotherapy.

ETIOPATHOGENESIS

DNA of HHV-8 has been identified in tissue samples of all variants of KS. There is seroepidemiologic evidence that this virus is involved in the pathogenesis.

CLASSIFICATION AND CLINICAL VARIANTS

CLASSIC OR EUROPEAN KS Occurs in elderly males of eastern European heritage (Mediterranean and Ashkenazi Jewish). Not so uncommon in eastern and southern Europe; rare in the United States. Males > females. Predominantly arises on the legs but also occurs in lymph nodes and abdominal viscera; slowly progressive.

AFRICAN-ENDEMIC KS Between 9% and 12.8% of all malignancies in Zaire. Two distinct age groups: young adults, mean age 35; and young children, mean age 3 years. Males > females. No evidence of underlying immunodeficiency. Four clinical patterns (see below).

IATROGENIC IMMUNOSUPPRESSION-ASSOCIATED KS Rare. Most commonly in solid-organ transplant recipients as well as individuals treated chronically with immunosuppressive drugs. Arises on average 16.5 months after transplantation. Resolves on cessation of immunosuppression.

HIV/AIDS-ASSOCIATED KS In HIV-infected individuals, the risk for KS is 20,000 times than that of the general population, 300 times than that of other immunosuppressed individuals. Despite a decline in recent years, KS is still the most common tumor in male homosexual patients with AIDS. Rarely women may have HIV/AIDS-associated KS. Associated with HIV infection, rapid progression, and extensive systemic involvement. At the time of initial presentation, one in six HIV-infected individuals with KS have CD4+ T cell counts of ≤500/μL. However, as of late, tumors have been reported significantly after reconstitution.

Rare variants have recently permeated the literature, in non-HIV-infected, non-mediterranean, non-iatrogenically immunosuppressed patients. Generally, young men appear over represented in these rare cohorts.

PATHOGENESIS

KS cells are likely derived from the endothelium of the blood/lymphatic microvasculature. KS lesions produce factors that promote their own growth as well as the growth of other cells, but it is not known how HHV-8 induces/promotes proliferation of endothelial cells.

CLINICAL MANIFESTATION

Mucocutaneous lesions are usually asymptomatic but are associated with significant cosmetic stigma. At times, lesions may ulcerate and bleed easily. Large lesions on the palms or soles may impede function. Lesions on the lower extremities that are tumorous, ulcerated, or associated with significant edema often give rise to moderate-to-severe pain. Urethral or anal canal lesions can be associated with obstruction. GI involvement rarely causes symptoms but can lead to obstruction and bleeding in late stages. Pulmonary KS can cause bronchospasm, intractable coughing, shortness of breath, and progressive respiratory failure.

SKIN LESIONS KS most often begins as an ecchymotic-like macule (Fig. 21-16). Macules evolve into patches, papules, plaques (Figs. 21-16 to 21-18), nodules, and tumors that are violaceous, red, pink, or tan and become purple-brownish (Figs. 21-16 and 21-19) with a greenish hemosiderin halo as they age. Often oval initially, and on the trunk often arranged parallel to skin tension lines (Fig. 21-20). Lesions may initially occur at sites of trauma, usually in the acral regions (Fig. 21-18). In time, individual lesions may enlarge and

FIGURE 21-16 Classic Kaposi sarcoma
Ecchymotic purple-brownish confluent macules
and a 1-cm nodule on the dorsum of the hand
of a 65-year-old male of Ashkenazi-Jewish extraction. The lesion was originally mistaken for a bruise
as were similar lesions on the feet and on the
other hand. The appearance of brownish nodules
together with additional macules prompted a referral of this otherwise completely healthy patient to
a dermatologist who diagnosed Kaposi sarcoma,
which was verified by biopsy. There is also onychomycosis of all fingernails.

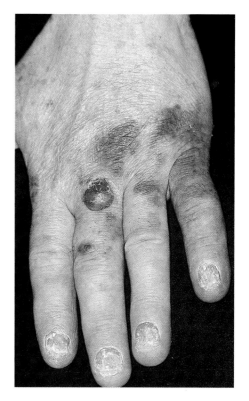

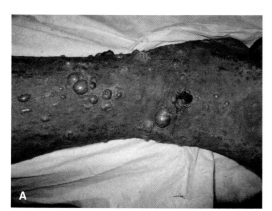

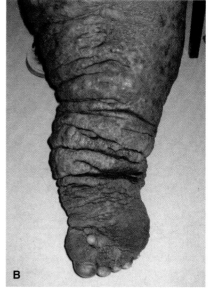

FIGURE 21-17 HIV/AIDS-associated Kaposi sarcoma (A) Multiple violaceous papules and nodules,
some coalescing and spontaneously ulcerative. Infiltration is noted surrounding the primary lesion. The
leg has become edematous caused by lymphatic involvement. **(B)** In more advanced cases, complete
obliteration of lymphatic vessels leads to an elephantiasis-like picture, often asymmetrical. Discrete violaceous papulo-nodules can still be seen (Used with permission from Adam Lipworth, MD).

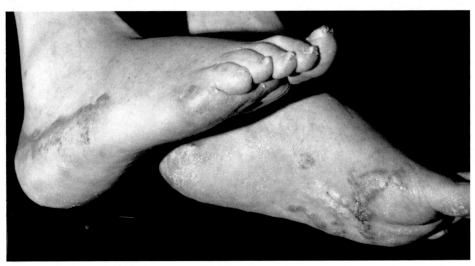

FIGURE 21-18 Classic Kaposi sarcoma of the feet Brownish to blue nodules and plaques, partially hyperkeratotic on the soles and lateral aspects of the feet. This is a typical localization of early classic KS.

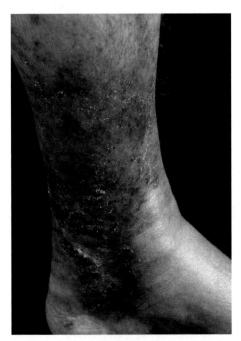

FIGURE 21-19 Classic Kaposi sarcoma Black confluent papules on the lower leg that are reminiscent of hyperpigmented stasis dermatitis in chronic venous insufficiency. Involvement of lymphatics has led to pronounced edema of the calf. This indicates that the disease process is further advanced.

become confluent, forming tumor masses. Secondary changes to larger nodules and tumors include erosion, ulceration, crusting, and hyperkeratosis.

Lymphedema usually occurs on the lower extremities (Figs. 21-17 and 21-19) and results from confluent masses of lesions caused by deeper involvement of lymphatics and lymph nodes. Distal edema may initially be unilateral but later becomes symmetric and involves not only the lower legs but also the genitalia and/or face.

Distribution. Widespread or localized. In classic KS, lesions almost always occur on the feet and legs or the hands, and slowly spread centripetally (Figs. 21-16 and 21-19). The tip of the nose (Fig. 21-17), periorbital areas, ears, and scalp as well as penis and legs may also be involved, but involvement of the trunk is rare. In HIV/AIDS-associated KS, there is early involvement of the face and widespread distribution on the trunk (Fig. 21-20).

MUCOUS MEMBRANES Oral lesions are the first manifestation of KS in 22% of cases; HIV/AIDS-associated KS is often a marker for CD4+ T cell counts of <200/μL but exceptions exist. Very common (50% of individuals) on the hard palate, appearing first as a violaceous stain, which evolves into papules and nodules with a cobblestone appearance (see Section 33).

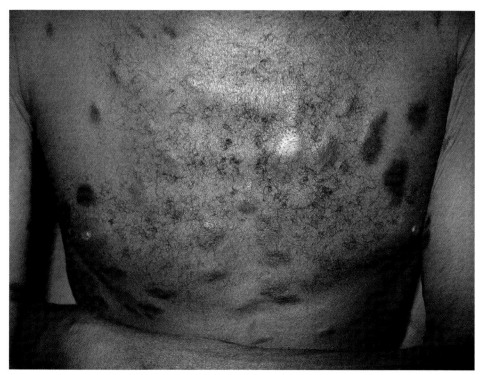

FIGURE 21-20 HIV/AIDS-associated Kaposi sarcoma Multiple purplish plaques and nodules on the chest of a homosexual AIDS patient. The patient had CD4+ T cell counts <200/μL. (Used with permission from Adam Lipworth, MD).

Lesions also arise on soft palate, uvula, pharynx, gingiva, and tongue. Conjunctival lesions are uncommon.

Special Features of African-Endemic KS (non-HIV associated). Four clinical patterns are recognized:

- Nodular type: Runs a rather benign course with a mean duration of 5 to 8 years and resembles classic KS.
- Florid or vegetating type: Characterized by more aggressive biologic behavior; it is also nodular but may extend deeply into the subcutis, muscle, and bone.
- Infiltrative type: Shows an even more aggressive course with florid mucocutaneous and visceral involvement.
- Lymphadenopathic type: Predominantly affects children and young adults. Frequently confined to lymph nodes and viscera, but

occasionally also involves the skin and mucous membrane.

GENERAL EXAMINATION *Viscera* KS lesions of the viscera, though common, are often asymptomatic. This is particularly true for classic KS. An autopsy of HIV-infected individuals with mucocutaneous KS, reveal that 75% have visceral involvement (bowel, liver, spleen, or lungs).

Lymph Nodes. Lymph nodes are involved in half of the cases of HIV/AIDS-associated KS and in all cases of African lymphadenopathic type KS.

Urogenital Tract. Prostate, seminal vesicles, testes, bladder, penis, and scrotum.

Lung. Pulmonary infiltrates, particularly in HIV-associated KS.

GI Tract. GI hemorrhage, rectal obstruction, protein-losing enteropathy can occur

Other. Heart, brain, kidney, and adrenal glands.

LABORATORY EXAMINATIONS

SKIN BIOPSY Vascular channels lined by atypical endothelial cells among a network of reticulin fibers and extravasated erythrocytes with hemosiderin deposition. In the *nodular stage*: Spindle cells in sheets and fascicles with mild-to-moderate cytologic atypia, single cell necrosis, trapped RBCs within an extensive network of slitlike vascular spaces. Stains against HHV-8 can be used in cases where diagnostic uncertainty exists.

IMAGING For internal organ involvement.

DIAGNOSIS AND DIFFERENTIAL DIAGNOSIS

Confirmed on lesional skin biopsy.

DIFFERENTIAL DIAGNOSIS Includes single pigmented lesions: Dermatofibroma, pyogenic granuloma, hemangioma, bacillary (epithelioid) angiomatosis, melanocytic nevus, ecchymosis, granuloma annulare, insect bite reactions, and stasis dermatitis.

COURSE AND PROGNOSIS

CLASSIC KS Average survival, 10 to 15 years; death usually from unrelated causes. Secondary malignancies arise in >35% of cases.

AFRICAN-ENDEMIC KS Mean survival in young adults, 5 to 8 years; young children, 2 to 3 years.

IATROGENIC IMMUNOSUPPRESSION-ASSOCIATED KS The course may be chronic or rapidly progressive; KS usually resolves after immunosuppressive drugs are discontinued.

HIV/AIDS-Associated KS (see also Section 27). HIV-infected individuals with high CD4+ T cell counts can have stable or slowly progressive disease for many years. Rapid progression of KS can occur after decline of CD4+ T cell counts to low values, prolonged systemic glucocorticoid therapy, or illness such as *Pneumocystis carinii* pneumonia. KS of the bowel and/or lungs is the cause of death in 10 to 20% of patients. Patients with only a few lesions, present for several months, without history of opportunistic infections, and CD4+ T cell counts >200/µL tend to respond better to therapy and have a better overall prognosis. At time of initial diagnosis, 40% of KS patients have GI involvement; 80% at autopsy. Reduced survival rate in patients with GI involvement.

Pulmonary KS has high short-term mortality rate, i.e., median survival <6 months.

MANAGEMENT

The goal of therapy for KS is to control symptoms of the disease, not cure. A number of local and systemic therapeutic modalities are effective in controlling symptoms. Classic KS responds well to radiotherapy of involved sites. African-endemic KS, when symptomatic, responds best to systemic chemotherapy. Immunosuppressive drug-associated KS regresses or resolves when drug dosages are reduced or discontinued. HIV/AIDS-associated KS usually responds to a variety of local therapies; for extensive mucocutaneous involvement or visceral involvement, chemotherapy is indicated. Of course, all this in addition to HAART, the most effective therapy.

Limited Intervention

RADIOTHERAPY Indicated for tumorous lesions, confluent lesions with a large surface area, large lesions on distal extremity, and large oropharyngeal lesions. **Cryosurgery.** Indicated for deeply pigmented, protruding nodules. **Laser Surgery.** Pulsed-dye laser effective for small superficial lesions. **Photodynamic Therapy.** For small superficial lesions.

ELECTROSURGERY Effective for ulcerated, bleeding nodular lesions. **Excisional Surgery.** Effective for selected small lesions. **Intralesional Cytotoxic Chemotherapy.** *Vinblastine, Vincristine, and Bleomycin.*

Aggressive Intervention

Single-Agent Chemotherapy. With adriamycin, vinblastine, lipid formulations of daunorubicin and doxorubicin. Paclitaxel (Taxol), thalidomide, and col-3. **Combination Chemotherapy.** Vincristine + bleomycin + adriamycin or interferon-α + zidovudine.

Type-Specific Therapy

- *Classic KS*: Any of the preceding.
- *African KS*: Any of the preceding.
- *Immunosuppression-related KS*: Reduction in immunosuppression, replacement of calcineurin inhibitors by rapamycin.
- *HIV/AIDS-related KS*: Any of the preceding, preferably liposomal anthracyclines intravenously plus HAART.

ANGIOSARCOMA ICD-10: C49.9

- Tumors are composed of cells lining blood vessels. Lymphangiosarcomas arise from cells lining lymphatic vessels. Cutaneous angiosarcomas can present anywhere on the skin but in elderly individuals, there is predilection for the scalp, face and neck. In the face may start as ecchymosis-like lesion (Fig. 21-21B). No racial predilection exists.
- When they occur at sites of chronic lymphedema, usually following radical mastectomy for treatment of breast cancer, the syndrome Stweart_Treves is diagnosed and often carries a worse prognosis.
- Clinically, tumors present as round blue or red nodules (Fig. 21-21A). In late presentations, several nodules may be noted, some with superficial erosion from rapid cell turnover.
- Histopathology shows a collection of jagged vessels, nuclear atypia and pleomorphism. In highly de-differentiated tumors, vascular markers such as CD31, CD34, factor VIII, and Ulex can be helpful.
- Treatment is difficult. Surgical excision is often indicated, depending on the clinical extent of the tumor. Surgical margin control is often difficult to obtain. Radiation therapy and chemotherapy are often used. Recurrences are common. Prognosis is poor, particularly in Stewart_Treves.

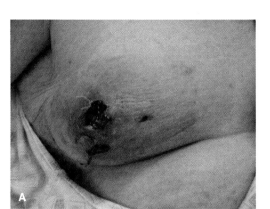
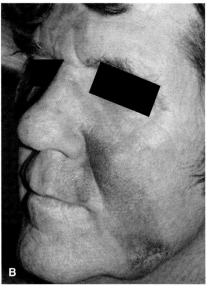

FIGURE 21-21 **Angiosarcoma** **(A)** This ulcerative plaque over an area of induration and erythema was noted over a previously radiated field. Radical surgery failed to control tumor growth and extension (Used with permission from Ruth Ann Vleugels, MD). **(B)** This unusual presentation resembling ecchymosis clearly follows a vascular pattern. Treatment is mostly palliative (Used with permission from Maryam Asgari, MD).

DERMATOFIBROSARCOMA PROTUBERANS (DFP) ICD10: C44.9

- Tissue sarcoma arising in the dermis and often penetrates into fat.
- Etiology is unknown but has been reported to arise in scars. It is caused by a translocation between chromosome 17 and 22.
- Incidence is low, approximately 1 to 5 people per million
- There appears to be a higher rate in African Americans compared to Caucasians and females are overrepresented. Tumor growth may be accelerated during pregnancy.
- Peak age of incidence is between 20 to 50 years of age
- The tumor may present as a non-specific plaque often resembling a keloid, with purplish to brownish coloration (**Fig. 21-22**). Other clinical variants include the Bednar tumor (pigmented) giant cell fibroblastoma (usually in children) and fribrosarcomatous DFSP which carries the highest risk of metastasis.
- Diagnosis is by histopathology, which shows a spindle cell proliferation often arranged as whorls (so-called herringbone pattern). Clinical distinction from dermatofirboma can be made by showing CD34 staining.
- Treatment is usually surgical. MOHS micrographic surgery has been used. Resulting from the molecular basis for this tumor, Imatinib has also been used, mostly to attempt decrease in tumor size prior to surgical intervention. Radiation is also an option.
- If cleared by resection, prognosis is good.

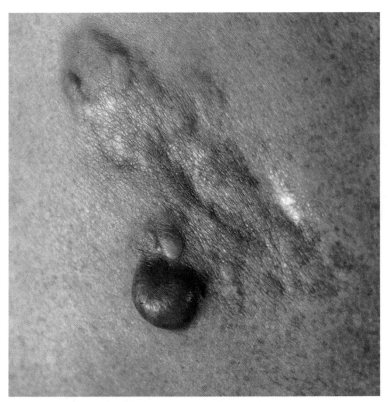

FIGURE 21-22 Dermatofibrosarcoma protuberans Tumors may present as nodules coalescing into plaques, often resembling a keloid. On the lower margin there is a reddish nodule representing exophytic growth. Though the tumor itself was slow-growing, peripheral infiltration into skin differentiates this lesion from a hypertrophic scar or keloid. The lesion was excised with wide margins and there was no recurrence.

ATYPICAL FIBROXANTHOMA (AFX) ICD01: C49.M12

- A not so rare, rapidly growing tumor of intermediate malignant potential.
- AFX is an asymptomatic, solitary papule, nodule, or plaque often resembling an SCC or BCC initially.
- Occurs in sun-damaged skin of older patients especially on the forehead, scalp (**Fig. 21-23**), nose, and ears.
- Histopathology may show highly atypical and "bizzare" cells that may be confused for more aggressive neoplasms
- Treatment is surgical.

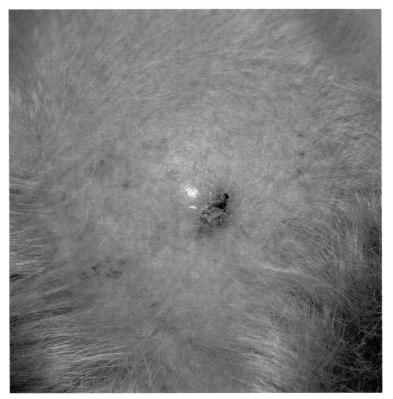

FIGURE 21-23 Atypical fibroxanthoma This is a 57-year old male with dermatoheliosis and a history of solar keratoses, invasive and in situ squamous carcinoma, and basal cell carcinoma. This nodule on the vertex was clinically atypical for either basal cell carcinoma or squamous cell carcinoma; histopathology revealed atypical fibroxanthoma.

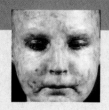

SECTION 22

SKIN DISEASES IN ORGAN AND BONE MARROW TRANSPLANTATION

Organ transplant recipients are chronically immunosuppressed and their T cell function is impaired. Ensuing diseases are mostly infections and are similar to those occurring in other conditions associated with T cell impairment, such as AIDS. In addition, organ transplant recipients are at great risk for developing nonmelanoma skin cancer and other cancers. Bone marrow and stem cell graft recipients are candidates for graft-versus-host disease (GVHD).

MOST COMMON INFECTIONS ASSOCIATED WITH ORGAN TRANSPLANTATION

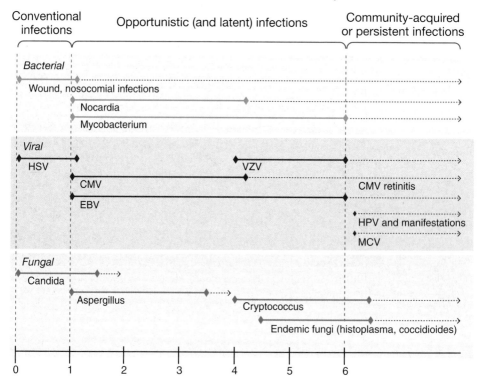

FIGURE 22-1 Timeline of common infections after transplantation.

SKIN CANCERS ASSOCIATED WITH ORGAN TRANSPLANTATION*

- Nonmelanoma skin cancer is the most common malignancy in adult solid organ transplant patients.
- The majority are squamous cell carcinomas (SCC) (Section 11).
- The risk of developing SCC increases exponentially with the length of immunosuppression.
- The cumulative incidence is 80% after 20 years of immunosuppression in renal transplantation. SCC in posttransplant patients are aggressive.
- HPV infection is implicated in the pathogenesis.
- Other epithelial proliferative lesions are actinic keratoses, keratoacanthomas, porokeratosis, appendage tumors, and Merkel cell carcinomas (Section 11).
- Children and adults with organ transplants may also be at higher risk for the development of melanoma (Section 12).
- Lymphoproliferative disorders are common in graft recipients and related to Epstein–Barr virus-mediated proliferation of B cells and most are lymphomas of B cell origin. Cutaneous T cell lymphomas account for 30% of cutaneous lymphomas in transplant patients (Section 21).
- Kaposi sarcoma occurs in immunosuppressed transplant recipients with an incidence of 0.5 to 5%. All cases are associated with Kaposi sarcoma-associated herpesvirus (KSHV) infection (Section 21).

*Clinical manifestations are discussed in their respective sections.

GRAFT-VERSUS-HOST DISEASE (GVHD) ICD-10: T86.0

- GVHD is the totality of organ dysfunction caused by the action of histoincompatible, immunocompetent donor cells against the tissues of an immunocompetent host.
- Graft-versus-host reaction (GVHR) is the expression of GVHD in a specific organ (e.g., cutaneous GVHR).
- Acute cutaneous GVHD, usually occurring 10 to 100 days after bone marrow transplantation (BMT). However, diagnosis now rests of clinical features, not the number of days following transplantation. It is the earliest and most frequent GVHR. Liver and GI tract GVHR are also common.
- Chronic cutaneous GVHD generally occurs >100 days after allogeneic BMT and manifests as lichenoid and sclerodermoid changes. Again, clinical features now define the diagnosis as opposed to days post-transplantation.
- **Incidence.** Allogeneic BMT: 20 to 80% of successful engraftments. Autologous BMT: Mild cutaneous GVHR occurs in 8%. Low incidence after blood transfusion in immunosuppressed patients, maternal-fetal transfer in immunodeficiency disease.

ACUTE CUTANEOUS GVHD

- During the first months after BMT (usually between 10 and 100 days but acute disease can occur even after development of chronic GVHD): mild pruritus, localized/generalized; pain on pressure of the palms and soles. Nausea/vomiting, abdominal pain; watery diarrhea. Jaundice; dark yellow urine.
- **Skin Lesions.** Initially, subtle, discrete macules and/or papules on the upper trunk, hands, and feet (Fig. 22-2), especially the palms and soles. Macules; confluent in the face, often erosive (Fig. 22-3). Painful. Mild edema with violaceous hue, periungual and on pinna. Erythema often in perifollicular array. If controlled/resolved, erythema diminishes with subsequent desquamation (Fig. 22-4) and postinflammatory hyperpigmentation. If it progresses, macules/papules become generalized, confluent, and evolve into erythroderma. Subepidermal bullae, especially over pressure/trauma sites of the palms and soles. Positive Nikolsky sign. If bullae widespread with rupture/erosion, TEN-like form of acute cutaneous GVHD can occur and portends a worse prognosis (see Section 8) (Fig. 22-5). For staging, see Table 22-1.
- **Mucosa.** Lichen planus-like lesions in buccal mucosa; erosive stomatitis, oral and ocular sicca-like syndrome; esophagitis/esophageal strictures. Keratoconjunctivitis.
- **General Findings.** Fever, jaundice, nausea, vomiting, right upper quadrant pain/tenderness, cramping, abdominal pain, diarrhea, serositis, pulmonary insufficiency, and dark urine.
- **Chemistry.** Elevated SGOT, bilirubin, and alkaline phosphatase.
- **Dermatopathology.** Focal vacuolization of basal cell layer, apoptosis of individual keratinocytes; mild perivenular mononuclear cell infiltrate. Apposition of lymphocytes to necrotic keratinocytes (satellitosis); vacuoles coalesce to form subepidermal clefts → subepidermal blister formation. Endothelial cell swelling. Immunocytochemistry: HLA-DR expression of keratinocytes precedes morphologic changes and thus represents important, early diagnostic sign.
- **Differential Diagnosis.** Exanthematous drug reaction, viral exanthem, TEN, and erythroderma.
- **Course and Prognosis.** Mild-to-moderate GVHR responds well to treatment. Prognosis of TEN-like GVHR is grave. Severe GVHD susceptible to infections—bacterial, fungal, and viral (CMV, HSV, VZV). Acute GVHD is primary or associated cause of death in 15 to 70% of BMT recipients.
- **Management Topical.** Glucocorticoids. PUVA, extracorporeal photopheresis. Systemic. Methylprednisolone, tacrolimus, sirulimus, cyclosporine, methotrexate, mycophenolate mofetil, etanercept, and infliximab.

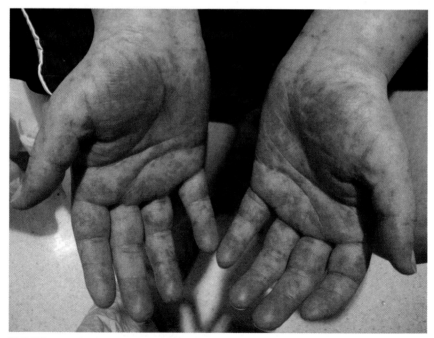

FIGURE 22-2 Acute cutaneous GVHD Discrete and confluent erythematous, blanching macules, and rarely elevated papules with indistinct borders involving both hands. The clinical picture evolved into disseminated disease, spreading from the acra to the central trunk. Prominent facial edema was eventually noted (Used with permission from Jennifer Tan, MD).

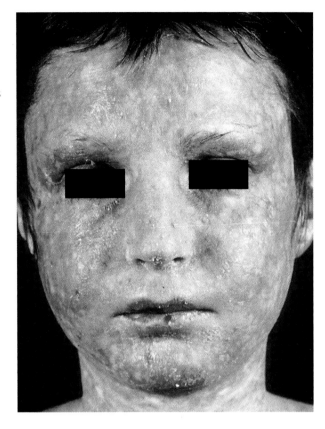

FIGURE 22-3 Acute cutaneous GVHD involving the face of a 10-year-old boy The individual lesions are confluent, there is slight desquamation, and there are erosions on the lips, cheeks, and chin. The mucous membranes were severely involved.

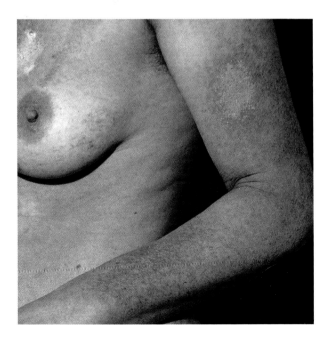

FIGURE 22-4 Acute cutaneous GVHD, remitting The maculo-papular lesions have acquired a brownish hue and there is slight scaling.

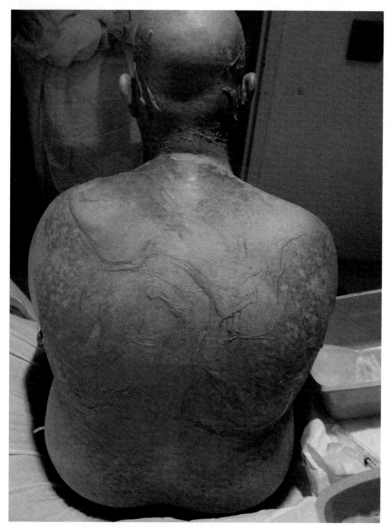

FIGURE 22-5 Acute GVHR, TEN-like Confluent epidermal necrosis with wrinkling and dislodgement of the necrotic epidermis. This severe reaction involved the entire skin and is indistinguishable from TEN. It occurred after allogeneic BMT and carries a high mortality (Used with permission from Jennifer Tan, MD).

TABLE 22-1 Clinical Staging of Acute Cutaneous GVHD

1. Erythematous maculopapular eruption involving <25% of body surface
2. Erythematous maculopapular eruption involving 25–50% of body surface
3. Erythroderma
4. Bulla formation

CHRONIC CUTANEOUS GVHD

- More than 100 days after BMT. Evolving from acute GVHR or arising de novo. Acute GVHR not always followed by chronic GVHR. Clinical classification thus distinguishes between quiescent onset, progressive onset, and de novo chronic cutaneous GVHD. Chronic GVHR occurs in 25% of recipients of marrow from an HLA-identical sibling who survives >100 days. It is the most common cause of non-relapse associated mortality.
- **Skin Lesions.** Flat-topped (lichen planus-like) papules of violaceous color, initially on distal extremities but later generalized (Fig. 22-6) and/or confluent areas of dermal sclerosis (Fig. 22-7A) with overlying scale resembling scleroderma mainly on the trunk, buttocks, hips, and thighs. With more severe disease, severe generalized sclerodermoid changes also involve the face (Fig. 22-7B) with necrosis and ulceration on acral and pressure sites. Hair loss; anhidrosis; nails: dystrophy (pterygium, ridging), anonychia; vitiligo-like hypopigmentation. Asteatotic, psoriasiform, and icthyosiform variants have also been reported.
- **Mucosa.** Like erosive/ulcerative lichen planus, glossitis, desquamation, and gingivitis.
- **General Findings.** Chronic liver disease, general wasting.
- **Chemistry.** Elevated ALT, AST, and γ-glutamyl-transferase.
- **Dermatopathology.** Like *lichen planus* or *scleroderma*.
- **Course and Prognosis.** Sclerodermoid GVHR with tight skin/joint contracture may result in impaired mobility and ulcerations. Permanent hair loss; xerostomia, xerophthalmia, corneal ulcers, and blindness. Malabsorption. Mild chronic cutaneous GVHD may resolve spontaneously. Chronic GVHR may be associated with recurrent and occasionally fatal bacterial infections.
- **Management.** *Topical* glucocorticoids, PUVA, and extracorporeal photopheresis. *Systemic immunosuppression* with prednisone, cyclosporine, azathioprine, mycophenolate mofetil, methotrexate, tacrolimus, and thalidomide. The most important concept in management is to treat symptoms without decreasing or impairing graft-versus-leukemia/leymphoma effects, and thus increase the possibility of disease remission. Clinical consultation with an oncologist is often required at this stage.

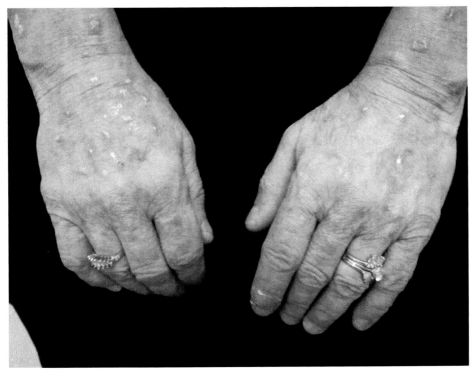

FIGURE 22-6 Chronic cutaneous GVHD, lichen planus-like   Erythematous lichenoid papules, often with psoriasiform scale (thus the term lichen-planus-like rather than lichenoid), over extensor surfaces in a 65-year-old female status post peripheral stem cell transplantation for acute myeloid leukemia.

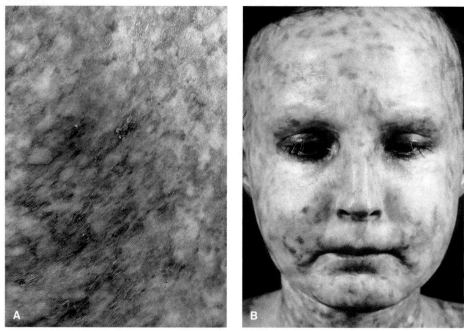

FIGURE 22-7 Chronic cutaneous GVHD, sclerodermoid (A) Close-up view of the back of a patient with poikilodermatous changes (hypo- and hyperpigmentation) and telangiectasias in the sclerotic skin. **(B)** Ebony-white bound down skin and telangiectasias in the 10-year-old boy shown in **Figure 22-3**. Skin looks and feels like severe scleroderma. In this case, acute GVHR evolved directly into chronic GVHR and involved the entire skin of the head, trunk, and extremities.

ADVERSE CUTANEOUS DRUG REACTIONS[1]

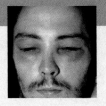

ADVERSE CUTANEOUS DRUG REACTIONS ICD:10: T88.7

- Adverse cutaneous drug reactions (ACDRs) are unpredictable They affect 2 to 3% of inpatients and lead to 0.1 to 0.3% of hospital fatalities.
- In the United States, adverse drug events account for up to 140,000 deaths and $136 billion in costs annually.
- Most reactions are mild, accompanied by pruritus, and resolve promptly after the offending drug is discontinued.
- *Drug eruptions can mimic virtually all the morphologic expressions in dermatology and must be the first consideration in the differential diagnosis of a suddenly appearing eruption.*
- Drug eruptions are caused by immunologic or nonimmunologic mechanisms and are provoked by systemic or topical administration of a drug.
- The majority are based on a hypersensitivity mechanism and are thus immunologic and may be of types I, II, III, or IV.

CLASSIFICATION

IMMUNOLOGICALLY MEDIATED ACDR
(see Table 23-1) It should be noted that in most reactions both cellular and humoral immune reactions are involved. Nonimmunologic reactions are summarized in Table 23-2.

GUIDELINES FOR ASSESSMENT OF POSSIBLE ACDRS

- Exclude alternative causes, especially infections (most commonly viral).
- Examine interval between introduction of a drug and onset of the reaction.
- Note any improvement after drug withdrawal.
- Determine whether similar reactions have been associated with the same compound.
- Note any reaction on readministration of the drug.

FINDINGS INDICATING POSSIBLE LIFE-THREATENING ACDR

- Skin pain.
- Confluent erythema.
- Facial edema or central facial involvement.
- Palmar/plantar painful erythema.
- Epidermal detachment and blisters.
- Positive Nikolsky sign.
- Mucous membrane erosions.
- Urticaria.
- Swelling of the tongue.
- High fever (temperature >40°C).
- Enlarged lymph nodes.
- Arthralgia.
- Shortness of breath, wheezing, and hypotension.
- Palpable purpura.
- Skin necrosis.

CLINICAL TYPES OF ADVERSE DRUG REACTIONS

ACDRs can be exanthematous and can manifest as urticaria/angioedema, anaphylaxis, and anaphylactoid reactions, or serum sickness. They can mimic other dermatoses and they can also present as cutaneous necrosis, pigmentation, alopecia, and hypertrichosis. They can induce nail changes. An overview is presented in Tables 23-3 and 23-4.

---

[1]Skin reactions or changes regularly occurring after high dose or prolonged administration of certain drugs like glucocorticoids, retinoids, cyclosporine, and others are not discussed in this section but throughout the book whenever these drugs are discussed in greater detail.

TABLE 23-1 Immunologically Mediated Adverse Cutaneous Drug Reactions*

Type of Reaction	Pathogenesis	Examples of Causative Drug	Clinical Patterns
Type I	IgE-mediated; immediate-type immunologic reactions	Penicillin, other antibiotics	Urticaria/angioedema of skin/mucosa, edema of other organs, and anaphylactic shock
Type II	Drug + cytotoxic antibodies cause lysis of cells such as platelets or leukocytes	Penicillin, sulfonamides, quinidine, isoniazid	Petechiae due to thrombocytopenic purpura, drug-induced pemphigus
Type III	IgG or IgM antibodies formed to drug; immune complexes deposited in small vessels activate complement and recruitment of granulocytes	Immunoglobulins, antibiotics, rituximab, infliximab	Vasculitis, urticaria, serum sickness
Type IV	Cell-mediated immune reaction; sensitized lymphocytes react with drug, liberating cytokines, which trigger cutaneous inflammatory response**	Sulfamethoxazole, anticonvulsants, allopurinol	Morbilliform exanthematous reactions, fixed drug eruption, lichenoid eruptions, Stevens–Johnson syndrome, toxic epidermal necrolysis

*After the Gell and Coombs classification of immune reactions.
**For contact sensitivity see Section 2.

TABLE 23-2 Nonimmunologic Drug Reactions

Idiosyncrasy	Reactions due to hereditary enzyme deficiencies
Individual idiosyncrasy to a topical or systemic drug	Mechanisms not yet known
Cumulation	Reactions are dose dependent, based on the total amount of drug ingested: pigmentation due to gold, amiodarone, or minocycline
Reactions due to combination of a drug with ultraviolet irradiation (photosensitivity)	Reactions have a toxic pathogenesis but can also be immunologic in nature (see Section 10)
Irritancy/toxicity of a topically applied drug	5-Fluorouracil, imiquimod
Atrophy by topically applied drug	Glucocorticoids

TABLE 23-3 Types of Clinical ACDRs

Type	Drugs	Comment
Basic Reactions		
Exanthematous reactions	Any	Most common; initial reaction usually <14 days after drug intake; recurs after rechallenge (see page 494);
Urticaria/ angioedema	See Table 23-4	Second most common; usually within 36 h after initial exposure; within minutes after rechallenge (see page 498) (Figs. 22-6 and 22-7)
Fixed drug eruptions	See Table 23-6	Third most common, see page 499
Anaphylaxis and anaphylactoid reactions	Antibiotics, extracts of allergens, radiocontrast media, monoclonal antibodies (see Table 23-5)	Most serious type of ACDR, within minutes and hours; more common with oral than parenteral drug administration. Intermittent administration of drug may predispose to anaphylaxis
Serum sickness	IVIg, antibiotics, bovine serum albumin (used for oocyte retrieval in in vitro fertilization), cefaclor, cefprozil, bupropion, minocycline, rituximab, infliximab	5–21 days after initial exposure *Minor form*: fever, urticaria, arthralgia *Major (complete) form*: fever, urticaria, angioedema, arthralgia, arthritis, lymphadenopathy, eosinophilia, ± nephritis, ± endocarditis.

TABLE 23-4 ACDR Mimicry of Other Dermatoses

Type	Drugs	Comment
Basic Reactions		
Acneiform eruption	Glucocorticoids, anabolic steroids, contraceptives, halogens, isoniazid, lithium, azathioprine, danazol, erlotinib	Mimics acne. See Section 1 and page 496
Bullous eruptions	Naproxen, nalidixic acid, furosemide, oxaprozin, penicillamine, piroxicam, tetracyclines	Mimics fixed drug eruption, drug-induced vasculitis, Stevens–Johnson syndrome (SJS), toxic epidermal necrolysis (TEN), porphyria, pseudoporphyria, drug-induced pemphigus, drug-induced pemphigoid, drug-induced linear IgA disease, bullae over pressure areas in sedated patients
Dermatomyositis-like reactions	Penicillamine, NSAIDs, carbamazepine, hydroxyurea	Mimics dermatomyositis. See Section 14
Drug hypersensitivity syndrome	Antiepileptic drugs, sulfonamides, and others	Mimics exanthematous reactions; systemic involvement (see page 501)

(continued)

TABLE 23-4 ACDR Mimicry of Other Dermatoses (*Continued*)

Type	Drugs	Comment
Eczematous eruptions	Ethylenediamine, antihistamines, aminophylline/aminophylline suppositories; procaine/benzocaine; iodides, iodinated organic compounds, radiographic contrast media/iodine; streptomycin, kanamycin, paromomycin, gentamicin/neomycin sulfate; nitroglycerin tablets/nitroglycerin ointment; disulfiram/thiuram	Systemic administration of a drug to an individual who has been previously sensitized to the drug by topical application can provoke a widespread eczematous dermatitis (systemic contact-type dermatitis, see Section 2) or urticaria
Erythema multiforme, SJS, TEN	Anticonvulsants, sulfonamides, allopurinol, NSAIDs (piroxicam)	See Sections 8 and 14
Erythema nodosum	Sulfonamides, other antimicrobial agents, analgesics, oral contraceptives, granulocyte colony-stimulating factor (G-CSF)	See Section 7
Exfoliative dermatitis and erythroderma	Sulfonamides, antimalarials, phenytoin, penicillin	See Section 8
Lichenoid eruptions (resemble lichen planus)	Gold, beta-blockers, ACE inhibitors, especially captopril; antimalarials, thiazide diuretics, furosemid, spironolactone, penicillamine, calcium-channel blockers, carbamazepine, lithium, sulfonylurea, allopurinol	See Section 14 May be extensive, occurring weeks to months after initiation of drug therapy; may progress to exfoliative dermatitis Adnexal involvement may result in alopecia, anhidrosis Resolution after discontinuation slow, 1–4 months; up to 24 months after gold
Lupus erythematosus (LE)	Procainamide, hydralazine, isoniazid, minocycline, acebutolol, Ca²⁺ channel blockers, ACE inhibitors, docetaxel	See Section 14 5% of cases of systemic LE are drug-induced Cutaneous manifestations, including photosensitivity; however, urticaria, erythema multiforme-like lesions, Raynaud phenomenon are not common
Necrosis	Warfarin, heparin, interferon-α, cytotoxic agents	See page 506
Photosensitivity	See Tables 10-4 to 10-6	See Section 10 Phototoxic, photoallergic, or photocontact

TABLE 23-4 ACDR Mimicry of Other Dermatoses (*Continued*)

Type	Drugs	Comment
Pigmentary disorders	Amiodarone, minocycline, antimalarials, cytotoxic agents	See page 502
Pityriasis rosea-like eruptions	Gold, captopril, imatinib, and others	For clinical appearance, see Section 3
Pseudolymphoma	Phenytoin, carbamazepine, allopurinol, antidepressants, phenothiazines, benzodiazepine, antihistamines, beta-blockers, lipid-lowering agents, cyclosporine, D-penicillamine	Papular eruptions with a histology mimicking lymphoma
Pseudoporphyria	Tetracycline, furosemide, naproxen	See Section 10 and page 505
Psoriasiform eruption	Antimalarials, beta-blockers, lithium salts, NSAIDs, interferon, penicillamine, methyldopa	See Section 3
Purpura	Penicillin, sulfonamides, quinine, isoniazid	See Section 20 Hemorrhage into morbilliform ACDR occurs not uncommonly on the legs Progressive pigmented purpura also reported associated with drugs (see Section 14)
Pustular eruptions	Ampicillin, amoxicillin, macrolides, tetracyclines, beta-blockers, Ca^{2+} channel blockers EGFR inhibitors (Fig. 23-4)	Acute generalized exanthematous pustulosis (AGEP, page 496) Must be differentiated from pustular psoriasis; eosinophil in the infiltrate suggests AGEP
Scleroderma-like reactions	Penicillamine, bleomycin, bromocriptine, Na-valproate, 5-hydroxytryptophan, docetaxel, gemcitabine, acetanilide-containing rapeseed cooking oil	See Section 14
Sweet syndrome	All-*trans* retinoic acid, contraceptives, G-CSF, granulocyte-macrophage CSF (GM-CSF), minocycline, imatinib, trimethoprim-sulfamethoxazole	See Section 7
Vasculitis	Propylthiouracil, hydralazine, G-CSF, GM-CSF, allopurinol, cefaclor, minocycline, penicillamine, phenytoin, isotretinoin	See Section 14

EXANTHEMATOUS DRUG REACTIONS ICD-10: T88.7

- An exanthematous drug reaction (EDR) (eruption) is an adverse hypersensitivity reaction to an ingested or parenterally administered drug that mimics a measles-like viral exanthem.
- Most common type of cutaneous drug reaction.
- Systemic involvement is low.
- *Drugs with a high probability of reaction* (3 to 5%): Penicillin and related antibiotics, carbamazepine, allopurinol, and gold salts (10 to 20%). *Medium probability:* Sulfonamides (bacteriostatic, antidiabetic, diuretic), nonsteroidal anti-inflammatory drugs (NSAIDs), hydantoin derivatives, isoniazid, chloramphenicol, erythromycin, and streptomycin. *Low probability* (<1%): Barbiturates, benzodiazepines, phenothiazines, and tetracyclines.
- **Prior Drug Sensitization.** Patients with a prior history of exanthematous drug eruption will most likely develop a similar reaction if rechallenged with the same drug.
- Sensitization occurs during administration or after completing the course of drugs; peak incidence is usually at ninth day after administration. However, EDR may occur at any time between the first day and 3 weeks after the beginning of treatment. Reaction to penicillin can begin ≥2 weeks after drug is discontinued. In previously sensitized patient, eruption starts within 2 or 3 days after readministration of drug.
- Usually quite pruritic. Painful skin lesions suggest development of a more serious ACDR, such as toxic epidermal necrolysis (TEN).
- **Systems Review.** ± Fever and chills.
- **Skin Lesions.** Macules and/or papules, a few millimeters to 1 cm in size (**Fig. 23-1**). Bright or "drug" red. In time, lesions become confluent forming large macules, polycyclic/gyrate erythema, reticular eruptions, sheet-like erythema (**Fig. 23-1**), or erythroderma; also erythema multiforme-like. Purpura may be seen in lesions of the lower legs. In individuals with thrombocytopenia, exanthematous eruptions can mimic vasculitis because of intralesional hemorrhage. Scaling and/or desquamation may occur with healing.
- **Distribution.** Symmetric (**Fig. 23-1**). Almost always occurs on the trunk and extremities. In children, it may be limited to the face and extremities.
- **Mucous Membranes.** Enanthem on buccal mucosa.
- **Laboratory.** Peripheral eosinophilia. Dermatopathology: Perivascular lymphocytes and eosinophils.
- Differential diagnosis includes all exanthematous eruptions: Viral exanthem, secondary syphilis, atypical pityriasis rosea, and early widespread allergic contact dermatitis.
- After discontinuation of the drug, the rash usually fades. However, it may worsen for a few days. The eruption may also begin after the drug has been discontinued. Eruption usually recurs with rechallenge.
- The definitive step in management is to identify the offending drug and discontinue it. Oral antihistamine can alleviate pruritus. **Glucocorticoids.** *Potent Topical Preparation, Oral or IV.* If the offending drug cannot be substituted or omitted, systemic glucocorticoids can be administered to treat the ACDR. **Prevention.** Patients must be aware of their specific drug hypersensitivity and that other drugs of the same class can cross-react. Wearing a medical alert bracelet is advised.

REACTIONS TO SPECIFIC DRUGS (SELECTED)

Allopurinol. Incidence: 5%. Begins on the face, spreads rapidly to all areas; may occur in photodistribution. Onset: 2 to 3 weeks after initiation of therapy. Associated findings: Facial edema; systemic vasculitis, especially involving kidneys. The rash may fade in spite of continued administration.

Ampicillin, Amoxicillin. In up to 100% of patients with EBV or CMV mononucleosis syndrome. Increased incidence of EDR to penicillins in patients taking allopurinol. Ten percent cross-react with cephalosporins.

Carbamazepine. Morphology: diffuse erythema; severe erythroderma may follow. Site: Begins on the face, then spreads rapidly to all areas; may occur in photodistribution. Onset: 2 weeks after initiation of therapy. Associated findings: Facial edema.

Hydantoin Derivatives. Macular → confluent erythema. Begins on the face, then spreads to trunk and extremities. Onset: 2 weeks after initiation of therapy. Associated findings: Fever, peripheral eosinophilia; facial edema; lymphadenopathy (can mimic lymphoma histologically).

Sulfonamides. Occurs in up to 50 to 60% of HIV/AIDS-infected patients (trimethoprim sulfamethoxazole). Patients sensitized to one sulfa-based drug may cross-react with another sulfa drug in 20%.

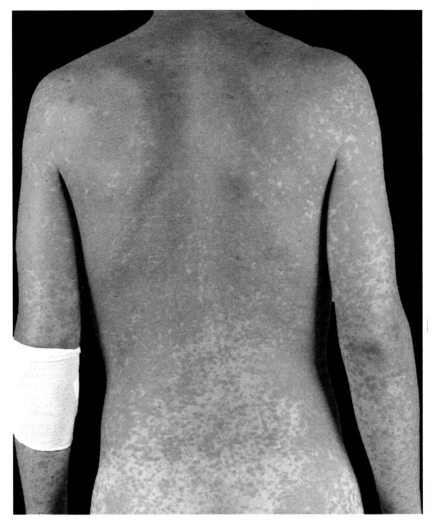

FIGURE 23-1 Exanthematous drug eruption: ampicillin Symmetrically arranged, brightly erythematous macules and papules, discrete in some areas, and confluent in others, on the trunk and the extremities.

PUSTULAR ERUPTIONS ICD-10: T88.7

- *Acute generalized exanthematous pustulosis* (AGEP) is an acute febrile eruption that is often associated with leukocytosis (Fig. 23-2). After drug administration, it may take 1 to 3 weeks before skin lesions appear. However, in previously sensitized patients, the skin symptoms may occur within 2 to 3 days.
- Onset is acute, most often following drug intake, but viral infections can also trigger the disease.
- AGEP typically presents with nonfollicular sterile pustules occurring on a diffuse, edematous erythema (Fig. 23-2).
- May be irregularly dispersed (Fig. 23-2) or grouped (Fig. 23-3), usually starting in the folds and/or the face.
- Fever and elevated blood neutrophils are common.
- Histopathology typically shows spongiform subcorneal and/or intraepidermal pustules; a marked edema of the papillary dermis; and eventually vasculitis, eosinophils, and/or focal necrosis of keratinocytes.
- Pustules resolve spontaneously in <15 days and generalized desquamation occurs approximately 2 weeks later.
- Differential diagnosis includes pustular psoriasis, the hypersensitivity syndrome reaction with pustulation, subcorneal pustular dermatosis (Sneddon–Wilkinson disease), and pustular vasculitis.
- *Acneiform pustular eruptions* (see Section 1) are associated with iodides, bromides, adrenocorticotropic hormone (ACTH), glucocorticoids, isoniazid, androgens, lithium, actinomycin D, and phenytoin. The EGFR tyrosine kinase inhibitors erlotinib, gefitinib, cetuximab, and panitumumab produce pustules that are acneiform but without comedos and erupt in the face (Fig. 23-4) but can erupt also in atypical areas, such as on the arms and legs, and are most often monomorphous.

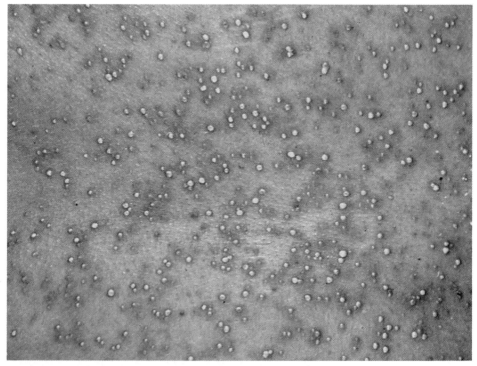

FIGURE 23-2 Pustular drug eruption: acute generalized exanthematous pustulosis (AGEP) Multiple tiny nonfollicular pustules against the background of diffuse erythema that first appeared in the large folds and then covered the entire trunk and the face.

FIGURE 23-3 **Pustular drug eruption: AGEP** Multiple sterile pustules surrounded by fiery-red erythema in a 58-year-old female who had fever and leukocytosis. In contrast to the disseminated pustules in Fig. 23-2, here the pustules show a tendency for grouping and confluence. Differential diagnosis of von Zumbusch pustular psoriasis (compare with Fig. 3-12).

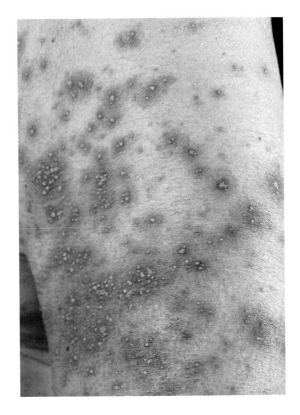

FIGURE 23-4 **Pustular drug eruption: erlotinib** This pustular eruption occurred in a patient who had received an anti-EGR monoclonal antibody for cancer of the colon localized to face. Differential diagnosis to acne and rosacea.

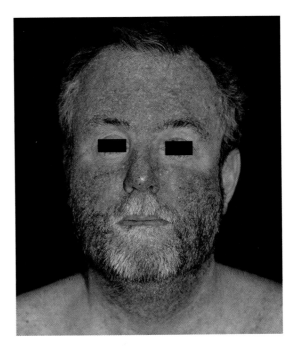

DRUG-INDUCED ACUTE URTICARIA, ANGIOEDEMA, EDEMA, AND ANAPHYLAXIS   (see also section 14)

- Drug-induced urticaria and angioedema occur, caused by a variety of mechanisms (see Table 23-1) and are characterized clinically by transient wheals (see Fig. 14-6) and angioedema causing extensive tissue swelling with involvement of deep dermal and subcutaneous tissues. Angioedema is often pronounced on the face (Fig. 23-5A) or mucous membranes (tongue, Fig. 23-5B).
- In some cases, cutaneous urticaria/angioedema is associated with systemic anaphylaxis, which is manifested by respiratory distress, vascular collapse, and/or shock.
- Drugs causing urticaria/angioedema and anaphylaxis are listed in Table 23-5.
- **Time from Initial Drug Exposure to Appearance of Urticaria**
- *IgE-Mediated.* Initial sensitization, usually 7 to 14 days. In previously sensitized individuals, usually within minutes or hours.
- *Immune Complex-Mediated.* Initial sensitization, usually 7 to 10 days, but as long as 28 days; in previously sensitized individuals, 12 to 36 h.
- *Analgesics/Anti-Inflammatory Drugs.* 20 to 30 min (up to 4 h).
- **Prior Drug Exposure.** *Radiographic Contrast Media.* 25 to 35% probability of repeat reaction in individuals with history of prior reaction to contrast media.
- **Skin Symptoms.** Pruritus, burning of palms, and soles with airway edema difficulties breathing.
- **Constitutional Symptoms.** IgE-mediated: Flushing, sudden fatigue, yawning, headache, weakness, and dizziness; numbness of tongue, sneezing, bronchospasm, substernal pressure, and palpitations; nausea, vomiting, crampy abdominal pain, diarrhea, and possibly arthralgia.

Drug-induced urticaria/angioedema usually resolves within hours, days, or weeks after the causative drug is withdrawn.

MANAGEMENT Identify and withdraw offending drugs. **Antihistamines.** H₁ blockers or H₂ blockers or combination. **Systemic Glucocorticoids** *Intravenous.* Hydrocortisone or methylprednisolone for severe symptoms. *Oral.* Prednisone, 70 mg, tapering by 10 or 5 mg daily over 1 to 2 weeks, is usually adequate. In **Acute Severe Urticaria/Anaphylaxis** *Epinephrine.* 0.3 to 0.5 mL of a 1:1000 dilution subcutaneously, repeated in 15 to 20 min. Maintain airway. Intravenous access. *Radiographic Contrast Media.* Avoid use of contrast media known to have caused prior reaction. If not possible, pretreat patient with antihistamine and prednisone (1 mg/kg) 30 to 60 min before contrast media exposure.

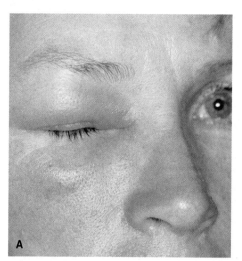
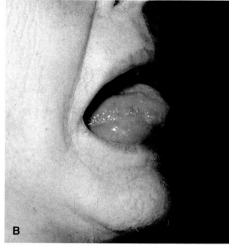

FIGURE 23-5 Drug-induced angioedema: penicillin (A) Angioedema has led to closure of right eye. **(B)** Sublingual angioedema in another patient interfered with breathing, talking, and eating and caused great concern.

TABLE 23-5 Drugs Causing Urticaria/Angioedema/Anaphylaxis

Drug Type	Specific Drugs
Antibiotics	Penicillins: ampicillin, amoxicillin, dicloxacillin, mezlocillin, penicillin G, penicillin V, ticarcillin. Cephalosporins, third-generation sulfonamides and derivatives
Cardiovascular drugs	Amiodarone, procainamide
Immunotherapeutics, vaccines	Antilymphocyte serum, levamisole, horse serum, monoclonal antibodies
Cytostatic agents	L-Asparaginase, bleomycin, cisplatin, daunorubicin, 5-fluorouracil, procarbazine, thiotepa
Angiotensin-converting enzyme inhibitors	Captopril, enalapril, lisinopril
Calcium-channel blockers	Nifedipine, diltiazem, verapamil
Drugs releasing histamine	Morphine, meperidine, atropine, codeine, papaverine, propanidid, alfaxalone, D-tubocurarine, succinylcholine, amphetamine, tyramine, hydralazine, tolazoline, trimethaphan camsylate, pentamidine, propamidine, stilbamidine, quinine, vancomycin, radiographic contrast media, and others

FIXED DRUG ERUPTION   ICD-10: T88.7

- A fixed drug eruption (FDE) is an adverse cutaneous reaction to an ingested drug, characterized by the formation of a solitary (but at times multiple) erythematous patch or plaque. The most commonly implicated agents are listed in Table 23-6.
- If the patient is rechallenged with the offending drug, the FDE occurs repeatedly at the identical skin site (i.e., fixed) within hours of ingestion.
- *Skin symptoms:* Usually asymptomatic. May be pruritic, painful, or burning.
- **Skin Lesions.** A sharply demarcated macule, round or oval in shape. Initially erythema, then dusky red to violaceous (Fig. 23-6A). Most commonly, lesions are solitary and can spread to become quite large, but they may be multiple (Fig. 23-7) with random distribution. Lesions may evolve to become a bulla (Fig. 23-6B) and then an erosion. Eroded lesions, especially on genitals or oral mucosa, are quite painful. After healing, dark brown with violet hue postinflammatory hyperpigmentation. Genital skin (see Section 34) is frequently involved site, but any site may be involved; perioral or periorbital (Fig. 23-6A). They occur in conjunctivae or oropharynx.
- **Dermatopathology.** Similar to findings in erythema multiforme and/or TEN.
- **Patch Test.** An inflammatory response occurs in only 30% of cases.
- FDE resolves within a few weeks of withdrawing the drug. Recurs within hours after ingestion of a single dose of the drug.
- **Management.** Withhold offending drug. Noneroded lesions: Potent topical glucocorticoid ointment. Eroded lesions: Antimicrobial ointment. For widespread, generalized, and highly painful mucosal lesions, oral prednisone 1 mg/kg body weight tapered over a course of 2 weeks.

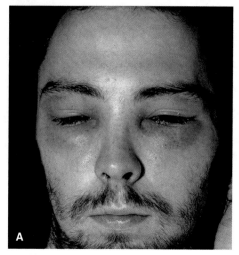
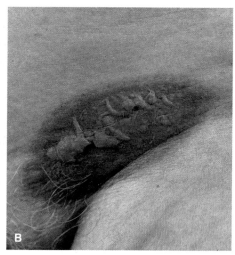

FIGURE 23-6 Fixed drug eruption (A) Tetracycline. Two well-defined periorbital plaques with edema. This was the second such episode following ingestion of a tetracycline. No other lesions were present. **(B)** Tylenol. A large oval violaceous lesion with blistering in the center. Erosive mouth lesions were also present.

TABLE 23-6 Most Commonly Implicated Agents in Fixed Drug Eruptions
Tetracyclines (tetracycline, minocycline, doxycycline)
Sulfonamides, other sulfa drugs
Metronidazole, nystatin, salicylates, NSAIDs, phenylbutazone, phenacetin
Barbiturates
Oral contraceptives
Quinine (including quinine in tonic water), quinidine
Phenolphthalein
Food coloring (yellow): in food or medications

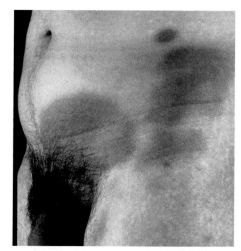

FIGURE 23-7 Fixed drug eruption Doxycycline. Multiple lesions. Similar violaceous plaques were also on the anterior and posterior trunk.

DRUG HYPERSENSITIVITY SYNDROME ICD.0: I88.7

- Drug hypersensitivity syndrome is an idiosyncratic adverse drug reaction that begins acutely in the first 2 months after initiation of the drug and is characterized by fever, malaise, and facial edema with lymphadenopathy or an exfoliative dermatitis. *Synonym:* Drug rash with eosinophilia and systemic symptoms (DRESS).

- **Etiology.** Most commonly: Antiepileptic drugs (phenytoin, carbamazepine, or phenobarbital; cross-sensitivity among the three drugs is common) and sulfonamides (antimicrobial agents, dapsone, or sulfasalazine). Less commonly: Allopurinol, gold salts, sorbinil, minocycline, zalcitabine, calcium-channel blockers, ranitidine, thalidomide, or mexiletine.

- Some patients have a genetically determined inability to detoxify the toxic arene oxide metabolic products of anticonvulsant agents. Slow *N*-acetylation of sulfonamide and increased susceptibility of leukocytes to toxic hydroxylamine metabolites are associated with a higher risk of hypersensitivity syndrome.

- **Skin Lesions.** *Early:* Morbilliform eruption (Fig. 23-8) on the face, upper trunk, and the upper extremities; cannot be distinguished from an exanthematous drug eruption. May progress to generalized exfoliative dermatitis/erythroderma, especially if the drug is not discontinued. Eruption becomes infiltrated with edematous follicular accentuation. Facial edema (especially periorbitally) is characteristic and may result in blister formation. Sterile pustules may occur. Eruption may become purpuric on legs. Scaling and/or desquamation may occur with healing.

- **Distribution.** Symmetric. Almost always on the trunk and extremities. Lesions may become confluent and generalized.

- **Mucous Membranes.** Cheilitis, erosions, erythematous pharynx, and enlarged tonsils.

- **General Examination.** Involvement of the liver, kindeys, lymph nodes, heart, lungs, joints, muscles, thyroid, and brain also occurs.

- **Eosinophilia** (30% of cases). Leukocytosis. Mononucleosis-like atypical lymphocytes. **Histology Skin.** Lymphocytic infiltrate, dense and diffuse or superficial and perivascular. ± Eosinophils or dermal edema. In some cases, bandlike infiltrate of atypical lymphocytes with epidermotropism, simulating cutaneous T cell lymphoma.

- **Proposed Diagnostic Criteria.** (1) Cutaneous drug eruption, (2) hematologic abnormalities (eosinophilia ≥1500/μL or atypical lymphocytes), and (3) systemic involvement [adenopathies ≥2 cm in diameter or hepatitis (SGOT ≥2 *N*) or interstitial nephritis, or interstitial pneumonitis or carditis]. Diagnosis is confirmed if three criteria are present.

- Course and prognosis: Rash and hepatitis may persist for weeks after the drug is discontinued. In patients treated with systemic glucocorticoids, rash and hepatitis may recur as glucocorticoids are tapered. Lymphadenopathy usually resolves when the drug is withdrawn; however, rare progression to lymphoma has been reported. Patients may die from systemic hypersensitivity such as with eosinophilic myocarditis (10%). Clinical findings recur if the drug is given again.

- **Management.** Identify and discontinue the offending drug. *Systemic.* Prednisone (0.5 mg/kg per day) usually results in rapid improvement of symptoms and laboratory parameters.

- **Prevention.** The individual must be aware of his or her specific drug hypersensitivity and that other drugs of the same class can cross-react. These drugs must never be readministered. Patient should wear a medical alert bracelet.

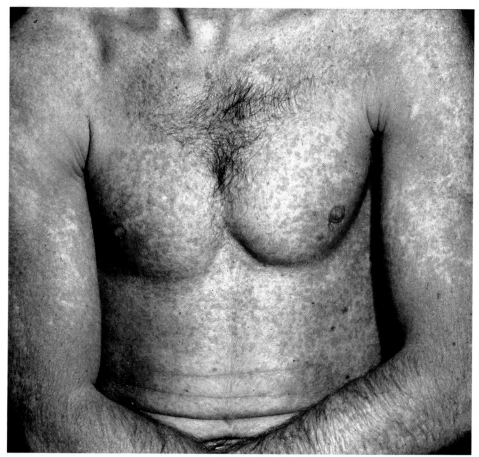

FIGURE 23-8 Drug hypersensitivity syndrome: phenytoin Symmetric, bright red, exanthematous eruption, confluent in some sites; the patient had associated lymphadenopathy and fever.

DRUG-INDUCED PIGMENTATION ICD-10: T88.7

- Drug-induced pigmentation is common and results from the deposition of a variety of endogenous and exogenous pigments in the skin.
- Drugs most commonly causing hyperpigmentation:
  - Antiarrhythmetic: amiodarone.
  - Antimalarial: Chloroquine, hydroxychloroquine, quinacrine, and quinine.
  - Antimicrobial: Minocycline, clofazimine, and zidovudine.
  - Antiseizure: Hydantoins.
  - Cytostatic: Bleomycin, cyclophosphamide, doxorubicin, daunorubicin, busulfan, 5-fluorouracil, and dactinomycin.
- Metals: silver, gold, and iron.
- Hormones: ACTH, estrogen or progesterone.
- Psychiatric: Chlorpromazine.
- Dietary: β-carotene.

CLINICAL MANIFESTATION

AMIODARONE More than 75% of patients after 40-g cumulative dose after >4 months of therapy. More common in skin phototypes I and II, and may be limited to the light-exposed areas in a small proportion (8%) of patients.

Dusky-red erythema and later, blue-gray dermal melanosis (Fig. 23-9) in exposed areas (the face and hands). Lipofuscin-type pigment deposited in macrophages and endothelial cells. ANTIMALARIALS *Cloroquine, hydroxychloroquine.* Occurs in 25% of individuals who take the drug for >4 months. Brownish,

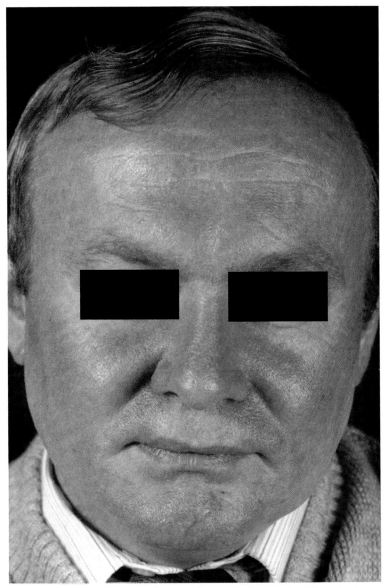

FIGURE 23-9 **Drug-induced pigmentation: amiodarone** A striking mix of a slate gray and brown pigmentation in the face. The bluish color is caused by the deposition of melanin and lipofuscin contained in macrophages and endothelial cells in the dermis. The brown color is caused by melanin. The pigmentation is reversible, but it may take up to a year or more to complete resolution.

gray-brown, and/or blue-black discoloration resulting from melanin or hemosiderin. Over shins; the face and nape of neck; hard palate; under finger- and toenails (see Section 32); may also occur in the cornea and retina. *Quinacrine*: Yellow, yellow-green skin, and sclerae (resembling icterus); yellow-green fluorescence of the nail bed with Wood lamp.

MINOCYCLINE Onset delayed, usually after total dose of >50 g, but may occur after a small dose. Not melanin but an iron-containing brown pigment. Blue-gray or slate-gray pigmentation (Fig. 23-10). Distributed on extensor legs, ankles, dorsa of the feet, the face, especially around eyes; sites of trauma or inflammation such as acne scars, contusions, abrasions; hard palate, teeth; nails.

CLOFAZIMINE Orange, reddish brown (range, pink to black) discoloration, ill-defined on light-exposed areas; conjunctivae; accompanied by red sweat, urine, feces. Subcutaneous fat is orange.

ZIDOVUDINE Brown macules on lips or oral mucosa; longitudinal brown bands in nails.

PHENYTOIN High dose over a long period of time (>1 year). *Discoloration* is spotty, resembling melasma, in light-exposed areas and is caused by melanin.

BLEOMYCIN Tan to brown to black and results from an increase in epidermal melanin at sites of minor inflammation, i.e., parallel linear streaks at sites of exoriations caused by scratching ("flagellate" pigmentation), most commonly on the back, elbows, small joints, and nails.

CYCLOPHOSPHAMIDE Brown. Diffuse or discrete macules on elbows; palms with Addisonian-like pigmentation (see Fig. 15-8) and macules.

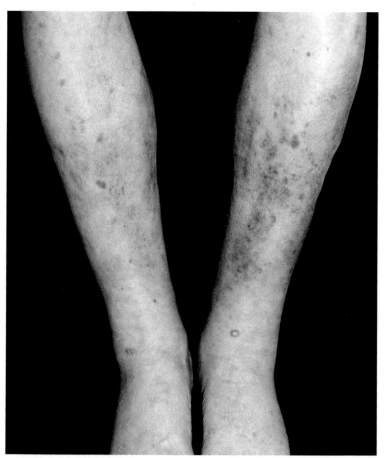

FIGURE 23-10 Drug-induced pigmentation: minocycline Striking, blue-gray pigmentation on the lower legs. This 75-year-old woman had been treated with minocycline for >1 year because of nontuberculous mycobacterial infection.

BUSULFAN Occurs in 5% of treated patients. Addisonian-like pigmentation. Face, axillae, chest, abdomen, and oral mucous membranes.

ACTH Addisonian pigmentation of skin and oral mucosa. First 13 amino acids of ACTH are identical to α-melanocyte-stimulating hormone (MSH) (see Fig. 15-11).

ESTROGENS/-PROGESTERONE Caused by endogenous and exogenous estrogen combined with progesterone, i.e., during pregnancy or with oral contraceptive therapy. Sunlight causes marked darkening of pigmentation. Tan/brown. Melasma (see Fig. 13-9).

SILVER (ARGYRIA OR ARGYROSIS) *Source*: Silver nitrate nose drops; silver sulfadiazine applied as an ointment. Silver sulfide (photographic film). Blue-gray discoloration. Primarily areas exposed to light, i.e., the face, dorsa of the hands, nails, and conjunctiva; also diffuse.

IRON *Source*: IM iron injections; multiple blood transfusions. Brown or blue-gray discoloration. Generalized; also local deposits at site of injection.

CAROTENE Ingestion of large quantities of β-carotene-containing vegetables; β-carotene tablets. Yellow-orange discoloration. Most apparent on the palms and soles.

PSEUDOPORPHYRIA ICD-10: E80.25

- Pseudoporphyria is a condition that clinically presents with cutaneous manifestations of porphyria cutanea tarda (PCT) (see Section 10) without the characteristic abnormal porphyrin excretion.
- Drugs causing pseudoporphyria are naproxen, nabumetone, oxaprozin, diflunisal, celecoxib, tetracyclines, ketoprofen, mefenamic acid, tiaprofenic acid, nalidixic acid, amiodarone, and furosemide.
- Develops on the dorsa of hands and feet with characteristic tense bullae that rupture and leave erosions (**Fig. 23-11**) and heal with scars and milia formation.
- It is characterized by subepidermal blistering with little or no dermal inflammation and, in contrast to true PCT, little or no deposition of immunoreactants around upper dermal blood vessels and capillary walls.
- A bullous dermatosis that is morphologically and histologically indistinguishable from pseudoporphyria also occurs in patients with chronic renal failure receiving maintenance hemodialysis (see Section 18).

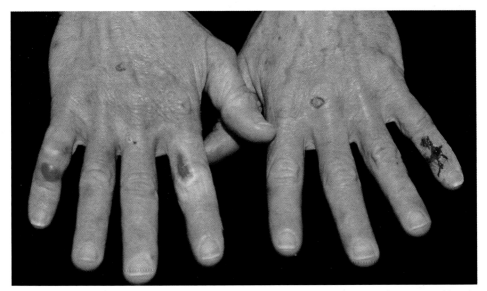

FIGURE 23-11 Pseudoporphyria: nonsteroidal anti-inflammatory agents In this 20-year-old male, blisters appeared on the dorsa of both hands that led to erosions, crusting, and were clinically indistinguishable from porphyria cutanea tarda. However, there was no urinary fluorescence, and porphyrin studies were negative. The patient had taken an NSAID for arthritis and had impaired kidney function.

ACDR-RELATED NECROSIS ICD-10: T88.7

- Drugs can cause cutaneous necrosis when given orally or at injection sites.
- *Warfarin-induced cutaneous necrosis* is a rare reaction with onset between the third and fifth days of anticoagulation therapy with the warfarin derivatives, manifested by cutaneous infarction.
- *Risk factors*: Higher initial dosing, obesity, female sex; individuals with hereditary deficiency of protein C, protein S, or antithrombin III deficiency.
- Lesions vary with severity of reaction: Petechiae to ecchymoses to tender hemorrhagic infarcts to extensive necrosis, which can be well demarcated, deep purple to black (**Fig. 22-12**). *Distribution*: Areas of abundant subcutaneous fat: breasts (**Fig. 23-12**), buttocks, abdomen, thighs, and calves; acral areas are spared.
- *Differential diagnosis*: Purpura fulminans (disseminated intravascular coagulation), hematoma/ ecchymosis/necrotizing soft tissue infection, vasculitis, or brown recluse spider bite.
- *Heparin* can cause cutaneous necrosis, usually at the site of the subcutaneous injection (**Fig. 23-13**).
- *Interferon-α* can cause necrosis and ulceration at injection sites, often in the lower abdominal panniculus or thighs (**Fig. 23-14**).
- Ergotamine-containing medications lead to acral gangrene; ergotamine-containing suppositories after prolonged use cause extremely painful anal and perianal black eschars which, after having been shed, leave deep painful ulcers (**Fig. 23-15**).
- *Embolia cutis medicamentosa*: Deep necrosis developing at the site of intramuscular injection of oily drugs inadvertently injected into an artery (**Fig. 23-16**).
- Necrosis also develops in obtunded or deeply sedated patients at pressure sites (**Fig. 23-17**).

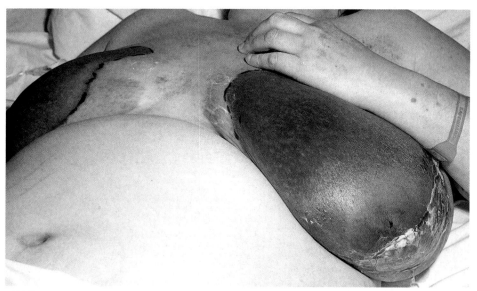

FIGURE 23-12   ACDR-related cutaneous necrosis: warfarin Bilateral areas of cutaneous infarction with purple-to-black coloration of the breast surrounded by an area of erythema occurred on the fifth day of warfarin therapy.

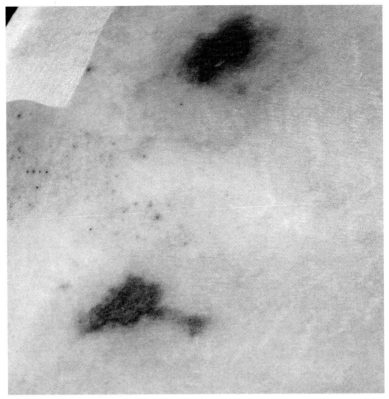

FIGURE 23-13 ACDR-related cutaneous necrosis: heparin Two lesions of irregular dark-red erythema with central hemorrhagic necrosis on the abdomen occurring postoperatively in a female injected with heparin.

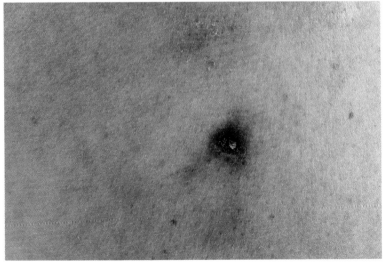

FIGURE 23-14 ACDR-related cutaneous necrosis: interferon-α An ulcer on the thigh at the site of interferon injection.

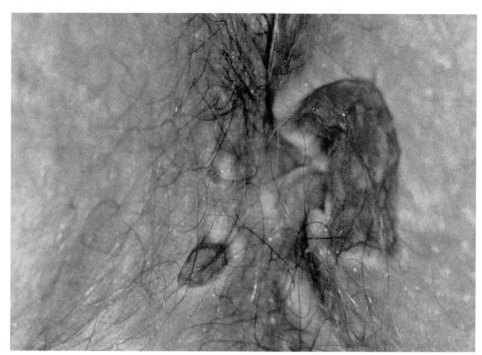

FIGURE 23-15 ACDR-related cutaneous necrosis: ergotamine This 60-year-old male had used ergot-containing suppositories for pain relief over many months. Painful black necrosis followed by ulceration developed on the anus and perianally and extended into the rectum.

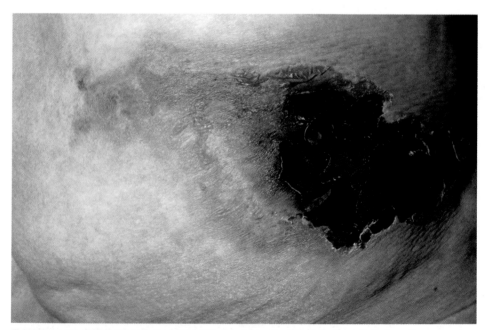

FIGURE 23-16 ACDR-related necrosis following intramuscular injection Embolia cutis medicamentosa. The drug (an oily preparation of testosterone) had been inadvertently administered intraarterially.

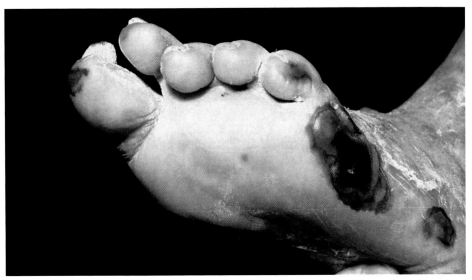

FIGURE 23-17 ACDR-related necrosis with hemorrhagic blistering after an overdose of barbiturates This patient had attempted suicide.

ACDR-RELATED TO CHEMOTHERAPY ICD-10: T88.7

- Chemotherapy may induce local and systemic skin toxicity with a wide range of cutaneous manifestations from benign to life threatening.
- The ACDR can be related to overdose, pharmacologic side effects, cumulative toxicity, delayed toxicity, or drug–drug interactions.
- Clinical manifestations range from alopecia (see Section 31) and nail changes (see Section 32) to mucositis and acral erythema, often with sensory abnormalities: Palmoplantar dysesthesia (capecitabine, cytarabine, doxorubicin, fluorouracil).
- Chemotherapeutic agents are also responsible for inflammation and ulceration at sites of extravasation of intravenous medications, such as doxorubicin or taxol, which can be followed by skin necrosis with ulceration.
- Other reactions are radiation recall or enhancement (as with methotrexate), erosion or ulceration of psoriasis caused by an overdose of methotrexate, inflammation and sloughing of actinic keratosis resulting from 5-fluorouracil or fludarabine, or erosions caused by cisplatin plus 5-fluorouracil (Fig. 23-18A).
- Table 23-7 lists newer chemotherapeutics including "biologicals" and their ACDR.

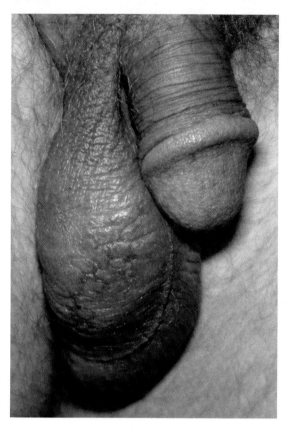

FIGURE 23-18 ACDR-related cellulitis *Erosions resulting from cisplatin and 5-fluorouracil (5FU).* This patient had received chemotherapy with cisplatin and 5FU. Painful erosive lesions appeared on the scrotum and there was also erosive mucositis.

TABLE 23-7 Newer Chemotherapeutic Agents and Their ACDR

Class	Agents	ACDR[a]
Spindle inhibitor	Taxanes: docetaxel, paclitaxel	Hand-foot skin reaction[b]; combined with sensory abnormalities: erythrodysesthesia; radiation recall urticaria, exanthems, mucositis, alopecia, nail changes (see Section 32); scleroderma-like changes on lower extremities; subacute cutaneous lupus erythematosus (SCLE), AGEP and fixed drug reaction (paclitaxel)
	Vinca alkaloids: vincristine, vinblastine, vinorelbine	Phlebitis, alopecia, acral erythema, extravasation reactions (including necrosis)
Antimetabolites	Fludarabine	Serpentine supravenous hyperpigmetnation, macular, papular exanthem, mucositis, acral erythema, paraneoplastic pemphigus, drug-induced SCLE
	Cladribine	Exanthem, TEN(?)
	Capecitabine	Hand-foot skin reaction[b] acral hyperpigmentation, palmoplantar keratoderma, pyogenic granuloma, inflammation of actinic keratoses

TABLE 23-7 Newer Chemotherapeutic Agents and Their ACDR (*Continued*)

Class	Agents	ACDR[a]
	Tegafur	Hand-foot skin reaction[b] acral hyperpigmentation; pityriasis lichenoides et varioliformis acuta, phototoxic reactions
	Gemcitabine	Mucositis, alopecia, maculopapular exanthem, radiation recall, linear IgA bullous dermatosis, pseudoscleroderma, lipodermatosclerosis, erysipelas-like plaques, pseudolymphoma, lymphomatoid papulosis
	Pemetrexed	Exanthema, radiation recall, urticarial vasculitis
Genotoxic agents	Carboplatin	Alopecia, hypersensitivity reaction (erythema, facial swelling, dyspnea, tachycardia, wheezing), palmoplantar erythema, facial flushing
	Oxaliplatin	Hypersensitivity reaction (see preceding); irritant extravasation reaction; radiation recall
	Liposomal doxorubicin	Acral erythema, palmoplantar erythrodysesthesia neutrophilic eccrine hidradenitis, hyperpigmentation (blue-gray), mucositis, alopecia, exanthems, radiation recall, ultraviolet light recall
	Liposomal daunorubicin	Alopecia, mucositis, extravasation reactions
	Idarubicin	Radiation recall; alopecia, acral erythema, mucositis, nail changes (transverse pigmented bands), extravasation reactions
	Topotecan	Maculopapular exanthem, alopecia, neutrophilic hidradenitis
	Irinotecan	Mucositis, alopecia, lichenoid reactions
Signal transduction inhibitors	EGFR antagonists: gefitinib, cetuximab, erlotinib, panitumumab	Papulopustular eruptions in seborrheic areas, erythematous plaques, telangiectasias; xerosis, paronychia; hair abnormalities (trichomegaly, curling, fragility, see Section 31) Usually start a week after initiation of drug. Can treat with topical antibiotics, retinoids (topical or systemic). Can also lead to paronychia, trichomegaly, leukocytocalstic vasculitis, urticaria, anaphylaxis and necrolytic migratory erythema.
	Multikinase inhibitors: Imatinib	Maculopapular exanthem (face, forearms, ankles), exfoliative dermatitis, graft-versus-host reaction-like reaction, erythema nodosum, vasculitis, SJS, AGEP; hypopigmentation, hyperpigmentation, darkening of hair, nail hyperpigmentation, lichen planus-like eruption (skin and oral mucosa), follicular mucinosis, pityriasis rosea-like eruption, Sweet syndrome, exacerbation of psoriasis, palmoplantar hyperkeratosis, porphyria cutanea tarda, primary cutaneous EBV-related B cell lymphoma

(*continued*)

TABLE 23-7 Newer Chemotherapeutic Agents and Their ACDR (*Continued*)

Class	Agents	ACDR[a]
	Dasatinib and nilotinib	Localized and generalized erythema, maculopapular exanthem, mucositis, pruritus, exfoliation, alopecia, xerosis "acne," urticaria, panniculitis, Sweet' syndrome.
	Sorafenib and sunitinib	Rash/desquamation, hand-foot skin reaction[b] pain, alopecia, mucositis, xerosis, flushing edema, seborrheic dermatitis, yellow skin coloration (sunitinib, one week after starting drug), subungual splinter hemorrhages, pyoderma gangrenosum, SCC (KA-type) and eruptive melanocytic lesions (sorafenib)
Proteasome inhibitor	Bortezomib	Erythematous nodules and plaques, morbilliform exanthem, ulceration, vasculitis and Sweet' syndrome
Immune Modulators	Ipilimumab (CTLA-4 AB)	Immune-mediated side effects: macular and papular eruption, pruritis, hepatitis, vitiligo, hypothyroidism, enterocolitis, hepatitis, SJS/TEN
	Pembrolizumab and Nivoluman (PD-1 receptor antibody)	Immune-mediated side effects: macular and papular eruption, pruritus, vitiligo, hypothyroidism, enterocolitis, hepatitis, mucositis
BRAF inhibitors	Vemurafinib	Rash (68%), arthralgias, photosensitivity (42%), SCC (23%, most occur in first few months)
	Dabrafenib	Pyrexia, headaches, rash

[a]Only cutaneous adverse reactions are listed here.
[b]Hand-foot skin reaction: erythema, hyperkeratotic with halo of erythema, tender, localized to areas of pressure on fingertips, toes, and heels.

Source: Collated from N Haidary et al. J Am Acad Dermatol. 2008;58:545. Please note that this table has also been supplemented by the authors.

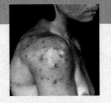

DISORDERS OF PSYCHIATRIC ETIOLOGY

BODY DYSMORPHIC SYNDROME (BDS) ICD-10: F45.2

- Patients with dysmorphic syndrome regard their image as distorted in the eyes of the public; this becomes almost an obsession.
- The patient with BDS does not generally consult a psychiatrist but a dermatologist or plastic surgeon. The typical patient with BDS is a single, female, young adult who is anxious.
- Common dermatologic complaints are facial (wrinkles, acne, scars, hypertrichosis, and dry lips), scalp (incipient baldness, increased hair growth), genital (normal sebaceous glands on the penis, red scrotum, red vulva, and vaginal odor), hyperhidrosis, and bromhidrosis.
- Management is a problem. One strategy is for the dermatologist to establish rapport; in a few visits, the complaint can be explored and further discussed.
- If the patient and physician do not agree that the complaint is a vastly exaggerated skin or hair change, then the patient should be referred to a psychiatrist; this latter plan is usually not accepted, in which case the problem may persist indefinitely.

DELUSIONS OF PARASITOSIS ICD-10: F22.0

- This rare disorder, which occurs in adults and is present for months or years, is associated with pain or paresthesia and is characterized by the presence of numerous skin lesions, mostly excoriations, which the patient truly believes are the result of a parasitic infestation (Fig. 24-1A).
- The onset of the initial pruritus or paresthesia may be related to xerosis or, in fact, to a previously treated infestation.
- Patients pick with their fingernails or dig into their skin with needles or tweezers to remove the "parasites" (Fig. 24-1B).
- It is important to rule out other causes of pruritus. This problem is serious; patients truly suffer and are opposed to seeking psychiatric help.
- The patient should see a psychiatrist for at least one visit and for recommendations of drug therapy: pimozide plus an antidepressant. Treatment is difficult and usually unsuccessful.

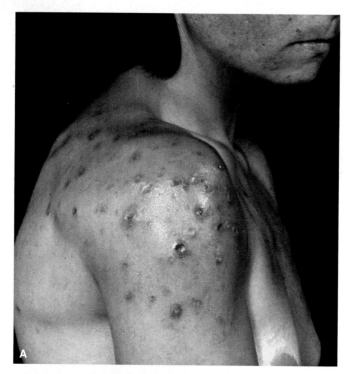

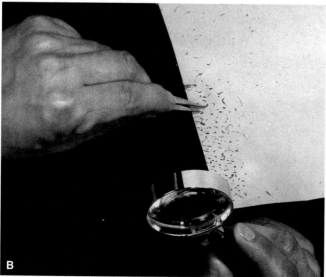

FIGURE 24-1 Delusions of parasitosis (A) Usually patients collect small pieces of debris from their skin by scratching with their nails or an instrument and submit them to the doctor for examination for parasites. In this case, pointed tweezers were used and the results are ulcers, crusted lesions, and scars. **(B)** Occasionally, this can progress to an aggressive behavior such as depicted in this case where the patient posed to demonstrate how she collects the "parasites" from her skin on a piece of paper. In the majority of cases, patients are not dissuaded from their monosymptomatic delusion.

NEUROTIC EXCORIATIONS AND TRICHOTILLOMANIA ICD-10: L98.1

- *Neurotic excoriations* are not an uncommon problem, occurring more in females than in males and in the third to fifth decades.
- They may relate the onset to a specific event or to chronic stress; patients deny picking and scratching.
- The clinical lesions are an admixture of several types of lesions, principally excoriations, all produced by habitual picking of the skin with the fingernails; most common on the face (**Fig. 24-2**), back (**Fig. 24-3**), and extremities but also at other sites. There may be depigmented atrophic or hyperpigmented macules → scars (**Fig. 24-3**).
- *The lesions are located only on sites that the hands can reach, thus often sparing the center of the back.*
- Psychiatric guidance may be necessary if the problem is not solved, as it can be very disfiguring on the face and disruptive to the patient and the family. The course is prolonged, unless life adjustments are made.
- Pimozide has been helpful but must be used with caution and with the advice and guidance of a psychopharmacologist. Also, antidepressant drugs may be used.
- **Trichotillomania** is a compulsive desire or habit to pluck hair. Can be on the scalp or any other hairy region (e.g., beard). Confluence of areas with very short sparse hairs, small bald areas, and normal area of scalp (**Fig. 24-4**). More pronounced on the side of the dominant hand. Can be combined with neurotic excoriations induced by vigorous plucking with tweezers. Microscopically, anagen hairs, bluntly broken hairs, and pigment casts. Treatment as for neurotic excoriations.

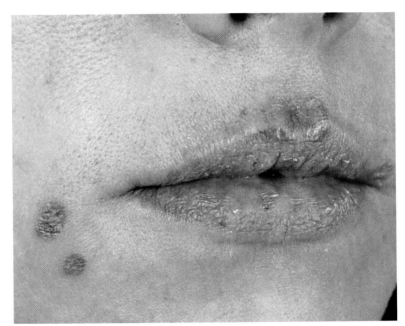

FIGURE 24-2 Neurotic excoriations Several erythematous and crusted macules and erosions on the lower cheek and upper lip of a 19-year-old female with mild facial acne. No primary lesions are seen. The patient, who is moderately depressed, has mild acneiform lesions, which she compulsively picks with her fingernails.

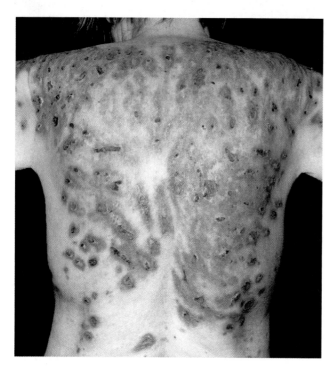

FIGURE 24-3 Neurotic excoriations: back Excoriations of the upper, mid-back, and (not shown) on gluteal areas and linear areas of postinflammatory hyperpigmentation, crusting, and scarring in a 66-year-old diabetic female. Lesions have been present for at least 10 years. The ulcerated crusted lesion resolved with cloth tape occlusion. Once the protection was removed, the patient resumed excoriating the sites.

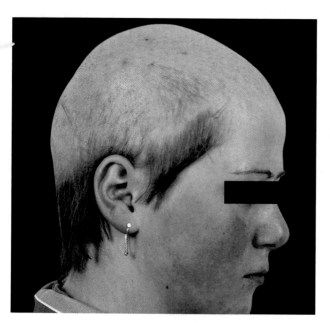

FIGURE 24-4 Trichotillomania This extensive alopecia has resulted from pulling and plucking hairs by the 17-year-old patient. She appeared balanced but mildly depressed and had considerable conflict with her parents. She admitted pulling hairs after considerable questioning.

FACTITIOUS SYNDROMES (MÜNCHHAUSEN SYNDROME) ICD-10: F 68.1

- The term *factitious* means "artificial," and in this condition, there is a self-induced dermatologic lesion(s); either the patient claims no responsibility or admits deliberately mutilating the skin.
- It occurs in young adults, females > males. The history of the evolution of the lesions is vague ("hollow" history).
- The lesions may be present for weeks to months to years (Fig. 24-5).
- The patient may be normal looking and act normally in every respect, although frequently there is a strange affect and bizarre personality.
- The skin lesions consist of cuts (Fig. 24-5), ulcers, and dense adherent necrotic eschar (Fig. 24-6). The shape of the lesions may be linear (Fig. 24-5), bizarre shapes, geometric patterns, single or multiple. The diagnosis can be difficult, but the nature of the lesions (bizarre geometric shapes) may immediately suggest an artificial etiology.
- It is important to rule out every possible cause—chronic infections, granulomas, and vasculitis—perform a biopsy before assigning the diagnosis of *dermatosis artefacta*, both for the benefit of the patient and because the physician may be at risk for malpractice if he or she fails to diagnose a true pathologic process.
- There is often serious personality and/or psychosocial stress, or a psychiatric disease.
- The condition demands the utmost tact on the part of the physician, who can avert a serious outcome (i.e., suicide) by attempting to gain enough empathy with the patient to ascertain the cause.
- The condition may persist for years in a patient who has selected his or her skin as the target organ of his or her conflicts. Consultation and management with a psychiatrist are mandatory.

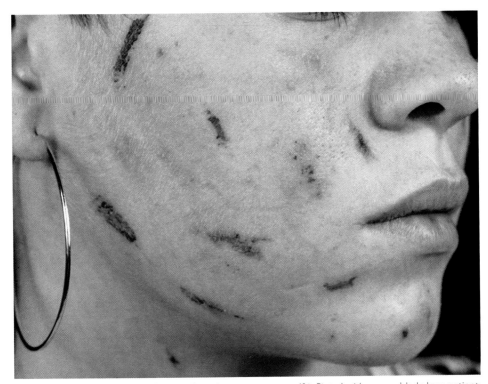

FIGURE 24-5 Factitious syndrome These linear cuts were self-inflicted with a razor blade by a patient with a borderline syndrome. Similar, much deeper cuts were on the forearms.

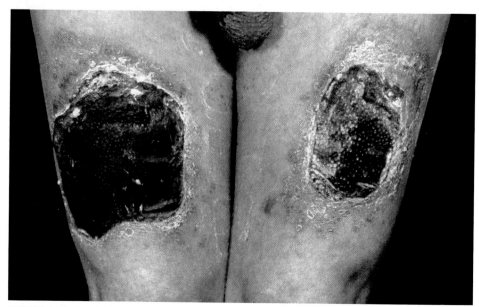

FIGURE 24-6 **Factitious syndrome** These necroses were self-inflicted by the covert application of diluted sulfuric acid and tightly fitting bandages. The patient appeared well adjusted and refused to see a psychiatrist.

CUTANEOUS SIGNS OF INJECTING DRUG USE

- Injecting drug users often develop cutaneous stigmata as a result of their habit, whether injecting subcutaneously or intravascularly.
- Cutaneous lesions range from foreign body response to injected material, infections, and scars.

CUTANEOUS INJECTION REACTIONS **Cutaneous Injury.** Multiple punctures at the sites of cutaneous injection, often linear over veins or linear scars (Fig. 24-7).

Tattoos. Carbon on needles (after flame sterilization) can result in inadvertent tattooing and pigmented linear scars (Fig. 24-8).

Foreign Body Granuloma. Subcutaneous injection of adulterants (talc, sugar, starch, baking soda, flour, cotton fibers, glass, etc.) can elicit a foreign body response ± cellulitis ± granuloma ± ulceration (Fig. 24-9).

INTRAVASCULAR INJECTION REACTIONS **Venous Injury.** Intravenous injection can result in thrombosis, thrombophlebitis, and septic phlebitis. Chronic edema of the upper extremity is common.

Arterial Injury. Chronic intra-arterial injection can result in injection site pain, cyanosis, erythema, sensory and motor deficits, and vascular compromise (vascular insufficiency/gangrene).

INFECTIONS **Transmission of Infectious Agents.** Injecting drug use can result in transmission of HIV, hepatitis B virus, and hepatitis C virus with subsequent life-threatening systemic infections.

Injection Site Infections. Local infections include cellulitis (Fig. 24-9), abscess formation, lymphangitis, and septic phlebitis/thrombophlebitis. The most common organisms are those from the drug users, e.g., *S. aureus* and GAS. Less common microbes: Enteric organisms, anaerobes, *Clostridium botulinum*, oral flora, fungi (*Candida albicans*), and polymicrobial infections.

Systemic Infections. Intravenous injection of microbes can result in an infection of vascular endothelium, most commonly heart valve with infectious endocarditis.

Atrophic Punched-Out Scars. Result from subcutaneous injections (i.e., "skin popping") after an inflammatory (sterile or infected) response to injected material (Fig. 24-7).

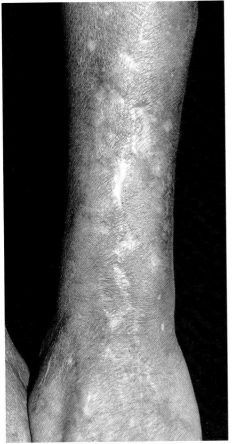

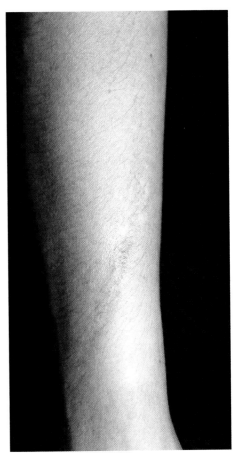

FIGURE 24-7 Injecting drug use: injection tracks over veins on the lower arms Linear tracks with punctures, fibrosis, and crusts were created by daily injections into the superficial veins.

FIGURE 24-8 Linear tattoos From carbon on needles resulted from intravenous injections.

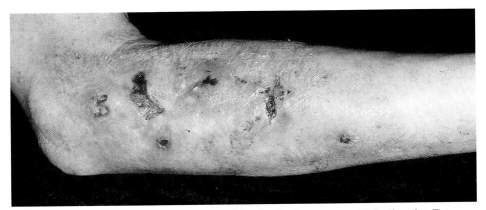

FIGURE 24-9 Injecting drug use: cellulitis and foreign body response at injection site The patient injected into the subcutaneous tissue as well as veins of the forearm, resulting in foreign body response and *S. aureus* cellulitis with associated bacteremia and infectious endocarditis.

PART III

Diseases Caused By Microbial Agents

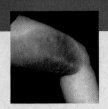

SECTION 25

BACTERIAL COLONIZATIONS AND INFECTIONS OF SKIN AND SOFT TISSUES

The human microbiome or microbiota represents diverse viral, bacterial, fungal, and other species that live on and within us. They are part of us and we are part of this complex ecosystem. The human body contains >10 times more microbial cells than human cells. Skin supports a range of microbial communities that live in distinct niches. Microbial colonization of skin is more dense in humid intertriginous and occluded sites such as axillae, anogenital regions, and webspaces of feet. An intact stratum corneum is the most important defense against invasion of pathogenic bacteria.

Coagulase-negative staphylococci normally colonize skin shortly after birth and are not considered to be pathogens when cultured from skin.

Overgrowth of flora in occluded areas often results in clinical syndromes of *erythrasma*, *pitted keratolysis*, and *trichomycosis*.

Pyoderma is an archaic term, literally "pus in the skin." Skin and soft-tissue infections, commonly caused by *Staphylococcus aureus* and group A streptococcus (GAS), have been referred to as "pyoderma." Pyoderma gangrenosum is a *noninfectious* inflammatory process, often associated with a systemic disorder such as inflammatory bowel disease.

S. aureus colonizes the nares and intertriginous skin intermittently, can penetrate the stratum corneum, and cause *skin infections*, e.g., impetigo, folliculitis. Deeper infection results in *soft-tissue infections*. Methicillin-resistant *S. aureus* (MRSA) is an important pathogen for community-acquired (CA-MRSA) and health-care-acquired (HA-MRSA) infections. MRSA strain USA300 is the major cause of skin and soft tissue as well as more invasive infections in community and health-care settings.

GAS usually colonizes the skin first and then the nasopharynx. Group B streptococcus (GBS; *Streptococcus agalactiae*) and group G β-hemolytic streptococci (GGS) colonize the perineum of some individuals and may cause superficial and invasive infections.

Cutaneous production of toxins by bacteria (*S. aureus and* GAS) causes systemic intoxications such as toxic shock syndrome (TSS) and scarlet fever.

ERYTHRASMA ICD-10: L08.1

- Etiology. *Corynebacterium minutissimum*, gram-positive (diphtheroid) bacillus; normally in human microbiome. Growth favored by humid cutaneous microclimate.

CLINICAL MANIFESTATION

Asymptomatic except for subtle discoloration.

Patches, sharply marginated (Fig. 25-1). Tan or pinkish; postinflammatory hyperpigmentation in more heavily pigmented individuals.

In webspaces of the feet, it may be macerated (Fig. 25-2). *Distribution*: Intertriginous skin, i.e., toe webs (Fig. 25-2), inguinal folds, axillae, and other occluded sites.

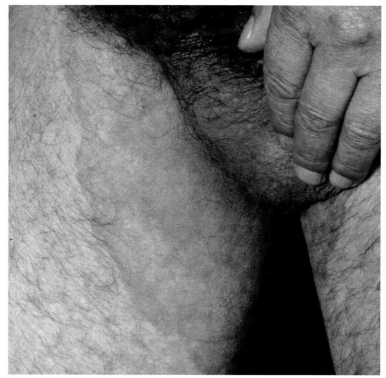

FIGURE 25-1 **Erythrasma: groins** Sharply marginated, tan patches in the genito-crural fold. Wood lamps demonstrates bright coral-red fluorescence differentiating erythrasma from intertriginous psoriasis. KOH preparation was negative for hyphae.

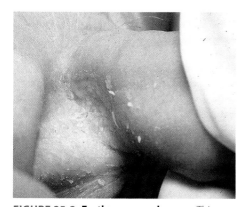

FIGURE 25-2 **Erythrasma: webspace** This macerated interdigital webspace appeared bright coral-red when examined with Wood's lamp; KOH preparation was negative for hyphae. The webspace is the most common site for erythrasma in temperate climates. In some cases, interdigital tinea pedis and/or pseudomonal intertrigo may coexist.

DIAGNOSIS

Wood's lamp examination demonstrates corral-red fluorescence. KOH negative; rules out epidermal dermatophytosis.

DIFFERENTIAL DIAGNOSIS

Intertriginous psoriasis, epidermal dermatophytosis, pityriasis versicolor, and Hailey–Hailey disease.

COURSE

Persists and recurs unless microclimate is altered.

TREATMENT

Usually controlled with benzoyl peroxide wash or sanitizing alcohol gel. Clindamycin lotion and erythromycin are beneficial.

PITTED KERATOLYSIS

- Etiology. *Kytococcus sedentarius.* One of human microbiome on plantar feet in the setting of hyperhidrosis; produces two extracellular proteases that can digest keratin.

CLINICAL MANIFESTATION

Punched out pits in stratum corneum, 1 to 8 mm in diameter (Fig. 25-3). Pits can remain discrete or become confluent, forming large areas of eroded stratum corneum. Lesions are more apparent with hyperhidrosis and maceration. Symmetric or asymmetric involvement of both feet. *Distribution:* Pressure-bearing areas, ventral aspect of toe, ball of foot, heel; interface of toes.

DIAGNOSIS

Clinical diagnosis. KOH to rule out tinea pedis.

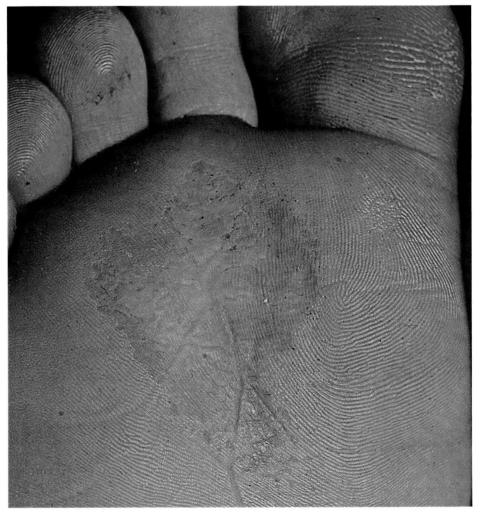

FIGURE 25-3 Pitted keratolysis: plantar The stratum corneum of the plantar skin shows confluent multiple, confluent "pits" (defects in the stratum corneum).

DIFFERENTIAL DIAGNOSIS

Concomitant tinea pedis, erythrasma, candidal intertrigo, and pseudomonal webspace infection may be present.

COURSE

Persists and recurs unless microclimate is altered.

TREATMENT

Usually controlled with benzoyl peroxide wash or sanitizing alcohol gel. Topical antibiotics, such as erythromycin and clindamycin, and aluminum chloride solution can also be helpful.

TRICHOMYCOSIS ICD-10: A48.8/L08.8

- Superficial colonization on hair shafts in sweaty regions, axillary and pubic.
- Etiology. *Corynebacterium tenuis* and other corynebacterial *species*; gram-positive diphtheroid. *Not* fungus.
- Malodorous granular concretions (yellow, black, or red) on hair shaft (Fig. 25-4). Hair appears thickened, beaded, and firmly adherent.
- Treatment. Usually controlled with benzoyl peroxide wash or sanitizing alcohol gel. Antiperspirants. Shaving area.

FIGURE 25-4 Trichomycosis axillaris
40-year-old obese male. Axillary hairs have cream-color encrustation. Some skin tags are also seen.

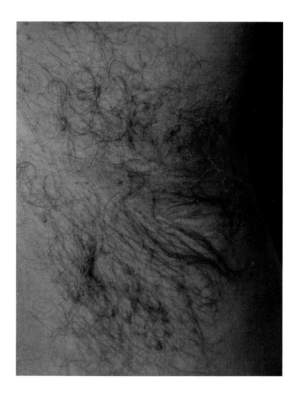

INTERTRIGO ICD-10: L30.4

- Intertrigo (Latin *inter*, "between"; *trigo*, "rubbing").
- Inflammation of opposed skin (inframammary regions, axillae, groins, gluteal folds, and redundant skin folds of obese persons). May represent inflammatory dermatosis or superficial colonization or infection.
- Dermatoses occurring in intertriginous skin include intertriginous psoriasis, seborrheic dermatitis, Hailey–Hailey disease, and Langerhans cell histiocytosis. *S. aureus* and streptococcus can cause secondary infection of these dermatoses.

INFECTIOUS INTERTRIGO

BACTERIAL
- Beta-hemolytic streptococci. Group A (Fig. 25-5), group B, and group G (Fig. 25-6). Streptococcal intertrigo can progress to soft-tissue infection (Fig. 25-6).
- *S. aureus.* Often gains entry into the skin via hair follicles, causing folliculitis and furuncles.
- *Pseudomonas aeruginosa* (Fig. 25-7).
- *C. minutissimum* (erythrasma) (Figs. 25-1 and 25-2).
- *K. sedentarius* (pitted keratolysis) (Fig. 25-3).

CLINICAL MANIFESTATION

Usually asymptomatic. Discomfort usually indicates infection rather than colonization. Soft-tissue infection can gain entry in *S. aureus* or streptococcal intertrigo.

DIAGNOSIS

Identify pathogen by bacterial culture, Wood's lamp examination, or KOH preparation.

TREATMENT

Identify and treat pathogen.

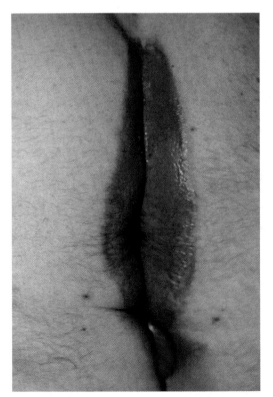

FIGURE 25-5 Intergluteal intertrigo: group A streptococcus A painful moist erythematous plaque in a male with inter-triginous psoriasis, with foul odor. Infection resolved with penicillin VK.

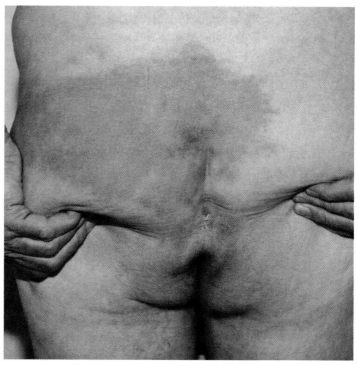

FIGURE 25-6 Erysipelas: group G streptococcus 65-year-old male with sharply marginated erythematous plaque on buttocks. Portal of entry of infection was intergluteal intertrigo.

FIGURE 25-7 Webspace intertrigo: P. *aeruginosa* Erosion of a webspace of the foot with a bright red base and surrounding erythema. Tinea pedis (interdigital and moccasin patterns) and hyperhidrosis were also present, which facilitated growth of *Pseudomonas.*

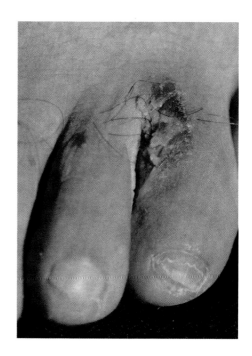

IMPETIGO ICD-10: B08.0

- Etiology. *S. aureus*; GAS.
- Portal of Entry. Impetigo occurs adjacent to the site of *S. aureus* colonization such as the nares. Secondary infection of (1) minor breaks in the epidermis (impetiginization), (2) preexisting dermatoses, (3) other infections such as eczema herpeticum, or (4) wounds.
- Clinical Manifestation. Honey-colored crusted erosions.
- Treatment
  - Reduced colonization.
  - Topical antibiotic to infected and colonized sites; systemic antibiotic.

EPIDEMIOLOGY AND ETIOLOGY

- *S. aureus*: Methicillin-sensitive (MSSA) and methicillin-resistant (MRSA). Bullous impetigo: Local production of epidermolytic toxin A–producing *S. aureus*, which also causes staphylococcal scalded skin syndrome.
- Beta-hemolytic streptococcus: group A.

S. aureus and GAS are not members of human skin *microbiome*. They may transiently colonize skin and cause superficial infections.

DEMOGRAPHY Secondary infections, any age. Primary infections most often occur in children.

PORTALS OF ENTRY OF INFECTION Minor breaks in the skin most commonly. Facial lesions usually associated with *S. aureus* colonization of nares. Dermatoses such as atopic dermatitis or Hailey–Hailey disease. Traumatic wounds. Bacterial infections occur in other cutaneous infections.

CLINICAL MANIFESTATION

Superficial infections often asymptomatic. Ecthyma may be painful and tender.

IMPETIGO Erosions with crusts (Figs. 25-8 and 25-9). Golden-yellow crusts are often seen in impetigo but are hardly pathognomonic; 1- to >3-cm lesions; central healing often apparent if lesions present for several weeks (Fig. 25-9). *Arrangement*: Scattered, discrete lesions;

without therapy, lesions may become confluent; satellite lesions occur by autoinoculation. Secondary infection of various dermatoses is common (Figs. 25-10 and 25-11).

BULLOUS IMPETIGO Superficial blisters containing clear yellow or slightly turbid fluid with erythematous halo, arising on normal-appearing skin. Bullous lesions rupture easily, revealing shallow moist *erosions* (Figs. 25-12 and 25-13). *Distribution*: More common in intertriginous sites.

ECTHYMA Ulceration with a thick adherent crust (Fig. 25-14). Lesions may be tender, indurated. Usually occurs at occluded sites (common in homeless or soldiers in trenches during combat who do not or cannot change boots).

DIFFERENTIAL DIAGNOSIS

IMPETIGO Excoriation, contact dermatitis, herpes simplex, epidermal dermatophytosis, and scabies.

INTACT BULLAE Acute contact dermatitis, insect bites, thermal burns, and porphyria cutanea tarda (PCT) (dorsa of hands).

ECTHYMA Excoriations, insect bites.

DIAGNOSIS

Clinical findings confirmed by culture: *S. aureus*, commonly; failure of oral antibiotic suggests MRSA. GAS.

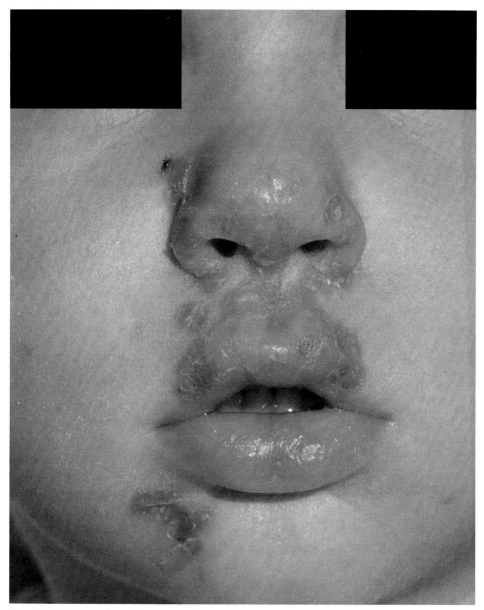

FIGURE 25-8 Impetigo: MSSA Crusted erythematous erosions becoming confluent on the nose, cheek, lips, and chin in a child with nasal carriage of *S. aureus*.

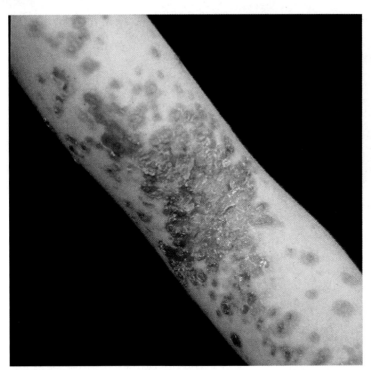

FIGURE 25-9 Impetigo: MSSA Crusted, erythematous erosions becoming confluent in the antecubital fossa, upper and lower arm in a child with atopic dermatitis.

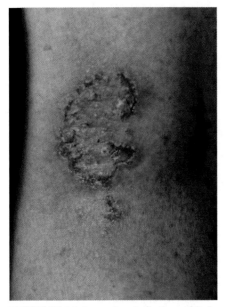

FIGURE 25-10 Secondary infection of Hailey–Hailey disease: MRSA 51-year-old female with Hailey–Hailey disease has chronic MRSA infection of cutaneous erosions on thigh.

COURSE

Untreated, lesions of impetigo become more extensive and develop into ecthyma. With adequate treatment, prompt resolution. Lesions can progress to deeper skin and soft-tissue infections. Nonsuppurative complications of GAS infection include guttate psoriasis, scarlet fever, and glomerulonephritis. Ecthyma may heal with scarring. Recurrent *S. aureus* or GAS infections can occur because of the failure to eradicate pathogen or by recolonization. Undiagnosed MRSA infection does not respond to usual oral antibiotics given for methicillin-sensitive *S. aureus*.

TREATMENT

PREVENTION Benzoyl peroxide wash. Check family members for signs of impetigo. Ethanol or isopropyl gel for hands and/or involved sites.

TOPICAL TREATMENT Mupirocin and retapamulin ointment is highly effective in eliminating *S. aureus* from the nares and cutaneous lesions.

SYSTEMIC ANTIMICROBIAL TREATMENT According to sensitivity of isolated organism.

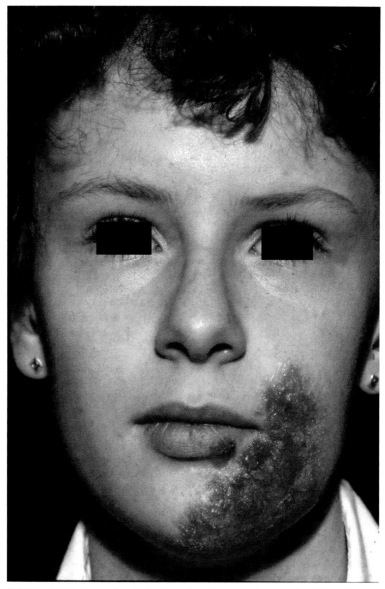

FIGURE 25-11 Secondary infection of mild atopic dermatitis: MRSA 11-year-old boy has yellowish crusted lesions on left cheek and chin.

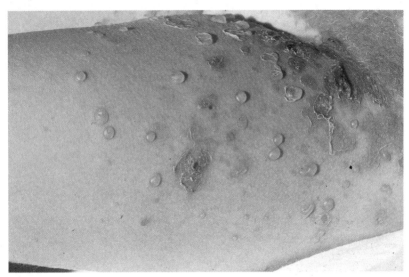

FIGURE 25-12 Bullous impetigo Scattered, discrete, intact, and ruptured thin-walled blisters on the inguinal area and adjacent thigh of a child; lesions in the groin have ruptured, resulting in superficial erosions.

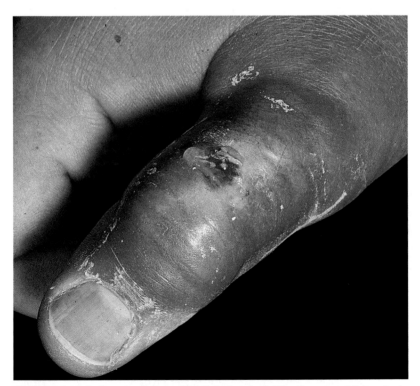

FIGURE 25-13 Bullous impetigo with blistering dactylitis: *S. aureus* A large, single bulla with surrounding erythema and edema on the thumb of a child; the bulla has ruptured and clear serum exudes.

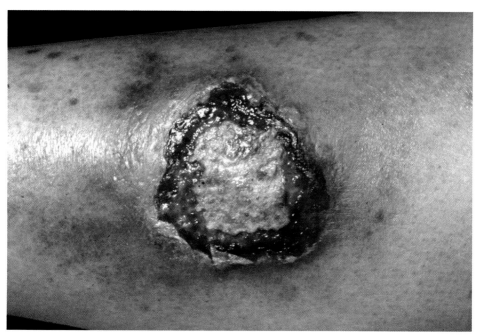

FIGURE 25-14 Ecthyma: MSSA Thickly crusted ulcer on the leg that had been present on the lower leg of a homeless who had not taken off his boots for weeks. The crust was adherent and the site bled with debridement.

ABSCESS, FOLLICULITIS, FURUNCLE, AND CARBUNCLE ICD-10: L02

- Deeper skin infections can follow traumatic inoculation into skin or the extension of infection into hair follicles.
- *Abscess*: Acute or chronic localized inflammation, associated with a collection of pus accumulated in a tissue. Inflammatory response to an infectious process or foreign material.
- *Folliculitis*: Infection of hair follicle with ± pus in the ostium of follicle.
- *Furuncle*: Acute, deep-seated, red, hot, tender nodule or abscess (boil) that evolves from a staphylococcal folliculitis.
- *Carbuncle*: Deeper infection composed of interconnecting abscesses usually arising in several contiguous hair follicles.

EPIDEMIOLOGY AND ETIOLOGY

S. aureus (MSSA, MRSA).
Other Organisms. Less common.

Sterile abscess can occur as a foreign-body response (splinter, ruptured inclusion cyst, injection sites). Cutaneous odontogenic sinus can appear anywhere on the lower face, even at sites distant from the origin (see Cutaneous Odontogenic (Dental) Abscess, Section 33).

Folliculitis, furuncles, and carbuncles represent a continuum of severity of *S. aureus* infection. Portal of entry: Ostium of hair follicle.

CLINICAL MANIFESTATION

ABSCESS May arise in any organ or tissue. Abscesses that present on the skin arise in the dermis, subcutaneous fat, muscle, or a variety of deeper structures. Initially, a tender red nodule forms. In time (days to weeks), pus collects within a central space (Fig. 25-15). A well-formed abscess is characterized by fluctuance of the central portion of the lesion. Arise at sites of trauma. Ruptured inclusion cyst on the back often presents as painful abscess. When arising from *S. aureus* folliculitis, it may be solitary or multiple.

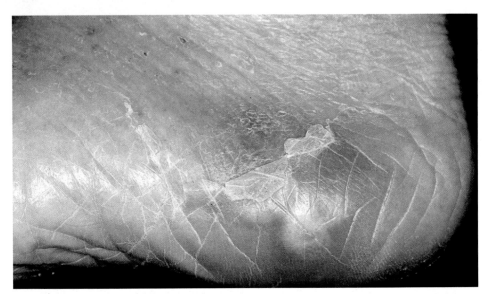

FIGURE 25-15 Abscess: MSSA A very tender abscess with surrounding erythema on the heel. The patient was a diabetic patient with sensory neuropathy; puncture by a sewing needle that was imbedded in the heel had provided a portal of entry. The foreign body was removed surgically.

FOLLICULITIS Begins in the upper portion of the hair follicle. Can arise from bacteria, fungi, virus and mites. Follicular papule, pustule, erosion or crust at the follicular infundibulum, and can extend deeper into the entire length of the follicle (sycosis). Usually nontender or slightly tender; may be pruritic. (Fig. 25-16). Predisposing factors include shaving hairy regions, occlusion of hair-bearing areas, topical corticosteroid preparations, systemic antibiotic promotes growth of gram-negative bacteria, diabetes mellitus, and immunosuppression. Extension of infection can progress to abscess or furuncle formation.

Bacterial agents: *S. aureus* (Bockhart impetigo); *Pseudomonas aeruginosa* (hot-tub); gram-negative folliculitis.
Viral: Herpetic, molluscum contagiosum (see Section 27).
Fungal: *Candida, Malassezia*, dermatophytes (see Section 26).
Other: Syphilitic (see Section 30), *Demodex* (see Section 28).

Variants

S. aureus Folliculitis can be either superficial folliculitis (infundibular) (Fig. 25-16) or deep (sycosis) (extension beneath infundibulum) (Fig. 25-17) with abscess formation. In severe cases (lupoid sycosis), the pilosebaceous units may be destroyed and replaced by fibrous scar tissue.

GRAM-NEGATIVE FOLLICULITIS Occurs in individuals with acne vulgaris treated with oral antibiotics. "Acne" typically worsens, having been in good control. Characterized by small follicular pustules and/or larger abscesses on the cheeks. **HOT-TUB FOLLICULITIS** *(Pseudomonas Aeruginosa)*. Occurs on the trunk following immersion in spa water (Fig. 25-18).

MANAGEMENT

FURUNCLE Initially, a firm tender nodule, up to 1 to 2 cm in diameter. In many individuals, furuncles occur in the setting of staphylococcal folliculitis. Nodule becomes fluctuant, with abscess formation ± central pustule. Nodule with cavitation remains after drainage of abscess. A variable zone of cellulitis may surround the furuncle. *Distribution:* Any hair-bearing region—Beard area, posterior neck and occipital scalp, axillae, buttocks. Solitary or multiple lesions (Figs. 25-19 to 25-23). **CARBUNCLE** Evolution is similar to that of furuncle. Composed of several to multiple, adjacent, and coalescing furuncles (Fig. 25-24). Characterized by multiple loculated dermal and subcutaneous abscesses, superficial pustules, necrotic plugs, and sieve-like openings draining pus.

FIGURE 25-16 Infectious folliculitis, superficial in axilla: MRSA A 25-year-old male with pruritic and tender axillary lesions for several weeks. Multiple follicular pustules and papules are seen in the vault of the shaved axilla. Shaving facilitates entry of *S. aureus* into the superficial hair follicle. The lesions resolved with minocycline.

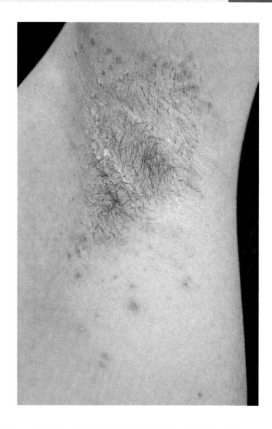

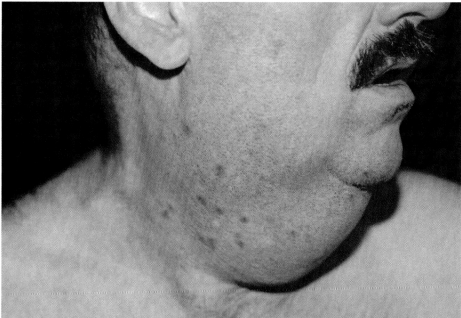

FIGURE 25-17 Infectious folliculitis A male patient with HIV/AIDS and persistent pruritic pustular and ruptured lesions on the cheek/beard for several months.

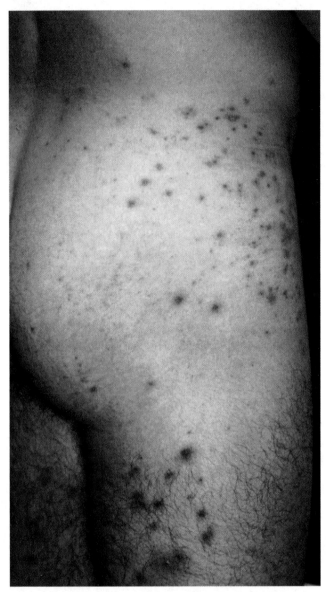

FIGURE 25-18 Infectious folliculitis ("hot tub"): *P. aeruginosa* A 31-year-old male with multiple painful follicular pustules 3 days after bathing in a hot tub. *P. aeruginosa* was isolated on culture from a lesion.

FIGURE 25-19 Furuncle: MSSA Abscess on the upper lip of a 35-year-old male. The lesion is crusted on the top and solid and extremely painful. The furuncle was incised and drained and treated with antibiotics.

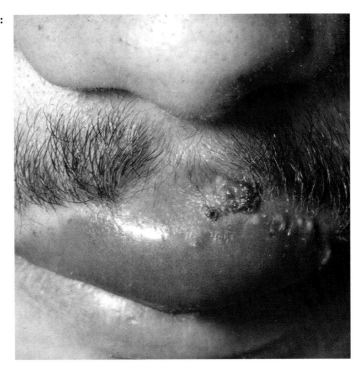

FIGURE 25-20 Furuncles and cellulitis: MRSA A 64-year-old male developed furuncles on the dorsum of the left hand **(A)** and forearm **(B)**. Infection was spreading from the abscess with cellulitis.

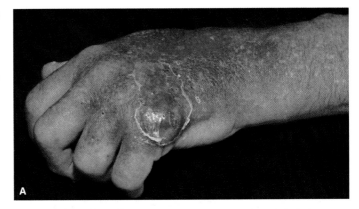

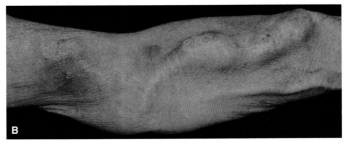

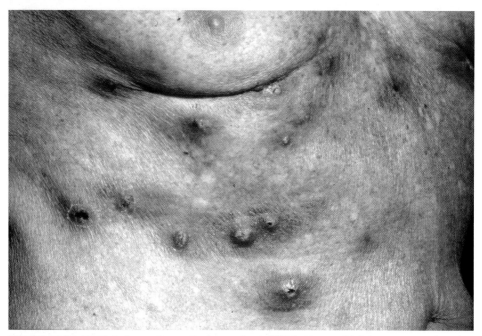

FIGURE 25-21 Multiple furuncles on the lower chest: MRSA 60-year-old diabetic nurse with multiple painful nodules. MRSA was isolated on culture of the nares and from an abscess. She was treated with clindamycin and mupirocin to nares. She was restricted from returning to work until culture sites were negative for *S. aureus* colonization.

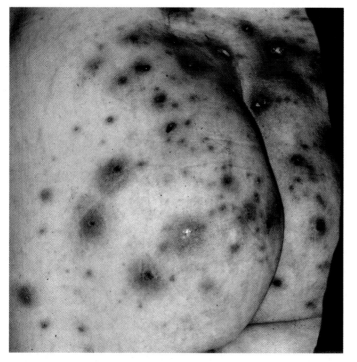

FIGURE 25-22 Multiple furuncles: MRSA Multiple painful nodules on the buttocks of a 52-year-old female with diabetes.

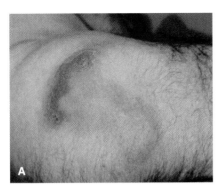
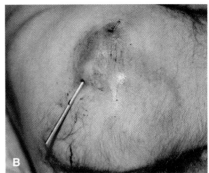
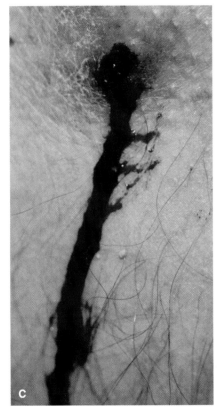

FIGURE 25-23 Chronic abscess, botryomycosis: MRSA 41-year old with HIV disease had an extensive abscess for months. **(A)** R-buttock abscess. **(B)** The abscess was drained and treated with linezolid. **(C)** The white grains noted in the drainage represent colonies of *S. aureus*.

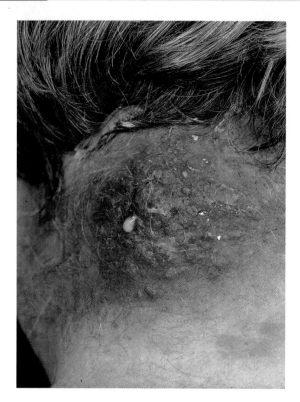

FIGURE 25-24 Carbuncle: MSSA
A very large, inflammatory plaque studded with pustules and draining pus on the nape of the neck. Infection extends down to the fascia and has formed from a confluence of many furuncles.

DIFFERENTIAL DIAGNOSIS

FOLLICULITIS Acneiform disorders (acne vulgaris, rosacea, or perioral dermatitis), HIV-associated eosinophilic folliculitis, chemical irritants (chloracne), acneiform adverse cutaneous drug reactions [epidermal growth factor receptor inhibitors (e.g., erlotinib), halogens, glucocorticoids, lithium], keloidal folliculitis, and pseudofolliculitis barbae.
PAINFUL DERMAL/SUBCUTANEOUS NODULE
Ruptured epidermoid or pilar cyst, hidradenitis suppurativa.

DIAGNOSIS

Clinical findings confirmed by findings on Gram staining and culture.

COURSE

Most cases of folliculitis and abscesses resolve with effective treatment. If diagnosis and treatment are delayed, furunculosis can be complicated by soft-tissue infection, bacteremia, and hematogenous seeding of viscera. Some individuals are subject to recurrent furunculosis, particularly diabetics.

TREATMENT

PROPHYLAXIS *Correct underlying predisposing condition.* Washing with antibacterial soap or benzoyl peroxide preparation or isopropyl/ethanol gel.
ANTIMICROBIAL THERAPY Bacterial Folliculitis.
Most will respond to natural penicillins but can consider dicloxacillin, amoxicillin, primary cephalosporins and clindamycin, usually for 7 to 10 days. Consider culture for resistant organisms. Minocycline, trimethoprim-sulfamethoxazole and quinolones may be necessary. There may be higher resistance to the erythromycin family.
Gram-Negative Folliculitis. Associated with systemic antibiotic therapy of acne vulgaris. Discontinue current antibiotics. Wash with benzoyl peroxide. In some cases, ampicillin (250 mg four times daily) or trimethoprim–sulfamethoxazole four times daily. Isotretinoin.

The treatment of an **abscess, furuncle,** or **carbuncle** is incision and drainage, with consideration of systemic antimicrobial therapy in immunocompromised patients or when there are signs of systemic infection.

SOFT-TISSUE INFECTION

- Characterized by inflammation of skin and adjacent subcutaneous tissues. Soft tissue refers to tissues that connect, support, or surround other structures and organs: skin, adipose tissue, fibrous tissues, fascia, tendon, ligaments.
- Syndromes. Cellulitis, erysipelas, lymphangitis, necrotizing fasciitis, or wound infection.
- Soft-tissue inflammation. Although often infectious, soft-tissue inflammation can be a manifestation of a noninfectious reaction pattern such as with neutrophilic dermatoses, erythema nodosum, and eosinophilic cellulitis.
- Cellulitis. Usually begins at a portal of entry in the skin, spreading proximally as an expanding solitary lesion. Uncommonly, soft-tissue infection can follow hematogenous dissemination with multiple sites of infection. Cellulitis is most often acute, caused by *S. aureus*.
- Acute Inflammation. Resulting from *cytokines* and bacterial *superantigens* rather than to overwhelming tissue infection.
- Chronic Soft-Tissue Infection. Nocardiosis, sporotrichosis, and phaeohyphomycosis.

CELLULITIS ICD-10: A46.0

- Acute, spreading infection of dermal and subcutaneous tissues. Characterized by a red, hot, and tender area of skin. Portal of entry of infection is usually apparent. Most common pathogen is *S. aureus*. Erysipelas is a variant of cellulitis involving cutaneous lymphatics, and is usually caused by beta-hemolytic streptococci.

EPIDEMIOLOGY AND ETIOLOGY

ETIOLOGY Adults: *S. aureus*, GAS.

Less commonly beta-homolytic streptococcus: Group B, C, or G. *Erysipelothrix rhusiopathiae* (erysipeloid); *P. aeruginosa*, *Pasteurella multocida*, *Vibrio vulnificus*; *Mycobacterium fortuitum* complex. In children: Pneumococci, *Neisseria meningitidis* group B (periorbital). *Haemophilus influenzae* type b (Hib) infections much less common because of Hib immunization.

Chronic Soft-Tissue Infections. Nocardia brasiliensis, Sporothrix schenckii, Madurella species, *Scedosporium* species, and nontuberculous mycobacteria (NTM).

Dog and Cat Saliva and Bites: P. multocida and other *Pasteurella* species. *Capnocytophaga canimorsus* (see Septic shock: ischemic necrosis of acral sites, p. 566).

PORTAL OF INFECTION Pathogens gain entry via any break in the skin or mucosa. Tinea pedis and leg and foot ulcers are common portals. Infections follow bacteremia/sepsis with cutaneous seeding.

RISK FACTORS Host defense defects, diabetes mellitus, drug and alcohol abuse, cancer and cancer chemotherapy, chronic lymphedema [postmastectomy, previous episode of cellulitis/erysipelas].

After entry, infection spreads to tissue spaces and cleavage planes (Fig. 25-25) as hyaluronidases break down polysaccharide ground substances, fibrinolysins digest fibrin barriers, and lecithinases destroy cell membranes. Local tissue devitalization is usually required to allow for significant anaerobic bacterial infection. The number of infecting organisms is usually small, suggesting that cellulitis may be more of a reaction to cytokines and bacterial superantigens than to overwhelming tissue infection.

CLINICAL MANIFESTATION

Symptoms of fever and chills can develop before cellulitis is clinically apparent. Higher fever (38.5°C) and chills usually associated with GAS infection. Local pain and tenderness. Necrotizing infections associated with severe pain and systemic symptoms.

Red, hot, edematous, and shiny plaque originating at the portal of entry. Enlarges with proximal extension (Figs. 25-26 and 25-27); borders usually sharply defined, irregular, and slightly elevated. Vesicles, bullae, erosions, abscesses, hemorrhage, and necrosis may form in plaque (Fig. 25-27). Lymphangitis. Lymph nodes can be enlarged and tender regionally.

DISTRIBUTION *Adults. Lower leg* most common site (Fig. 25-27). *Arm:* In young male, consider

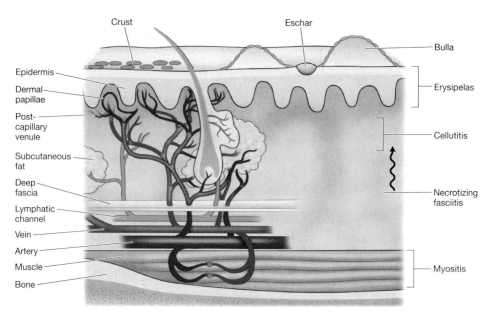

FIGURE 25-25 **Structural components of the skin and soft tissue, superficial infections, and infections of the deeper structures** The rich capillary network beneath the dermal papillae plays a key role in the localization of infection and in the development of the acute inflammatory reaction. (Reproduced with permission from Stevens DL. Infections of the skin, muscles, and soft tissues. In: Longo DL, Fauci AS, Kasper DL, et al, eds. *Harrison's Principles of Internal Medicine.* 18th ed. New York, NY: McGraw-Hill; 2012.)

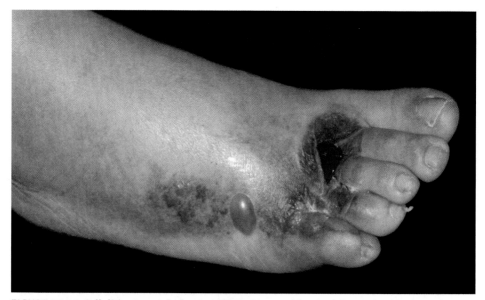

FIGURE 25-26 **Cellulitis at portal of entry: MSSA** 51-year-old male with interdigital tinea pedis noted pain on the dorsum of his foot. KOH preparation was positive for dermatophytic hyphae. Methicillin-sensitive *S. aureus* was isolated on culture of the webspace.

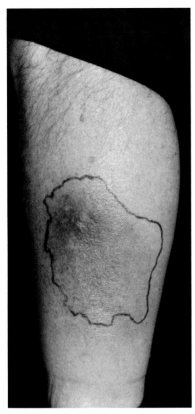

FIGURE 25-27 Cellulitis lower leg: MRSA 70-year-old male with increasing erythema and edema of the lower leg associated with fever.

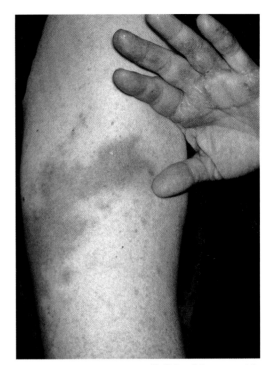

FIGURE 25-28 Recurrent cellulitis of the arm with chronic lymphedema: MSSA Right breast cancer had been treated with mastectomy and lymph node excision 10 years previously. Lymphedema of the right arm followed. Hand dermatitis was secondarily infected with MSSA. Cellulitis occurred repeatedly in the setting of chronic lymphedema.

IV drug use; in female, postmastectomy (Fig. 25-28). *Trunk*: Operative wound site. *Face*: Following rhinitis, conjunctivitis, pharyngitis; associated with colonization of nares by *S. aureus* and of pharynx by GAS.

VARIANTS OF CELLULITIS BY PATHOGEN

S. aureus: Portal of entry is usually apparent; cellulitis is an extension of focal infection. Toxin syndromes: Scalded-skin syndrome, TSS. Endocarditis may follow bacteremia.

Beta-hemolytic streptococci GAS (*Streptococcus pyogenes*) colonize skin and oropharynx. GBS and GGS colonize anogenital region. Beta-hemolytic streptococcal soft-tissue infections spread rapidly along superficial cutaneous lymphatic vessels, presenting tender red expanding plaques, i.e., erysipelas (Figs. 25-29

and 25-30). Following childbirth, known as *puerperal sepsis*; infection can extend into pelvis. GBS cellulitis occurs in neonates; high morbidity and mortality. GAS infection with necrotizing fasciitis and streptococcal TSS has high morbidity and mortality.

E. rhusiopathiae: Erysipeloid occurs in individuals who handle swine, sheep, poultry, or fish. *Painful, inflamed plaque* with sharply defined irregular raised border occurring at the site of inoculation, i.e., the fingers or hand (Fig. 25-31), spreading to the wrist but not to forearm. Color: Purplish red acutely; brownish with resolution. Enlarges peripherally with central fading. Usually no systemic symptoms.

Ecthyma gangrenosum: Rare variant of necrotizing soft-tissue infection caused by *P. aeruginosa in ill patients*. Clinically characterized by infarcted center with erythematous halo,

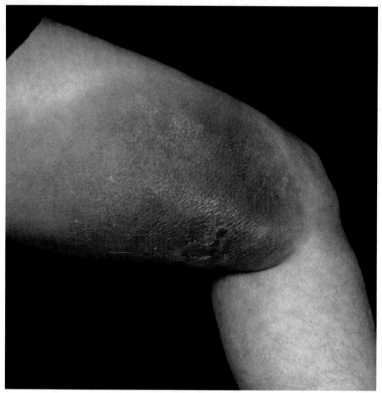

FIGURE 25-29 Erysipleas of thigh: group B streptococcus 52-year-old female with fever. Portal of entry was an insect bite in the popliteal fold. Lesion was very painful.

expanding rapidly without effective treatment (Fig. 25-32). *Distribution:* Most commonly in the axilla, groin, or perineum. Prognosis depends on prompt diagnosis, treatment, and restoration of host defense defects, usually correction of neutropenia.

H. influenzae: Occurs mainly in children <2 years. Cheek, periorbital area, head, and neck are most common sites. Clinically, swelling, characteristic violaceous erythema hue. Use of Hib vaccine has dramatically reduced incidence.

V. vulnificus, V. cholerae non-01 and non-0139. Underlying disorders: Cirrhosis, diabetes, immunosuppression, hemochromatosis, and thalassemia. Follows ingestion of raw/undercooked seafood, gastroenteritis, bacteremia with seeding of skin; also exposure of skin to seawater. Characterized by bulla formation, necrotizing vasculitis (Fig. 25-33). Usually on the extremities; often bilateral.

Aeromonas hydrophila: Water-associated trauma; preexisting wound. Immunocompromised host. Lower leg. Necrotizing soft-tissue infection.

C. canimorsus. Immunosuppression or asplenia; exposure to dog saliva or bite. Causes fulminant sepsis and disseminated intravascular coagulation (see Septic shock: ischemic necrosis of acral sites, p. 567).

P. multocida: Most common cause of infection following animal bite; soft-tissue infection.

Clostridium species. Associated with trauma; contamination by soil or feces; malignant intestinal tumor. Infection characterized by gas production (crepitation on palpation), marked systemic toxicity. Necrotizing infection.

Nontuberculous mycobacteria. History of recent surgery, injection, penetrating wound, systemic corticosteroid therapy. Low-grade cellulitis. Multiple sites of infection. Systemic findings lacking.

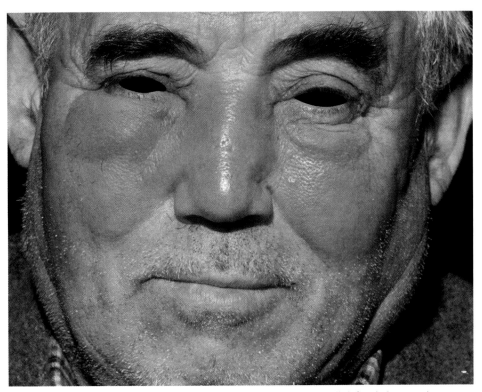

FIGURE 25-30 Erysipelas of face: group A streptococcus Painful, well-defined, shiny, erythematous, edematous plaques involving the central face of an otherwise healthy male. On palpation, the skin is hot and tender. There is fever (39.5°).

FIGURE 25-31 Erysipeloid of hand A well demarcated, violaceous, cellulitic plaque (without epidermal changes of scale or vesiculation) on the dorsa of the hand and fingers, occurred following cleaning fish; the site was somewhat painful, tender, and warm.

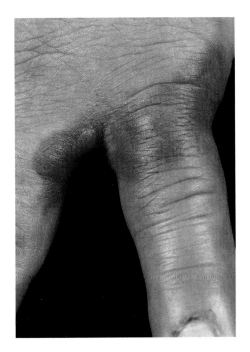

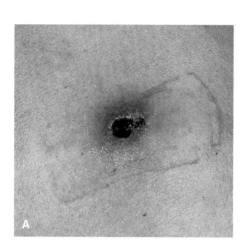
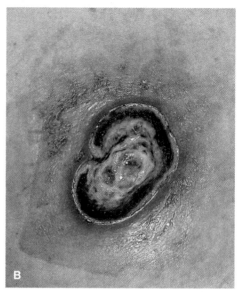

FIGURE 25-32 *Ecthyma gangrenosum* of buttock: *P. aeruginosa* A 30-year-old male with HIV disease and neutropenia. **(A)** An extremely painful, infarcted area with surrounding erythema present for 5 days. This primary cutaneous infection was associated with bacteremia. **(B)** Two weeks later, the lesion had progressed to a large ulceration. The patient died 3 months later of *P. aeruginosa pneumonitis* associated with chronic neutropenia.

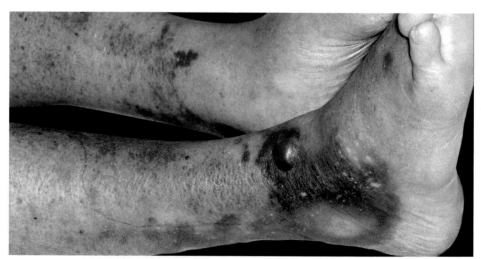

FIGURE 25-33 Bilateral cellulitis of legs: *V. vulnificus* Bilateral hemorrhagic plaques and bullae on the legs, ankles, and feet of an older diabetic with cirrhosis. Unlike other types of cellulitis in which microorganisms enter the skin locally, which is caused by *V. vulnificus*, usually follows a primary enteritis with bacteremia and dissemination to the skin. Most cases initially diagnosed as bilateral cellulitis are inflammatory (eczema, stasis dermatitis, psoriasis) rather than infectious.

Cryptococcus neoformans: Immunocompromised. Red, hot, tender, edematous plaque on extremity. Rarely multiple noncontiguous sites.

Mucormycosis: Usually occurring in individuals with uncontrolled diabetes.

Nocardiosis: *See* Cutaneous Nocardia Infections, p. 559.

Eumycetoma: *See* Section 26.
Chromoblastomycosis: *See* Section 26.

DIFFERENTIAL DIAGNOSIS

ERYSIPELAS/CELLULITIS Deep vein thrombophlebitis, urticaria, insect bite (hypersensitivity response), fixed drug eruption, erythema nodosum, acute gout, and erythema migrans (EM). NECROTIZING STIS Vasculitis, occlusive vasculopathy, peripheral vascular disease, calciphylaxis, warfarin necrosis, traumatic injury, cryoglobulinemia, pyoderma gangrenosum, and brown recluse spider bite.

DIAGNOSIS

Clinical diagnosis is based on morphologic features of lesion and the clinical setting, i.e., underlying diseases, travel history, animal exposure, history of bite, and age. Confirmed by culture in only 29% of cases in immunocompetent patients. Suspicion of necrotizing fasciitis (see below) requires immediate deep biopsy and tissue culture.

COURSE

With timely diagnosis and treatment, soft-tissue infection resolves with oral or parenteral antibiotic treatment.

Dissemination of infection (lymphatics, hematogenously), with metastatic sites of infection occurring, if effective treatment is delayed. In immunocompromised patients, prognosis depends on prompt restoration of altered immunity, usually on correction of neutropenia.

TREATMENT

Systemic high dose antibiotic treatment according to type and sensitivity of microbial organism.

NECROTIZING SOFT-TISSUE INFECTIONS   ICD-10: M72.510

- Characterized by rapid progression of infection with extensive necrosis of soft tissues and overlying skin. Necrotizing fasciitis.
- Etiology. Usually polymicrobial, historically beta-hemolytic GAS. Necrotizing soft-tissue infections also caused by *P. aeruginosa* and *Clostridium* species.
- Portal of Entry. May begin deep at site of nonpenetrating minor trauma (bruise, muscle, or strain). Minor trauma, laceration, needle puncture, or surgical incision on an extremity.
  Clinical variants of necrotizing soft-tissue infection differ with causative organism, anatomic location of infection, or underlying conditions. *Streptococcal necrotizing myositis* occurs as a primary myositis. *Streptococcal TSS* may occur with necrotizing fasciitis. GBS causes necrotizing fasciitis in episiotomy incisions.
- Diagnosis. Imperative in understanding pathogenesis and deciding on the appropriate antimicrobial and surgical therapies.
- When skin necrosis is not obvious, *diagnosis must be suspected if there are signs of* sepsis and/or some of the following local symptoms/signs: severe pain, indurated edema, bullae, cyanosis, skin pallor, skin hypesthesia, crepitation, muscle weakness, or foul smelling exudates.

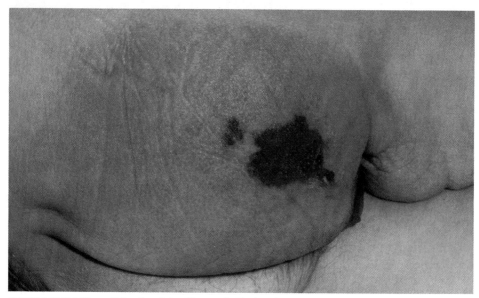

FIGURE 25-34 Necrotizing fasciitis of buttock Black eschar within an erythematous, edematous plaque involving the entire buttock with rapidly progressive area of necrosis.

CLINICAL MANIFESTATION

Local redness, edema, warmth, pain in the involved site, typically on an extremity.

Characteristic findings appear within 36 to 72 h after onset: Involved soft tissue becomes *dusky blue* in color; *vesicles or bullae* appear. Infection spreads rapidly along fascial planes (Fig. 25-34). Extensive, cutaneous soft-tissue *necrosis* develops. Involved tissue may be *anesthetic*. Necrosis manifests as a *black eschar* with surrounding irregular border of erythema. *Fever* and other constitutional symptoms are prominent as the inflammatory process extends rapidly over the next few days. *Metastatic abscesses* may occur as a consequence of bacteremia. Secondary thrombophlebitis occurs. Without surgical debridement necrotizing fasciitis is fatal.

DIFFERENTIAL DIAGNOSIS

Pyoderma gangrenosum, calciphylaxis, purpura fulminans, warfarin necrosis, pressure ulcer, and brown recluse spider bite.

TREATMENT

SURGICAL DEBRIDEMENT Requires early and complete surgical debridement of necrotic tissue in combination with high-dose antimicrobial agents.

LYMPHANGITIS ICD-10: 189–1

- An inflammatory process involving the subcutaneous lymphatic channels.
- Etiology.
  - Acute lymphangitis: GAS; *S. aureus*; other bacteria. Herpes simplex virus.
  - Subacute to chronic nodular lymphangitis: *Mycobacterium marinum*, other NTM, *Sporotrix schenkii*, and *N. brasiliensis*.

CLINICAL MANIFESTATION

ACUTE LYMPHANGITIS Portal of entry: Break in skin, wound, *S. aureus* paronychia, and primary andherpes simplex infection. Pain and/or erythema proximal to break in skin. Red linear streaks and palpable lymphatic cords, up to several centimeters in width, extend from the local lesion toward the regional lymph nodes (Fig. 25-35), which are usually enlarged and tender.

Subacute and chronic lymphangitis; nodular lymphangitis; see discussion on *Nocardiosis* (p. 559), NTM infection (p. 583), and sporotrichosisi (see Section 26).

DIFFERENTIAL DIAGNOSIS

LINEAR LESIONS ON EXTREMITIES Phyto-allergic contact dermatitis (poison ivy or oak), phytophotodermatitis, and superficial thrombophlebitis.
NODULAR LYMPHANGITIS *M. marinum, N. brasiliensis*, and *S. schenckii* infection.

DIAGNOSIS

The combination of an acute peripheral lesion with proximal tender/painful red linear streaks leading toward regional lymph nodes is diagnostic of lymphangitis. Isolate *S. aureus* or GAS from portal of entry.

COURSE

Resolves with correct diagnosis and treatment. Bacteremia with metastatic infection uncommon with adequate treatment.

TREATMENT

Systemic antibiotic depending on causative organism.

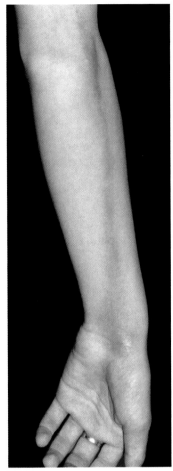

FIGURE 25-35 Acute lymphangitis of forearm *S. aureus* A small area of the cellulitis on the volar wrist with a tender linear streak extending proximally up the arm; the infection spreads from the portal of entry within the superficial lymphatic vessels.

WOUND INFECTION

- Wound. Injury in which skin is surgically incised or traumatically injured (open wound) or in which blunt force trauma causes a contusion (closed wound). Wound infection: Skin and all wounds are colonized by bacteria and other microbes, i.e., *cutaneous microbiome*. Infection is characterized by pain, tenderness, purulence, erythema, warmth, and must be diagnosed on clinical as well as culture findings.

ETIOLOGY AND EPIDEMIOLOGY

CLASSIFICATION *Traumatic wounds:* Open or closed wounds (Fig. 25-36). *Surgical wounds:* Infection in surgical incisions (Fig. 25-37). *Burn wounds:* Burn wound may become superficially colonized with *S. aureus*; open burn-related surgical wound infection; burn wound cellulitis; invasive infection in debrided burn wounds (Fig. 25-38). *Chronic ulcers:* Arterial insufficiency; venous insufficiency; neuropathic ulcers/diabetes mellitus; pressure ulcers (bedsores) (Figs. 25-39 to 25-41). *Bites:* Animal; human; insect.

EPIDEMIOLOGY *S. aureus* in the most common pathogen in wound infections, MSSA, and increasingly MRSA. Surgical wound infection is up to 10 times more likely among patients who harbor *S. aureus* in nares. Hospital-acquired (nosocomial) or health-care–associated infections (most commonly surgical wound infections) are the most common complication affecting hospitalized patients.

PATHOGENESIS Wounds are initially colonized by skin flora or introduced organisms. In some cases, these organisms proliferate, causing a host inflammatory response.

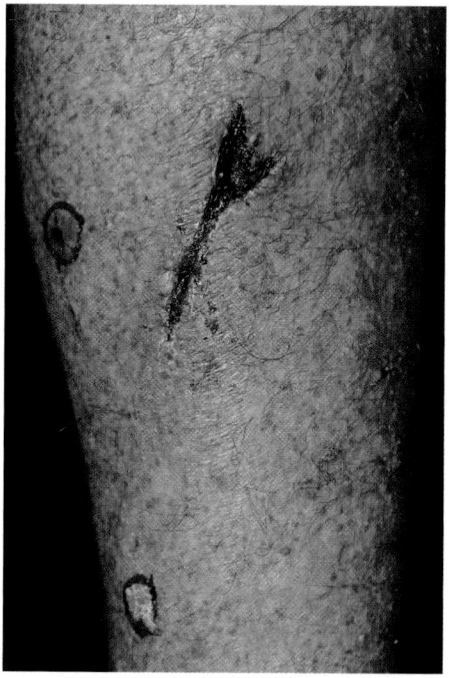

FIGURE 25-36   Laceration infection in renal transplant recipient: MRSA 60-year-old male immunosuppressed renal transplant recipient was unaware of a laceration on the calf. Erythema and induration are seen around the crusted wound. MRSA was isolated on culture. Two circled invasive squamous cell carcinomas are also seen on the calf.

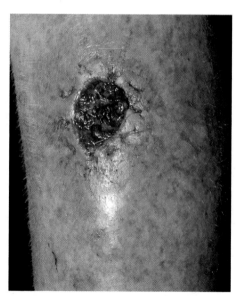

FIGURE 25-37   Surgical excision wound infection: MSSA Surgical wound became painful and tender 7 days after excision of squamous cell carcinoma; soft tissue (cellulitis) is seen adjacent to the wound margin. Necrotic tissue is seen in the base.

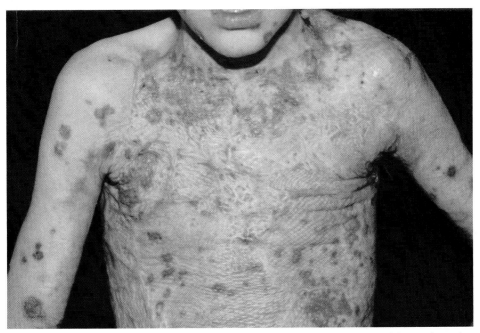

FIGURE 25-38 Burn wound infection: MSSA 10-year-old male with extensive third degree thermal burn treated with autologous skin grafting has extensive new crusted erosions. MSSA was cultured from the infected site.

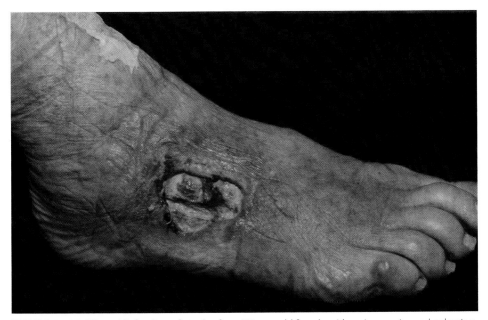

FIGURE 25-39 Wound infection of stasis ulcer 75-year-old female with varicose veins and enlarging stasis ulcer infected with MRSA and *Pseudomonas aeruginosa*. IV antibiotics were administered. Incompetent veins were treated with endovascular laser ablation. The ulcer healed with minimal scar.

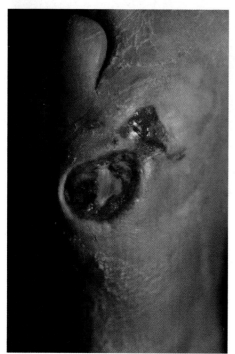

FIGURE 25-40 Infection of diabetic ulcer: MRSA 86-year-old male with diabetes mellitus type 2 had a chronic neuropathic ulcer on the R-lateral foot. The ulcer rapidly enlarged associated with fever and glucose of 450 mg/dL. MSSA was isolated from the wound. He was hospitalized and treated with IV antibiotics. He died 3 months later.

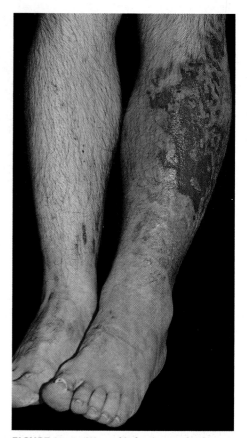

FIGURE 25-41 Wound infection and cellulitis: MRSA 53-year-old male with obsessive-compulsive disorder excoriates extremities in the evening. MRSA infection has occurred repeatedly. Ulcers resolved with doxycycline, doxepin, and unna boots applied weekly.

CLINICAL MANIFESTATION

LOCAL INFECTION Tenderness of wound area, erythema, hot, purulent drainage, and induration. Invasive infection: Malaise, anorexia, sweats, fever, or chills. Sepsis syndrome: Fever and hypotension.

TYPES OF SURGICAL INFECTIONS Superficial infection of wound, wound infection with soft-tissue infection, i.e., cellulitis and erysipelas, soft-tissue abscess, necrotizing soft-tissue infection, and tetanus.

DIFFERENTIAL DIAGNOSIS

Allergic contact dermatitis (e.g., neomycin), pyoderma gangrenosum, and vasculitis.

DIAGNOSIS

Because all open wounds are colonized with microorganisms, diagnosis of infection relies on the clinical characteristics of the wound. Wound culture identifies the potential pathogen(s).

TREATMENT

Although all wounds require treatment, only infected lesions require antimicrobial therapy.

DISORDERS CAUSED BY TOXIN-PRODUCING BACTERIA

- Bacteria colonize skin and mucosa (mucocutaneous *microbiome*), replicate locally, and elaborate toxins that cause local mucocutaneous and systemic disorders.
- Clinical syndromes caused by these toxins:
  - *S. aureus.*
    - *Bullous impetigo* (see **Figs. 25-12** and **25-13**).
    - Staphylococcal scalded-skin syndrome. Generalized form with extensive epidermolysis, followed by desquamation.
    - TSS. Abortive form, staphylococcal scarlet fever.
  - GAS.
    - *Scarlet fever.*
    - *Streptococcal TSS.*
    - *Bacillus anthracis:* Anthrax.
    - *Corynebacterium diphtheriae:* Diphtheria.
- *Clostridium tetani:* Tetanus.

STAPHYLOCOCCAL SCALDED-SKIN SYNDROME ICD-10: L00

- Etiology. *S. aureus* producing exfoliative toxins. Occurs in neonates and young children.
- Pathogenesis. Illness develops after toxin synthesis and the subsequent toxin-initiated host response. Exotoxins (Exfoliatin) cleave desmoglein-1 in epidermal granular cell-layer, resulting in its separation.

CLINICAL MANIFESTATION

LOCALIZED FORM See "Bullous Impetigo" in Figures 25-12 and 25-13. Intact flaccid purulent bullae, clustered. Rupture of the bullae results in moist red and/or crusted erosive lesions. Lesions are often clustered in an intertriginous area.

GENERALIZED FORM Exfoliative toxin-induced changes: *macular scarlatiniform rash* (staphylococcal scarlet fever syndrome) or diffuse, ill-defined erythema and a fine, stippled, sandpaper appearance occur initially. In 24 h, erythema deepens and involved skin becomes tender. Initially, periorificially on face, neck, axillae, groins; becoming more widespread in 24 to 48 h. Superficial epidermis is most pronounced peri-orificially on face; in flexural areas on neck, axillae, groins, and antecubital areas; back (pressure points). With epidermolysis, epidermis appears wrinkled and can be removed by gentle pressure (skin resembles wet tissue paper) (*Nikolsky sign*) (Fig. 25-42). In some infants, flaccid bullae occur. Unroofed epidermis forms erosions with red, moist base (Fig. 25-43A). Desquamation occurs with healing (Fig. 25-43B).

Mucous membrane, uninvolved. TSS, in comparison, manifests with mucosal erythema.

DIFFERENTIAL DIAGNOSIS

Kawasaki syndrome, adverse cutaneous drug eruption, or scarlet fever.

DIAGNOSIS

Clinical findings confirmed by bacterial cultures from bullous impetigo or nares. Erosions from epidermolytic toxin may not yield bacteria.

COURSE

With adequate antibiotic treatment, superficially denuded areas heal in 3 to 5 days associated with generalized desquamation; there is no scarring.

TREATMENT

Systemic antibiotic to treat infection and stop toxin production.

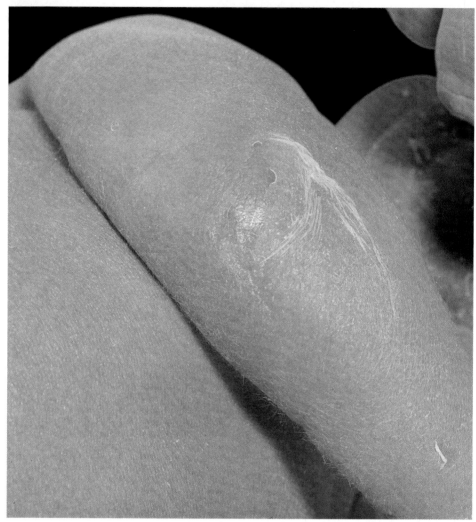

FIGURE 25-42 Staphylococcal scalded-skin syndrome: Nikolsky sign The skin of this infant is diffusely erythematous; gentle pressure to the skin of the arm has sheared off the epidermis, which folds like tissue paper.

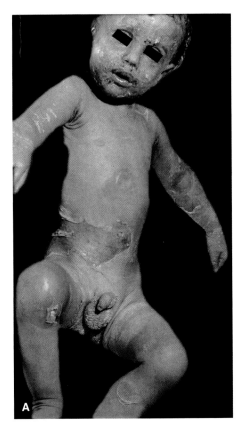

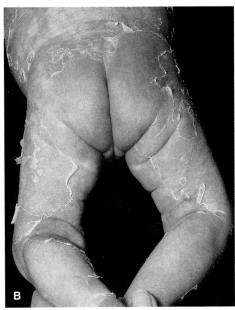

FIGURE 25-43 Staphylococcal scalded-skin syndrome: sloughing and desquamation in this infant, painful, tender, diffuse erythema was followed by generalized epidermal sloughing and erosions. *S. aureus* had colonized the nares with perioral impetigo, the site of exotoxin production. **(A)** Extensive desquamation is seen on buttocks and legs **(B)**.

TOXIC SHOCK SYNDROME ICD-10: A48.3

- Etiology. Exotoxin (TSST-1)-producing *S. aureus*; less commonly GAS.
- Staphylococcal TSS.
  - Menstrual TSS (MTSS).
  - Nonmenstrual TSS (NMTSS) occurs secondary to a wide variety of primary and secondary *S. aureus* infections of underlying dermatoses.
- Streptococcal TSS. Skin or soft-tissue infection with toxin production.
- Clinical manifestations. Rapid onset of fever, hypotension, and multisystem failure. Rash. Generalized and blanching scarlatiniform erythroderma "painless sunburn," most intense around infected areas. Fades within 3 days of appearance. Edema. Mucosal erythema/ulcers. Desquamation one week after onset of rash. Begins with the torso, face and extremities, followed by the hands and feet.
- Course. Streptococcal TSS 25 to 50% mortality. NMTSS 6.4% mortality; MTSS 2.5% mortality.
- Treatment. Systemic antibiotic to treat infection and stop toxin production. Supportive.

SCARLET FEVER ICD-10: A38

- Etiology.
- Group A β-hemolytic streptococcus (GAS) (*S. pyogenes*), erythrogenic toxin-producing strains.
- Exfoliative toxin (ET)-producing *S. aureus*.
- Clinical Manifestation. Infection: pharyngitis, tonsillitis, infected wound, or dermatoses.

  Toxin Syndrome (Scarlet Fever). Acutely ill with high fever, fatigue, sore throat, headache, nausea, vomiting, and tachycardia. Anterior cervical lymphadenitis associated with pharyngitis/tonsillitis. Scarlatiniform exanthema occurs in nonimmune persons.

  Exanthem. Face flushed with perioral pallor. Finely punctate erythema is first noted on the upper part of the trunk (Fig. 25-44); may be accentuated in skin folds such as the neck, axillae, groin, antecubital, and popliteal fossae; linear petechiae (Pastia sign) occur in body folds. The palms and soles are usually spared. Initial punctate lesions become confluently erythematous, i.e., *scarlatiniform*. *Exanthem fades* within 4 to 5 days, followed by *desquamation* on the body and extremities and by sheet-like exfoliation on the palms and fingers as well as the soles and toes. In subclinical or mild infections, exanthem and pharyngitis may pass unnoticed.

  Enanthem. Pharynx beefy red. *Forchheimer spots*: Small red macules on soft palate. Punctate petechiae may occur in the palate. *White tongue*: Initially is white with scattered red, swollen papillae (white strawberry tongue) (Fig. 25-45). Red strawberry tongue: By the fourth or fifth day, the hyperkeratotic membrane is sloughed, and the lingular mucosa appears bright red (Fig. 25-45).

- Complications. Acute rheumatic fever 1 to 4 weeks after onset of pharyngitis (incidence markedly decreased over past five decades), acute glomerulonephritis more common after impetigo with nephritogenic strain of GAS (types 2, 4, 12, 49 and 60), guttate psoriasis (see Section 3) and erythema nodosum (see Section 7).
- Differential Diagnosis. Viral exanthema, adverse cutaneous drug eruption, Kawasaki syndrome, and infectious mononucleosis.
- Diagnosis. Rapid direct antigen tests: Used to detect GAS antigens in throat swab specimens. Isolate GAS on culture of specimen from throat or wound. Blood cultures are rarely positive. *Centor criteria* for diagnosis of acute streptococcal pharyngitis: History of fever; tonsillar exudates; tender anterior cervical adenopathy; absence of cough.
- Treatment. Systemic penicillin is the drug of choice; alternatives are erythromycin, clindamycin, clarithromycin, or cephalosporins.

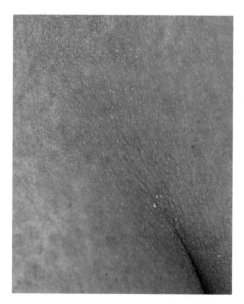

FIGURE 25-44 Scarlet fever: exanthem Finely punctated erythema has become confluent (scarlatiniform); petechiae can occur and have a linear configuration within the exanthem in body folds (Pastia line).

FIGURE 25-45 Scarlet fever: white and red strawberry tongue The white patches at the back of the tongue represent residua of the initial white strawberry tongue.

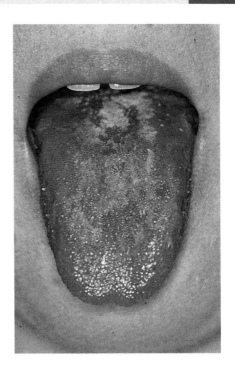

CUTANEOUS ANTHRAX ICD-10: A22.000

- Etiology. *B. anthracis*, a nonmotile, gram-positive, aerobic rod. Zoonosis. Spores can remain dormant in the soil for decades. Low-level germination occurs at the primary site, resulting in local edema and necrosis. Primary infection: Skin, pulmonary, and GI. Pathogenesis: Toxin mediated.
- Transmission. Zoonosis of mammals, especially herbivores. Human infections result from contact with contaminated wild and domestic animals or animal products. Human-to-human transmission does not occur. At risk: Farmers, herders; slaughterhouse, textile workers.
- Cutaneous anthrax. Accounts for 95% of anthrax cases in the United States.
  - Cut or abrasion on exposed sites of head, neck, extremities. Nondescript, painless, pruritic papule (resembling insect bite) appears 3 to 5 days after introduction of endospores. In 1 to 2 days, evolves to vesicle(s) ± hemorrhage + necrosis. Vesicles rupture to form *ulcers with extensive local edema* (Fig. 25-46), ultimately forming dry eschars (1 to 3 cm). Satellite lesions can form in a *nodular lymphangitis* proximally on edematous extremity (Fig. 25-46).
- Differential Diagnosis, Ecthyma, brown recluse spider bite, ulceroglandular tularemia, orf, or glanders.
- Diagnosis. Isolation of *B. anthracis* from skin lesions, blood, or respiratory secretions, or by measuring specific antibodies in blood of persons with suspected symptoms.
- Course and Treatment. Mortality rate in untreated persons with cutaneous anthrax is about 20%. Systemic penicillin is the drug of choice; alternatives are erythromycin, azathioprin, clarithromycin, or cephalosporins.

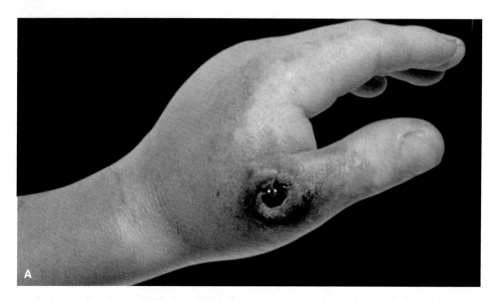

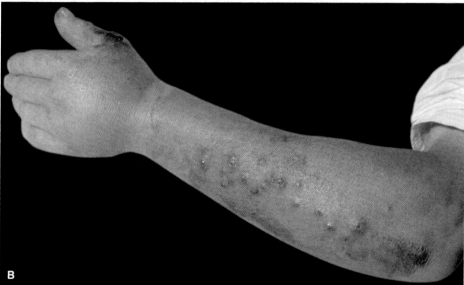

FIGURE 25-46 A cutaneous anthrax A 40-year-old farmer with anthrax. **(A)** A black eschar at the site of inoculation with a central hemorrhagic ulceration on the thumb associated with massive edema of the hand. **(B)** A nodular lymphangitis extending proximally from the primary lesion on the thumb.

CUTANEOUS DIPHTHERIA ICD-10: A30

- Etiology. *Corynebacterium diphtheria*. Cases in industrialized countries extremely rare.
- Pathogenesis. Localized infection caused by toxigenic and nontoxigenic strains. Acute infection may involve any mucous membrane or skin wound. Toxin causes myocarditis and *peripheral neuropathy*.
- Clinical Manifestations. Cutaneous: Nonspecific wound. Thick gray membrane in the pharynx. Mycarditis, arrhythmias. Polyneuritis involving cranial nerves: Diplopia, slurred speech, or difficulty swallowing.
- Diagnosis. Made by isolation of *C. diphtheria* on the culture of the wound.
- Treatment. Penicillin, erythromycin, or antitoxin.
  Vaccination. Immunity to vaccine wanes over time. Decennial boosters are recommended.

CUTANEOUS *NOCARDIA* INFECTIONS

- Etiology. *Nocardia* species of bacteria. Saprophytic gram-positive anaerobic actinomycetes living in soil. Actinomyces were mistakenly classified as fungi. *N. brasiliensis* is usually associated with disease limited to the skin. Infection follows traumatic inoculation into the skin on extremity.
- Clinical Manifestation. **Cellulitis.** Inflammation 1 to 3 weeks following traumatic inoculation. Expanding erythema, induration; firm, nonfluctuant. Untreated, infection can progress to involve adjacent muscles, tendons, bones, and joints. Dissemination is rare, and occurs in people with host defense defects.
  Nodular Lymphangitis. Begins as a nodule at the inoculation site. Untreated, infection extends into lymphatic vessels with linear subcutaneous nodules.
  Cutaneous Nocardiosis. Nodule occurs at the site of inoculation (Fig. 25-47), most commonly at the feet or hands. Untreated, infection expands forming plaques with *sinus tracts* and *fistula* formation (Fig. 25-48). As with eumycetoma, grains (dense masses of bacterial filaments extending radially from a central core) may be seen in discharging pus and tissue. After years, deformity of extremity may occur with involvement of adjacent anatomical structure.
- Diagnosis. Grains and organism in purulent discharge. Isolate and speciate *Nocardia* in pus, exudate, or tissue. Sensitivities determined on isolated organism.
- Differential Diagnosis. **Nodular Lymphangitis.** Sporotrichosis, NTM infection.
  Actinomycetoma. Eumycetoma.
- Course. Tends to relapse, especially with defective host defenses.
- Treatment. Trimethoprim/sulfamethoxazole is the preferred antimicrobial agent. Minocycline or linezolid. Surgical excision/debridement.

FIGURE 25-47 Cutaneous nocardiosis A 23-year-old female from Central America with a painful lesion for 6 months. Confluent erythematous violaceous nodules on the right prepatellar area arising in an abrasion. *Nocardia brasiliensis* isolated on culture of biopsy specimen. The lesion resolved with trimethoprim–sulfamethoxazole.

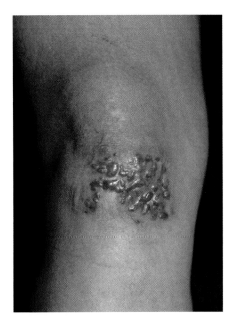

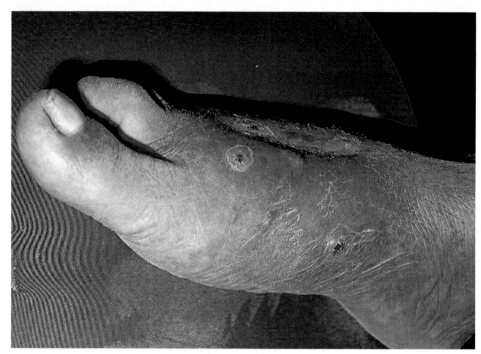

FIGURE 25-48 Chronic cutaneous nocardiasis Swelling, multiple sinus tracts, and involvement of the foot. (Used with permission from Amor Khachemoune, MD and The Ronald O. Perelman Department of Dermatology, NYU School of Medicine.)

RICKETTSIAL DISORDERS

- Rickettsiae. Gram-negative bacteria. Coccobacilli/short bacilli; obligate intracellular.
- Transmitted to humans by arthropods; tick, mite, flea, louse; mammalian reservoirs; humans are incidental hosts.
- Rickettsial Disorders. Spotted fever group, typhus group, and scrub typhus group.

CLINICAL MANIFESTATION

Exposure to vectors or animal reservoirs, travel to or residence in endemic locations (http://www.cdc.gov/ncidod/diseases/submenus/sub_typhus.htm).

Tâche noire (black spot or stain). Coin-like lesion with central eschar and a red halo at the site of the vector-feeding bite site.

EXANTHEM Macules–papules. Exception: Rickettsialpox with papules–vesicles.

LATER FINDINGS VARYING WITH PATHOGEN May become hemorrhagic with vasculitis.

DIAGNOSIS

Confirmed by paired serum samples after convalescence or demonstration of rickettsiae.

DERMATOPATHOLOGY Rickettsiae multiply in endothelial cells of small blood vessels and produce vasculitis with necrosis and thrombosis.

COURSE

Rickettsiae can cause life-threatening infections. Order of decreasing case-fatality rate: *R. rickettsii* [Rocky Mountain spotted fever (RMSF)]; *R. prowazekii* (epidemic louse-borne typhus); *Orientia tsutsugamushi* (scrub typhus); *R. conorii* (Mediterranean spotted fever); *R. typhi* (endemic murine typhus); in rare cases, other spotted fever group organisms.

TREATMENT

Doxycycline is the drug of choice, 100 mg BID orally. Alternates: Ciprofloxacin or chloramphenicol.

TICK SPOTTED FEVERS ICD-10: A77.0

- Characteristic exanthema: macules and papules.
- RMSF *R. rickettsia*.
- Boutonneuse fever *R. conorii*. Siberian tick typhus *R. sibirica*, Australian tick typhus *R. autralis*, oriental spotted fever *R. japonica*, African tick bite fever *R. africae*, etc.
- Rickettsialpox *R. akari*.
- Transmission. *Vector: Dermatocentor andersoni/variablis* (American dog tick), *Amblyomma american-num* (lone star tick), *Rhipicephalus sanguineus* (Brown dog tick), *Ixodes holocyclus/tasmani*. Worldwide distribution. Attachment often unnoticed.
- Inoculation. *Bite*; contact vector feces with open wound. *Travel history*: Recent travel to or living in endemic region.

CLINICAL MANIFESTATION

Incubation period: Average 7 days after tick bite. Onset sudden of symptoms in 50% of patients. Most common: Headache, fever; also chills, myalgias, arthralgias, malaise, or anorexia.

Tâche noire at inoculation site. An inoculation eschar: papule forms at the bite site and evolves to a painless, black-crusted ulcer with red halo (Fig. 25-49) in 3 to 7 days. Occurs in all spotted fevers except RMSF.

EXANTHEM About 3 to 4 days after appearance of *tâche noire*, an erythematous macules and papules appear on trunk; may subsequently disseminate, involving face, extremities, and the palms or soles. Density of eruption heightens during next few days. In severe cases, lesions may become hemorrhagic.

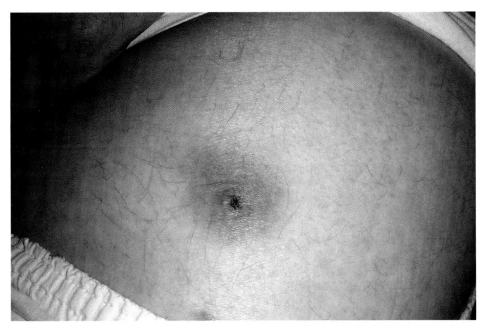

FIGURE 25-49 African spotted fever: tache noir 65-year-old female, who had recently returned from trip to South Africa, noted a lesion on the thigh and reported flu-like symptoms. A central dark crust (tache noir) with halo of erythema is seen at the site of tick bite. Paired serologies confirmed the diagnosis of African spotted fever. Symptoms resolved with doxycycline.

DISTRIBUTION Similar pattern of spread and distribution in all spotted fevers—trunk, extremities, face (centrifugal)—*except* RMSF, which first appears at wrists and ankles and spreads centripetally.

SYSTEMIC FINDINGS Conjunctivitis, pharyngitis, photophobia. Central nervous system (CNS) symptoms: Confusion, stupor, delirium, seizures, coma; common in RMSF but not seen in other spotted fevers.

DIFFERENTIAL DIAGNOSIS

Viral exanthems, drug eruption, vasculitis.

DIAGNOSIS

Clinical, epidemiologic, and convalescent serologic data establish the diagnosis of a spotted fever–group rickettsiosis.

COURSE

In France and Spain, mortality rate is similar to that of RMSF. Spotted fevers are usually milder in children. Morbidity and mortality rates are higher (up to 50%) in individuals with diabetes mellitus, cardiac insufficiency, and alcoholism.

ROCKY MOUNTAIN SPOTTED FEVER ICD-10: A77

- Etiology. *Rickettsia rickettsii.*
- Transmission. Bite of infected tick; only 60% of patients are aware prior tick bite. Most common in springtime in the southeastern United States; >2000 reported cases of RMSF in the United States annually.

CLINICAL MANIFESTATION

Abrupt onset of symptoms. Fever, chills, shaking rigor. Anorexia, nausea, vomiting. Malaise, irritability. Severe headache. Myalgia. Can mimic acute abdomen, acute cholecystitis, and acute appendicitis. *Tâche noire* uncommon in RMSF.

Early exanthem: 2 to 6 mm, pink, blanchable macules (Figs. 25-50 and 25-51). In 1 to 3 days, evolves to deep red papules (Fig. 25-52). Characteristically, rash begins on wrists, forearms, and ankles and somewhat later on the palms and soles. Within 6 to 18 h, the rash spreads centripetally to the arms, thighs, trunk, and face.

Later exanthem: In 2 to 4 days, become hemorrhagic, no longer blanchable. Local edema. Petechiae may occur on the palms and soles. Necrosis occurs in acral extremities following prolonged hypotension. Pedal edema.

Spotless fever: ≤10% of cases. Associated with higher mortality rate because of the delay in diagnosis.

DIAGNOSIS

Clinical and epidemiologic considerations are more important than a laboratory diagnosis in early RMSF. Suspect in febrile children, adolescents, and men >60 years of age with

tick exposure in endemic areas. Diagnosis made clinically and confirmed later. Only 3% of patients with RMSF present with the triad of rash, fever, and history of tick bite during the first 3 days of illness.

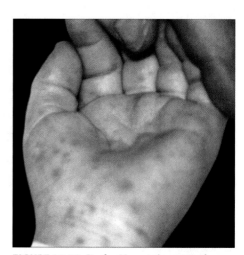

FIGURE 25-50 Rocky Mountain spotted fever: early Erythematous macules and papules appeared initially on the wrists of a young child. The lesions are not completely blanchable with pressure, indicating early hemorrhage of dermal blood vessels.

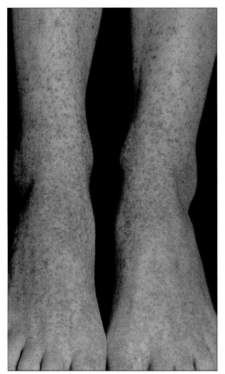

FIGURE 25-51 Rocky Mountain spotted fever: early Erythematous and hemorrhagic macules and papules appeared initially on the ankles of an adolescent.

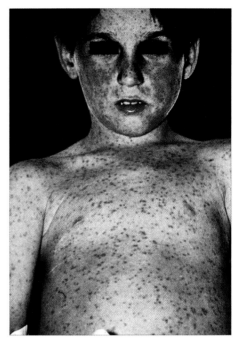

FIGURE 25-52 Rocky Mountain spotted fever: late Disseminated hemorrhagic macules and papules on the face, neck, trunk, and arms on the fourth day of febrile illness in an older child. The initial lesions were noted on the wrists and ankles, subsequently extending centripetally.

COURSE

Severe course is associated with older age, delay in diagnosis, delay in or no treatment and is more common in men, darker-skinned individuals, and those with alcoholism or G6PD deficiency. Fatality rate: 0.5%. Fulminant RMSF defined as a fatal disease whose course is unusually rapid (i.e., 5 days from onset to death) and usually characterized by early onset of neurologic signs and late or absent rash. In uncomplicated cases, defervescence usually occurs within 48 to 72 h after initiation of therapy.

TREATMENT

Doxycycline is preferred treatment. Chloramphenicol.

RICKETTSIALPOX ICD-10: A79.1

- Epidemiology. *R. akari.* Vector: Mice mite (*Liponyssoides sanguineus*), other mites; transovarian transmission. Geography: United States, Europe, Russia, South Africa, Korea, and Europe.

CLINICAL MANIFESTATION

Tâche noire (Fig. 25-53). At tick bite site. EXANTHEM 2 to 6 days after the onset of nonspecific symptoms, red macules and papules appear. May evolve to characteristic vesicles (pox); crusted erosions occur. Lesions usually heal without scarring.

COURSE

Fever resolves in 6 to 10 days without treatment with doxycycline.

DIFFERENTIAL DIAGNOSIS

Viral exanthems, varicella, and pityriasis lichenoides et varioliformis acuta.

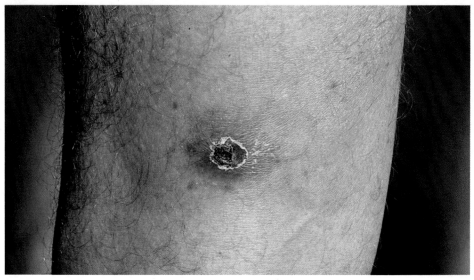

FIGURE 25-53 Rickettsialpox: tâche noire A crusted, ulcerated papule (eschar) with a red halo resembling a cigarette burn at the site of a tick bite.

INFECTIVE ENDOCARDITIS ICD-10: I33

- Inflammation of endocardium. Infective and noninfective. Usually of heart valve. Characterized by vegetations that are made up of fibrin, platelets, and inflammatory cells (also microcolonies of microorganism if infective endocarditis).
- *Infective endocarditis.* Occurs at sites on altered endothelium or endocardium. The primary event is *bacterial adherence* to damaged valves during transient bacteremia. Bacteria grow within the cardiac lesion(s), i.e., *vegetations*, with local extension and cardiac damage. Subsequently, *septic embolization* occurs to skin, kidney, spleen, brain, etc. *Circulating immune complexes* may result in glomerulonephritis, arthritis, or various mucocutaneous manifestations of vasculitis. Embolization of vegetative fragments results in *infection/infarction of remote tissues.*
  - Acute bacterial endocarditis rapidly damages cardiac structures, hematogenously seeds extracardiac sites, and may progress to death in a few weeks.
  - Subacute bacterial endocarditis (SBE) causes structural damage slowly, rarely causes metastatic infection, and is gradually progressive unless complicated by a major embolic event or ruptured mycotic aneurysm.
- Noninfective endocarditis: Occurs on previously undamaged valves. Hypercoagulable state. Marantic endocarditis. Libman-Sacks endocarditis.
- Diagnosis: Based on clinical features, echocardiogram, and blood cultures.

CLINICAL MANIFESTATION

SEPTIC ARTERIAL EMBOLI Common with acute *S. aureus* endocarditis. Hematogenously seeded focal infection (Fig. 25-54). Apparent in up to 50% of patients.

OSLER NODES Painful, erythematous nodules most commonly found on the pads of the fingers and toes of some patients with infective endocarditis.

JANEWAY LESIONS Nontender, erythematous, and nodular lesions most commonly found on the palms and soles (Fig. 25-55) of some patients with infective endocarditis.

SPLINTER HEMORRHAGES A small linear longitudinal subungual hemorrhage, initially red then brown. Middle third of nail bed in SBE.

PETECHIAL LESIONS Small, nonblanching, reddish-brown macules. Occur on extremities, upper chest, mucous membranes [conjunctivae

FIGURE 25-54 Septic vasculitis associated with bacteremia Dermal nodule with hemorrhage and necrosis on the dorsum of a finger. This type of lesion occurs with bacteremia (e.g., *S. aureus*, gonococcus) and fungemia (e.g., *Candida tropicalis*).

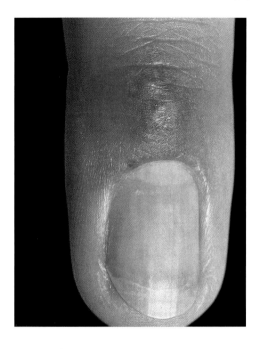

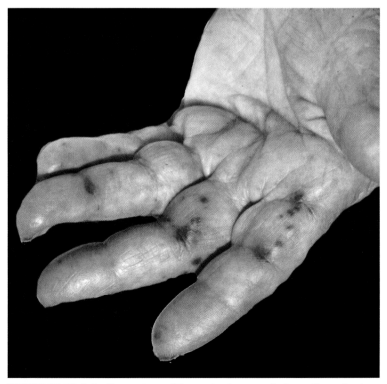

FIGURE 25-55 Infective endocarditis, acute: Janeway lesions Hemorrhagic, infarcted papules on the volar fingers in a patient with *S. aureus* endocarditis.

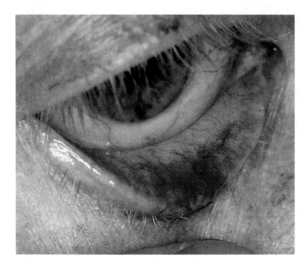

FIGURE 25-56 Infective endocarditis, acute: subconjunctival hemorrhage Submucosal hemorrhage of the lower eyelid in an elderly diabetic with enterococcal endocarditis; splinter hemorrhages in the midportion of the nail bed and Janeway lesions were also present on the volar fingers. Infection followed urosepsis.

(Fig. 25-56), palate]. Occur in crops. Fade after a few days (20 to 40%).

ROTH SPOTS White spot in the retina close to the optic disk, often surrounded by hemorrhages; also seen in pernicious anemia and leukemia.

SEPTIC EMBOLISM Painful, hemorrhagic macules, papules, or nodules, usually acral location.

COURSE AND TREATMENT

Varies with underlying cardiac disease and baseline health of the patient, as well as with the complications that occur. Complications: Congestive heart failure, stroke, other systemic embolizations, or septic pulmonary embolization. Aortic valve involvement has a higher risk of death or need for surgery. Antibiotics.

SEPSIS ICD: A40

- Sepsis is a whole-body inflammatory state, in response to infection. Can be complicated by multiple organ dysfunction.
- Characterized by fever or hypothermia, tachypnea, tachycardia, and, in severe cases, multiple organ dysfunction syndrome.
- Epidemiology. >1 million cases in the United States annually; >200,000 deaths. Two-thirds of cases occur in persons hospitalized for other illnesses. Incidence is increasing. Risk factors: Chronic disease and immunosuppression.

CLINICAL MANIFESTATION

Cutaneous infections as source of sepsis:
Superficial skin infections, soft-tissue infections, wounds. *E. gangrenosum* (Fig. 25-32): *P. aeruginosa* most commonly.

EXANTHEM See meningococcemia and RMSF (Fig. 25-50).

PETECHIAE Cutaneous/oropharyngeal location suggests meningococcal infection; less commonly, *H. influenzae*. In patient with tick bite living in endemic area, RMSF (Figs. 25-51 and 25-52).

HEMORRHAGIC BULLOUS LESIONS *V. vulnificus* in patient (diabetes mellitus, liver disease)

with history of eating raw oysters or clams (Fig. 25-33).

Disseminated intravascular coagulation. See Section 20.

Severe prolonged hypotension with acral necrosis *of the fingers, hands, and feet* (Fig. 25-57).

COURSE AND TREATMENT

Early sepsis is reversible; septic shock has high mortality/morbidity. High dose antibiotics plus treatment of disseminated intravascular coagulation.

FIGURE 25-57 Septic shock: ischemic necrosis of acral sites *Capnocytophaga canimorsus* sepsis (dog bite) with prolonged hypotension and hypoperfusion resulted in infarction of fingers and nose.

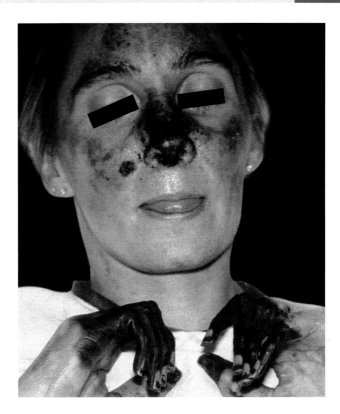

MENINGOCOCCAL INFECTION ICD-10: A39

- Etiology. *N. meningitidis,* colonizes nasopharynx. Infects only humans; no animal reservoirs. Spread by persons-to-person contact through respiratory droplets.
- Demography. The disease occurs sporadically throughout the world. The highest burden of the disease is caused by the cyclic epidemics occurring in the African "meningitis belt."

CLINICAL MANIFESTATIONS

Small pink blanchable *macules* and *papules* occur soon after onset of disease (Fig. 25-58). With vascular friability and hemorrhage, *petechiae* and *ecchymoses* occur; first seen on the ankles, wrists, axillae, mucosal surfaces, and conjunctivae. A cluster of petechiae may be seen at pressure points, e.g., where a blood pressure cuff has been inflated. *Ecchymoses* and *purpura* may progress to hemorrhagic bullae, undergo necrosis, and ulcerate. Confluent necrotic hemorrhagic lesions may have bizarre-shaped, grayish to black necrosis, i.e., *purpura fulminans*) associated with disseminated intravascular coagulation (DIC) in fulminant disease (Fig. 25-59).
MENINGOCOCCEMIA SEPTICEMIA Meningococci enter the bloodstream and multiply, damaging the walls of the blood vessels and causing bleeding into the skin and organs. Characterized by development of shock and multiorgan failure. Peripheral gangrene may occur, requiring amputation in those who survive.
WATERHOUSE–FRIDERICHSEN SYNDROME Fulminant meningococcal septicemia characterized by high fever, shock, widespread purpura, disseminated intravascular coagulation, thrombocytopenia, and adrenal insufficiency.
MENINGOCOCCAL MENINGITIS Bacteremia can result in the seeding of many organs, especially the meninges. The symptoms of meningococcal meningitis are those of typical bacterial meningitis, namely, fever, headache, stiff neck, and polymorphonuclear neutrophils (PMNs) in spinal fluid.

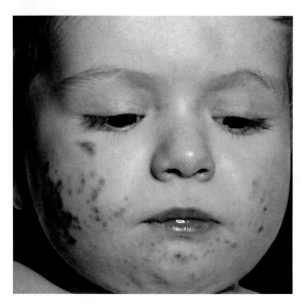

FIGURE 25-58 Acute meningococcemia: early exanthem Discrete, pink-to-purple macules and papules as well as purpura on the face of this young child. These lesions represent early disseminated intravascular coagulation with its cutaneous manifestation, purpura fulminans.

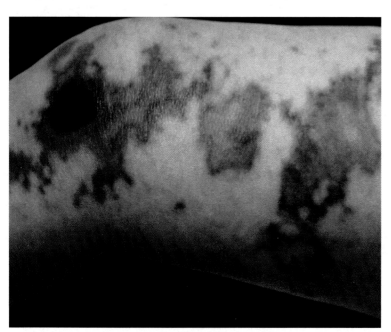

FIGURE 25-59 Acute meningococcemia: purpura fulminans Maplike, gray-to-black areas of cutaneous infarction of the leg in a child with NM meningitis and disseminated intravascular coagulation with purpura fulminans.

CHRONIC MENINGOCOCCEMIA Intermittent bacteremia. Slow replication seeds various organs: meninges, pericardium, large joints, and skin. Host inflammatory reaction limited to seeded site.

DIFFERENTIAL DIAGNOSIS

Adverse cutaneous drug eruptions, vasculitis, RMSF, and infective endocarditis.

DIAGNOSIS

Definitive etiologic diagnosis requires isolation of meningococci from blood or local site of infection.

COURSE

Onset of symptoms is sudden and death can follow within hours. In as many as 10 to 15% of survivors, there are persistent neurological defects, including hearing loss, speech disorders, loss of limbs, mental retardation, and paralysis.

TREATMENT

High dose antibiotic therapy and treatment of DIC.
PROPHYLAXIS Several vaccines are available to control the disease.

BARTONELLA INFECTIONS

- Etiology. *Bartonella* spp.; tiny gram-negative bacilli that can adhere to and invade mammalian cells such as endothelial cells and erythrocytes.
- Transmission. Cat scratch or bite. Body louse or sandfly bite.

CLINICAL MANIFESTATION

Vary with the immune status of the host.
Bartonella henselae. Immunocompetent host: *cat-scratch disease*. HIV disease: *bacillary angiomatosis*.
B. bacilliformis. Nonimmune, nonresidents of endemic area: *Oroya fever* with severe febrile illness, profound anemia. With immunity after convalescence: *verruga peruana* with red-purple cutaneous lesions (peruvian warts; resemble angiomatous lesions of bacillary angiomatosis).

B. quintana. *Trench fever* presenting as a febrile systemic illness with prolonged bacteremia; no cutaneous manifestations.
Diseases caused by *Bartonella* species:

- Cat-scratch disease: *B. henselae*.
- Bacillary angiomatosis: *B. henselae*, *B. quintana*.
- Bacillary peliosis: *B. henselae*.
- Trench fever: *B. quintana*.
- Bartonellosis (Carrión disease); Oroya fever and verruga peruana: *B. bacilliformis*.

CAT-SCRATCH DISEASE (CSD) ICD-10: A28.1

- Etiology. *B. henselae*. Reservoir: Domestic cat.
- Transmission. Associated with exposure to young cats. Blood cultures of kittens are frequently positive for *B. henselae*. Cat flea *Ctenocephalides felis* transmit infection between cats.
- Demography/Age of Onset. Majority of cases occur in children.
- Pathogenesis. *B. henselae* causes granulomatous inflammation in healthy individuals (CSD) and angiogenesis in immunocompromised persons.

CLINICAL MANIFESTATION

INOCULATION SITE Innocuous-looking, small (0.5 to 1 cm) papule, vesicle, or pustule; may ulcerate; skin color pink to red; firm, at times

tender (Fig. 25-60). Residual linear cat scratch. Persists for 1 to 3 weeks. *Distribution*: Exposed skin of the face and hands.
CONJUNCTIVAE If portal of entry is the conjunctiva, 3- to 5-mm whitish-yellow granulation on

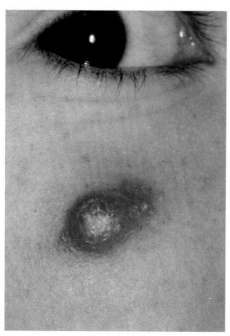

FIGURE 25-60 Bartonellosis: cat-scratch disease with primary lesion Erythematous nodule of the cheek of a 9-year-old girl at the site of cat scratch. Diagnosis was made on the histologic findings of the excised specimen.

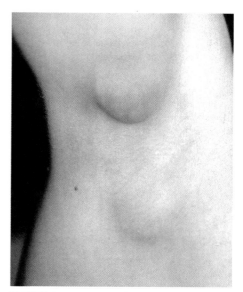

FIGURE 25-61 Bartonellosis: cat-scratch disease with axillary adenopathy Acute, very tender, axillary lymphadenopathy in a child; cat scratches were present on the dorsum of the ipsilateral hand. (Used with permission from Howard Heller, MD.)

palpebral conjunctiva associated with tender preauricular and/or cervical lymphadenopathy (*Parinaud oculoglandular syndrome*).

Uncommonly urticaria, transient maculopapular eruption, or erythema nodosum.

REGIONAL LYMPHADENOPATHY (Fig. 25-61) Evident within 2 to 3 weeks after inoculation in 90% of cases; primary lesion, if present, may have resolved by the time lymphadenopathy occurs. Nodes are often solitary, moderately tender, and freely movable. Involved lymph nodes: epitrochlear, axillary, pectoral, and cervical. Nodes may suppurate. Usually resolved within 3 months. Generalized lymphadenopathy or involvement of the lymph nodes of more than one region is unusual.

DIFFERENTIAL DIAGNOSIS

Chancriform syndrome. Suppurative bacterial lymphadenitis, NTM infection, sporotrichosis, and tularemia.

OTHER CAT-ASSOCIATED INFECTIONS Bite infections caused by *P. multocida* and *C. canimorsus*,

sporotrichosis; *Microsporum canis* dermatophytosis.

DIAGNOSIS

Suggested by regional lymphadenopathy developing over 2 to 3 weeks in an individual with cat contact and a primary lesion at the site of contact; confirmed by identification of *B. henselae* from tissue or serodiagnosis.

COURSE

Self-limiting, usually within 1 to 2 months. Uncommonly, prolonged morbidity with persistent high fever, suppurative lymphadenitis, and severe systemic symptoms. May be confused with lymphoma. Uncommonly, cat-scratch encephalopathy occurs. Antibiotic therapy has not been very effective in altering the course of the infection.

TREATMENT

In the immunocompromised, azithromycin; in immunocompetent, spontaneous resolution occurs.

BACILLARY ANGIOMATOSIS (BA) ICD-10: A44.8

- Etiology. *B. henselae*, *B. quintana*. Both cause cutaneous angiomas. *B. quintana* causes subcutaneous nodules and lytic bone lesion.
- Demography. Occurs in advanced HIV disease. Incidence decreased with antiretroviral therapy (ART) and prophylaxis of opportunistic infections.
- Risk Factors. *B. henselae*: contact with cats and/or cat fleas (*C. felis*). *B. quintana*: low income, home-lessness, body louse (*P. humanis corporis*) infestation.

CLINICAL MANIFESTATION

Papules or nodules resembling *angiomas* (bright red, violaceous, or skin colored) (Fig. 25-62); up to 2 to 3 cm in diameter; usually situated in dermis with thinning or erosion of overlying epidermis. Larger lesions may ulcerate. *Subcutaneous nodules*, 1 to 2 cm in diameter, resembling cysts. Uncommonly, abscess formation. Papules/nodules range from solitary lesions to >100. Firm, nonblanching.

DISTRIBUTION Any site, but palms and soles are usually spared. Occasionally, lesions occur at the site of a cat scratch. A solitary lesion may present as *dactylitis*.

MUCOUS MEMBRANES Angioma-like lesions of lips and oral mucosa. Laryngeal involvement with obstruction.

SYSTEMIC FINDINGS Infection may spread hema-togenously or via lymphatics to become sys-temic, commonly involving the liver (peliosis hepatitis) and spleen. Lesions may also occur in the heart, bone marrow, lymph nodes, muscles, soft tissues, and CNS.

DIFFERENTIAL DIAGNOSIS

Kaposi sarcoma, pyogenic granuloma, and cherry angioma.

DIAGNOSIS

Clinical findings confirmed by demonstration of *Bartonella* bacilli on the Warthin-Starry silver stain of lesional biopsy specimen, culture, or antibody studies.

COURSE AND TREATMENT

Rarely seen in persons with HIV disease suc-cessfully treated with ART. Untreated systemic infection causes significant morbidity and mortality. With effective antimicrobial therapy (erythromycin is treatment of choice; alterna-tively, doxycycline), lesions resolve within 1 to 2 weeks. As with other infections occurring in HIV disease, relapse may occur and require lifelong secondary prophylaxis.

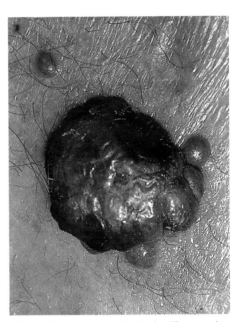

FIGURE 25-62 Bartonellosis: bacillary angio-matosis 3- to 5-mm cherry hemangioma-like papules and a larger pyogenic granuloma-like nodule on the shin of a male with advanced HIV disease. Subcutaneous nodular lesions were also present. Lesion promptly resolved with oral eryth-romycin, but required secondary prophylaxis for recurrent lesions.

TULAREMIA ICD-10: A21

- Etiology: *Francisella tularensis,* types A and B. After inoculation into skin, mucous membrane, lung (inhalation), or GI tract, *F. tularensis* reproduces and spreads through lymphatic channels to the lymph nodes and bloodstream.
- Transmission. *Bite of insect vector* (ticks, deer flies, body lice, or other arthropods). Handling flesh of infected animals; inoculation of conjunctiva; ingestion of infected food; inhalation. Most US cases occur in June to September when arthropod transmission is most common.
- Animal Reservoir. Rabbits, hares, muskrats, squirrels, voles, and beavers.
- Incidence. Rare; <200 cases reported in the United States per year; underdiagnosed, underreported.

CLINICAL MANIFESTATION

About 48 h after inoculation, pruritic papule develops at the site of trauma or insect bite followed by enlargement of the regional lymph nodes. Fever to 41°C.

Inoculation site: Erythematous tender papule evolving to a vesicopustule, enlarging to crusted ulcer with raised, sharply demarcated margins (96 h) (Fig. 25-63). Depressed center that is often covered by a black eschar (chancriform). Primary lesion on the finger or hand at the site of trauma or insect bite; groin or axilla after tick bite.

OTHER CUTANEOUS FINDINGS *Exanthem* may occur after bacteremia on the trunk and extremities with macules, papules, and petechiae. Erythema multiforme. Erythema nodosum.

CONJUNCTIVAE In oculoglandular tularemia, *F. tularensis* is inoculated into conjunctiva, causing a purulent conjunctivitis with pain, edema, and congestion. Small yellow nodules occur on conjunctivae and ulcerate.

REGIONAL LYMPH NODES As the ulcer develops, nodes enlarge and become tender, i.e., chancriform syndrome (Fig. 25-63). If untreated, they become suppurating buboes.

DIFFERENTIAL DIAGNOSIS

Acute cutaneous ulcer: Furuncle, paronychia, anthrax, *P. multocida* infection, sporotrichosis, and *M. marinum* infection. *Chancriform syndrome:* Herpes simplex virus lymphadenitis, plague, and cat-scratch disease.

DIAGNOSIS

Clinical diagnosis in a patient with chancriform syndrome with appropriate animal or insect exposure.

COURSE

Untreated, mortality rate for ulceroglandular form is 5%; 1% if therapy is initiated promptly.

TREATMENT

Streptomycin is the treatment of choice. Also gentamycin, chloramphenicol, doxycycline, and ciprofloxacin.

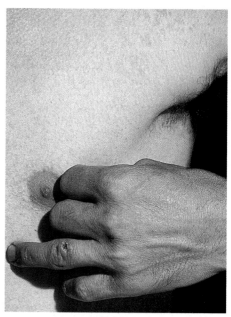

FIGURE 25-63 Tularemia: primary lesion and regional adenopathy A crusted ulcer at the site of inoculation is seen on the dorsum of the left ring finger with associated axillary lymph node enlargement (chancriform syndrome). The infection occurred after the patient killed and skinned a rabbit.

CUTANEOUS *PSEUDOMONAS AERUGINOSA* INFECTIONS

- *P. aeruginosa:* Nonfastidious, motile; produce pyocyanin and pyoverdine, pigments that cause yellow to dark green to bluish color.
- Ecology. Widespread in nature, inhabiting water, soil, plants, and animals, preferring moist environments. In healthy individuals, carriage rate of skin is low; pseudomonas is minimally invasive.
- Transmission. Most invasive infections are hospital acquired. Entry sites wounds, ulcers, and thermal burns; foreign bodies (IV or urinary catheter), and aspiration/aerosolization into respiratory tract.

CLINICAL MANIFESTATIONS

GREEN NAILS *P. aeruginosa* grows as a biofilm on ventral or dorsal surface of abnormal nails. Onycholytic nails, e.g., psoriasis and onychomycosis, create a moist environment for *Pseudomonas* to colonize. Less commonly, *Pseudomonas* can colonize the dorsal surface of fingernails associated with chronic paronychia. The onycholytic nail plate can be trimmed to eliminate the abnormal space.

INTERTRIGO Gram-negative webspace intertrigo presents as macerated and eroded skin on interdigital toes. *Pseudomonas* is the most common cause. Usually occurs in the setting of hyperhidrosis and hydration of stratum corneum. Interdigital tinea pedis and erythrasma may also be present. Superficial intertrigo can progress with interdigital ulceration and soft-tissue infection.

EXTERNAL OTITIS *Swimmer's ear:* Moist environment of external auditory canal provides medium for superficial infection, presenting as pruritus, pain, and discharge; usually self-limited. Malignant external otitis occurs in elderly diabetic patients most commonly; may progress to deeper invasive infection.

HOT TUB FOLLICULITIS *P. aeruginosa* can infect multiple hair follicles during exposure in hot tubs or physiotherapy pools, presenting as multiple follicular pustules on the trunk (Fig. 25-18). Infection is self-limited.

COLONIZATION OF WOUNDS Thermal burns, stasis ulcers, pressure ulcers, and surgical wounds are more commonly colonized with *Pseudomonas* (Fig. 25-39) after prior treatment of *S. aureus* with systemic antibiotics, diabetes, and other host defense defects. Soft-tissue infection can occur in colonized wounds.

SOFT-TISSUE INFECTION AND *E. GANGRENOSUM* Superficial infection can progress to cellulitis. *E. gangrenosum* is a necrotizing soft-tissue infection associated with blood vessel invasion, septic vasculitis, vascular occlusion, and necrosis (Fig. 25-32).

PSEUDOMONAL BACTEREMIA Hematogenous dissemination of *P. aeruginosa* can seed the dermis, resulting in multiple tender subcutaneous nodules.

DIAGNOSIS

Clinical suspicion confirmed by culture of skin lesion.

TREATMENT

Antibiotic according sensitivity of microbes. Surgical debridement.

MYCOBACTERIAL INFECTIONS

Mycobacteria are rod-shaped or coccobacilli acid-fast bacilli (AFB). More than 120 species identified. Relatively few associated with human disease:

- Hansen disease (leprosy).
- Tuberculosis.
- Non Tuberculous Mycobacterium (NTM) infections.
- Buruli or Bairnsdale ulcer disease is the third most common mycobacterial disease globally.

HANSEN DISEASE (LEPROSY) ICD-10: A30

- Etiology. *Mycobacterium leprae.*
- Chronic granulomatous disease principally acquired during childhood or young adulthood.
- Sites of infection. Skin, peripheral nervous system, upper respiratory tract, eyes, and testes.
- Clinical manifestations, natural history, and prognosis of leprosy are related to the host response: Various types of leprosy (tuberculoid, lepromatous, etc.) represent the spectra of the host's immunologic response (cell-mediated immunity).

Source: http://www.cdc.gov/nczved/divisions/dfbmd/diseases/hansens_disease/technical.html/.

CLASSIFICATION

Based on clinical, immunologic, and bacteriologic findings.

- *Tuberculoid (TL):* Localized skin involvement and/or peripheral nerve involvement; few organisms.
- *Lepromatous (LL):* Generalized involvement including skin, upper respiratory mucous membrane, reticuloendothelial system, adrenal glands, and testes; many bacilli.
- *Borderline (or "dimorphic") (BL):* Has features of both TL and LL. Usually many bacilli present, varied skin lesions: macules, plaques; progresses to TL or regresses to LL.
- *Indeterminate forms.*
- *Transitional forms:* See "Pathogenesis," in the following discussion.

ETIOLOGY AND EPIDEMIOLOGY

Mycobacterium leprae: Obligate intracellular acid-fast bacillus; reproduces optimally at 27 to 30°C. Organism cannot be cultured in vitro. Infects skin and cutaneous nerves (Schwann cell basal lamina). In untreated patients, only 1% of organisms are viable. Grows best in cooler tissues (skin, peripheral nerves, anterior chamber of eye, upper respiratory tract, and testes), sparing warmer areas of the skin (axilla, groin, scalp, and mid-line of back). Humans are main reservoirs of *M. leprae.* Wild armadillos (southern United States) as well as mangabey monkeys and chimpanzees are naturally infected with *M. leprae;* armadillos can develop lepromatous lesions.

Incidence rate peaks at 10 to 20 years; prevalence peaks at 30 to 50 years. More common in males than in females. Inverse relationship between skin color and severity of disease; in black Africans, susceptibility is high, but there is predominance of milder forms of the disease, i.e., TL vis-à-vis LL.

TRANSMISSION Uncertain. Likely spread from person to person in respiratory droplets.

DEMOGRAPHY Disease of the developing world. In 2010, 228,474 new cases detected worldwide; 294 in the United States. The vast majority were from Angola, Bangladesh, Brazil, China, Congo, Ethiopia, Indonesia, Madagascar, Mozambique, Myanmar, Nepal, Nigeria, Phillipines, Sudan, and Sri Lanka. Risk groups: Close contact with patients with untreated, active, predominantly multibacillary disease, and persons living in countries with highly endemic disease. Most individuals have natural immunity and do not develop disease.

PATHOGENESIS Clinical spectrum of leprosy depends exclusively on variable limitations in host's capability to develop effective cell-mediated immunity to *M. leprae.* Organism is capable of invading and multiplying in peripheral nerves and infecting and surviving in endothelial and phagocytic cells in many organs. Subclinical infection with leprosy is common among residents in endemic areas. Clinical expression of leprosy is development of a *granuloma;* patient may develop a *"reactional state,"* which may occur in some form in >50% of certain groups of patients.

GRANULOMATOUS SPECTRUM OF LEPROSY

- High-resistance tuberculoid response (TT).
- Low- or absent-resistance lepromatous pole (LL).
- Dimorphic or borderline region (BB).
- Two intermediary regions.
  - Borderline lepromatous (BL).
  - Borderline tuberculoid (BT).

In order of decreasing resistance, the spectrum is TT, BT, BB, BL, and LL.

IMMUNOLOGIC RESPONSES Immune responses to *M. leprae* can produce several types of reactions associated with a sudden change in the clinical status.

Lepra Type 1 Reactions. Acute or insidious tenderness and pain along affected nerve(s), associated with loss of function.

Lepra Type 2 Reactions. Erythema nodosum leprosum (ENL). Seen in half of LL patients, usually occurring after initiation of antilepromatous therapy, generally within the first 2 years of treatment. Massive inflammation with erythema nodosum–like lesions. *Lucio Reaction.* Individuals with diffuse LL develop shallow, large polygonal sloughing ulcerations on the legs. The reaction appears to be either a variant of ENL or secondary to arteriolar occlusion.

CLINICAL MANIFESTATION

Incubation period is 2 to 40 years (most commonly 5 to 7 years). Onset is insidious and painless; first affects peripheral nervous system with persistent or recurrent painful paresthesias and numbness without any visible clinical signs. At this stage, there may be transient macular skin eruptions; blister, but lack of awareness of trauma. Neural involvement leads to muscle weakness, muscle atrophy,

severe pain, and contractures of the hands and feet.

TUBERCULOID LEPROSY (TT, BT) Few well-defined *hypopigmented hypesthetic macules* (Fig. 25-64) with raised edges and varying in size from a few millimeters to very large lesions covering the entire trunk. Erythematous or purple border and hypopigmented center. Sharply defined, raised; often annular; enlarge peripherally. Central area becomes atrophic or depressed. Advanced lesions are anesthetic, devoid of skin appendages (sweat glands or hair follicles). Any site including the face. *TT:* Lesions may resolve spontaneously; not associated with lepra reactions. *BT:* Does not heal spontaneously; type 1 lepra reactions may occur.

Nerve Involvement: May be a thickened nerve on the edge of the lesion; large peripheral nerve enlargement frequent (ulnar, posterior auricular, peroneal, and posterior tibial nerves). Skin involvement is absent in *neural leprosy.* Nerve

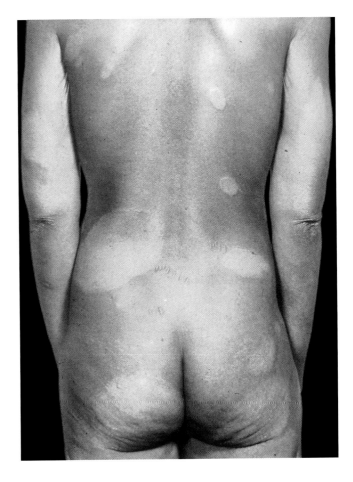

FIGURE 25-64 Leprosy: tuberculoid type Well-defined, hypopigmented, slightly scaling, anesthetic macules and plaques on the posterior trunk.

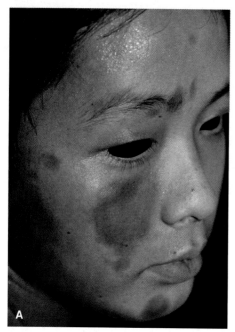
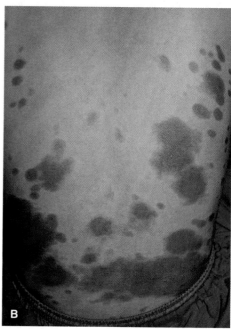

FIGURE 25-65 Leprosy: borderline-type A 26-year-old Vietnamese male. **(A)** Well-demarcated, infiltrated, erythematous plaques on the face. **(B)** Identical red plaques on the lower back.

involvement is associated with hypesthesia (pinprick, temperature, or vibration) and myopathy.
BORDERLINE BB LEPROSY Lesions are intermediate between tuberculoid and lepromatous and are composed of macules, papules, and plaques (Fig. 25-65). Anesthesia and decreased sweating are prominent in the lesions.
LEPROMATOUS LEPROSY (LL, BL) Skin-colored or slightly erythematous papules or nodules. Lesions enlarge; new lesions occur and coalesce. Later, symmetrically distributed nodules, raised plaques, diffuse dermal infiltrate, which on the face results in loss of hair (lateral eyebrows and eyelashes) and leonine facies (lion's face; Fig. 25-66). *Diffuse lepromatosis*, occurring in western Mexico, Caribbean, presents as diffuse dermal infiltration and thickened dermis. Bilaterally symmetric involving the earlobes, face, arms, and buttocks, or less frequently the trunk and lower extremities. Tongue: Nodules, plaques, or fissures.

Nerve Involvement: More extensive than in TT.

Other Involvement: Upper respiratory tract, anterior chamber of eye, and testes.

Reactional States

Immunologically mediated inflammatory states, occurring spontaneously or after initiation of therapy.

Lepra Type 1 Reactions: Skin lesions become acutely inflamed, associated with edema and pain; may ulcerate. Edema is most severe on the face, hands, and feet.

Lepra Type 2 Reactions (ENL): Present as painful red skin nodules arising superficially and deeply. In contrast the tru erythema nodosum lesions form abscesses or ulcerate; they occur most commonly on the face and extensor limbs.

Lucio Reaction: Occurs in patients from Mexico or Caribbean with diffuse LL. Presents as irregularly shaped erythematous plaques; lesions may resolve spontaneously or undergo necrosis with ulceration.

General Findings

Extremities: Sensory neuropathy, plantar ulcers, secondary infection; ulnar and peroneal palsies (Fig. 25-67), Charcot joints. Squamous cell carcinoma can arise in chronic foot ulcers (Fig. 11-13).

Nose: Chronic nasal congestion, epistaxis; destruction of cartilage with saddle-nose deformity (Fig. 25-67).

Eyes: Cranial nerve palsies, lagophthalmos, and corneal insensitivity. In LL, anterior chamber can be invaded with uveitis, glaucoma, and cataract formation. Corneal damage can occur

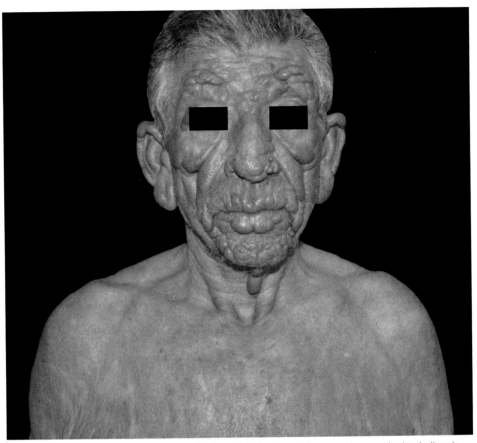

FIGURE 25-66 Diffuse skin infiltration, multiple nodular lesions, and sensory loss are the key hallmarks of **lepromatous leprosy (LL)**. This patient presented lesions on the upper part of the thorax, forehead, ears, nose, lips, perilabial, and mentonian regions, as well as lax skin of the malar and palpebral superior regions, with muscle force impairment on the left side. Superciliary and ciliary madarosis were also present. Ulnar and tibial posterior nerves were enlarged. A Ziehl–Neelsen stained skin smear had a 6+ bacterial index for acid-fast bacilli in clumps, and ELISA titration for anti-PGL-1 IgM was 3.445 (cutoff 0.295). The 12-month World Health Organization multidrug therapy regimen and prednisone were prescribed, with significant improvement. LL is the anergic form of leprosy; it generates an exacerbated but inefficient humoral immune response, leading to highly infectious patients. Mycosis fungoides, neurofibromatosis, sarcoidosis, amyloidosis, syphilis, anergic leishmaniasis, and lobomycosis are among diseases in the differential diagnosis. (Used with permission from Claudio G. Salgado, MD, PhD and Josafá G. Barreto, PhD, Pará Federal University, Brazil.)

secondary to trichiasis and sensory neuropathy, secondary infection, and muscle paralysis.

Testes: May be involved in LL with resultant hypogonadism.

Complications of Leprosy: *Squamous cell carcinoma* can arise in chronic neurotrophic ulcers on the lower extremities (see Fig. 11-13). The tumors are usually low-grade malignancies but can metastasize to regional lymph nodes and cause death. *Secondary amyloidosis* with hepatic and renal abnormalities.

DIFFERENTIAL DIAGNOSIS

Hypopigmented lesions with granulomas.
Sarcoidosis, leishmaniasis, NTM infection, lymphoma, syphilis, and granuloma annulare.

LABORATORY EXAMINATIONS

SLIT-SKIN SMEARS A small skin incision is made; the site is then scraped to obtain tissue fluid from which a smear is made and examined after

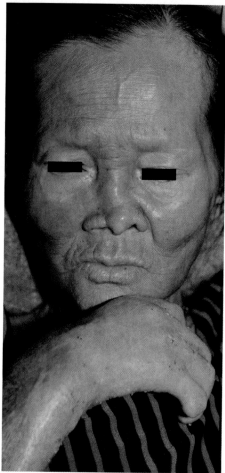

FIGURE 25-67 Leprosy: lepromatous type
A 60-year-old Vietnamese female with treated advanced disease. Ulnar palsy, loss of digits on right hand, and saddle-nose deformity associated with loss of nasal cartilage are seen.

Ziehl–Neelsen staining. Specimens are usually obtained from multiple sites (both earlobes, elbows, knees, and active lesions). High Bacterial Index (BI) is seen in LL, low/negative BI can be seen in paucibacillary cases, treated cases, and cases examined by an inexperienced technician.
CULTURE *M. leprae* has not been cultured in vitro; however, it does grow when inoculated into the mouse foot pad. Routine bacterial cultures to rule out secondary infection.
PCR *M. leprae* DNA detected by this technique makes the diagnosis of early paucibacillary leprosy and identifies *M. leprae* after therapy.

SEROLOGY Measure IgM antibodies to phenolic glycolipid-1 (PGL-1).
DERMATOPATHOLOGY TL shows epithelioid cell granulomas forming around dermal nerves; AFB are sparse or absent. LL shows an extensive cellular infiltrate separated from the epidermis by a narrow zone of normal collagen. Skin appendages are destroyed. Macrophages are filled with *M. leprae,* having abundant foamy or vacuolated cytoplasm (lepra cells or Virchow cells).

DIAGNOSIS

Made if one or more of the cardinal findings are detected: Patient from endemic area, skin lesions characteristic of leprosy with diminished or loss of sensation, enlarged peripheral nerves, finding of *M. leprae* in skin or, less commonly, other sites.

COURSE

After the first few years of drug therapy, the most difficult problem is management of the changes secondary to neurologic deficits; contractures and trophic changes in the hands and feet. Uncommonly, secondary amyloidosis with renal failure can complicate long-standing leprosy. Lepra type 1 reactions last 2 to 4 months in individuals with BT and up to 9 months in those with BL. Lepra type 2 reactions (ENL) occur in 50% of individuals with LL and 25% of those with BL within the first 2 years of treatment. ENL may be complicated by uveitis, dactylitis, arthritis, neuritis, lymphadenitis, myositis, and orchitis. Lucio reaction occurs secondary to vasculitis with subsequent infarction.

TREATMENT

General principles of treatment:

- Tuberculoid: Dapsone plus rifampin.
- Lepromatous: Dapsone plus clofazimine plus rifampin.
- Eradicate infection with antilepromatous therapy.
- Prevent and treat reactions (prednisone or thalidomide).
- Reduce the risk of nerve damage.
- Educate patient to deal with neuropathy and anesthesia.
- Treat complications of nerve damage.
- Rehabilitate patient into society.

Management involves a broad multidisciplinary approach including orthopedic surgery, podiatry, ophthalmology, and physical therapy.

CUTANEOUS TUBERCULOSIS ICD-10: A18.4

- Etiology. *Mycobacterium tuberculosis* complex. Commonly infects lungs; rarely skin.
- Transmission. Airborne spread of droplet nuclei from those with infectious pulmonary Tb to lungs.
- Cutaneous Infection. Exogenous inoculation into skin. Direct extension from deeper tissues such as joint; lymphatic spread to skin; hematogenous spread to skin.

CLASSIFICATION

EXOGENOUS INOCULATION TO SKIN Primary inoculation tuberculosis (PIT), i.e., *tuberculous chancre*: Occurs at inoculated site in nonimmune host. *Tuberculosis verrucosa cutis* (TVC): Occurs at inoculated site in individual with prior tuberculosis infection.

Tuberculosis may also result from bacille Calmette-Guérin (BCG) immunization.

ENDOGENOUS SPREAD TO SKIN Lymphatics, hematogenous, and bodily fluids (sputum, feces, or urine). *Lupus vulgaris. Scrofuloderma.* Metastatic tuberculosis abscess. Acute miliary tuberculosis. *Orificial tuberculosis.*

PATHOGENESIS

Type of clinical lesion depends on route of cutaneous inoculation and immunologic status of the host.

- Cutaneous inoculation results in a *tuberculous chancre* in the nonimmune host and *TVC* in the immune host.
- Direct extension from underlying tuberculous infection, i.e., lymphadenitis or tuberculosis of bones and joints, results in *scrofuloderma*.
- Lymphatic spread to skin results in *lupus vulgaris*.
- Hematogenous dissemination results in *acute miliary tuberculosis, lupus vulgaris,* or *metastatic tuberculosis abscess.*
- Autoinoculation from body fluids such as sputum, urine, and feces results in *orificial tuberculosis*.

Globally, the incidence of cutaneous tuberculosis is increasing, associated with HIV disease. Problem of multidrug resistance (MDR) is also common in persons with HIV disease.

CLINICAL MANIFESTATION

PIT Initially, papule occurs at the inoculation site 2 to 4 weeks after inoculation. Lesion enlarges to a painless ulcer, *tuberculous chancre* (Fig. 25-68) with shallow granular base. Older ulcers become indurated with thick crusts.

Deeper inoculation results in *subcutaneous abscess*. Most common on exposed skin at sites of minor injuries. Oral ulcers on gingiva or palate occur after ingestion of bovine bacilli in nonpasteurized milk. *Regional lymphadenopathy* occurs several weeks after appearance of the ulcer (*chancriform syndrome*) (Fig. 25-68).

TVC Initial papule with violaceous halo. Evolves to *hyperkeratotic, warty, or firm plaque* (Fig. 25-69). Clefts and fissures occur from which pus and keratinous material can be expressed. Border often irregular. Lesions are usually single, but multiple lesions occur. Most commonly on the dorsolateral hands and fingers. In children, on the lower extremities, knees. No lymphadenopathy.

LUPUS VULGARIS Initial papule ill-defined and soft, evolves into *well-defined, irregular plaque* (Fig. 25-70). Reddish-brown. Diascopy (glass slide pressed against skin) shows an *"apple jelly" color* (i.e., orange-tan). Lesions are characteristically soft and friable. Surface is initially smooth or slightly scaly but may become hyperkeratotic. Hypertrophic forms result in soft tumorous nodules. Ulcerative forms present as punched-out, often serpiginous ulcers surrounded by soft, brownish infiltrate. Usually solitary, but several sites may occur. *Most lesions on the head and neck*, most often on nose, ears, or scalp. Lesions on ears or nose can result in destruction of underlying cartilage. *Scarring is prominent.* Characteristically new brownish infiltrates occur within atrophic scars.

SCROFULODERMA Firm subcutaneous nodule that initially is freely movable; lesion then becomes doughy and evolves into irregular, *deep-seated node or plaque* that liquefies and perforates (Fig. 25-71). Ulcers and irregular sinuses, usually of linear or serpiginous shape, discharge pus or caseous material. Edges are undermined, inverted, with dissecting subcutaneous pockets alternating with soft, fluctuating infiltrates and bridging scars. Most often occurs in the *parotid, submandibular,* and *supraclavicular regions*; lateral neck, scrofuloderma most often results from contiguous spread from affected lymph nodes or tuberculous bones (phalanges, sternum, or ribs) or joints.

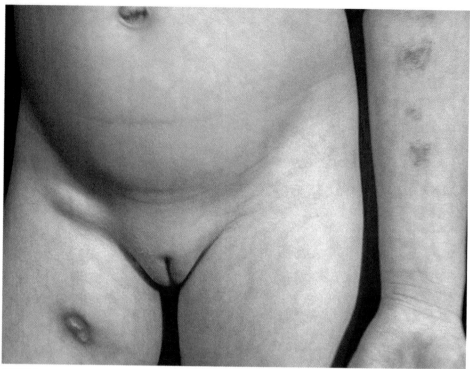

FIGURE 25-68 Primary inoculation tuberculosis A large, ulcerated nodule at the site of *Mycobacterium* tuberculosis inoculation on the right thigh associated with inguinal lymphadenopathy. The erythematous papules on the left forearm occurred at the site of tuberculin testing.

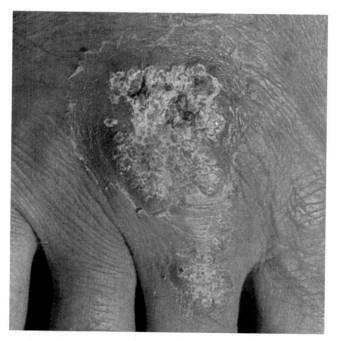

FIGURE 25-69 Tuberculosis verrucosa cutis A 40-year-old male with warty and crusted plaques on the dorsum of the hand for 6 months. (Reproduced with permission from Sethi A. Tuberculosis and infections with atypical Mycobacteria. In: Goldsmith LA, Katz SI, Gilchrest BA, et al, eds. *Fitzpatrick's Dermatology in General Medicine.* 8th ed. New York, NY: McGraw-Hill; 2012.)

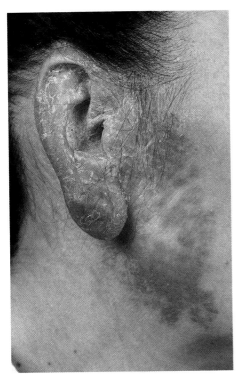

FIGURE 25-70 Lupus vulgaris Reddish-brown plaque, which on diascopy exhibits the diagnostic yellow-brown apple-jelly color. Note nodular infiltration of the earlobe, scaling of the helix, and atrophic scarring in the center of the plaque.

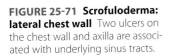

FIGURE 25-71 Scrofuloderma: lateral chest wall Two ulcers on the chest wall and axilla are associated with underlying sinus tracts.

METASTATIC TUBERCULOSIS ABSCESS Subcutaneous abscess, nontender, "cold," and fluctuant. Coalescing with overlying skin, breaking down and forming fistulas and ulcers. Single or multiple lesions, often at sites of previous trauma.

ACUTE MILIARY TUBERCULOSIS Exanthem. *Disseminated lesions* are minute macules and papules or purpuric lesions. Sometimes vesicular and crusted. Removal of crust reveals umbilication. Disseminated on all parts of the body, particularly the trunk.

ORIFICIAL TUBERCULOSIS Small yellowish nodule on mucosa breaks down to form *painful circular or irregular ulcer* (Fig. 25-72) with undermined borders. Surrounding mucosa swollen, edematous, and inflamed. Since orifical tuberculosis results from autoinoculation of mycobacteria from progressive tuberculosis of internal organs, it is usually found on the oral, pharyngeal (pulmonary tuberculosis), vulvar (genitourinary tuberculosis), and anal (intestinal tuberculosis) mucous membranes. Lesions may be single or multiple, and in the mouth most often occur on the tongue, soft and hard palate, or lips.

DIAGNOSIS

Clinical findings, tuberculin skin testing (Fig. 25-73), dermatopathology, confirmed by isolation of *M. tuberculosis* on culture or by PCR.

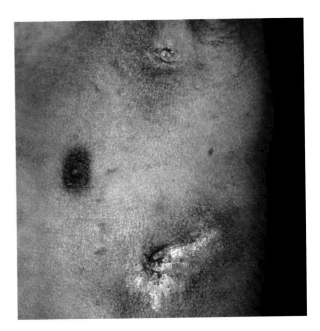

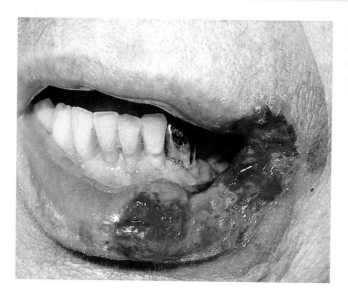

FIGURE 25-72 Orificial tuberculosis: lips A large, very painful ulcer on the lips of this patient with advanced cavitary pulmonary tuberculosis.

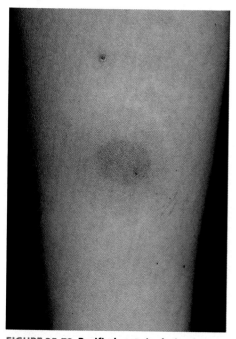

FIGURE 25-73 Purified protein derivative or Mantoux test: positive test A 31-year-old Taiwanese female with psoriasis, with a negative skin test 1 year previously, was retested prior to beginning etanercept. She had become infected while visiting her father, who had pulmonary tuberculosis, in Taiwan. A red plaque with surrounding erythema is seen at the test site.

COURSE

The course of cutaneous tuberculosis is quite variable, depending on the type of cutaneous infection, amount of inoculum, extent of extracutaneous infection, age of the patient, immune status, and therapy.

TREATMENT

Only PIT and TVC are limited to the skin. All other patterns of cutaneous tuberculosis are associated with systemic infection that has disseminated secondarily to skin. As such, therapy should be aimed at achieving a cure, avoiding relapse, and preventing emergence of drug-resistant mutants.

ANTITUBERCULOUS THERAPY Prolonged antituberculous therapy with at least two drugs is indicated for all cases of CTb except for TVC that can be excised.

- Standard antituberculous therapy:
  - Isoniazid (5 mg/kg daily).
  - Rifampin (600 mg/kg daily).
- Supplemented in initial phases with:
  - Ethambutol (25 mg/kg daily) and/or
  - Streptomycin (10 to 15 mg/kg daily) and/or
  - Pyrazinamide (15 to 30 mg/kg daily).

Isoniazid and rifampin for at least 9 months; can be shortened to 6 months if four drugs are given during the first 2 months.

MULTIDRUG RESISTANT (MDR) TB Incidence is increasing.

NONTUBERCULOUS MYCOBACTERIAL INFECTIONS ICD-10: A31.1

- Nontuberculous mycobacteria (NTM) defined as mycobacteria other than *M. tuberculosis* complex and *M. leprae*. Occur naturally in the environment: *M. marinum, M. ulcerans, M. fortuitum* complex, *M. abscessus, M. avium-intracellulare,* and *M. haemophilum.*
- Infection. Capable of causing primary infections in otherwise healthy individuals and more serious infection with host defense defects such as:
  - Immunocompetent individuals: primary cutaneous infections at sites of inoculation. Nodules, lymphocutaneous lesions, or nodular lymphangitis.
  - Immunocompromised host: disseminated mucosal and cutaneous lesions.
- Diagnosis. Detection of mycobacteria histochemically or by culture on specific media. New molecular techniques based on DNA amplification accelerate diagnosis, identify common sources of infection, and reveal new types of NTM.
- Treatment. Clarithromycin, rifampicin, fluoroquinolones, and minocycline.

MYCOBACTERIUM MARINUM INFECTION

- Etiology. *M. marinum*, an environmental nontuberculous mycobacterium. Infection usually follows traumatic inoculation in aqueous environment, i.e., fish tank, unchlorinated water.
- Demography. Healthy adults. More invasive or disseminated infections with host defense defects.

CLINICAL MANIFESTATION

INCUBATION PERIOD Variable: Usually weeks to months after inoculation. Lesions may be asymptomatic or tender.

INOCULATION SITE Papule(s) enlarging to inflammatory (Fig. 25-74), red to red-brown *nodule* or *plaque* 1 to 4 cm in size on the dominant hand. Surface of lesions may be *hyperkeratotic* or *verrucous* (Fig. 25-75). May become *ulcerated* with superficial crust, granulation tissue base, ± serosanguineous, or purulent discharge. In some cases, small satellite papules and draining sinuses may develop. Usually solitary, over bony prominence. More extensive soft-tissue infection may occur with host defense defects. Atrophic scarring follows spontaneous regression or successful therapy.

NODULAR LYMPHANGITIS Deep-seated nodules in a linear configuration on hand and forearm exhibit lymphocutaneous spread (Fig. 25-76). Boggy inflammatory reaction may mimic bursitis, synovitis, or arthritis about the elbow, wrist, or interphalangeal joints. Tenosynovitis, septic arthritis, and osteomyelitis. Host defense defects.

DISSEMINATED INFECTION Rare. May occur with host defense defects. Regional lymphadenopathy uncommon.

DIAGNOSIS

History of trauma in an aqueous environment, clinical findings, confirmed by isolation of *M. marinum* on culture. *M. marinum* grows at 32°C (but not at 37°C) in 2 to 4 weeks. Early lesions yield numerous colonies. Lesions 3 months or older generally yield few colonies.

LABORATORY FINDINGS

LESIONAL BIOPSY Acid-fast stain demonstrates *M. marinum* only in approximately 50% of cases.

COURSE

Usually self-limited but can remain active for a prolonged period. Single papulonodular lesions resolve spontaneously within 3 months to 3 years; nodular lymphangitis can persist for years. With host defense defects, more extensive deep infection can occur.

TREATMENT

Drug of first choice: Clarithromycin and either rifampin or ethambutol for 1 to 2 months after lesions have resolved (3 to 4 months). Minocycline alone may be effective.

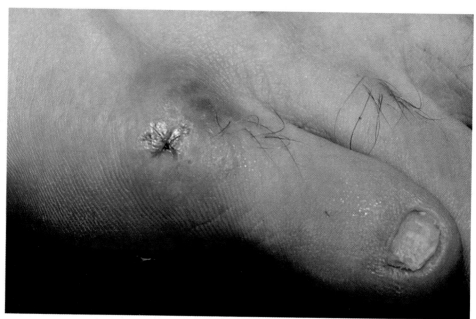

FIGURE 25-74 *M. marinum*: inoculation site infection on the foot A 31-year-old male with painful indurated plaque on the lateral dorsal foot. The lesion arose at the site of a small blister 1 year ago while in Afghanistan. Three previous biopsies and tissue cultures had been unsuccessful at making a diagnosis. After intralesional injection of triamcinolone 1.5 mg/mL, acid–fast bacilli were identified in the biopsy specimen and *M. marinum* isolated on culture. He was successfully treated with four antimycobacterial agents.

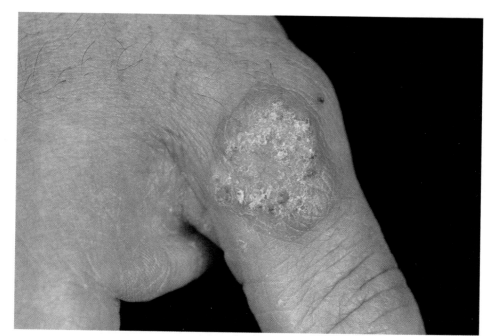

FIGURE 25-75 *M. marinum* infection: verrucous plaque A red-violet, verrucous plaque on the dorsum of the right thumb of a fish tank hobbist at the site of an abrasion.

FIGURE 25-76 *M. marinum*: soft-tissue infection and lymphangitis beginning on finger A 48-year-old female with painful swelling of the right middle finger for 4 months. She recalled cleaning a fish tank several weeks before the distal digital became red and tender. The finger and hand became progressively more inflamed and red nodules appeared on the forearm. Slight enlargement of axillary nodes was detected.

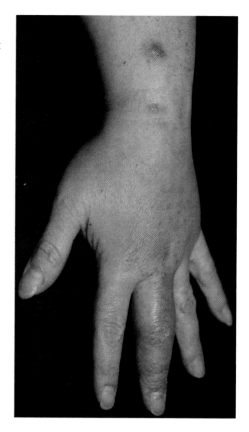

MYCOBACTERIUM ULCERANS INFECTION ICD-10: A31.1

- *Synonyms:* Buruli ulcer or Buruli ulcer disease in Africa. Bairnsdale or Daintree ulcer in Australia.
- Etiology. *M. ulcerans.* An environmental habitat for the organism has not been established. Incidence: Third most common mycobacterial infection after tuberculosis and leprosy.
- Transmission. Inoculation probably via minor trauma occurring in wet, marshy, or swampy sites. Bites of aquatic insects; *M. ulcerans* replicates in insect salivary glands; in endemic areas, 5 to 10% of aquatic insects have microbe in salivary gland.
- Demography. Occurs in >30 countries. Tropical regions of West Africa; Australia, Papua New Guinea; Central Mexico.
- Pathogenesis. *M. ulcerans* produces polypeptide toxin (mycolactone), which suppresses immune response to microbe.

CLINICAL MANIFESTATION

Incubation period approximately 3 months. The early nodule at the site of trauma and subsequent ulceration are usually painless. Fever, constitutional findings are usually absent.

Painless subcutaneous swelling occurs at the site of inoculation. Papule(s), nodule(s), and plaques are often overlooked. Lesion enlarges and *ulcerates*. The ulcer extends into the subcutaneous fat and its margin is deeply undermined (Fig. 25-77). Ulcerations may enlarge to involve an entire extremity. Legs more commonly involved, sites of trauma. Any site may be involved. Soft tissue and bony involvement can occur. As ulcerations healed, scarring and disabling deformities may occur. Osteomyelitis may occur.

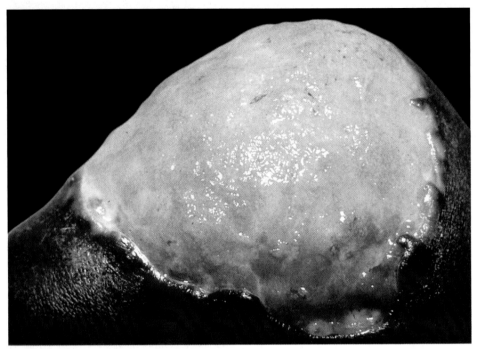

FIGURE 25-77 *M. ulcerans*: Buruli ulcer A 15-year-old Ugandan male with a huge ulcer with a clean base and undermined margins extends into the subcutaneous tissue. (Used with permission from Dr. Manfred Dietrich.)

DIAGNOSIS

Identification of microbe on culture or by PCR.

LABORATORY FINDINGS

DERMATOPATHOLOGY Necrosis originates in interlobular septa of subcutis. Poor inflammatory response despite clusters of extracellular bacilli. Granulation with giant cells but no caseation necrosis. AFB are always demonstrable.

DIFFERENTIAL DIAGNOSIS

Sporotrichosis, nocardiosis, phaeohyphomycosis, and squamous cell carcinoma.

COURSE

Because of delay in diagnosis and treatment, lesions are often extensive. Ulcerations persist for months to years. Spontaneous healing occurs eventually in some patients; scarring, contracture of the limb, and lymphedema. Malnutrition and anemia delay healing.

TREATMENT

ANTIMYCOBACTERIAL DRUG THERAPY Rifampicin and streptomycin combined with surgery. Combination of rifampicin and ciprofloxacin may be effective.
SURGERY Excision followed by grafting.

MYCOBACTERIUM FORTUITUM COMPLEX INFECTIONS ICD-10: A31.1

- Etiology. *M. fortuitum, M. chelonae, M. abscessus.* Organisms are widely distributed in soil, dust, and water.
- Natural Reservoirs. Nosocomial environments: Municipal water supplies, moist areas in hospitals, contaminated biological agents.
- Cutaneous infections account for 60% of infections.
- Transmission. Inoculation via traumatic puncture wounds, percutaneous catheterizations or injections. Whirlpool footbaths in nail salons (*M. fortuitum*).

CLINICAL MANIFESTATION

Incubation period usually within 1 month (range 1 week to 2 years).

SKIN AND SOFT-TISSUE INFECTIONS Nodular on lower legs following foot baths at nail salons. Furunculosis (Fig. 25-78); shaving legs provides a portal of entry. Wound infections at surgical sites or sites of trauma. Multiple nodules, abscesses, and crusted ulcers with host defense defects (Figs. 25-79 and 25-80).

DIAGNOSIS

Lesional skin biopsy specimen or identify by PCR.

LABORATORY EXAMINATIONS

DERMATOPATHOLOGY Necrosis is often present without caseation; AFB can be seen within microabscesses.

COURSE

The infection becomes chronic unless treated with antimycobacterial therapy, ± surgical debridement.

TREATMENT

Antimycobacterial chemotherapy. Surgical debridement with delayed closure for localized infections.

FIGURE 25-78 *M. fortuitum infection* A 45-year-old female with erythematous tender nodules on the lower legs. The lesions occurred several weeks after a pedicure in a foot care salon. Shaving of legs may have facilitated the infection. *M. fortuitum* was isolated on culture of lesional biopsy specimen.

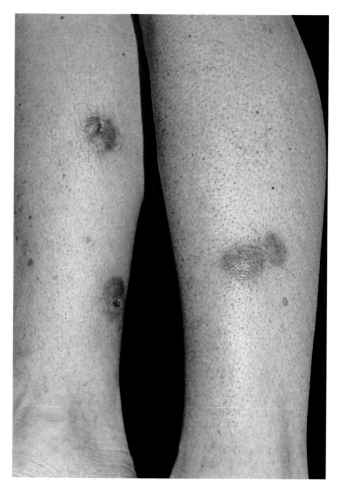

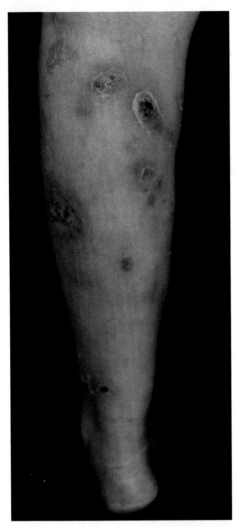

FIGURE 25-79 Multiple sites of soft-tissue infection lower leg: *Mycobacterium chelonae*
A 74-year-old female with chronic progressive lung disease treated with prednisone and azathioprine developed soft-tissue infections with multiple abscesses on hands, lower legs, and feet. *M. chelonae* was isolated on culture of biopsy specimen.

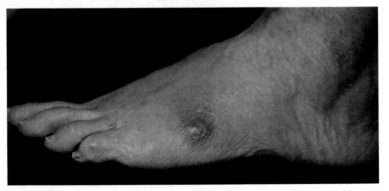

FIGURE 25-80 *M. chelonae* abscess on L-dorsolateral foot A 74-year-old female treated with prednisone and azathioprine. *M. chelonae* isolated on lesional biopsy specimen.

LYME DISEASE ICD-10: A69.2

- Etiologic agent: *Borrelia* spirochetes. Transmitted to humans by the bite of an infected Ixodes scapularis (US) or *Ixodes ricinus* (Europe) tick (deer tick).
- *Stage 1 early localized disease*: Up to 30 days post tick bite. Erythematous plaque at the tick bite site, *erythema migrans* (EM), noted in 70 to 80% of cases. Acute illness syndrome (fever, chills, myalgia, headache, weakness, and photophobia). *Lymphocytoma*.
- *Stage 2 early disseminated disease*: Days to weeks post tick bite. *Secondary lesions*. Meningitis, *cranial neuritis* (8%), radiculoneuritis (4%), peripheral neuritis. *Carditis*: AV nodal block (1%). *Migratory musculoskeletal pain* (33%), *arthralgias*.
- *Stage 3 late disseminated disease*: Persistent infection, developing months or years later: Intermittent or *persistent arthritis*, chronic encephalopathy or polyneuropathy, acrodermatitis chronica atrophicans (ACA).
- Posttreatment Lyme disease syndrome: 10 to 20% of treated patients have persistent symptoms.

ETIOLOGY AND EPIDEMIOLOGY

ETIOLOGIC AGENT US: *Borrelia burgdorferi,* recently *Borrelia mayonii* (Midwestern US). Europe: B. afzelii, B. garinii.

VECTOR Infected nymph Ixodes tick. Three stages of tick development: *larva, nymph, adult*; each stage requires blood meal. Preferred host of adult *Ixodes* is the white-tailed deer.

SEASON In the Midwestern and Eastern United States, most cases occur late May through early autumn.

RISK FOR EXPOSURE Strongly associated with prevalence of tick vectors and proportion of those ticks that carry *B. burgdorferi*. In the northeastern United States with endemic disease, the infection rate of the nymph *I. scapularis* tick with *B. burgdorferi* is 20 to 35%.

INCIDENCE LD is the most common vector-borne infection in the United States, with 25,359 cases reported in 2014. Cases reported in all 50 states except Hawaii.

PATHOGENESIS After inoculation into the skin, spirochetes replicate and migrate centrifugally, producing the *EM* lesion, and invade vessels, spreading hematogenously to other organs. The spirochete has a particular trophism for tissues of the skin, nervous system, and joints. The organism persists in affected tissues during all stages of the illness. The immune response to the spirochete develops gradually. Specific IgM antibodies peak between the third and sixth weeks after disease onset. The specific IgG response develops gradually over months. Proinflammatory cytokines, TNF-α, and IL-1 are produced in affected tissues.

CLINICAL MANIFESTATION

Incubation period for *EM*: 3 to 32 days after tick bite. *Cardiac manifestations* 35 days (3 weeks to >5 months after tick bite). *Neurologic manifestations*: Average 38 days (2 weeks to months) after tick bite. *Rheumatologic manifestations*: 4 days to 2 years after bite.

PRODROME With disseminated infection (stage 2), malaise, fatigue, lethargy, headache, fever, chills, stiff neck, arthralgia, myalgia, backache, anorexia, sore throat, nausea, dysesthesia, vomiting, abdominal pain, and photophobia.

HISTORY Because of the small size (*poppy seed*) of nymph tick, most patients are unaware of tick bite; adults are *sesame seed* size. Bites are asymptomatic. Removal of the nymphal tick within 36 h of attachment may preclude transmission. EM may be associated with burning sensation, itching, or pain. Only 75% of patients with Lyme disease exhibit EM. Joint complaints more common in North America. Neurologic involvement more common in Europe. With persistent disease, chronic fatigue.

STAGE 1 LOCALIZED INFECTION *EM*. Initial erythematous macule or papule expanding centrifugally within days to form a lesion with a distinct red border at the bite site (Fig. 25-81). Maximum median diameter is 15 cm. As EM expands, site may remain uniformly erythematous, or several rings of varying shades of red with concentric rings (*targetoid* or *bull's eye* lesions). When occurring on the scalp, only a linear streak may be evident on the face or neck (Fig. 25-82). *Multiple EM lesions* are seen with multiple bite sites. Most common sites: thigh, groin, and axilla. Center may become indurated, vesicular, ecchymotic, or necrotic. As EM evolves, postinflammatory hyperpigmentation, transient alopecia, and desquamation may occur.

Borrelial Lymphocytoma (BL). Mainly seen in Europe. Usually arises at the site of tick bite.

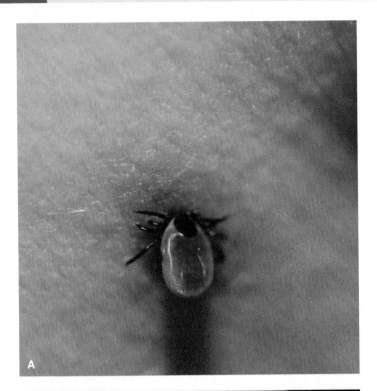

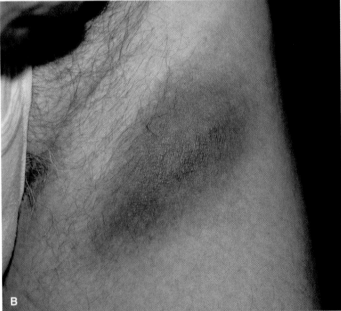

FIGURE 25-81 Lyme borreliosis: erythema migrans (EM) on upper thigh (A). Attachment of Ixodes tick **(B)**; oval erythema, slowly increasing (i.e., migrans). Will later resolve in the center, forminig a ring.

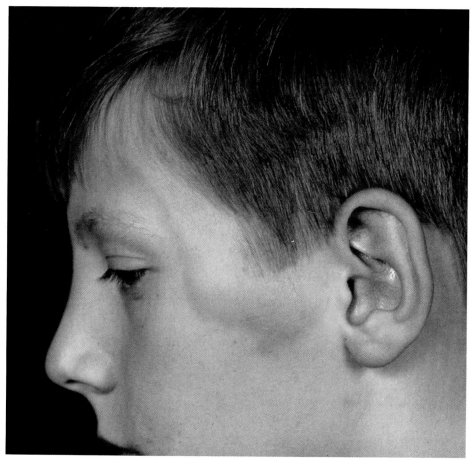

FIGURE 25-82 Lyme borreliosis: erythema migrans on face Serpiginous erythematous lesion on the forehead represents the margin of a large lesion occurring on the scalp.

Some patients have a history of EM; others may show concomitant EM located around or near the lymphocytoma. Usually presents as a solitary bluish-red nodule (Fig. 25-83). Sites of predilection: Earlobe (children), nipple/areola (adults), areola, scrotum; 3 to 5 cm in diameter. *Other Cutaneous Findings.* Malar rash, diffuse urticaria, and subcutaneous nodules (panniculitis).

STAGE 2 DISSEMINATED INFECTION *Secondary Lesions.* Secondary lesions resemble EM but are smaller, migrate less, and lack central induration and may be scaly. Lesions occur at any site except the palms and soles. A few or dozens of lesions may occur; can become confluent.

STAGE 3 PERSISTENT INFECTION *Acrodermatitis chronica atrophicans* (ACA) associated with

B. afzelii infection in Europe and Asia. More common in elderly women. Initially, diffuse or *localized violaceous erythema*, usually on one extremity, accompanied by mild to prominent edema. Extends centrifugally over several months to years, leaving central areas of atrophy, veins, and subcutaneous tissue become prominent (Fig. 25-84). Localized fibromas and plaques are seen as subcutaneous nodules around the knees and elbows.

DIFFERENTIAL DIAGNOSIS

ERYTHEMA MIGRANS Insect bite (annular erythema caused by ticks, mosquitoes, or Hymenoptera), epidermal dermatophytoses, allergic contact dermatitis, herald patch of pityriasis rosea, and fixed drug eruption.

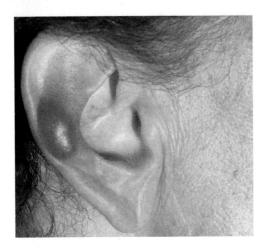

FIGURE 25-83 Lyme borreliosis: lympho-cytoma cutis Solitary, red-purple nodule on the ear.

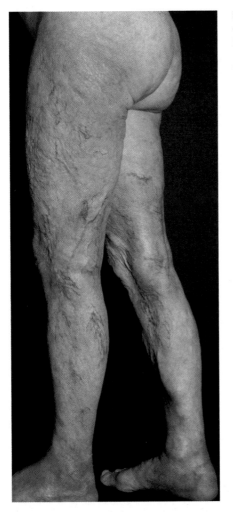

FIGURE 25-84 Lyme borreliosis: acrodermatitis chronica atrophicans: end stage Advanced atrophy of the epidermis and dermis with associated violaceous erythema of legs and feet; the visibility of the superficial veins is striking.

Lyme disease-like illness with exposure in Midwest and southern United States transmitted by Lone Star tick (*Amblyomma americanum*); referred to as *southern tick-associated rash illness*.

SECONDARY LESIONS Secondary syphilis, pityriasis rosea, erythema multiforme, and urticaria.

LABORATORY EXAMINATIONS

Skin Biopsy of EM. Deep and superficial perivascular and interstitial infiltrate containing lymphocytes and plasma cells with some degree of vascular damage (mild vasculitis or hypervascular occlusion). Spirochetes can be demonstrated in up to 40% of EM biopsy specimens.

DIAGNOSIS

The CDC recommends a two-step approach: http://www.cdc.gov/lyme/diagnosis treatment/LabTest/TwoStep/.

Diagnosis of early LB made on *characteristic clinical findings* in a person living in or having visited an endemic area; does not require laboratory confirmation. Diagnosis of *late LB* confirmed by specific serologic tests.

COURSE

After adequate treatment, early lesions resolve within 2 weeks and late manifestations are prevented. Late manifestations identified early usually clear after adequate antibiotic therapy. However, delay in diagnosis may result in permanent joint or neurologic disabilities. EM (short duration of infection) treated with antimicrobial agents does not confer protective immunity. If LB goes untreated for months, immunity may develop that protects against reinfection for years.

TREATMENT

Doxycycline 100 mg twice daily for 14 to 21 days is the treatment of choice for early localized and disseminated disease. Late stage Lyme disease should be treated for 14 to 28 days. Amoxicillin, cefuroxime, ceftriaxone, cefotaxime, and penicillin can be used in children under 8, pregnant woman, and doxycycline-allergic patients.

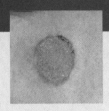

FUNGAL INFECTIONS OF THE SKIN, HAIR, AND NAILS

INTRODUCTION

- **Superficial Fungal Infections.** Caused by fungi that are capable of colonizing (cutaneous microbiome) and superficially invading skin and mucosal sites:
  - *Candida* species.
  - *Malassezia* species.
  - Dermatophytes.
- **Deeper, Chronic Cutaneous Fungal Infections.** Occur after percutaneous inoculation:
  - *Phaeohyphomycosis* (*eumycetoma, chromoblastomycosis*).
  - *Sporotrichosis.*
- **Systemic Fungal Infections with Cutaneous Dissemination.** Occur most often with host defense defects. Primary lung infection disseminates hematogenously to multiple organ systems, including the skin: Cryptococcosis, histoplasmosis, North American blastomycosis, coccidioidomycosis, and penicilliosis.

SUPERFICIAL FUNGAL INFECTIONS ICD-10: B36

- **Superficial fungal infections** are the most common mucocutaneous infections, often caused by an imbalanced overgrowth of mucocutaneous microbiome.
- **Candida Species.** Require a warm humid environment.
- **Malassezia Species.** Require lipids for growth.
- **Dermatophytes.** Infect keratinized epithelium, hair follicles, and nail apparatus. *Trichosporon, Microsporum,* and *Epidermophyton* species.
- ***Hortaea werneckii.* Causes tinea nigra.**

CANDIDIASIS ICD-10: B37.0

- **Etiology.** Most commonly caused by the yeast *Candida albicans*. Less often by other *Candida* species.

CLINICAL MANIFESTATION

MUCOSAL CANDIDIASIS Otherwise healthy individuals: Oropharynx and genitalia. Host defense defects occur in the esophagus and tracheobronchial tree.

CUTANEOUS CANDIDIASIS Intertriginous and occluded skin.
DISSEMINATED CANDIDEMIA Host defense defects, especially neutropenia. Usually after invasion of the gastrointestinal (GI) tract.

EPIDEMIOLOGY AND ETIOLOGY

ETIOLOGY *C. albicans, C. tropicalis, C. parapsilosis, C. guilliermondi, Candida krusei, C. kefyr, C. zeylanoides, C. glabrata.*

ECOLOGY Candida spp. frequently colonize the GI tract and can be transmitted via the birth canal. Approximately 20% of healthy individuals are colonized. Antibiotic therapy increases the incidence of colonization.

Ten percent of women are colonized vaginally; antibiotic therapy, pregnancy, oral contraception, and intrauterine devices increase incidence. *C. albicans* may transiently be present on the skin and infection is usually endogenous. *Candida* balanitis may be transmitted from sexual partner. The young and old are more likely to be colonized.

HOST FACTORS Host defense defects, diabetes mellitus, and obesity; hyperhidrosis, warm climate, and maceration; polyendocrinopathies; glucocorticoids; chronic debilitation.

LABORATORY EXAMINATIONS

DIRECT MICROSCOPY KOH preparation visualizes pseudohyphae and yeast forms (Fig. 26-1).

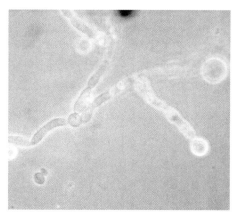

FIGURE 26-1 *Candida albicans:* **KOH preparation** Budding yeast forms and sausage-like pseudohyphal forms.

CULTURE Identifies species of *Candida*. However, the presence in the culture of *C. albicans* does not make the diagnosis of candidiasis. Sensitivities to antifungal agents can be performed on isolated cases of recurrent infection. Rule out bacterial secondary infection.

CUTANEOUS CANDIDIASIS

- Cutaneous candidiasis occurs in moist, occluded sites.
- Many patients have predisposing factors.

See Section 32 for candidiasis of the nail.

Clinical Manifestation

CANDIDAL INTERTRIGO Pruritus, tenderness, and pain. Initial pustules on erythematous base become eroded and confluent. Subsequently, fairly sharply demarcated, polycyclic, erythematous, eroded patches with small pustular lesions at the periphery (*satellite pustulosis*). Distribution: Inframammary or submammary axillae, groins (Figs. 26-2 or 26-3), perineal, and intergluteal cleft.

INTERDIGITAL Most common in obese elderly. Initial pustule becomes eroded, with formation of superficial erosion or fissure (Fig. 26-4). May be associated with *Candida* paronychia. *Distribution*: Webspace usually between third and fourth fingers (Fig. 26-4); feet: Maceration in webspace.

DIAPER DERMATITIS Irritability, discomfort with urination, defecation, and changing diapers. Beefy-red plaques with papular and pustular lesions; erosions, collarette-like scaling at the margins of lesions. *Distribution:* Genital and perianal skin, inner aspects of thighs and buttocks, involves intertriginous areas, unlike irritant dermatitis (Fig. 26-5).

OCCLUDED SKIN Under occlusive dressing, under cast, on back in hospitalized patient.

FOLLICULAR CANDIDIASIS Small, discrete pustules in ostia of hair follicles. Usually in occluded skin.

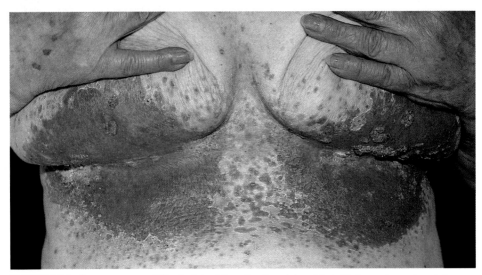

FIGURE 26-2 Cutaneous candidiasis: intertrigo Small peripheral "satellite" papules and pustules that have become confluent centrally, creating a large eroded area in the submammary region.

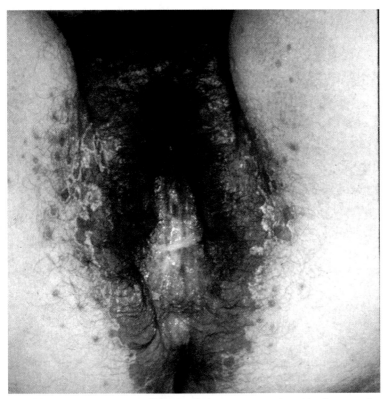

FIGURE 26-3 Cutaneous candidiasis: Erythematous papules with a few pustules and scaling, becoming confluent in the perigenital and perianal region.

FIGURE 26-4 Cutaneous candidiasis: interdigital intertrigo A 55-year-old female with sore and pruritic site in the webspace of the hand. Erosion with erythema and maceration is seen in the webspace between two fingers.

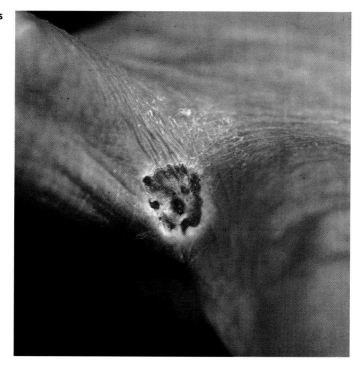

FIGURE 26-5 Candidiasis: diaper dermatitis Confluent erosions, marginal scaling, and "satellite pustules" in the area covered by a diaper in an infant. Atopic dermatitis or psoriasis also occurs in this distribution and may be concurrent.

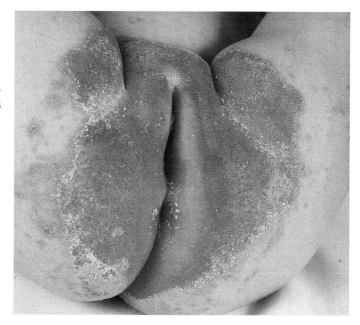

DIFFERENTIAL DIAGNOSIS

INTERTRIGO/OCCLUDED SKIN Intertriginous psoriasis, erythrasma, dermatophytosis, pityriasis versicolor, and streptococcal intertrigo.
DIAPER DERMATITIS Atopic dermatitis, psoriasis, irritant dermatitis, and seborrheic dermatitis.
FOLLICULITIS Bacterial (*Staphylococcus aureus, Pseudomonas aeruginosa*) folliculitis, *Pityrosporum* folliculitis, and acne.

DIAGNOSIS

Clinical findings confirmed by direct microscopy or culture.

TREATMENT

PREVENTION Keep intertriginous areas dry, wash with benzoyl peroxide bar, and use antifungal powder.
TOPICAL ANTIFUNGALS Nystatin, azole, or imidazole cream or powder.
ORAL ANTIFUNGALS Nystatin (suspension, tablet) eradicates bowel colonization. May be effective in recurrent cutaneous candidiasis.
SYSTEMIC ANTIFUNGAL AGENTS Fluconazole tablets, oral suspension, and IV infusion. Itraconazole capsules, oral solution; voriconazole; amphotericin B IV for severe disease.

OROPHARYNGEAL CANDIDIASIS ICD-10: B38.0

- Occurs with minor variations in host factors. Antibiotic therapy; glucocorticoid therapy (topical or systemic); age (very young, very old); host defense defects.

EPIDEMIOLOGY

INCIDENCE Often mucosal candidiasis occurs in otherwise healthy individuals. In advanced HIV disease, oropharyngeal candidiasis is common, relapses after treatment, and may be associated with esophageal and tracheobronchial candidiasis.

CLASSIFICATION OF MUCOSAL CANDIDIASIS

OROPHARYNGEAL CANDIDIASIS

- Pseudomembranous candidiasis or thrush.
- Erythematous or atrophic candidiasis.
- Candidal leukoplakia or hyperplastic candidiasis.
- Angular cheilitis.

ESOPHAGEAL AND TRACHEOBRONCHIAL CANDIDIASIS Occurs in states of severe host defense defects. AIDS-defining conditions.

CLINICAL MANIFESTATION

OROPHARYNGEAL CANDIDIASIS Often asymptomatic. Burning or pain on eating spices/acidic foods, diminished taste sensation. Cosmetic concern about white curds on tongue. Odynophagia. In HIV disease, this may be the initial presentation.

- *Pseudomembranous Candidiasis.* See Figures 26-6 through 26-8. White cottage cheese-like flecks (colonies of *Candida*) on any mucosal surface; vary in size from 1 to 2 mm to extensive and widespread. Removal with a dry gauze pad leaves an erythematous mucosal surface. *Distribution:* Dorsum of tongue, buccal mucosa, hard/soft palate, and pharynx extending down into the esophagus and tracheobronchial tree.
- *Erythematous or Atrophic Candidiasis.* Dorsum of the tongue is smooth, red, and atrophic (Fig. 26-8). Areas of thrush may also be present.
- *Candidal Leukoplakia.* White plaques that cannot be wiped off but regress with anticandidal therapy. Distribution: Buccal mucosa, tongue, and hard palate.
- *Angular Cheilitis.* Intertrigo at the angles of lips (Fig. 26-9). Erythema; slight erosion. White colonies of *Candida* in some cases. Can be associated with oropharyngeal colonization with *Candida*.

ESOPHAGEAL AND TRACHEOBRONCHIAL CANDIDIASIS Occurs in HIV disease when CD4+ cell count is low and is an AIDS-defining condition. Odynophagia, resulting in difficulty eating and malnutrition. Pseudomembranous lesions are seen on endoscopy.

INVASIVE DISSEMINATED CANDIDIASIS In individuals with severe prolonged neutropenia. Portal of entry of *Candida*: GI tract, invading submucosa, and blood vessels; intravascular catheter. Candidemia: hematogenous dissemination to skin and viscera. Disseminated red papules (Disseminated Candidiasis, p. 605)

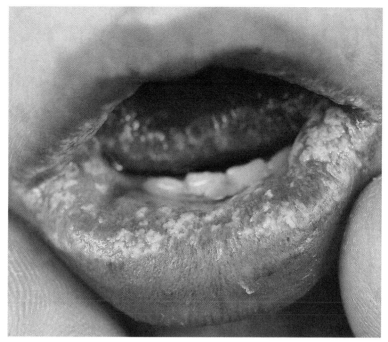

FIGURE 26-6 Oral candidiasis: thrush White curd-like material on the mucosal surface of the lower lip of a child; the material can be abraded with gauze (pseudo-membranous), revealing underlying erythema.

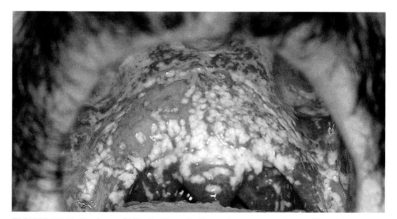

FIGURE 26-7 Oral candidiasis: thrush Extensive cottage cheese-like plaques, colonies of *Candida* that can be removed by rubbing with gauze (pseudomembra-nous), on the palate and uvula of an individual with advanced HIV/AIDS. Patches of erythema between the white plaques represent erythematous (atrophic) candidiasis. Involvement may extend into the esophagus and become associated with dysphagia.

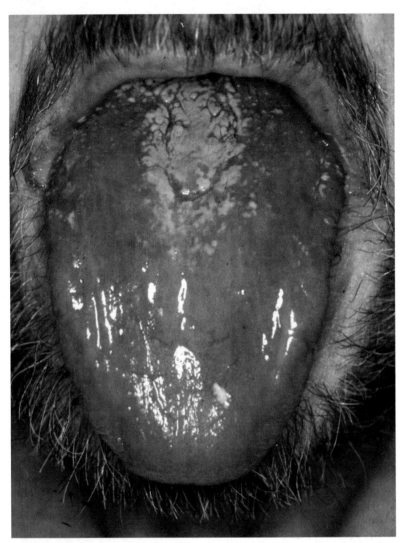

FIGURE 26-8 Oral candidiasis: atrophic and pseudomembranous A 48-year-old male with HIV disease. The surface of the tongue is shiny and red; posterior tongue has a white coating (thrush).

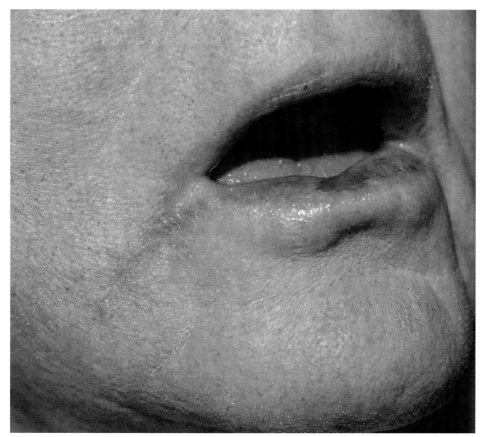

FIGURE 26-9 Angular cheilitis A 55-year-old male. The angle of the lips is moist and red. KOH preparation revealed candida pseudohyphae. Oral candidiasis was also present.

DIFFERENTIAL DIAGNOSIS

PSEUDOMEMBRANOUS CANDIDIASIS Oral hairy leukoplakia, condyloma acuminatum, geographic tongue, hairy tongue, lichen planus, and bite irritation.
ATROPHIC CANDIDIASIS Lichen planus, poor nutrition, and vitamin deficiency.

DIAGNOSIS

Clinical suspicion confirmed by KOH preparation of scraping from mucosal surface. Endoscopy to document esophageal and/or tracheobronchial candidiasis.

COURSE

Most cases respond to correction of the precipitating cause. Topical agents effective in most cases. Clinical resistance to antifungal agents may be related to patient noncompliance, severe immunocompromised, and drug–drug interaction (rifampin–fluconazole).

TREATMENT

TOPICAL THERAPY Nystatin or clotrimazole.
SYSTEMIC THERAPY Oral fluconazole and echinocandins (caspofungin, micafungin, or anidulafungin).

GENITAL CANDIDIASIS ICD-10: B37.3/B37.4

- Occurs on the nonkeratinized genital mucosa.
  - Vulva and vagina.
  - Preputial sac of the penis.
- Usually represents overgrowth of *Candida* in mucocutaneous microbiome.

EPIDEMIOLOGY

More than 20% of women have vaginal colonization by *Candida*. *C. albicans* accounts for 80 to 90% of genital isolates.

INCIDENCE Most vaginal candidiasis occurs in the healthy population. Seventy-five percent of women experience at least one episode; 40 to 45% experience two or more episodes. Often associated with vulvar candidiasis, i.e., vulvovaginal candidiasis.

RISK FACTORS Diabetes mellitus and HIV disease. Females: Often none, but pregnancy. Males: uncircumcised.

CLINICAL MANIFESTATION

VULVITIS/VULVOVAGINITIS Onset often abrupt, usually the week before menstruation. Symptoms may recur before each menstruation. Pruritus, vaginal discharge, vaginal soreness, vulvar burning, dyspareunia, and external dysuria.

Vulvitis. Erosions, edema, erythema (Fig. 26-10), swelling, and removable curd-like material. Pustule on lateral vulva and adjacent skin (see also Fig. 26-3).

Vulvovaginitis. Vaginal erythema and edema; white plaques that can be wiped off vaginal and/or cervical mucosa. May be associated with candidal intertrigo of inguinal folds and perineum. Subcorneal pustules at periphery with fringed, irregular margins. In chronic cases, vaginal mucosa glazed and atrophic.

Balanoposthitis, balanitis glans, and preputial sac: Papules, pustules, and erosions (Fig. 26-11). Maculopapular lesions with diffuse erythema. Edema, ulcerations, and fissuring of prepuce, usually in diabetic men; white plaques under foreskin.

DIFFERENTIAL DIAGNOSIS

VULVOVAGINAL CANDIDIASIS Trichomoniasis (caused by *T. vaginalis*), bacterial vaginosis (caused by replacement of normal vaginal flora by an overgrowth of anaerobic microorganisms and *Gardnerella vaginalis*), lichen planus, and lichen sclerosus et atrophicus.

BALANOPOSTHITIS Psoriasis, eczema, and lichen planus

DIAGNOSIS

Clinical suspicion confirmed by KOH preparation of scraping from mucosal surface.

TREATMENT

AZOLE CREAMS OR SUPPOSITORY Treat sexual partners and consider systemic therapy (as for mucocutaneous candidiasis, p. 598) if recurrent.

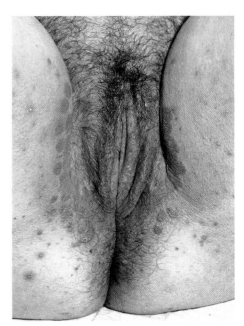

FIGURE 26-10 Candidiasis: vulvitis and intertrigo Psoriasiform, erythematous lesions becoming confluent on the vulva with erosions and satellite pustules on the thighs.

FIGURE 26-11 Candidiasis: balanoposthitis
A 52-year-old uncircumcised male. Erythema and a curd-like matter is seen on the glans penis and foreskin.

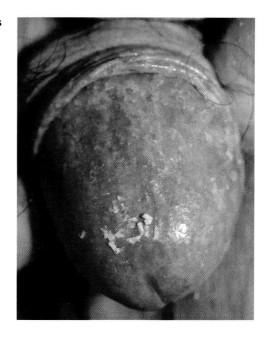

CHRONIC MUCOCUTANEOUS CANDIDIASIS ICD-10: B37.7

- Characterized by persistent or recurrent Candida infections of the oropharynx, skin, and nail apparatus.
- **Inheritance.** Usually autosomal recessive or sporadic.
- **Host Defense Defect.** Various specific and global defects in cell-mediated immunity.
- **Onset.** Usually in infancy or early childhood.

CLINICAL MANIFESTATION

OROPHARYNGEAL CANDIDIASIS Refractory to conventional therapy. Relapsing after successful therapy. Chronic infection results in hypertrophic (leukoplakic) candidiasis.

Cutaneous candidiasis manifests as:
Intertrigo Widespread infection (Figs. 26-12 and 26-13) of the face, trunk, and/or extremities. Lesions become hypertrophic in chronic untreated cases. Infection of the nail apparatus is universal: *Chronic paronychia; nail plate infection and dystrophy*; eventually total nail dystrophy.

Many patients also have *dermatophytosis* and cutaneous warts.

Six Types of Chronic Mucocutaneous Candidiasis

- Chronic oral candidiasis.
- Chronic candidiasis with endocrinopathy.
- Chronic candidiasis without endocrinopathy.
- Chronic localized mucocutaneous candidiasis.
- Chronic diffuse candidiasis.
- Chronic candidiasis with thymoma.

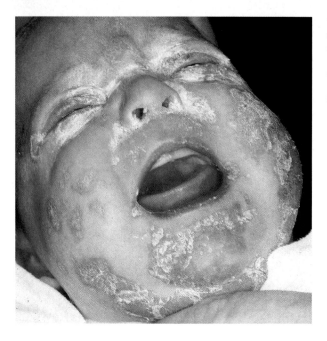

FIGURE 26-12 Mucocutaneous candidiasis Persistent candidiasis in an immunocompromised infant manifesting as erosions covered by scales and crusts, oropharyngeal candidiasis, and widespread infection of the trunk.

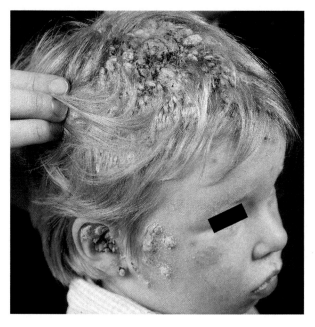

FIGURE 26-13 Mucocutaneous candidiasis A 3-year-old child with hypothyroidism had thrush, intertriginous candidiasis, warty hyperkeratoses, and crusts on the scalp and face; KOH preparation revealed candida colonies. There was also candidal onychomycosis.

DISSEMINATED CANDIDIASIS ICD-10: B37

- **Etiology.** *C. albicans, C. glabrata, C. parapsilosis,* and other non-*albicans* species.
- **Incidence.** Fourth most common cause of nosocomial bloodstream infections in the United States.
- **Risk Factors.** Neutropenia. Venous access catheters. Hospitalization.
- **Pathogenesis.** *Candida* enters the blood stream having colonized venous access catheters or penetrated the intestinal mucosa. Candidemia seeds the skin and internal organs, i.e., hepatosplenic candidiasis.

CLINICAL MANIFESTATION

CUTANEOUS LESIONS Small disseminated erythematous cutaneous papules (Fig. 26-14). Lesions may occur acutely or chronically. SYSTEMIC DISSEMINATION Eye with retinal changes. Liver, spleen, and CNS.

DIFFERENTIAL DIAGNOSIS

Malassezia folliculitis, which occurs on the trunk of healthy individuals.

DIAGNOSIS

Lesional biopsy specimen: *Candida* yeast forms are visualized in the dermis; *Candida* species isolated on culture.

COURSE

Candidemia has high associated morbidity and mortality.

TREATMENT

Echinocandins, fluconazole, and amphotericin B.

FIGURE 26-14 Invasive candidiasis with candidemia Multiple, erythematous papules on the hand of a febrile patient with granulocytopenia associated with treatment of acute myelogenous leukemia. The usual source of the infection is the gastrointestinal tract. *C. tropicalis* was isolated on blood culture; candidal forms were seen on lesional skin biopsy.

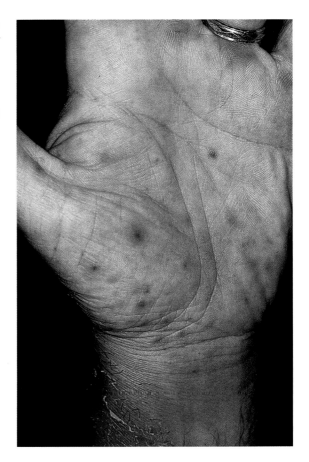

TINEA VERSICOLOR ICD-10: B36.0

- **Etiology.** Associated with the superficial overgrowth of *Malassezia furfur and M. globosa*. Lipophilic yeast that normally resides in the keratin of skin (Fig. 26-15) and hair follicles of individuals at puberty and beyond. Also implicated in the pathogenesis of seborrheic dermatitis *Malassezia* folliculitis. *Malassezia* infections are not contagious; *o*vergrowth of resident cutaneous flora (cutaneous microbiome) occurs under certain favorable conditions.
- **Clinical Findings.** Chronic. Well-demarcated patches with fine scale. Variable pigmentation: Hypo- and hyperpigmented; pink. Most commonly on the trunk.
- **Demography.** Young adults. Less common when sebum production is reduced or absent; tapers off during fifth and sixth decades.
- **Predisposing Factors.** *Sweating*. Warm season or climates; tropical climate. Hyperhidrosis; aerobic exercise. Oily skin. Temperate zones: More common in the summertime; 2% prevalence in temperate climates; up to 50% in tropics. Application of lipids such as cocoa butter.
- **Pathogenesis.** *Malassezia* changes from a yeast to hyphal form under the influence of predisposing factors. Produces dicarboxylic acid, which inhibits tyrosinase in epidermal melanocytes and leads to hypomelanosis

CLINICAL MANIFESTATION

Usually asymptomatic. Cosmetic concerns about dyspigmentation. Lesions present for months or years.

Macules, sharply marginated (Figs. 26-16 to 26-19) round or oval in shape, varying in size. Fine scaling is best appreciated by gently abrading lesions. Treated or resolved lesions lack scale. Some patients have findings of *Malassezia* folliculitis and seborrheic dermatitis.

Color. In nontanned skin, lesions are *light brown* (Fig. 26-18) or pink. On tanned skin, *hypopigmented* (Fig. 26-19). In brown- or black-skinned persons, *dark brown macules* (Fig. 26-20). Brown of varying intensities and hues (Fig. 26-18). In time, individual lesions may enlarge and merge, forming extensive *geographic areas*.

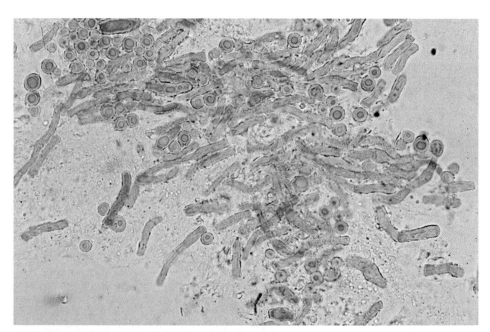

FIGURE 26-15 *Malassezia furfur:* **KOH preparation** Round yeast and elongated pseudohyphal forms, so-called "spaghetti and meatballs."

FIGURE 26-16 Pityriasis versicolor A 39-year-old white female with orange-tan lesions of the neck and upper chest. Sharply marginated scaling macules.

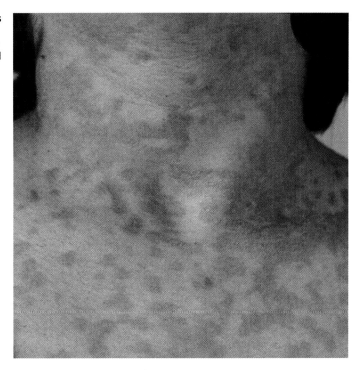

FIGURE 26-17 Pityriasis versicolor: groin A 23-year-old obese male with discoloration of the entire chest, axillae, abdomen and groin for 1 year. Sharply marginated brown confluent macules with fine scaling, KOH preparation showed "spaghetti and meat balls."

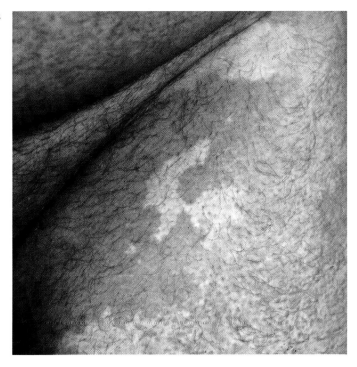

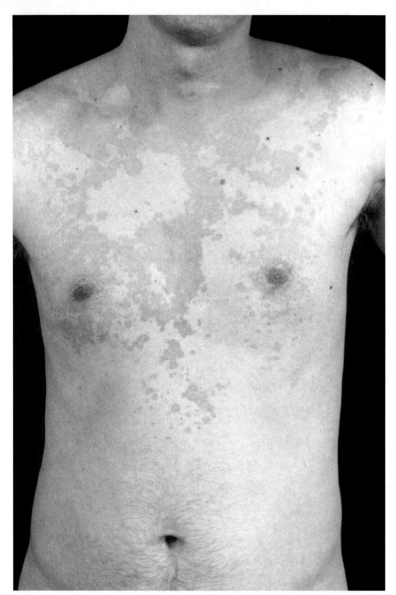

FIGURE 26-18 Pityriasis versicolor: chest, neck, and shoulders A 22-year-old
male with pigmented patches on chest and neck for several years. Multiple pink to
tan, well-demarcated scaling macules becoming confluent on the neck, chest, flank,
and arm.

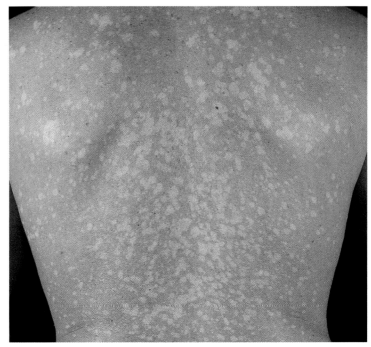

FIGURE 26-19 Pityriasis versicolor: back Multiple, small-to-medium-sized, well-demarcated hypopigmented macules on the back of a tanned individual with white skin.

Distribution. Upper trunk, upper arms, neck, abdomen, axillae, groins, thighs, genitalia. Facial, neck, or scalp lesions occur in persons applying creams or ointments, or topical gluco-corticoid preparations.

DIFFERENTIAL DIAGNOSIS

HYPOPIGMENTED MACULES Vitiligo, pityriasis alba, postinflammatory hypopigmentation.
SCALING LESIONS Tinea corporis, seborrheic dermatitis, and cutaneous T cell lymphoma.

LABORATORY EXAMINATIONS

DIRECT MICROSCOPIC EXAMINATION OF SCALES PREPARED WITH KOH Filamentous hyphae and globose yeast forms, termed *spaghetti and meatballs* are seen (Fig. 26-15).
WOOD'S LAMP Blue-green fluorescence of scales; may be negative in individuals who have showered recently because the fluorescent chemical is water soluble. Vitiligo appears as depigmented, white, and has no scale.

DERMATOPATHOLOGY Budding yeast and hyphal forms in the most superficial layers of the stratum corneum, seen best with periodic acid–Schiff (PAS) stain. Variable hyperkeratosis, psoriasiform hyperplasia, and chronic inflammation with blood vessel dilatation.

DIAGNOSIS

Clinical findings confirmed by positive KOH preparation findings.

COURSE

Infection persists for years if predisposing conditions persist. Dyspigmentation persists for months after infection has been eradicated.

TREATMENT

Topitcal agents. Selenium sulfide (2.5%) lotion or shampoo. Ketoconazole shampoo. Azole creams (ketoconazole, econazole, micronazole, or clotrimazole). Terbinafine 1% solution.

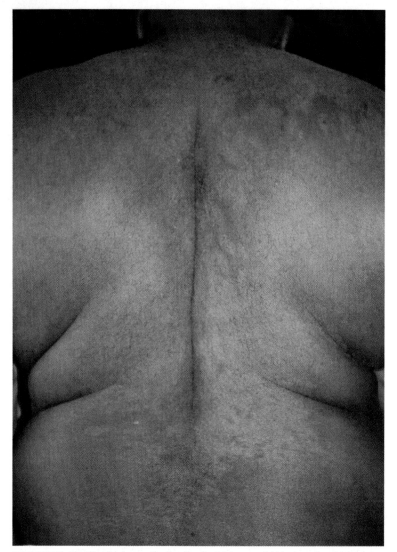

FIGURE 26-20 Pityriasis versicolor: back A 28-year-old black male with hyper-pigmented scaling patches on his torso. He had been applying olive oil to his skin.

Systemic therapy *Fluconazole* 300 mg weekly × 3 weeks. *Itraconazole* 400 mg (single dose).

Secondary prophylaxis. Topical agents weekly or systemic agents monthly.

MALASSEZIA FOLLICULITIS More common in subtropical and tropical climates. Pruritic, monomorphic eruption characterized by

follicular papules and pustules on the trunk, most often on the back (Fig. 26-21), upper arms, and less often on the neck and face; excoriated papules. Absence of comedones differentiates it from acne vulgaris). *Synonym:* Pityrosporum folliculitis.

SEBORRHEIC DERMATITIS See "Seborrheic Dermatitis," in Section 2.

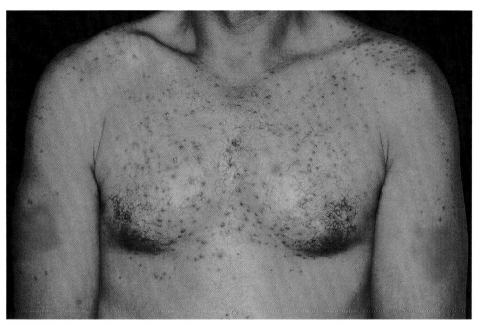

FIGURE 26-21 Infectious folliculitis: *Malassezia furfur* A 41-year-old Hispanic male with multiple, discrete, and follicular papulopustules on the chest.

TRICHOSPORON INFECTIONS

- **Etiology.** *Trichosporon* species of yeasts. Soil inhabitants. Microbiome of skin and GI tracts.
- **Treatment.** Topical or systemic azoles, liposomal amphotericin B.

CLINICAL MANIFESTATION

PIEDRA Asymptomatic superficial fungal biofilm/colonization on the *hair shaft*. Incidence is high in tropical regions with high temperature and humidity.

- *White piedra.* White to beige nodules on hair shaft; soft; easily removed. Pubic, axillary, beard, and eyebrow or eyelash hair.

- *Black piedra.* Darkly pigmented, firmly attached nodules (up to a few millimeters) on the hair shaft; weakens hair shaft with hair breakage. Scalp hair.

DISSEMINATED TRICHOSPORONOSIS Emerging opportunistic infection. Associated with neutropenia. Dissemination occurs to the skin (erythematous or purpuric tender papules), lungs, kidneys, and spleen. Similar to disseminated candidiasis.

TINEA NIGRA ICD-10: B36.1

- Superficial fungal colonization of the stratum corneum.
- **Etiology.** *Hortaea werneckii*, a dematiaceous or pigmented fungus.
- **Epidemiology.** More common in tropical climates. Transmitted by direct inoculation onto the skin from contact with decaying vegetation, wood, or soil seems to be the mode of acquisition.
- **Clinical Manifestation.** Brown to black macule(s) with well-defined borders (**Fig. 26-22**) that resemble silver nitrate stains. *Distribution:* Palm: tinea nigra palmaris. Sole: tinea nigra plantaris.
- **Diagnosis.** Direct microscopy, visualizing abundant branching septate hyphae.
- **Management.** Topical azole or alcohol gel sanitizer.

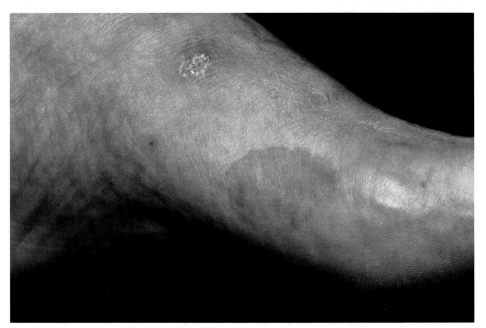

FIGURE 26-22 Tinea nigra Uniformly tan macule on the plantar foot, present for several years. KOH preparation showed hyphae.

DERMATOPHYTOSES ICD-10: B35.0-B36

- **Dermatophytes** are a unique group of fungi capable of infecting nonviable keratinized cutaneous structures including stratum corneum, nails, and hair. Arthrospores can survive in human scales for 12 months. Dermatophytosis denotes an infection caused by dermatophytes.
- **Clinical Infection by Structure Involved.** Epidermal dermatophytosis. Dermatophytosis of hair and hair follicles. *Onychomycosis or tinea unguium*: Dermatophytosis of the nail apparatus.
- **Pathogenesis** of dermatophytosis leading to different clinical manifestations is schematically depicted in Figures 26-23 and 26-24.
- The term *tinea* is best used for dermatophytoses and is modified according to the anatomic site of infection, e.g., tinea pedis.
- "Tinea" versicolor is referred to as *pityriasis versicolor* except in the United States; it is not a dermatophytosis but rather an infection caused by the yeast *Malassezia* (see p. 606).
- Tinea nigra is caused by a pigmented or dematiaceous fungus, not a dermatophyte (see p. 612).

EPIDEMIOLOGY AND ETIOLOGY

ETIOLOGY Three genera of dermatophytes ("skin plants"): *Trichophyton, Microsporum,* and *Epidermophyton.* More than 40 species are currently recognized; approximately 10 spp. are common causes of human infection.

- *Trichophyton rubrum* is the most common cause of epidermal dermatophytosis and onychomycosis in industrialized nations. Currently, 70% of the United States population experiences at least one episode of tinea pedis.

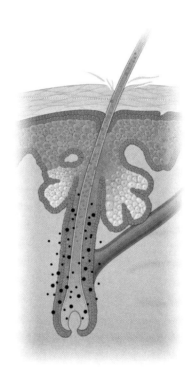

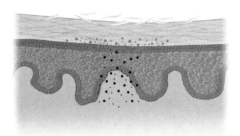

FIGURE 26-23 Epidermal dermatophyte infections Dermatophytes (green dots and lines) within the stratum corneum disrupt the horny layer and thus lead to scaling; also elicit an inflammatory response (black dots symbolize inflammatory cells), which may then manifest as erythema, papulation, and vesiculation.

FIGURE 26-24 Hair follicle dermatophyte infections Hair shaft is involved (green dots) resulting in the destruction and breaking off of the hair. If the dermatophyte infection extends farther down into the hair follicle, it will elicit a deeper inflammatory response (black dots) and this manifest as deeper inflammatory nodules, follicular pustulation, and abscess formation.

AGE OF ONSET Children have scalp infections (*Trichophyton, Microsporum*). Young and older adults have intertriginous infections. The incidence of onychomycosis is correlated directly with age; in the United States, up to 50% of individuals over 70 years have onychomycosis.

GEOGRAPHY Some species have a worldwide distribution; others are restricted to particular continents or regions. *T. concentricum,* the cause of tinea imbricata, is endemic to the South Pacific, India, and Central America.

TRANSMISSION Dermatophyte infections can be acquired from three sources:

■ Most commonly from another person [usually by fomites, less so by direct skin-to-skin contact (tinea gladiatorum)].
■ From animals such as dogs or cats.
■ Least commonly from soil.

CLASSIFICATION OF DERMATOPHYTES Based on their ecology, dermatophytes classified:

■ *Anthropophilic*: Person-to-person transmission by fomites and by direct contact.
■ *Zoophilic*: Animal-to-human by direct contact or by fomites.
■ *Geophilic*: Environmental.

PREDISPOSING FACTORS *Atopic diathesis*: Cell-mediated immune deficiency for *T. rubrum*. *Topical immunosuppression* by application of glucocorticoids: Tinea incognito. *Systemic immunocompromised*: Patients have a higher incidence and more intractable dermatophytoses; follicular abscesses and granulomas may occur (Majocchi granuloma).

CLASSIFICATION

In vivo, dermatophytes grow only on or within keratinized structures and as such involve the following:

■ Epidermal dermatophytosis. Tinea facialis, tinea corporis, tinea cruris, tinea manus, and tinea pedis.
■ Dermatophytoses of nail apparatus. Tinea unguium (toenails and fingernails). Onychomycosis (more inclusive term, including nail infections caused by dermatophytes, yeasts, and molds).
■ Dermatophytoses of hair and hair follicle. Dermatophytic folliculitis, Majocchi granuloma, tinea capitis, and tinea barbae.

PATHOGENESIS

Dermatophytes synthesize keratinases that digest keratin and sustain existence of fungi in keratinized structures. Cell-mediated immunity and antimicrobial activity of polymorphonuclear leukocytes restrict dermatophyte pathogenicity. *Host factors that facilitate dermatophyte infections*: Atopy, topical and systemic glucocorticoids, ichthyosis, and collagen vascular disease. *Local factors favoring dermatophyte infection*: Sweating, occlusion, and occupational exposure, geographic location, high humidity (tropical or semitropical climates). The clinical presentation of dermatophytoses depends on several factors: Site of infection, immunologic response of the host, and species of fungus. Dermatophytes (e.g., *T. rubrum*) that initiate little inflammatory response are better able to establish chronic infection. Organisms such as *Microsporum canis* cause an acute infection associated with a brisk inflammatory response and spontaneous resolution. In some individuals, infection can involve the dermis, as in kerion and Majocchi granuloma.

LABORATORY EXAMINATIONS

Direct Microscopy

See Figure. 26-25.

SAMPLING

■ *Skin*: Collect scale with a no. 15 scalpel blade, edge of a glass microscope slide, and brush (tooth or cervical brush). Scales are placed on the center of the microscope slide, swept into a small pile, and covered with a coverslip. Recent application of cream/ointment or powder often makes identification of fungal element difficult or impossible.
■ *Nails*: Keratinaceous debris is collected with a no. 15 scalpel blade or small curette. Distal lateral subungual onychomycosis (DLSO): Debride from the undersurface of the nail of most proximally involved site or nail bed; avoid nail plate. Superficial white onychomycosis: Superficial nail plate. Proximal subungual onychomycosis (PSO): Undersurface of proximal nail plate; obtain sample by using a small punch biopsy tool, boring through involved nail plate to undersurface; obtain keratin from undersurface of the involved nail plate.

FIGURE 26-25 Dermatophytes: KOH preparation Multiple, septated, tubelike structures (hyphae or mycelia) and spore formation in scales from an individual with tinea pedis.

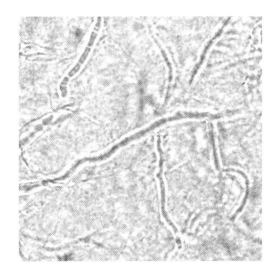

- *Hair*: Remove hairs, preferably broken, with a needle holder or forceps. Place on microscope slide and cover with glass coverslip. Skin scales from involved hairy site can be obtained with a brush (tooth or cervical).

Preparation of sample potassium hydroxide 5 to 20% solution is applied at the edge of the coverslip. Capillary action draws solution under the coverslip. The preparation is gently heated with a match or lighter until bubbles begin to expand, clarifying the preparation. Excess KOH solution is blotted out. Condenser should be "racked down." Epidermal dermatophytosis: Positive unless patient has been effectively treated. 90% of cases positive. Variations in KOH with fungal stains: Swartz–Lamkin stain and chlorazol black E stain.

Microscopy Dermatophytes are recognized as septated, tubelike structures (hyphae or mycelia; Fig. 26-25).

Wood's lamp examination: Hairs infected with *Microsporum* spp. fluoresce blue-green.

FUNGAL CULTURES Specimens collected from scaling skin lesions, hair, and nails into fungal culture plate or specimen container. Culture on Sabouraud's glucose medium.

Dermatopathology DLSO. PAS or methenamine silver stains are more sensitive than KOH preparation or fungal culture in identification of fungal elements in DLSO.

TREATMENT

Topical agents for epidermal dermatophytoses: Imidazoles (clotrimazole, miconazole, ketoconazole, econazole, oxiconazole, sulconazole, or sertaconazole); allylamines (naftifine, terbinafine); naphthionates (tolnaftate); substituted pyridine (ciclopirox olamine).

Systemic Antifungal Agents

- Terbinafine 250-mg tablet. Allylamine. Most effective oral antidermatophyte antifungal; low efficacy against other fungi. Approved for onychomycosis in the United States.
- Itraconazole 100-mg capsules; oral solution (10 mg/mL): Intravenous. Triazole. Needs acid gastric pH for dissolution of capsule. Raises levels of digoxin and cyclosporine. Approved for onychomycosis in the United States.
- Fluconazole 100-, 150-, 200-mg tablets; oral suspension (10 or 40 mg/mL); 400 mg IV.

Dermatophytoses of Epidermis

Epidermal dermatophytoses are the most common dermatophytic infection. May be associated with dermatophytic infection of hair or hair follicles and/or the nail apparatus. *Synonym*: Ringworm.

TINEA PEDIS ICD-10: B35.3

- Dermatophytic infection of the feet.
- **Clinical Findings.** Erythema, scaling, maceration, and/or bulla formation. Infections at other sites such as tinea cruris usually associate initial tinea pedis.
- **Course.** Provides breaks in the integrity of the epidermis through which bacteria such as *S. aureus* or group A streptococcus (GAS) can invade, causing skin or soft-tissue infection.
- **Synonyms.** Athlete's foot. Jungle rot.

EPIDEMIOLOGY

AGE OF ONSET Late childhood or young adult life. Most common, 20 to 50 years.
PREDISPOSING FACTORS Hot, humid climate; occlusive footwear; hyperhidrosis.

CLINICAL MANIFESTATION

Duration: Months to years to lifetime. Often, prior history of tinea pedis, and tinea unguium of toenails. Usually asymptomatic. Pruritus. Pain with secondary bacterial infection (Fig. 25-26).
INTERDIGITAL TYPE Two patterns: dry scaling (Fig. 26-27); maceration, scaling, fissuring of toe webs (Fig. 26-28). Hyperhidrosis common. Most common site: Between fourth and fifth toes. Infection may spread to adjacent areas of feet.

MOCCASIN TYPE Well-demarcated scaling with erythema with minute papules on margin, fine white scaling, and hyperkeratosis (Figs. 26-29 and 26-30) (confined to heels, soles, or lateral borders of feet). *Distribution*: Sole, involving area covered by a *ballet slipper*. One or both feet may be involved with any pattern; bilateral involvement more common.
INFLAMMATORY/BULLOUS TYPE Vesicles or bullae filled with clear fluid (Fig. 26-31). Pus usually indicates secondary bacterial infection. After rupturing, erosions with ragged ringlike border. May be associated with "id" reaction (autosensitization or dermatophytid). *Distribution*: Sole, instep, and webspaces.
ULCERATIVE TYPE Extension of interdigital tinea pedis onto plantar and lateral foot. May be secondarily by *S. aureus*.

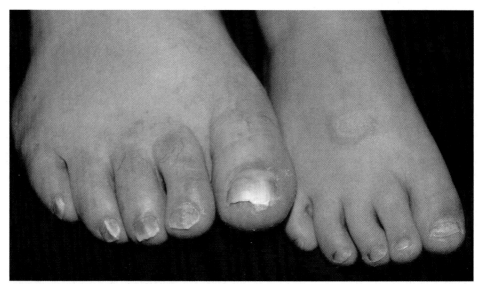

FIGURE 26-26 Tinea pedis and onychomycosis in father and son The foot of a 5-year-old male with tinea pedis (ringworm lesion) and toenail dystrophy shown with his father's foot with similar, but more advanced findings. The son most likely became infected with dermatophyte from fomite in his home. Both father and son had atopic diathesis with history of atopic dermatitis.

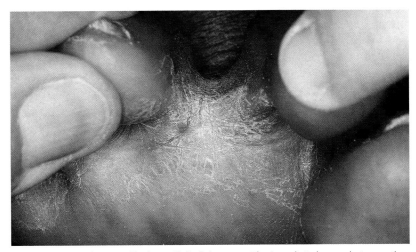

FIGURE 26-27 Tinea pedis: interdigital dry type The interdigital space between the toes shows erythema and scaling; the toenail is thickened, indicative of associated distal subungual onychomycosis.

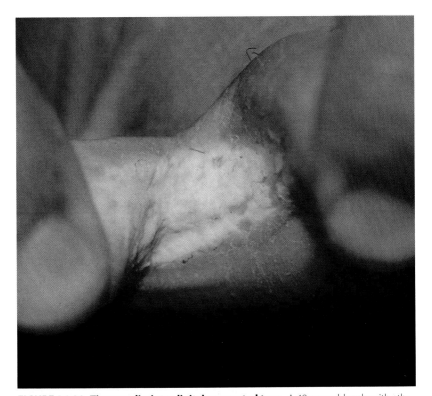

FIGURE 26-28 Tinea pedis: interdigital macerated type A 48-year-old male with athlete's foot and hyperhidrosis for years. The skin of the webspace between the fourth and fifth toes is hyperkeratotic and macerated (hydration of the stratum corneum). The KOH+ preparation shows septated hyphae, confirming the diagnosis of dermatophytosis. Wood's lamp demonstrated coral-red fluorescence confirming concomitant erythrasma. *P. aeruginosa* was isolated on bacterial culture. This explains the greenish discoloration of the macerated lesion.

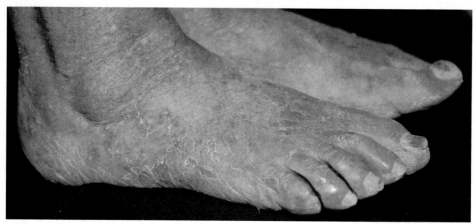

FIGURE 26-29 Tinea pedis: moccasin type A 65-year-old female with scaling feet for years. Sharply marginated erythema of the foot with a mild keratoderma associated with distal/lateral subungual onychomycosis, typical of *T. rubrum* infection.

DIFFERENTIAL DIAGNOSIS

INTERDIGITAL TYPE Erythrasma and pitted keratolysis.
MOCCASIN TYPE Psoriasis, eczematous dermatitis (dyshidrotic, atopic, allergic contact), and pitted keratolysis.

Inflammatory/bullous type. Bullous impetigo, allergic contact dermatitis, dyshidrotic eczema, and bullous disease.

LABORATORY EXAMINATIONS

Direct Microscopy (Fig. 26-25). In bullous type, examine scraping from the inner aspect of bulla roof for detection of hyphae.
WOOD'S LAMP Negative fluorescence usually rules out erythrasma in interdigital infection. Erythrasma and interdigital tinea pedis may coexist.
CULTURE Dermatophytes can be isolated in 11% of normal-appearing interspaces and

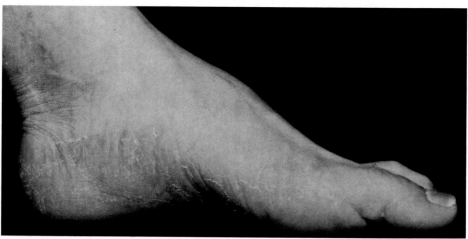

FIGURE 26-30 Tinea pedis: moccasin type A 63-year-old male with scaling feet for years. Sharply marginated erythema of the medial foot with a mild keratoderma. Tinea corporis was also present on the forearms and dorsum of hands.

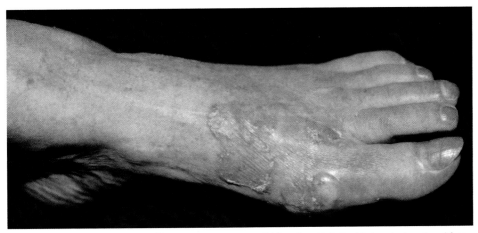

FIGURE 26-31 Tinea pedis: bullous types A 34-year-old female with itchy blisters on her dorsal foot.

31% of macerated toe webs. *Candida* spp. may be copathogens in webspaces. In individuals with macerated interdigital space, *S. aureus, P. aeruginosa,* and diphtheroids are commonly isolated. *S. aureus* causes secondary infection.

DIAGNOSIS

Demonstration of hyphae on direct microscopy, isolation of dermatophyte on culture.

COURSE

Tends to be chronic. May provide portal of entry for soft-tissue infections, especially in patient's venous stasis. Without secondary prophylaxis, recurrence is the rule.

TREATMENT

See, p. 615, this Section.

TINEA MANUUM CD-10: B35.2

- Chronic dermatophytosis of the hand(s).
- Often unilateral, most commonly on the dominant hand.
- Usually associated with tinea pedis.

CLINICAL MANIFESTATION

Frequently symptomatic. Pruritus. *Dyshidrotic type*: Episodic symptoms of pruritus.

Well-demarcated scaling patches, hyperkeratosis, and fissures on palmar hand (Fig. 26-32). Borders well demarcated; central clearing. May extend onto dorsum of hand with follicular papules, nodules, and pustules with dermatophytic folliculitis. *Dyshidrotic type*: Papules, vesicles, bullae (uncommon on the margin of lesion) on palms and lateral fingers, and similar to lesions of bullous tinea pedis. *Secondary changes*: Lichen simplex chronicus, prurigo nodules, secondary *S. aureus* infection. *Distribution: Diffuse* hyperkeratosis of the palms with pronounced involvement of palmar creases or patchy scaling on the dorsa and sides of fingers; 50% of patients have unilateral involvement. Usually associated with tinea pedis (Fig. 26-32) and tinea cruris. If chronic, often associated with tinea unguium of fingernails and toenails (Fig. 26-33).

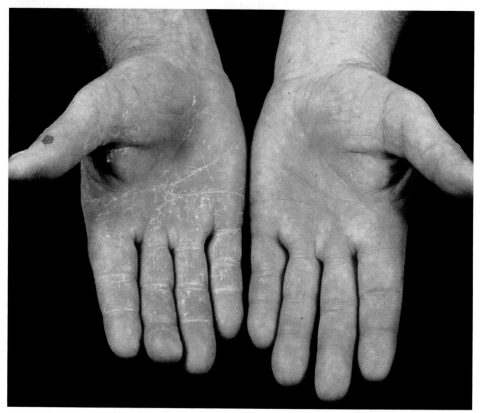

FIGURE 26-32 Tinea manuum Erythema and scaling of the right hand, which was associated with bilateral tinea pedis; the "one-hand, two-feet" distribution is typical of epidermal dermatophytosis of the hands and feet. In time, distal/lateral subungual onychomycosis occurs on the fingernails (see Fig. 26-33).

DIFFERENTIAL DIAGNOSIS

Atopic dermatitis, lichen simplex chronicus, allergic contact dermatitis, irritant contact dermatitis, and psoriasis vulgaris.

COURSE

Chronic, does not resolve spontaneously. After treatment, recurs unless onychomycosis of fingernails, feet, and toenails is eradicated. Fissures and erosions provide portal of entry for bacterial infections.

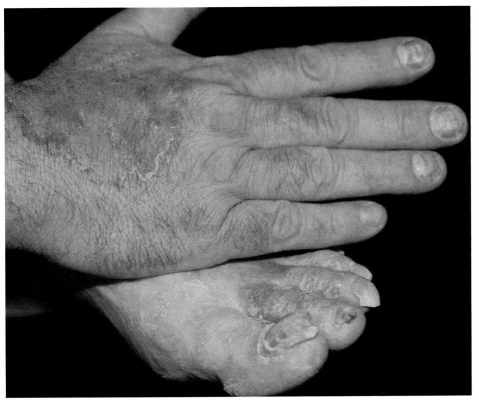

FIGURE 26-33 Tinea manuum, tinea pedis, and onychomycosis A 57-year-old male immunosuppressed renal transplant recipient with extensive epidermal dermatophytosis of hands, feet, and nail. The feet are initially infected; infection spreads to hands, arms, and nails.

TREATMENT

Must eradicate tinea unguium of fingernails as well as toenails; also tinea pedis and tinea cruris, otherwise, tinea manuum will recur.

Oral agents eradicate dermatophytoses of hands, feet, and nails: *Terbinafine*: 250 mg daily for 14 days. *Itraconazole*: 200 mg daily for 7 days. *Fluconazole*: 150 to 200 mg daily for 2 to 4 weeks. *Note*: Eradication of fingernail onychomycosis requires longer use.

TINEA CRURIS ICD-10: B35.6

■ Subacute or chronic dermatophytosis of the upper thigh and adjacent inguinal and pubic regions. Usually associated with tinea pedis, the source of the infection.

CLINICAL MANIFESTATION

Months to years duration. Often, history of long-standing tinea pedis and prior history of tinea cruris.

Large, scaling, well-demarcated dull red/tan/brown plaques (Fig. 26-34). Central clearing. Papules, pustules may be present at margins: Dermatophytic folliculitis. Treated lesions: lack scale; postinflammatory hyperpigmentation in darker-skinned persons. In atopics, chronic scratching may produce secondary changes of lichen simplex chronicus. *Distribution.* Groins and thighs; may extend to buttocks

(Figs. 26-34 to 26-36). Scrotum and penis are rarely involved.

DIFFERENTIAL DIAGNOSIS

Erythrasma, *Candida* intertrigo, intertriginous psoriasis, tinea, or pityriasis versicolor.

TREATMENT

PREVENTION After eradication minimize reinfection with shower shoes and antifungal powders.
ANTIFUNGAL AGENTS See p. 615.

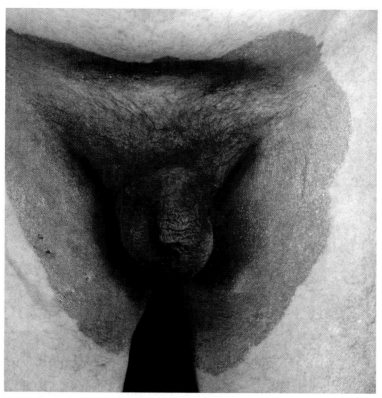

FIGURE 26-34 Tinea cruris (inguinalis): acute A 65-year-old male with pruritic inguinal red rash for several weeks. He was being treated with prednisone for poly-arthritis. KOH preparation revealed a thick network of hyphae.

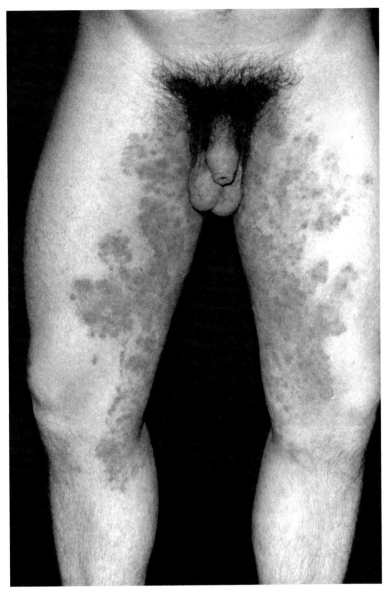

FIGURE 26-35 Tinea cruris (inguinalis): subacute A 24-year-old male with pruritic inguinal rash that spread to thighs down to popliteal regions for several months. He was a college wrestler. Concomitant dermatophyte infection was also present on the feet and trunk, and face. He was treated with oral terbinafine.

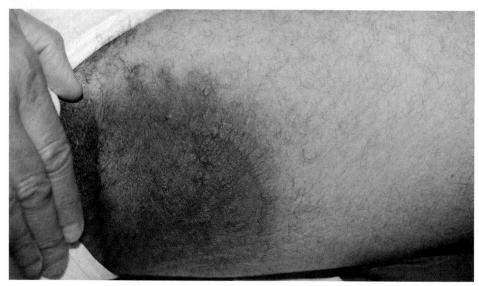

FIGURE 26-36 Tinea cruris (inguinalis): chronic A 65-year-old male with pruritic inguinal rash for many months. The skin of the proximal thigh is lichenified from chronic rubbing and scratching. He had applied topical corticosteroid to the site. He also had tinea pedis and onychomycosis.

TINEA CORPORIS ICD-10: B35.4

- **Dermatophyte.** Infections of the trunk, legs, arms, and/or neck, *excluding* the feet, hands, and groin.
- **Etiology.** Most commonly caused by *T. rubrum*. Also *T. tonsurans, M. canis*

CLINICAL MANIFESTATION

Scaling, sharply marginated plaques. Peripheral enlargement and central clearing (Figs. 26-37 through 26-40) produce annular configuration with concentric rings or arcuate lesions; fusion of lesions produces gyrate patterns. Single and occasionally scattered multiple lesions.

Psoriasiform plaques. Lesions of zoophilic infection (contracted from animals) are more inflammatory, with marked vesicles, pustules, crusting at margins. Papules, nodules, pustules: Dermatophytic folliculitis, i.e., Majocchi granuloma (see Fig. 26-41).

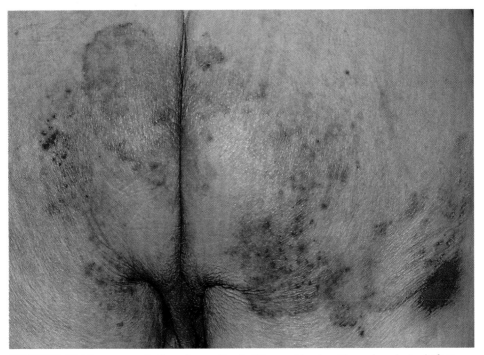

FIGURE 26-37 Tinea corporis: tinea incognito An 80-year-old male with a rash on buttocks for 1 year. Erythematous patches on the buttocks, some with sharp margination, others with clearing, and excoriations. He had been treating the pruritus with topical corticosteroid. Tinea cruris, tinea pedis, and onychomycosis were also present.

DIFFERENTIAL DIAGNOSIS

Allergic contact dermatitis, atopic dermatitis, annular erythemas, psoriasis, seborrheic dermatitis, pityriasis rosea, pityriasis alba, tinea versicolor, erythema migrans, subacute lupus erythematosus, and cutaneous T cell lymphoma.

DIAGNOSIS

See "Direct Microscopy (Fig. 26-25)," and culture.

TREATMENT

See p. 615.

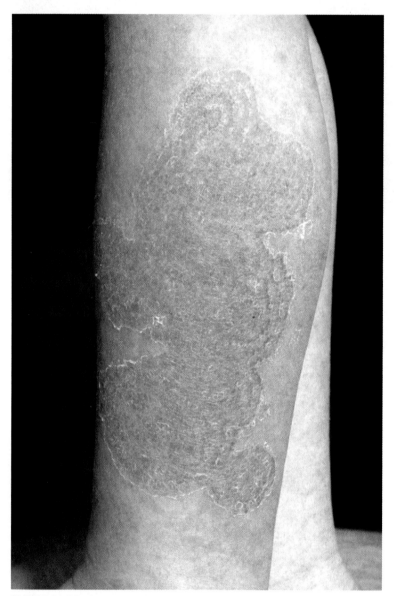

FIGURE 26-38 Tinea corporis A 13-year-old girl with red, scaling lesions on the lower leg. Lesions are sharply marginated, multicentric, and scaly. Corticosteroid has been applied to the site for pruritus.

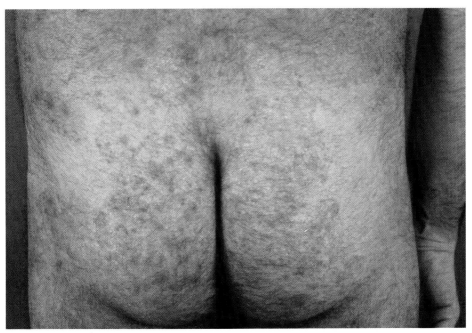

FIGURE 26-39 Tinea corporis Annular scaly erythematous patches on the buttocks, upper thighs, and abdomen. KOH preparation showed septated hyphae.

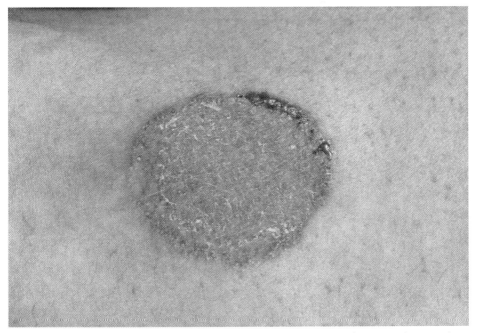

FIGURE 26-40 Tinea corporis: inflammatory A 13-year-old female with inflammatory lesion on the arm for 1 week. Other siblings were also affected. Acutely inflamed edematous exudative annular plaque with vesiculation at the margins on the lower arm. Similar lesions were present on the trunk. The children had been playing with guinea pigs which were infected.

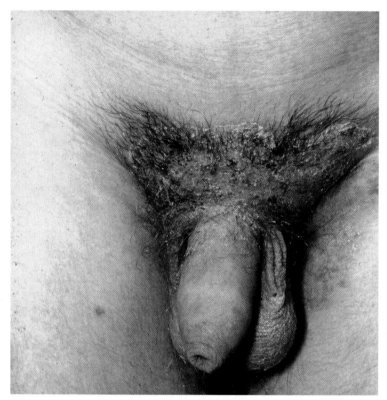

FIGURE 26-41 Dermatophytic folliculitis: *Trichophyton rubrum* Trichophyton rubrum A 31-year-old male with a pruritic rash in the pubic region for 1 year; topical glucocorticoids had not been effective. Multiple follicular papules, scaling erythema and pustules are seen in the pubic area and groins; tinea pedis was also present. KOH preparation showed septated hyphae. The lesions resolved with oral terbinafine.

TINEA FACIALIS

- Dermatophytosis of the glabrous facial skin. Well-circumscribed erythematous patch. More commonly misdiagnosed than any other dermatophytosis.
- *Synonym*: Tinea faciei.
- **Etiology.** *T. tonsurans* in America. *T. mentagrophytes*, *T. rubrum* in Europe and Asia.

CLINICAL MANIFESTATION

Well-circumscribed macule to plaque of variable size; elevated border and central regression (Figs. 26-42 and 26-43). Scaling is often minimal. Pink to red; in black patients, hyperpigmentation. Any area of face but usually not symmetric.

DIFFERENTIAL DIAGNOSIS

Seborrheic dermatitis, contact dermatitis, erythema migrans, lupus erythematosus, polymorphous light eruption, phototoxic drug eruption, and lymphocytic infiltrate.

DIAGNOSIS

See "Direct Microscopy," and culture.

TREATMENT

See p. 615.

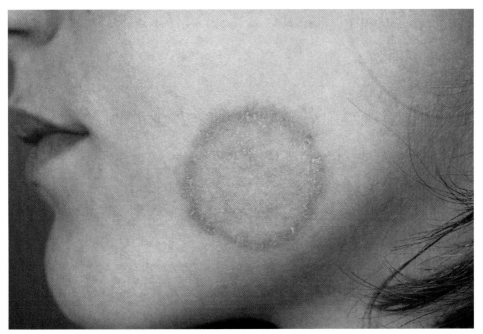

FIGURE 26-42 Tinea facialis A 12-year-old girl with inflammatory lesion in the mandibular area. Papules are dermatophytic folliculitis of vellus hairs. Note sharp margination. The site has previously been treated with hydrocortisone cream.

FIGURE 26-43 Tinea facialis A 83-year-old immunosuppressed male with a history of prednisone treatment for polymyalgia rheumatica and chronic lymphatic leukemia. Note the well-demarcated erythema and scaling in the beard area. SCC in situ is also present on the left eyebrow.

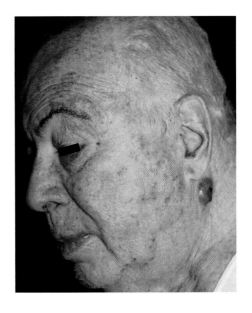

TINEA INCOGNITO

- Epidermal dermatophytosis, often associated with dermatophytic folliculitis.
- Occurs after the topical application of a glucocorticoid preparation to a site colonized or infected by dermatophyte.

CLINICAL MANIFESTATION

Variably inflamed patches. Occurs when an inflammatory dermatophytosis is mistaken for psoriasis or an eczematous dermatitis (Figs. 26-35 to 26-39 and 26-43). Involved sites often have exaggerated features of epidermal dermatophytoses, being a deep red or violaceous. Scaling is often not apparent. Papules or pustule within involved sites is *dermatophytic folliculitis. Epidermal atrophy* caused by chronic glucocorticoid application may be present.

TREATMENT

Systemic antifungal therapy may be indicated caused by deep involvement of the hair apparatus.

DERMATOPHYTOSES OF HAIR

- Dermatophytes are capable of invading hair follicles and hair shafts causing:
    - Tinea capitis.
    - Tinea barbae.
    - Dermatophytic folliculitis.
    - Majocchi granuloma.
- Two types of hair involvement are seen (see Fig. 26-44).

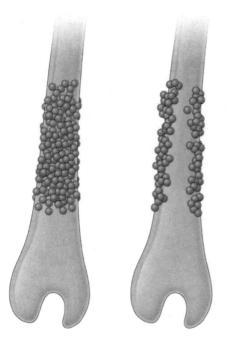

FIGURE 26-44 Dermatophytic folliculitis
Ectothrix type: mycelia and arthroconidia are seen on the surface of the hair follicle (extrapilary, right). Endothrix type: hyphae and arthroconidia occur within the hair shaft (intrapilary, left).

TINEA CAPITIS ICD-10: B35.0

- Dermatophytic trichomycosis of the scalp, predominantly in preadolescent children.
- Clinical presentations vary widely:
  - Noninflammatory scaling.
  - Scaling and broken-off hairs.
  - Severe, painful inflammation with painful, boggy nodules that drain pus (kerion) and result in scarring alopecia.
- *Synonyms*: Ringworm of the scalp, tinea tonsurans.

EPIDEMIOLOGY AND ETIOLOGY

Toddlers and school-age children (6 to 10 years of age) are most commonly affected. Much more common in blacks than in whites in the United States. Etiology varies from country to country and from region to region. Species change in time resulting from immigration. Infections can become epidemic in schools and institutions, especially with overcrowding. United States: Random fungal cultures in urban study detected a 4% infection rate and a 12.7% colonization rate among black children.

- *North and Central America.* 90% of cases of tinea capitis caused by *T. tonsurans*. Less commonly, *M. canis.*
- *Europe: M audouinii, M canis, T violaceum.*
- *Asia: T violaceum* and *M canis.*
- *Africa: T. violaceum, T schoenleinii,* and *M canis.*

TRANSMISSION Person-to-person, animal-to-person, via fomites. Spores are present on asymptomatic carriers, animals, or inanimate objects.
PATHOGENESIS Scalp hair traps fungi from the environment or fomites. Asymptomatic colonization is common. Trauma assists inoculation. Dermatophytes initially invade stratum corneum of scalp, which may be followed by hair shaft infection. Spread to other hair follicles then occurs.

CLASSIFICATION

- Ectothrix infection. Occurs outside the hair shaft. Hyphae fragment into arthroconidia, leading to cuticle destruction. Caused by *Microsporum* spp. (*M. audouinii* and *M. canis*) (Fig. 26-44).
- Endothrix infection. Occurs within the hair shaft without cuticle destruction (Fig. 26-44). Arthroconidia found within the hair shaft. Caused by *Trichophyton* spp. (*T. tonsurans* in North America; *T. violaceum* in Europe, Asia, parts of Africa).

- *"Black dot" tinea capitis.* Variant of endothrix resembling seborrheic dermatitis.
- *Kerion.* Variant of endothrix with boggy inflammatory plaques.
- *Favus.* Variant of endothrix with arthroconidia and airspaces within hair shaft. Very uncommon in Western Europe and North America. However, in some parts of the world (Middle East and South Africa) it is still endemic.

CLINICAL MANIFESTATION

NONINFLAMMATORY INFECTION Scaling. Diffuse or circumscribed alopecia. Occipital or posterior auricular adenopathy.

"Gray patch" tinea capitis (Fig. 26-45). Partial alopecia, often circular in shape, showing numerous broken-off hairs, and dull gray from their coating of arthrospores. Fine scaling with fairly sharp margin. Hair shaft becomes brittle, breaking off at or slightly above scalp. Small patches coalesce, forming larger patches. Inflammatory response minimal, but massive scaling. Several or many patches, randomly arranged, may be present. *Microsporum* species may show green fluorescence with Wood's lamp. Differential *diagnosis*: Seborrheic dermatitis, psoriasis, atopic dermatitis, lichen simplex chronicus, and alopecia areata.
"BLACK DOT" TINEA CAPITIS Broken-off hairs near the scalp give the appearance of "dots" (Fig. 26-46) (swollen hair shafts) in dark-haired patients. Dots occur as affected hair breaks at surface of scalp. Tends to be diffuse and poorly circumscribed. Low-grade folliculitis may be present. Resembles seborrheic dermatitis. Usually caused by *T. tonsurans, T. violaceum*. *Differential diagnosis*: Seborrheic dermatitis, psoriasis, atopic dermatitis, lichen simplex chronicus, chronic cutaneous lupus erythematosus, and alopecia areata.
KERION Inflammatory mass in which remaining hairs are loose. Characterized by boggy, purulent, inflamed nodules, and plaques

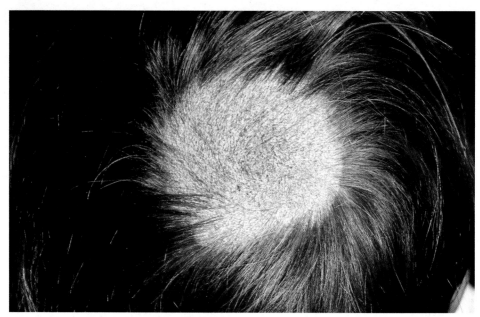

FIGURE 26-45 Tinea capitis: "gray patch" type A large, round, hyperkeratotic plaque of alopecia caused by breaking off of hair shafts close to the surface, giving the appearance of a mowed wheat field on the scalp of a child. Remaining hair shafts and scales exhibit a green fluorescence when examined with Wood's lamp. *M. canis* was isolated on culture.

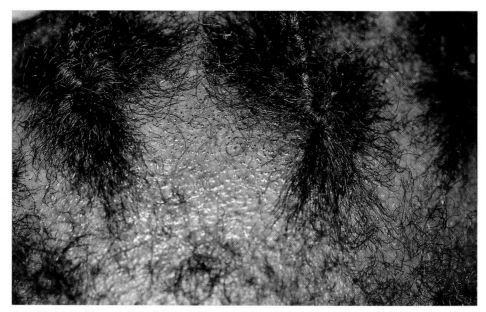

FIGURE 26-46 Tinea capitis: "black dot" variant A subtle, asymptomatic patch of alopecia resulting from breaking off of hairs on the frontal scalp in a 4-year-old black child. The lesion was detected because her infant sister presented with tinea corporis. *T. tonsurans* was isolated on culture.

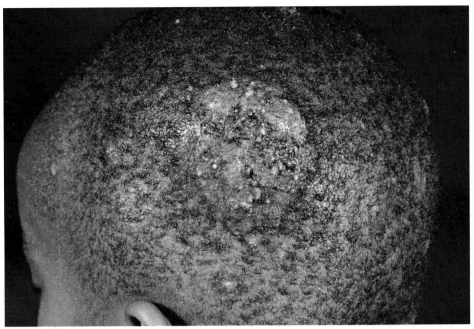

FIGURE 26-47 Kerion A 5-year-old black boy with an inflammatory very painful mass on the scalp unresponsive to oral antibiotics. The boggy swelling with multiple pustules and postauricular lymphadenopathy. *T. tonsurans* was isolated on fungal culture. He was successfully treated with oral terbinafine for 4 weeks. (Used with permission from Laura Proudfoot, PhD and Rachael Morris-Jones, PhD. See also Proudfoot LE, Morris-Jones R. Kerion celsi. *N Engl J Med.* 2012;366:1142.)

(Fig. 26-47). Usually painful; drains pus from multiple openings, like honeycomb. Hairs do not break off but fall out and can be pulled without pain. Follicles may discharge pus; sinus formation; mycetoma-like grains. Thick crusting with matting of adjacent hairs. A single plaque is usual, but multiple lesions may occur with involvement of the entire scalp. Frequently, associated lymphadenopathy is present. Usually caused by zoophilic (*T. verrucosum, T. mentagrophytes* var. *mentagrophytes*) or geophilic species. Heals with scarring alopecia.

FAVUS Latin for honeycomb. Early cases show perifollicular erythema and matting of hair. Later, thick yellow adherent crusts (scutula) composed of skin debris and hyphae that are pierced by remaining hair shafts (Fig. 26-48). Fetid odor. Shows little tendency to clear spontaneously. Often results in scarring alopecia. *Differential diagnosis:* Impetigo, ecthyma, and crusted scabies.

LABORATORY EXAMINATIONS

WOOD'S LAMP *T. tonsurans* does not fluoresce. *M. canis* fluoresces blue-green.
DIRECT MICROSCOPY Skin scales contain hyphae and arthrospores. *Ectothrix*: arthrospores can be seen surrounding the hair shaft in the cuticle. *Endothrix*: Spores within hair shaft. *Favus*: Loose chains of arthrospores and airspaces in hair shaft.
FUNGAL CULTURE Growth of dermatophytes usually seen in 10 to 14 days.
BACTERIAL CULTURE Rule out bacterial infection, usually *S. aureus* or GAS.

COURSE AND TREATMENT

Chronic untreated kerion and favus, especially if secondarily infected with *S. aureus*, result in scarring alopecia. Regrowth of hair is the rule if treated with systemic antifungal agents (see p. 615).

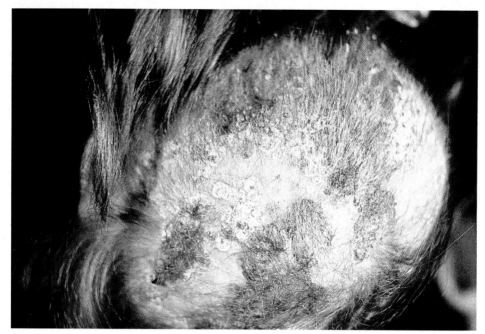

FIGURE 26-48   Tinea capitis: favus Extensive hair loss with atrophy, scarring, and so-called scutula, i.e., yellowish adherent crusts present on the scalp; remaining hairs pierce the scutula. *T. schoenleinii* was isolated on culture.

TINEA BARBAE ICD-10: B35.0

■ Dermatophytic folliculitis involving the androgen-sensitive beard and moustache areas. Resembles tinea capitis, with invasion of the hair shaft.

ETIOLOGY

T. verrucosum, T. mentagrophytes var. *mentagrophytes*, most commonly. May be acquired through animal exposure. *T. rubrum* is an uncommon cause, but occurs.

CLINICAL MANIFESTATION

Pustular folliculitis (Fig. 26-49), i.e., hair follicles surrounded by red inflammatory papules, pustules, nodules, or plaques. Involved hairs are loose and easily removed. With less follicular involvement, there are scaling, circular, reddish patches (tinea facialis) in which hair is broken off at the surface. Papules may coalesce to inflammatory plaques topped by pustules.

Kerion: Boggy purulent nodules and plaques as with tinea capitis (Fig. 26-50). Beard and moustache areas, rarely, eyelashes, and eyebrows.

Regional lymphadenopathy, especially if of long duration and if superinfected.

DIFFERENTIAL DIAGNOSIS

S. aureus folliculitis, furuncle, carbuncle, acne vulgaris, rosacea, and pseudofolliculitis.

LABORATORY EXAMINATIONS KOH preparation and culture.

TREATMENT

Topical agents ineffective. Systemic antifungal therapy required (see p. 615).

FIGURE 26-49 Tinea barbae A 63-year-old male with pustules in beard area for several months. A large pustule in an inflammatory nodule is seen on the moustache area. Extensive subtle tinea facialis was also present. Tinea pedis, onychomycosis, and tinea cruris were present as well. KOH preparation was positive; *T. rubrum* was detected on dermatophyte culture. Bacterial culture was negative for pathogens. Facial lesions resolved with oral terbinafine.

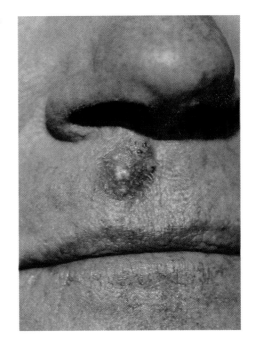

FIGURE 26-50 Tinea barbae with kerion and tinea facialis Confluent, painful papules, nodules, and pustules on the upper lip (kerion). Epidermal dermatophytosis (tinea facialis) with sharply marginated erythema and scaling is present on the cheeks, eyelids, eyebrows, and forehead. *T. mentagrophytes* was isolated on culture. In this case, the organism caused two distinct clinical patterns (epidermal involvement, tinea facialis versus follicular inflammation, tinea barbae), depending on whether glabrous skin or hairy skin was infected.

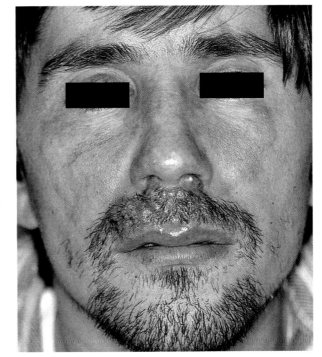

MAJOCCHI GRANULOMA

- Dermatophytic folliculitis with foreign-body granuloma occurring in response to keratin in dermis and immune reaction to dermatophyte.
- **Etiology.** Most commonly *T. rubrum, T. tonsurans*
- **Risk Factors.** Topical glucocorticoid application. Host defense defects

CLINICAL MANIFESTATION

Follicular type with local immunosuppression (topical glucocorticoid use).

Subcutaneous nodular type with systemic immunocompromised (Fig. 26-51). Solitary or multiple.

- Folliculocentric papules and pustules arise within an area of epidermal dermatophytosis such as tinea incognito (Fig. 26-41).

DISTRIBUTION Any hair-bearing area; the scalp, face, forearms (Fig. 26-52), dorsum of hands or feet, and shaved legs.

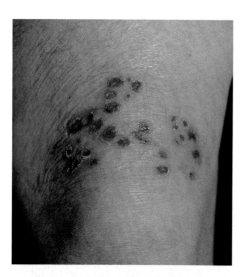

FIGURE 26-51 Majocchi granuloma A 55-year-old diabetic male renal transplant recipient with painful nodules on left lower thigh. Eroded papules with crusting above the knee. Tinea pedis and onychomycosis were also present. *T. rubrum* was isolated on dermatophyte culture. He was treated with voriconazole.

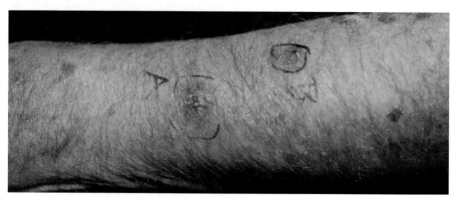

FIGURE 26-52 Majocchi granuloma An 87-year-old male with two nodules on the L-forearm for 6 weeks. Initial impression was cutaneous malignancies. Diagnosis of Majocchi granuloma was made on lesional biopsy. Systemic terbinafine was given.

INVASIVE AND DISSEMINATED FUNGAL INFECTIONS

SUBCUTANEOUS MYCOSES ICD-10: B48.8

- A heterogeneous group of fungal infections that develop at the sites of transcutaneous trauma.
- Sporotrichosis.
- Phaeohyphomycoses:
  - Eumycetoma.
  - Chromoblastomycosis.
- Etiology. Fungi resident on plants or in soil.
  - Melanin-producing (dematiaceous or pigmented): brown to black.
  - Nonpigmented (hyaline).
- Clinical Manifestations. Slowly enlarging plaques with verrucous lesions, fistulae, sinuses, and scarring, most commonly on lower extremity; can occur at any site of inoculation.
- Host Defense Defect. Infections more extensive. Can disseminate.
- Diagnosis. Clinical findings, demonstration of grains or Medlar bodies on dermatopathology, culture of organism.

SPOROTRICHOSIS ICD-10: B42

- Etiology. *Sporothrix schenckii.* Infection follows accidental inoculation of skin.
- Clinical Manifestations.
  - Nodule or plaque at inoculation site infection.
  - Lymphangitis. Chronic nodular lymphangitis (sporotrichoid lymphocutaneous syndrome).
  - Subcutaneous swelling occurs proximal to inoculation site.
- Disseminated infection can occur from skin or pulmonary infection with host defense defects.

ETIOLOGY AND EPIDEMIOLOGY

ETIOLOGY S. schenckii, a thermally dimorphic fungus. Lives as a saprophyte on plants. Worldwide distribution. More common in temperate and tropical zones.

DEMOGRAPHY Occupational exposure important: Agricultural and forest workers, gardeners, farmers, lawn laborers, florists, paper manufacturers, and gold miners.

TRANSMISSION Cutaneous puncture or small abrasion. Rarely transmitted from cats; armadillos.

PATHOGENESIS After subcutaneous inoculation, S. schenckii grows locally and can extend proximally to *nodular lymphangitis*.

CLINICAL MANIFESTATION

Incubation period ranges from, 3 days to 12 weeks after trauma or injury to site of lesion. Lesions are painless. Afebrile.

FIXED CUTANEOUS (PLAQUE) SPOROTRICHOSIS Dermal papule, pustule, or nodule appears at inoculation site several weeks after injury. May enlarge to verrucous plaque or ulcer with induration. Draining lymph nodes become inflamed and enlarged (chancriform syndrome). *Distribution:* Primary lesion most common on dorsum of hand or finger. Fixed plaque: Face in children; upper extremities in adults.

NODULAR LYMPHANGITIS Follows proximal lymphatic extension from inoculation site. *Distribution:* Inoculation nodule on the hand/fingers with nodular lymphangiitis extending proximally the on arms (Figs. 26-53 and 26-54).

DISSEMINATED SPOROTRICHOSIS From pulmonary sporotrichosis, disseminates hematogenously to skin, as well as joints, eyes, and meninges.

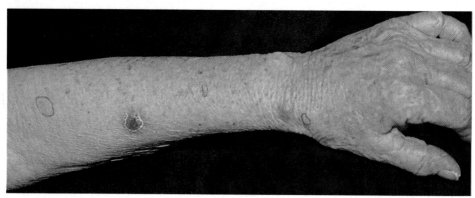

FIGURE 26-53 Sporotrichosis: nodular lymphangitic type A 78-year-old gardener with tender nodules on hand and arm for 4 weeks. Erythematous nodules in a linear array in lymphatic channels on the dorsum of the hand and forearm. *S. schenckii* was isolated on a culture of a lesional biopsy specimen.

DIFFERENTIAL DIAGNOSIS

NODULAR LYMPHANGITIS *Mycobacterium marinum, Nocardia brasiliensis, Leishmania brasiliensis.*
CHANCRIFORM SYNDROME Syphilis, nocardiosis, cutaneous tularemia, and cutaneous anthrax.

DIAGNOSIS

Clinical suspicion and isolation of organism on culture.

COURSE

Shows little tendency to resolve spontaneously. Responds well to therapy; may relapse.

TREATMENT

Itraconazole is the preferred treatment for cutaneous and lymphocutaneous sporotrichosis. Saturated potassium iodide solution has been used for cutaneous lesions.

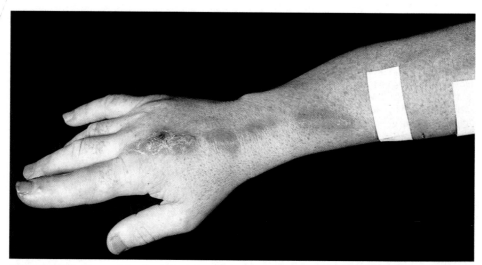

FIGURE 26-54 Sporotrichosis: chronic lymphangitic type An erythematous papule at the site of inoculation on the index finger with a linear arrangement of erythematous dermal and subcutaneous nodules extending proximally in lymphatic vessels of the dorsum of the hand and arm.

PHAEOHYPHOMYCOSES ICD-10 B47

Chronic skin and soft tissue infections caused by pigmented and hyaline nonpigmented molds: *eumycetoma* and *chromoblastomycosis*. Follows traumatic inoculation, most often on the foot.

ETIOLOGY AND EPIDEMIOLOGY

ETIOLOGIC AGENTS Opportunistic pathogens. Residents in soil or on plants.
Nocardiosis (actinomycotic mycetomas). Caused by *Nocardia. Phaeohyphomycoses.* Caused by fungi.

- Eumycetomas: *Madurella* (pigmented or dematiaceous) species most common. Organisms produce melanin. *Scedosporium* species (nonpigmented or hyaline) molds.
- Chromoblastomycosis: *Fonsecaea* and *Cladophialophora* species are most common.

TRANSMISSION Cutaneous inoculation of organism: Thorn prick, wood splinter, and stone cut, contaminated with soil or plant debris.

DEMOGRAPHY Occur in tropical and subtropical areas; most common in male rural laborers. Most occur on lower legs also hands, arms. Risk factor: poverty.

CLINICAL MANIFESTATIONS

EUMYCETOMA Characterized by swelling, development of sinus tracts and fistulae, draining pus with grains (colonies of fungi discharged from the sinus tract). Tissue becomes greatly distorted (Fig. 26-55). Central clearing gives older lesions an annular shape. *Distribution:* Unilateral on the leg, foot, and hand. *Complications:* Regional lymphadenopathy; bacterial secondary infections; extension into fascia, muscle, bone; loss of function and disfigurement.

CHROMOBLASTOMYCOSIS Smaller lesions coalesce to form nodular, verrucous, or plaque-like lesions (Fig. 26-56). Gradually enlarge into contiguous skin and soft tissue. Infection can also spread along lymphatics and by autoinoculation. *Complications:* Bacterial superinfection; chronic edema, elephantiasis; squamous cell carcinoma (Marjolin ulcer); hematogenous dissemination.

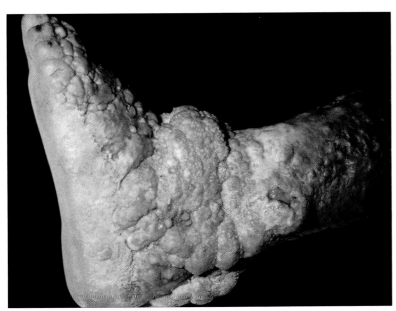

FIGURE 26-55 Eumycetoma The foot, ankle, and leg are grossly distorted with edema and confluent subcutaneous nodules, cauliflower-like tumors, and ulcerations.

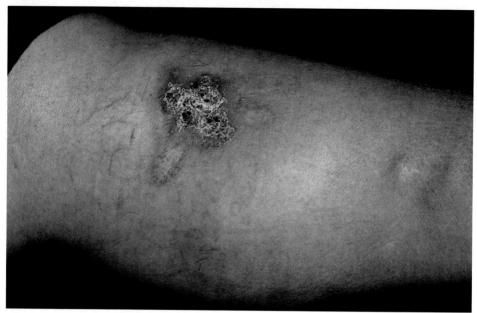

FIGURE 26-56 Chromoblastomycosis Hyperkeratotic and crusted plaque with old scars on the leg had been present for several decades.

Chromoblastomycosis, tumoral form. Chronic disease led to elephantiasis and involvement of the entire lower limb.

DIAGNOSIS

Isolation of mold in culture, CT scan, and echosonography define the extent of involvement. X-ray of bone shows multiple osteolytic lesions (cavities).
EUMYCETOMA Lesion with swelling, sinus tracts, and grains. Rule out nocardiosis.
CHROMOBLASTOMYCOSIS Medlar bodies (sclerotic cells or 'copper pennies'): thick-walled pigmented septated fungal hyphal forms, resembling large yeasts seen in lesional scraping (KOH), and/or biopsy specimen; isolation of organism on culture.

DIFFERENTIAL DIAGNOSIS

Sporotrichosis, blastomycosis, nontuberculous cutaneous mycobacterial infection, foreign body granuloma, pyoderma gangrenosum, and squamous cell carcinoma.

TREATMENT

Involves both surgical extirpation of lesions and administration of systemic antifungal agents such as itraconazole. Most effective earlier in course. Pigmented fungi may be more resistant to medication than hyaline species.

Systemic Fungal Infections with Dissemination to Skin

Systemic fungal infections with cutaneous dissemination occur most often with host defense defects.

Primary or reactivated fungal lung infection can disseminate hematogenously to multiple organ systems, including the skin.

GI tract or intravascular catheter can be the source of candidemia and disseminated candidiasis. See disseminated candidiasis (see page 605).

CRYPTOCOCCOSIS ICD-10: B45.0

■ Cryptococcosis. Primary pulmonary infection. With host defense defects, hematogenous dissemination to meninges and skin.

ETIOLOGY AND EPIDEMIOLOGY

Cryptococcus neoformans. Yeast found in soil and dried bird droppings. Worldwide, ubiquitous. Polysaccharide capsule is major virulence factor; basis for antigen testing.

INCIDENCE Globally, cryptococcosis (usually meningitis) is the most common invasive mycosis in HIV disease, occurring in up to 9% of persons with advanced untreated HIV disease in the United States and up to 30% in Africa.

PATHOGENESIS Primary pulmonary focus of infection may remain localized or disseminate. Reactivation of latent infection in the immunocompromised host may result in hematogenous dissemination to meninges, kidneys, and skin; 10 to 15% of patients have skin lesions.

CLINICAL MANIFESTATIONS

CUTANEOUS LESIONS Usually asymptomatic. CNS: Headache (80%) and mental confusion. **PAPULE(S) OR NODULE(S)** With surrounding erythema. Lesion may break down and exude mucinous fluid. In HIV disease, lesions occur most commonly on face/scalp. *Molluscum contagiosum-like lesions* occur in HIV disease (Fig. 26-57). *Acneiform. Cryptococcal cellulitis* mimics bacterial cellulitis, i.e., red, hot, tender, and edematous plaque on extremity; possibly multiple noncontiguous sites.

ORAL MUCOSA Nodules/ulcers.

FIGURE 26-57 Cryptococcosis: disseminated Multiple, skin-colored papules and nodules on the face in a person with advanced HIV disease. *Cryptococcus* disseminated hematogenously from pulmonary infection to skin and meninges. The lesions resemble molluscum contagiosum, which is common in HIV disease. (Used with permission from Loïc Vallant, MD.)

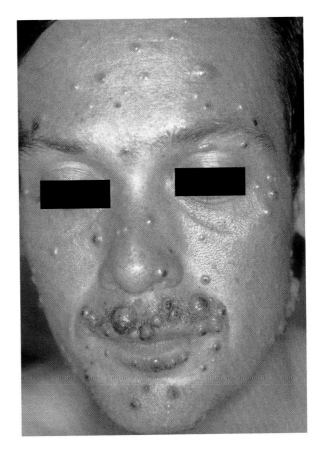

DIFFERENTIAL DIAGNOSIS

Molluscum contagiosum, disseminated histoplasmosis, acne, and sarcoidosis.

DIAGNOSIS

Confirmed by skin biopsy and fungal cultures.

COURSE

In HIV disease in the absence of immune reconstitution, cryptococcal meningitis relapses in 30% of cases after amphotericin B therapy (plus or minus flucytosine); lifelong secondary prophylaxis with fluconazole 200 mg/day reduces relapse rate to 4 to 8%.

TREATMENT

PRIMARY PROPHYLAXIS In some centers, fluconazole is given to HIV/AIDS-infected individuals with low CD4+ cell counts; the incidence of disseminated infection is reduced, but there is no effect on the mortality rate.

THERAPY OF MENINGITIS Amphotericin B (plus or minus flucytosine) for 2 to 6 weeks depending on severity. In uncomplicated cases and for 6 weeks in complicated cases.

INFECTION LIMITED TO SKIN Fluconazole, 400 to 600 mg daily. Itraconazole, 400 mg daily.

SECONDARY PROPHYLAXIS In HIV disease (without immune reconstitution), lifelong secondary prophylaxis is given with fluconazole, 200 to 400 mg daily or itraconazole 200 to 400 mg/daily.

HISTOPLASMOSIS ICD-10: B39

ETIOLOGY AND EPIDEMIOLOGY

ETIOLOGY *Histoplasma capsulatum* var. *capsulatum,* an unencapsulated dimorphic fungus. In Africa, *H. capsulatum* var. *duboisii.*

DEMOGRAPHY Endemic areas: Ohio/Mississippi River valleys. Equatorial Africa. Caribbean Islands.

TRANSMISSION Inhalation of microconidia in soil contaminated with bird or bat droppings. Acute pulmonary outbreaks may occur from occupational or recreational exposure.

PATHOGENESIS In HIV disease, can present as either primary histoplasmosis or reactivation of latent infection.

CLINICAL MANIFESTATION

PRIMARY PULMONARY INFECTION Accompanied or followed by hypersensitivity reactions: erythema nodosum and erythema multiforme.

CUTANEOUS INFECTION Hematogenous dissemination occurs with host defense defects. Papules or nodules (Fig. 26-58A); erythematous, necrotic, or hyperkeratotic. These can ulcerate spontaenously (Fig. 26-58B). Other morphologies: Guttate psoriasis-like papulosquamous lesions, pustules, and acneiform papules; chronic ulcers; vegetative plaques; panniculitis. Diffuse infiltration of skin (Fig. 26-59). Erythroderma. Diffuse hyperpigmentation with Addison disease secondary to adrenal infection.

OROPHARYNGEAL LESIONS Nodules, vegetations, painful ulcerations of soft palate, oropharynx, and epiglottis. Nasal vestibule.

DISSEMINATED DISEASE Hepatosplenomegaly, lymphadenopathy, and meningitis.

DIFFERENTIAL DIAGNOSIS

Miliary tuberculosis, disseminated coccidioidomycosis or cryptococcosis, leishmaniasis, and lymphoma.

DIAGNOSIS

Clinical suspicion, confirmed by culture.

COURSE

Prognosis linked to underlying condition, e.g., HIV disease.

TREATMENT

PREVENTION Protective clothing when working in areas contaminated with bird/bat droppings.

SYSTEMIC ANTIMYCOTIC THERAPY *Life-threatening and meningeal infection:* IV amphotericin B, followed by itraconazole for at least a year. *Non-life-threating infection:* Oral fluconazole 800 mg daily for 12 weeks. Oral itraconazole, 400 mg twice daily for 12 weeks. Documented maculopathy should be treated with the addition of steroids.

SECONDARY PROPHYLAXIS In HIV disease without immune restoration itraconazole, 200 mg daily or fluconazole, 400 mg daily.

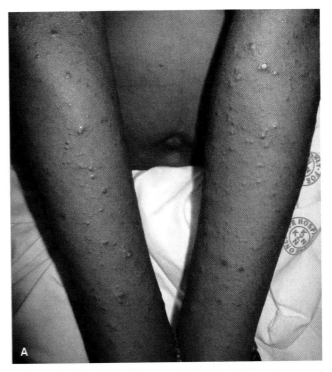

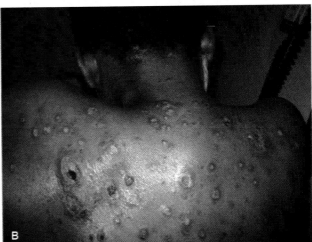

FIGURE 26-58 Histoplasmosis, disseminated to skin (A) In this child with HIV/AIDS, lesions appear as non-follicularly based papules that can coalesce into plaques. Violaceous hue is noted. **(B)** In progressive HIV disease/AIDS, lesions may spontaneously ulcerate, showing peripheral hyperpigmentation almost resembling neurotic excoriations at sites the patient cannot reach. The ears and the nose are often involved. Note the extent of neck lymphadenopathy. The patient expired soon after this picture from complications related to meningitis (Used with permission from Adam Lipworth, MD.)

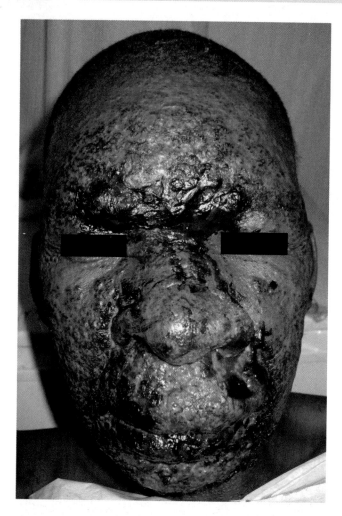

FIGURE 26-59 Histoplasmosis, disseminated to skin A 35-year-old African male presented with subacute febrile illness. Diffuse infiltration of the face with crusted erosions is seen. HIV disease with histoplasmosis was diagnosed. The patient died shortly after presentation. (Used with permission from Adam Lipworth, MD.)

BLASTOMYCOSIS ICD-10: B40.0

- Etiologic Agent. Blastomyces dermatitidis.
- Endemic in southeastern and Great Lakes area of United States.
- Primary pulmonary infection, which in some cases is followed by hematogenous dissemination to skin and other organs.

ETIOLOGY AND EPIDEMIOLOGY

ETIOLOGIC AGENT *Blastomyces dermatitidis*, a dimorphic fungus. Natural habitat: Wood debris. Lakes, river, and wetlands subject to flooding.
DEMOGRAPHY United States: Most cases occur in the southeastern, central, and Great Lakes areas. Canada: Toronto area.

PATHOGENESIS Asymptomatic primary pulmonary infection usually resolves spontaneously. Hematogenous dissemination may occur to the skin, skeletal system, prostate, epididymis, or mucosa of the nose, mouth, or larynx. Risk factors for dissemination: Host defense defects.

CLINICAL MANIFESTATIONS

PRIMARY PULMONARY INFECTION Accompanied or followed by hypersensitivity reactions: erythema nodosum, erythema multiforme. See Sections 7 and 14.

Cutaneous infection following hematogenous dissemination. Initial lesion, inflammatory nodule that enlarges and ulcerates (Fig. 26-60), with many small pustules on surface. Subsequently, verrucous and/or crusted plaque with sharply demarcated serpiginous borders. Peripheral border extends on one side, resembling a one-half to three-quarter moon. Pus exudes when crust is lifted. Central healing with thin geographic atrophic scar. Widespread lesions in HIV disease. *Distribution:* Usually symmetrically on trunk; also on the face, hands, arms, and legs; multiple lesions in one-half of patients.

MUCOUS MEMBRANES 25% of patients have oral or nasal lesions; one-half of those have contiguous skin lesions. Laryngeal infection.

DIFFERENTIAL DIAGNOSIS

Squamous cell carcinoma, pyoderma gangrenosum, tumor stage of mycosis fungoides, tuberculosis verrucosa cutis.

DIAGNOSIS

Clinical suspicion, confirmed by culture.

COURSE AND TREATMENT

Cutaneous infection usually occurs months or years after primary pulmonary infection. Skin most common site of extrapulmonary infection. Cure rate with itraconazole, 95%. Treat life-threatening infections with IV amphotericin B 0.7 to 1 mg/kg/day to a total dose of 2 g.

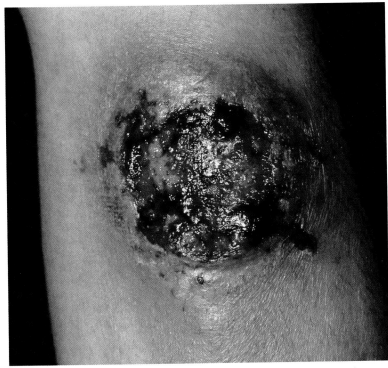

FIGURE 26-60 North American blastomycosis: disseminated Ulcerated, inflammatory plaque with surrounding erythema, edema, and fibrosis on the leg results from dissemination from pulmonary blastomycosis via blood to skin. The lesion must be differentiated from pyoderma gangrenosum. (Used with permission from Elizabeth M. Spiers, MD.)

COCCIDIOIDOMYCOSIS ICD-10: B38.0

- Etiologic Agent. *Coccidioides*.
- Endemic to desert areas of southwestern United States, northern Mexico, and Central and South America.
- Primary pulmonary infection usually resolves spontaneously.
- Can disseminate hematogenously resulting in chronic, progressive, granulomatous infection in skin, lungs, bone, and meninges.
- Cutaneous lesions in coccidioidomycosis.
  - Acute coccidioidomycosis.
    - Toxic erythema (diffuse erythema, morbilliform, urticaria).
    - Erythema nodosum.
    - Erythema multiforme (see Sections 7 and 14 for EN and EM).
  - Disseminated coccidioidomycosis.
    - Papules, nodules, and verrucous plaques.
- *Synonyms:* San Joaquin Valley fever, valley fever, and desert fever.

ETIOLOGY AND EPIDEMIOLOGY

ETIOLOGIC AGENTS *Coccidioides*, a dimorphic fungus; form arthroconidia, which become airborne. In a susceptible host, arthroconidia enlarges to become spherules, which contain endospores. Rarely, percutaneous.

DEMOGRAPHY More common in blacks and Filipinos. Risk of dissemination greater in males and pregnant females. Endemic in Arizona and southern California in San Joaquin Valley. Primary pulmonary coccidioidomycosis occurs in individuals living in these regions (endemic) or in visitors to the regions (nonendemic).

CLASSIFICATION Acute self-limited pulmonary coccidioidomycosis. Disseminated coccidioidomycosis (cutaneous, osteoarticular, and meningeal).

PATHOGENESIS Spores inhaled, resulting in primary pulmonary infection that is asymptomatic or accompanied by symptoms of coryza. Dissemination outside thoracic cavity occurs in <1% of infections associated with host defense defects.

CLINICAL MANIFESTATION

PRIMARY PULMONARY INFECTION Accompanied or followed by hypersensitivity reactions: "toxic erythema," erythema nodosum, and erythema multiforme.

PRIMARY CUTANEOUS INOCULATION SITE (RARE) Nodule eroding to ulcer. May have nodular lymphangitis or regional lymphadenitis.

HEMATOGENOUS DISSEMINATION TO SKIN Initially, papule (Fig. 26-61) evolving with formation of pustules, plaques, and nodules. Abscess formation, multiple draining sinus tracts, and ulcers; subcutaneous cellulitis; verrucous plaques; granulomatous nodules. Scars. Distribution: Face, especially the nasolabial fold, which is the preferential site; extremities.

DIFFERENTIAL DIAGNOSIS

Cryptococcosis, molluscum contagiosum.

DIAGNOSIS

Detection of *Coccidioides* spherules in the sputum, pus, and skin/tissue biopsy specimen. Isolation of *Coccidioides* on culture.

COURSE

In untreated HIV disease, mortality rate is high; relapse rate is also very high. In transplant patients, previously resolved infections reactivate 10% per year.

TREATMENT

Fluconazole, itraconazole, amphotericin B.

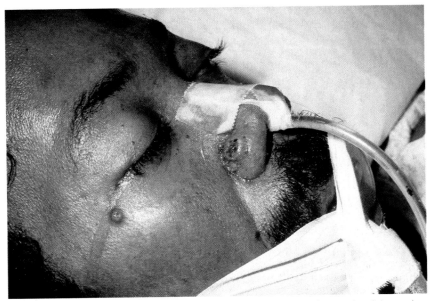

FIGURE 26-61 Coccidioidomycosis: disseminated Ulcerated and crusted nodules on the cheek and nose of an individual with pulmonary coccidioidomycosis with dissemination to the skin. (Used with permission from Francis Renna, MD.)

PENICILLIOSIS ICD-10: B44.9

- Etiology. *Penicillium marneffei*, dimorphic fungus.
- Demography. Occurs in the setting of HIV disease in those living in or traveling to Southeast Asia. With HIV disease, incidence similar to infections with *Cryptococcus neoformans* and *Mycobacterium tuberculosis*.
- Pathogenesis. Primary portal of entry is the lung. Hematologic dissemination with host defense defects.

CLINICAL MANIFESTATIONS

PRIMARY PULMONARY INFECTION Fever, chills, weight loss, anemia, generalized lymphadenopathy, and hepatomegaly.
DISSEMINATED PENICILLIOSIS TO SKIN Diffuse disseminated papular lesion (Fig. 26-62).

DIAGNOSIS

Histopathologic examination of tissue and blood smear; culture of clinical specimens.

TREATMENT

Amphotericin B.

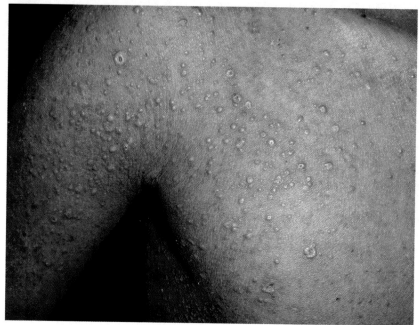

FIGURE 26-62 Penicilliosis in HIV disease: disseminated skin lesions A 27-year-old Vietnamese male with advanced untreated HIV disease presented with fever, weight loss, and disseminated umbilicated skin-colored papules. Hundreds of skin-colored papules of varying sizes, many umbilicated or with central erosion and crust. (Used with permission from Hoang Van Minh, M.D.)

SECTION 27

VIRAL DISEASES OF SKIN AND MUCOSA

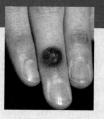

INTRODUCTION

Viral infections of skin and mucosa produce a wide spectrum of local and systemic manifestations.

- Human papillomavirus (HPV) and molluscum contagiosum virus (MCV) colonize the epidermis of most individuals without causing any clinical lesions. Benign epithelial proliferations such as warts and molluscum occur in some colonized persons, are transient, and eventually resolve without therapy. In immunocompromised individuals, however, these lesions may become extensive, persistent, and refractory to therapy.
- Primary infections with many viruses cause acute systemic febrile illnesses and exanthems, are usually self-limited, and convey lifetime immunity. Smallpox caused severe morbidity and mortality, but no longer occurs because of worldwide immunization.
- Eight human herpesviruses (HHV) often have asymptomatic primary infection but lifelong latent infection. With host defense defects, herpes viruses can become active and cause disease with significant morbidity and mortality.

POXVIRUS DISEASES

- Poxvirus family is a diverse group of epitheliotropic viruses that infect humans and animals. Only smallpox virus and molluscum contagiosum virus (MCV) cause natural disease in humans. Smallpox virus causes systemic infection with exanthema, i.e., smallpox or variola. MCV causes localized skin lesions. Human orf and milker's nodules are zoonoses that can occur in humans, given exposure to infected sheep or cattle. Other poxviruses zoonoses occurring in monkeys, cows, buffalo, sheep, and goats can also infect humans.

MOLLUSCUM CONTAGIOSUM ICD-10: B08.1

- Molluscum contagiosum is a self-limited epidermal viral infection.
- **Clinical Manifestation.** Firm pearly papules; often umbilicated. Few to myriads of lesions. Host defense defects: large nodules with confluence.
- **Course.** In healthy persons, resolves spontaneously.

ETIOLOGY AND EPIDEMIOLOGY

ETIOLOGY MCV with four discrete viral subtypes, I, II, III, IV; type I is responsible for >90% cases. Not distinguishable from other poxviruses by electron microscopy. MCV colonizes the epidermis and infundibulum of hair follicle. Transmitted by skin-to-skin contact.

DEMOGRAPHY More common in children and sexually active adults. In advanced human immunodeficiency virus (HIV) disease, hundreds of small mollusca or giant mollusca occur on the face and other sites.

PATHOGENESIS A subclinical carrier state of MCV probably exists in many healthy adults. Unique among poxviruses, MCV infection results in epidermal tumor formation; other human poxviruses cause a necrotic "pox" lesion. Rupture and discharge of infected cells occur in the umbilication/crater of the lesion.

CLINICAL MANIFESTATION

Papules, nodules, and tumors with central umbilication or depression (Figs. 27-1 to 27-4). Skin-colored. Round, oval, hemispherical. Isolated single lesion; multiple, scattered discrete lesions; or confluent mosaic plaques. Larger mollusca may have a central keratotic plug, which gives the lesion a central dimple or umbilication. Gentle pressure on a molluscum extrudes the central plug.

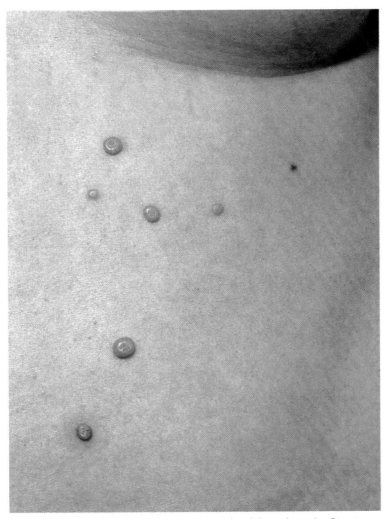

FIGURE 27-1 Molluscum contagiosum Typical umbilicated papules. Discrete, solid, skin-colored papules 3 to 5 mm on the chest of an adolescent female. The lesion with red halo is regressing spontaneously.

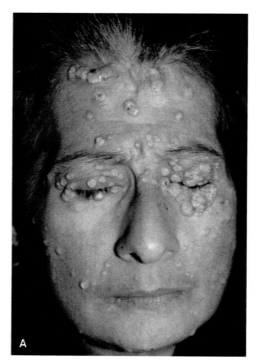
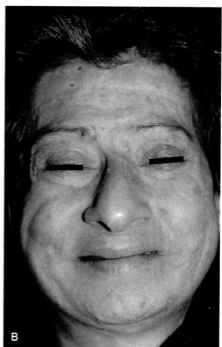

FIGURE 27-2 Molluscum contagiosum: face (A), large lesions on the face of a HIV+ woman. **(B)** Lesions resolved with electrodessication.

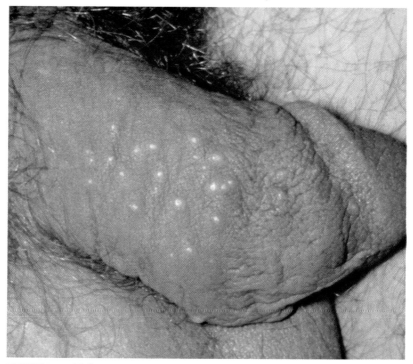

FIGURE 27-3 Molluscum contagiosum: penis Multiple, small shiny papules on penile shaft.

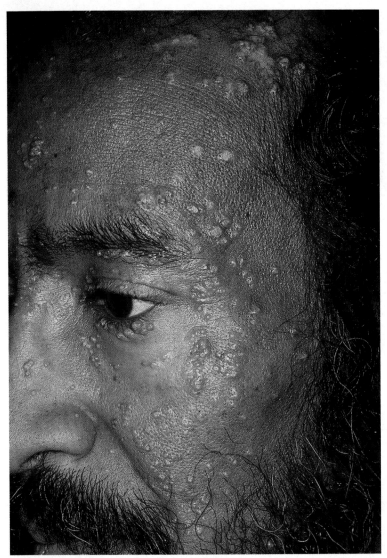

FIGURE 27-4 Molluscum contagiosum: face A 52-year-old male with HIV disease. Discrete and confluent umbilicated papules on the face.

Autoinoculation can occur by scratching or touching a lesion (Fig. 27-2).

Host immune response to viral antigen results in an inflammatory halo around mollusca (Fig. 27-2) and heralds spontaneous regression.

Host defense defects MC can be extensive with immunosuppressive therapy and HIV disease (Figs. 27-3 and 27-4).

In individuals with darker skin, significant postinflammatory hyperpigmentation may occur after treatment or spontaneous regression.

Distribution. Any site may be infected, especially naturally occluded sites, i.e., axillae, antecubital, popliteal fossae, and anogenital folds. Autoinoculation spreads lesions. Mollusca may be widespread in areas of atopic dermatitis. In adults with sexually transmitted mollusca: groins, genitalia, thighs, and the lower abdomen. Multiple facial mollusca (Fig. 27-4) suggest host defense defect.

Mollusca can occur in the conjunctiva, causing a unilateral conjunctivitis.

DIFFERENTIAL DIAGNOSIS

MULTIPLE SMALL PAPULES Flat warts, condylomata acuminata, syringoma, and sebaceous hyperplasia.
LARGE SOLITARY MOLLUSCUM Squamous cell carcinoma (SCC), basal cell carcinoma, and epidermal inclusion cyst.
MULTIPLE FACIAL MOLLUSCA IN HIV DISEASE Disseminated invasive fungal infection, i.e., cryptococcosis, histoplasmosis, coccidioidomycosis, and penicilliosis (see Section 26).

LABORATORY FINDINGS

DERMATOPATHOLOGY Infected cells contain large intracytoplasmic inclusions called Henderson-Patterson bodies, which appear as ovoid eosinophilic structures.

DIAGNOSIS

Usually made on clinical findings. Biopsy lesion in HIV disease if disseminated invasive fungal infection is in the differential diagnosis.

COURSE

In the normal host, mollusca often persist up to 6 months and then undergo spontaneous regression without scarring. In HIV disease, mollusca persist and proliferate even after aggressive local therapy. Mollusca are usually symptomatic, and can cause cosmetic disfigurement and concern about transmission of mollusca to a sexual partner.

TREATMENT

Office-based treatments include curettage, cryosurgery, cantharidin, and electrodessication. Imiquimod 5% cream may be effective.

HUMAN ORF ICD-10: B08.02

- **Zoonosis.** Caused by a dermatotropic parapoxvirus that commonly infects ungulates (sheep, goats, deer, etc.); it is transmitted to humans through contact with an infected animal or fomites. Most common in farmers, veterinarians, and sheep shearers. Only newborn animals lacking viral immunity are susceptible. Manifested as erythematous, exudative nodules around the mouth that heal spontaneously, resulting in permanent immunity.
- **Transmission to Humans.** Humans are infected by inoculation of virus by direct contact with lambs and indirectly by fomites. Human-to-human infection does not occur. Exposure occurs at the time of slaughter of lambs for Easter or the Muslim holiday Eid al-Adha.

CLINICAL MANIFESTATION

MACULES, PAPULES, AND NODULES AT SITE OF INOCULATION Most commonly occur on the hands, arms, legs, and face (Figs. 27-5 and 27-6). Lesions may appear edematous or bullous. Immune reconstitution inflammatory syndrome (IRIS) or target lesions occur. Color is pink to red to blanched. Lesions evolve to crusted erosions or ulcers. Healing occurs spontaneously in 4 to 6 weeks without scarring.
OTHER FINDINGS Ascending lymphangitis and lymphadenopathy. More extensive infection may occur with host defense defects.

DIFFERENTIAL DIAGNOSIS

Impetigo, furuncles, and milker's nodules.

DIAGNOSIS

Clinical findings with the appropriate history. Can be confirmed by detection of orf virus DNA by quantitative polymerase chain reaction (qPCR).

COURSE

Resolves spontaneously in 4 to 6 weeks, healing without scar formation. Erythema multiforme-like eruptions (see Section 14) have been reported in human orf. Widespread lesions spread by autoinoculation may occur in atopic dermatitis. In humans, lasting immunity is conferred by infection.

TREATMENT

No effective antiviral treatment. Treat bacterial secondary infection.

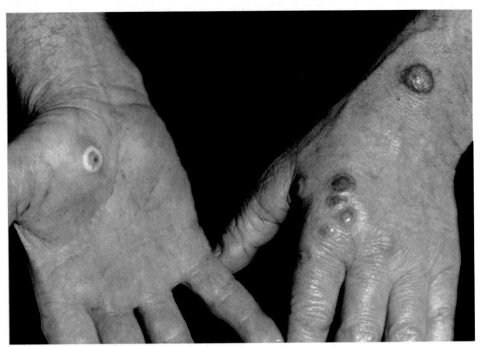

FIGURE 27-5 Human orf: multiple lesions on hands Multiple blisters with target/IRIS patterns in lesions on the hands of a sheep herder.

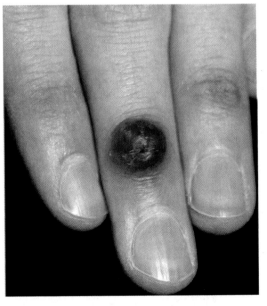

FIGURE 27-6 Human orf: finger A 19-year-old male of Greek heritage; lesions appeared 10 days after Greek Easter and was associated with slaughter of a lamb for the Easter feast.

MILKERS' NODULES ICD-10: B08.03

■ **Zoonosis.** Parapoxvirus infection. Papular lesions occur on muzzles and oral cavity of calves and on teats of cows. Virus transmitted to humans by contact with bovine lesions or teat cups of milking machines; most common in dairy farmers. Clinical findings and course are similar to human orf.

CLINICAL MANIFESTATION

Solitary or multiple red-purple nodules (Fig. 27-7) occur at the site of inoculation. Usually on exposed sites such as hands; may occur in burn wounds.

OTHER FINDINGS Lymphadenopathy.

DIFFERENTIAL DIAGNOSIS

Orf, furuncle, herpes simplex virus (HSV) infection, and pyogenic granuloma.

DIAGNOSIS

Usually made on history of bovine exposure and clinical findings.

COURSE

Resolves spontaneously.

TREATMENT

No effective antiviral treatment. Treat bacterial secondary infection.

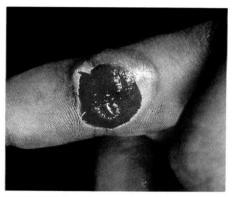

FIGURE 27-7 Milker's nodule: finger A single beefy eroded nodule on the finger of a dairy farmer at the site of inoculation.

SMALLPOX ICD-10: B03

■ Smallpox is a viral infection unique to humans. The disease has been eradicated caused by a global immunization program, with the last case having been reported in 1977.
http://www.bt.cdc.gov/agent/smallpox/overview/disease-facts.asp
http://www.who.int/csr/disease/smallpox/en/
■ **Etiology.** *Variola major* and *Variola minor*. Humans are only host. DNA virus replicates in cell cytoplasma. Transmitted by respiratory droplets. **Variola major** has a 30 to 50% mortality.
■ **Pathogenesis.** Enters respiratory tract, passing rapidly into local lymph nodes, and producing viremia. Infection with smallpox confers lifelong immunity.
■ **Clinical manifestation.** Acute onset of fever, followed by exanthem. Small red *macules* evolve to *papules* over 1 to 2 days. Initially, on the face, forearms and mouth, then gradually becomes disseminated. In 1 to 2 more days, papules become *vesicles*. Vesicles evolve to *pustules* about 4 to 7 days after onset of the rash (Fig. 27-8), and lasts for 5 to 8 days. Followed by *umbilication* and *crusting* (Fig. 27-8). Lesions are generally all at the same stage of development. Pockmarks/pitted scars occur in 65 to 85% of severe cases, especially on the face (Fig. 27-9). Secondary *Staphylococcus aureus* infection with abscesses and cellulitis may occur in smallpox lesions. Enanthema (tongue, mouth, or oropharynx) precedes exanthem by a day.
■ **Differential Diagnosis.** Severe chicken pox (varicella lesions are in different stages of development), measles, secondary syphilis (great pox), hand-foot-and-mouth disease (HFMD) (coxsackievirus A-16), cowpox, monkeypox, and tanapox.
■ **Treatment.** Report possible smallpox to public health officials; diagnosis confirmed in a Biological Safety Level 4 laboratory where staff members have been vaccinated. Cidofovir may be effective.

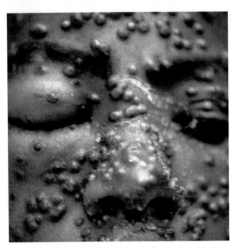

FIGURE 27-8 Smallpox: variola major Multiple pustules becoming confluent on the face.

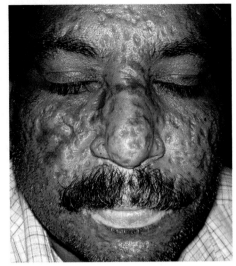

FIGURE 27-9 Smallpox: scarring on face A 50-year-old Indian male with a history of smallpox as a child has multiple depressed scars on face 40 years after smallpox infection. (Used with permission from Atul Taneja, MD.)

HUMAN PAPILLOMAVIRUS INFECTIONS ICD-10: B97.7

- HPV are ubiquitous in humans, causing:
    - Subclinical infection.
    - Wide variety of benign clinical lesions on skin and mucous membranes.
    - Cutaneous and mucosal premalignancies (Table 27-1): Squamous cell carcinoma in situ (SCCIS); invasive SCC.
- More than 150 types of HPV have been identified and are associated with various clinical lesions and diseases. Papillomaviruses infect all mammalian species as well as birds, reptiles, and others.
    - Cutaneous HPV infections occur commonly in the general population:
    - *Common warts*: Represent approximately 70% of all cutaneous warts, occurring in up to 20% of all school-age children.
    - *Butcher's warts*: Common in butchers, meat packers, and fish handlers.
    - *Plantar warts*: Common in older children and young adults, accounting for 30% of cutaneous warts.
    - *Flat warts*: Occur in children and adults, accounting for 4% of cutaneous warts.
    - Oncogenic HPV can cause SCCIS and invasive SCC with host defense defects.
- *Epidermodysplasia verruciformis (EDV)*.
- Anogenital HPV infections.
- *External genital wart*: Most prevalent sexually transmitted infection (see Section 30).
- Squamous Cell Carcinoma. Some HPV types have a major etiologic role in the pathogenesis of in situ as well as invasive SCC of the anogenital epithelium.
- During delivery, maternal genital HPV infection can be transmitted to the neonate, resulting in anogenital warts and respiratory papillomatosis after aspiration of the virus into the upper respiratory tract.

TABLE 27-1 Correlation of Human Papillomavirus Type with Disease

Disease	Associated HPV Types
Plantar warts	1,* 2,† 4, 63
Myrmecia	60
Common warts	1,* 2,* 4, 26, 27, 29, 41,† 57, 65, 77
Common warts of meat handlers	1, 2,* 3, 4, 7,* 10, 28
Flat warts	3,* 10,* 27, 38, 41,† 49, 75, 76
Intermediate warts	10,* 26, 28
Epidermodysplasia verruciformis	2,* 3,* 5,*† 8,*† 9,* 10,* 12,* 14,*† 15,* 17,*† 19, 20,† 21, 22, 23, 24, 25, 36, 37, 38,† 47, 50
Condyloma acuminatum	6,* 11,* 30,† 42, 43, 44, 45,† 51,† 54, 55, 70
Intraepithelial neoplasias Unspecified Low-grade High-grade	 30,† 34, 39,† 40, 53, 57, 59, 61, 62, 64, 66,† 67, 69, 71 6,* 11,* 16,† 18,† 31,† 33,† 35,† 42, 43, 44, 45,† 51,† 52,† 74 6, 11, 16,*† 18,*† 31,† 33,† 34, 35,† 39,† 42, 44, 45,† 51,† 52,† 56,† 58,† 66,†
Cervical carcinoma	16,*† 18,*† 31,† 33,† 35,† 39,† 45,† 51,† 52,† 56,† 58,† 66,† 68, 70
Laryngeal papillomas	6,* 11*
Focal epithelial hyperplasia of Heck	13,* 32*
Conjunctival papillomas	6,* 11,* 16*†
Others	6, 11, 16,† 30,† 33,† 36, 37, 38,† 41,† 48,† 60, 72, 73

*Most common associations.
†High malignant potential.

Note: Additional information on new HPV types can be found on the HPV Sequence Data Base through the Internet (*hpv-web.lanl.gov*).

ETIOLOGY

Papillomaviruses are double-stranded DNA viruses of the papovavirus class, which infect most vertebrate species with exclusive host and tissue specificity. Infections are restricted to squamous epithelia of skin and mucous membranes. Clinical lesions induced by HPV and their natural history are largely determined by HPV type, which are grouped according to their pathologic associations and tissue specificity, either as cutaneous or mucosal. Mucosal-associated HPV can be further subgrouped according to their risk of malignant transformation. New types of HPV are defined as possessing <90% homology to known types in six specified early and late genes.

HUMAN PAPILLOMAVIRUS: CUTANEOUS DISEASES

- Certain human HPV types commonly infect keratinized skin.
- Cutaneous warts are:
  - Discrete benign epithelial hyperplasia with varying degrees of surface hyperkeratosis.
  - Manifested as minute papules to large plaques.
- Lesions may become confluent, forming a mosaic.
- The extent of lesions is determined by the immune status of the host.

EPIDEMIOLOGY

TRANSMISSION Skin-to-skin contact. Minor trauma with breaks in stratum corneum facilitates epidermal infection.

DEMOGRAPHY Host defense defects are associated with an increased incidence of and more widespread cutaneous warts: HIV disease, iatrogenic immunosuppression with solid organ transplantation.

EPIDERMODYSPLASIA VERRUCIFORMIS Autosomal-recessive hereditary disorder. Acquired EDV-like lesions as seen in HIV disease.

CLINICAL MANIFESTATION

Common Wart or Verruca Vulgaris

Firm papules, 1 to 10 mm or larger (Figs. 27-10 to 27-14), hyperkeratotic, clefted surface, with vegetations. Isolated lesion, scattered discrete lesions. Occur at sites of trauma: hands, fingers, and knees. Palmar lesions disrupt the normal line of fingerprints. Return of fingerprints is a sign of resolution of the wart. *Characteristic* "red or brown dots," best visualized with dermatoscope, are pathognomonic, representing thrombosed dermal papilla capillary loops.

Linear arrangement: Inoculation by scratching.

Annular warts: At sites of prior therapy.

Butcher's warts: Large cauliflower-like lesions on hands of meat handlers.

Filiform warts have relatively small Δbases, extending out with elongated cap (see Fig. 27-18).

Plantar Warts (Verruca Plantaris)

Early small, shiny, sharply marginated papule (Fig. 27-15) → plaque with rough hyperkeratotic surface, studded with brown-black dots (thrombosed capillaries). As with palmar warts, normal dermatoglyphics are disrupted. Return of dermatoglyphics is a sign of resolution of the wart. Warts heal without scarring. Therapies such as cryosurgery and electrosurgery can result in scarring at treatment sites. Tenderness may be marked, especially in certain acute types and in lesions over sites of pressure.

Mosaic warts: Confluence of many small warts. "Kissing" warts: Lesion may occur on opposing surface of two toes (Fig. 27-16). Plantar foot, often solitary but may be three to six or more. Pressure points, heads of metatarsal, heels, and toes.

Flat Warts (Verruca Plana)

Sharply defined, flat papules (1 to 5 mm); "flat" surface; the thickness of the lesion is 1 to 2 mm (Fig. 27-17). Skin-colored or light brown. Round, oval, polygonal, linear lesions (inoculation of virus by scratching). Occur on face, beard area (Fig. 27-18), dorsa of hands, and shins.

Epidermodysplasia Verruciformis

Mostly autosomal-recessive, but can be acquired in patients with impaired immunity. Flat-topped papules. Tinea versicolor-like

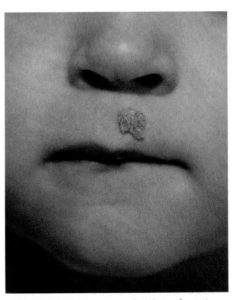

FIGURE 27-10 Verruca vulgaris on face A 3-year-old boy with common wart on the moustache area.

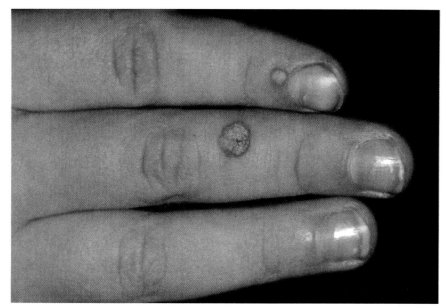

FIGURE 27-11 Verruca vulgaris: fingers A 20-year-old female with hyperkeratotic, verrucous papules on the index and middle fingers. The lesions resolved with electrodessication, having failed to respond to cryosurgery.

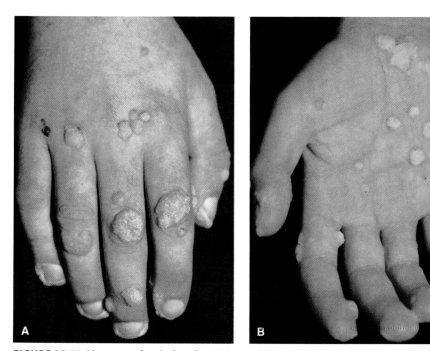

FIGURE 27-12 Verruca vulgaris: hands A 20-year-old immunosuppressed male with nephrotic syndrome. Multiple verrucae on the **(A)** dorsum and **(B)** palm of the hand.

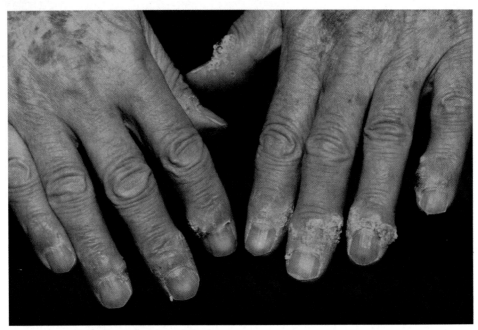

FIGURE 27-13 Periungual warts A 77-year-old male with extensive periungual warts. He was depressed and picked at periungual skin folds created portal of entry for HPV. Lesions resolved with hyperthermia.

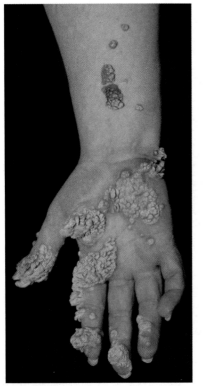

FIGURE 27-14 Giant warts on hand and forearm A 51-year-old female with recalcitrant warts on hands for 2 years. Immunodeficiency was suspected but not detected.

FIGURE 27-15 Verruca plantaris: plantar foot A 71-year-old male with chronic lymphatic leukemia. Large and painful on pressure, warts are seen on the plantar foot. After many failed therapeutic modalities, he was successfully treated with electron beam radiation.

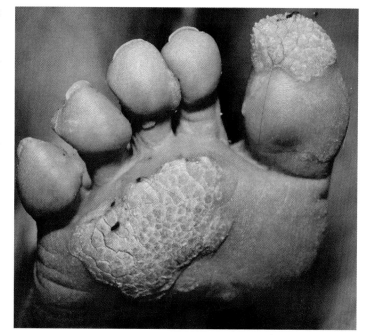

FIGURE 27-16 Extensive verrucae A 49-year-old male with HIV disease has confluent warts on the hands and feet. The large warts on opposing toes are referred to as "kissing warts."

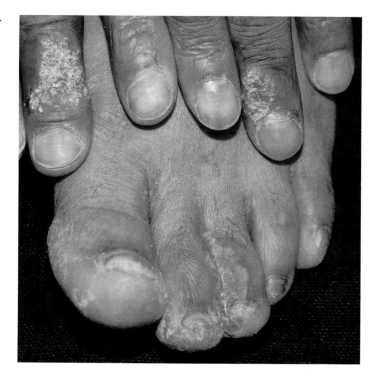

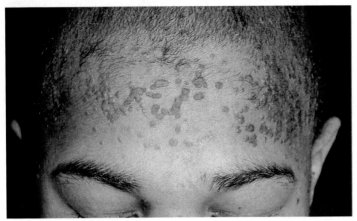

FIGURE 27-17 Verrucae planae A 12-year-old male kidney transplant recipient. Multiple brown keratotic papules are seen on the forehead and scalp.

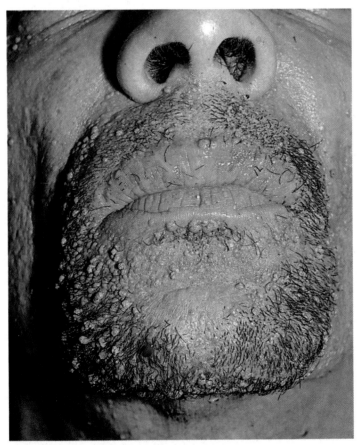

FIGURE 27-18 Filiform and flat warts A 38-year-old male with HIV disease has a confluence of lesions on face and beard area. Lesions resolved after successful antiretroviral therapy.

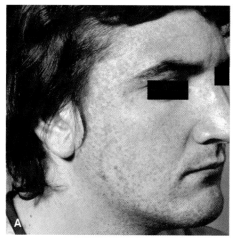
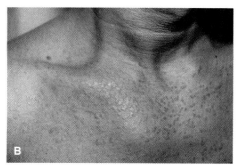

FIGURE 27-19 Epidermodysplasia verruciformis on face (A) A 35-year-old male had extensive EDV on face and neck: There are multiple barely visible tan flat papules. **(B)** Another patient with flat warts on neck and chest.

lesions, particularly on the trunk. Color: Skin-colored, light brown, pink, and hypopigmented. Lesions may be numerous, large, and confluent. Seborrheic keratosis-like and actinic keratosis-like lesions. Linear arrangement after traumatic inoculation. *Distribution*: Face, dorsa of hands, arms, legs, and anterior trunk (Fig. 27-19). Premalignant and malignant lesions arise most commonly on face. SCC: In situ and invasive.

Host Defense Defects

(HIV disease, iatrogenic immunosuppression). HPV-induced warts are common and may be difficult to treat successfully. Some have atypical histologic features and may progress to in situ and invasive SCC.

Human Papillomavirus: Oropharyngeal Diseases

HPV infects mucosal epithelial cells of the mouth, nose, and airways (Fig. 27-20). Oral infections may be subclinical or cause benign or malignant oral neoplasms. In respiratory or laryngeal papillomatosis, HPV 6 and 11 are acquired during vaginal delivery and cause warts of the oropharynx and upper airways. Laryngeal lesions cause major morbidity. SCC occurs in some persons.

Human Papillomavirus: Anogenital Infections

See Section 30, "Sexually Transmitted Diseases."

DIFFERENTIAL DIAGNOSIS

Verruca vulgaris: Molluscum contagiosum, seborrheic keratosis, actinic keratosis, keratoacanthoma, SCCIS, and invasive SCC.

- Verruca plantaris: Callus, corn, or keratosis.
- Verruca plana: Syringoma (facial) and molluscum contagiosum.
- Epidermodysplasia verruciformis: Pityriasis versicolor, actinic keratoses, seborrheic keratoses, SCCIS, and basal cell carcinoma.

LABORATORY FINDINGS

DERMATOPATHOLOGY Acanthosis, papillomatosis, hyperkeratosis. Characteristic feature is foci of vacuolated cells (koilocytosis), vertical tiers of parakeratotic cells, and foci of clumped keratohyaline granules.
DIAGNOSIS Usually made on clinical findings. With host defense defects, HPV-induced SCC at periungual sites or anogenital region should be ruled out by lesional biopsy.

COURSE

In immunocompetent individuals, cutaneous HPV infections usually resolve spontaneously, without therapeutic intervention. With host defense defects, cutaneous HPV infections may be very resistant to all modalities of therapy. With EDV, lesions first occur at 5 to 7 years

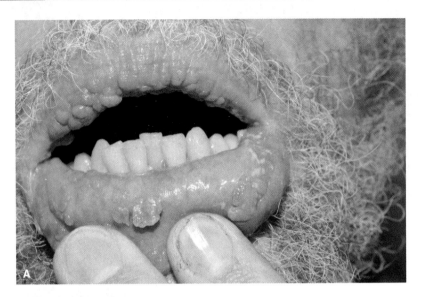

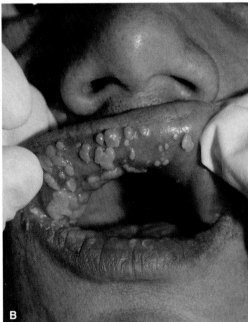

FIGURE 27-20 Multiple oral condylomata in HIV disease. **(A** and **B)** Lesions resolved with antiretroviral therapy.

of age and increase in numbers progressively, becoming widespread in some. About 30 to 50% of individuals with EDV develop malignant cutaneous lesions on areas of skin exposed to sunlight.

TREATMENT

GOAL Aggressive therapies, which are often quite painful and may be followed by scarring, are usually to be avoided because the natural history of cutaneous HPV infections is for spontaneous resolution in months or a few years. Plantar warts that are painful because of their location warrant more aggressive therapies.

PATIENT-INITIATED THERAPY Minimal cost; no/minimal pain. 17 to 40% salicylic acid daily for up to twelve weeks.

IMIQUIMOD CREAM At sites that are not thickly keratinized, apply three times per week. Persistent warts may require occlusion. Hyperkeratotic lesions on palms/soles should be debrided frequently.

HYPERTHERMIA FOR VERRUCA PLANTARIS Hyperthermia with hot water [45°C (113°F)]

immersion for 20 minutes or three times weekly for up to 16 treatments has been reported to be helpful in some patients.

CLINICIAN-INITIATED THERAPY Costly and painful.

CRYOSURGERY If patients have tried home therapies and liquid nitrogen is available, light cryosurgery using a cotton-tipped applicator or cryospray, freezing the wart and 1 to 2 mm of surrounding normal tissue can be effective. Freezing destroys the infected tissue but not HPV. Cryosurgery is usually repeated about every 3 weeks until the warts have disappeared.

ELECTROSURGERY Can also be effective, but associated with scarring. EMLA cream can be used for anesthesia for flat warts. Lidocaine injection is usually required for thicker warts, especially palmar/plantar lesions.

CO_2 LASER SURGERY May be effective for recalcitrant warts, but no better than cryosurgery or electrosurgery in the hands of an experienced clinician.

SURGERY Single, nonplantar verruca vulgaris: Curettage after freezing; surgical excision of cutaneous HPV infections is not indicated in that these lesions are epidermal infections.

SYSTEMIC VIRAL INFECTIONS WITH EXANTHEMS

- Primary systemic infections often present with characteristic mucocutaneous rashes: Exanthems and enanthems.
- Exanthem and enanthem. An exanthem is eruptive rash associated with a systemic disorder; enanthem, mucosal lesions are signs of a systemic disorder often associated with an exanthem. Often caused by viral agents but can also be associated with other infections: (bacterial, parasitic infections, sexually transmitted disease), adverse cutaneous reactions to drugs or toxin, and autoimmune disease.

ETIOLOGY AND EPIDEMIOLOGY

RNA Viruses. Picornaviridae: Poliovirus, coxsackieviruses, echovirus, enterovirus, hepatitis A virus, and rhinovirus. Togaviridae: Rubella virus, attenuated rubella virus in vaccine, and Chikungunya virus. Flaviviridae: Dengue, hepatitis C virus, and Zika virus. Paramyxoviridae: Measles and mumps. Orthomyxoviridae: Influenza A, B, and C viruses. Retroviridae: Human T-lymphotropic virus types I and II as well as HIV types 1 and 2 (acute HIV syndrome).

DNA Viruses. Parvoviridae: Parvovirus B19 (erythema infectiosum). Hepadnaviridae hepatitis B virus. Adenoviridae. Herpesviridae: HSV types 1 and 2, varicella zoster virus (VZV), cytomegalovirus (CMV), Epstein–Barr virus (EBV), HHV 6 and 7 (exanthem subitum, roseola infantum), Kaposi sarcoma (KS)-associated virus (HHV-8). Poxviridae: Variola (smallpox) virus, orf virus, and MCV.

Bacteria. Group A streptococcus: Scarlet fever and toxic shock syndrome. *S. aureus*:

Toxic shock syndrome. *Legionella, Leptospira, Listeria,* and Meningococci, *Treponema pallidum.*
Mycoplasmal Mycoplasma pneumoniae Rickettsiae Rocky Mountain spotted fever. Tick-borne spotted fevers. Rickettsialpox. Murine typhus. Epidemic typhus. *Miscellaneous Strongyloides, Toxoplasma.*

PATHOGENESIS Skin lesions may be produced by the following:

- Direct effect of microbial replication in infected cells.
- Host response to the microbe.
- Interaction of these two phenomena.

CLINICAL MANIFESTATION

PRODROME Acute infection syndrome: Fever, malaise, coryza, sore throat, nausea, vomiting, diarrhea, abdominal pain, and headache.
Exanthematous Eruption. Resembles the exanthem occurring with measles or morbilli, i.e., measles-like or "morbilliform." Also referred to as maculopapular. Characterized by initially discrete, often becoming confluent pink macules and papules (Fig. 27-21). Usually central, i.e., head, neck, trunk, and proximal extremities. Most often progresses centrifugally. Lesions can become hemorrhagic with petechiae and hemorrhagic measles.

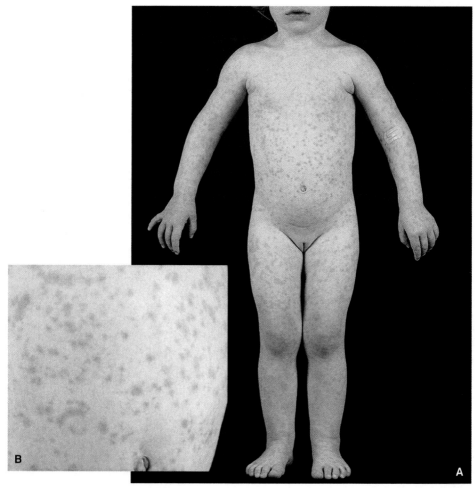

FIGURE 27-21 Measles-like exanthema Disseminated erythematous macules and papules, typical of the cutaneous changes with many viral infections. Differential diagnosis of an exanthematous or morbilliform adverse cutaneous drug eruption. **(A)** Typical distribution of lesions on the trunk and extremities. **(B)** Closeup of pink macules and papules becoming confluent in some areas.

Scarlatiniform Eruption. Diffuse erythema.
Vesicular Eruptions. Initially, vesicles with
clear fluid. May evolve to pustules. In a few
days to a week, roof of vesicle sloughs, resulting
in erosions. In varicella, lesions are disseminated and may involve oropharynx. In hand
foot and mouth disease, vesicles/erosion occur
in the oropharynx; tender vesicles on the
palms/soles.
Oropharyngeal Lesions. Enanthem. Koplik spots in measles. Petechiae on soft palate
(*Forchheimer sign*). Microulcerative lesions in
herpangina resulting from coxsackievirus A
(see Herpangina, p. 673). Palatal petechiae in
mononucleosis syndrome of primary EBV or
CMV infection. Aphthous ulcer-like lesions
occur with primary HIV infection.

CONJUNCTIVITIS Occurs with measles.
GENITALIA External aphthous ulcer-like lesion
with primary HIV infection.
SYSTEMIC FINDINGS Lymphadenopathy. Hepatomegaly. Splenomegaly.

DIFFERENTIAL DIAGNOSIS

Adverse cutaneous drug eruption (ACDE),
systemic lupus erythematosus, Kawasaki
syndrome.

DIAGNOSIS

Usually made on history and clinical findings. Serology: Acute and convalescent titers
most helpful in specific diagnosis. Cultures: If
practical.

RUBELLA ICD-10: B06

- **Etiologic Agent.** Rubella virus, an RNA togavirus.
- **Clinical Manifestation.** Characteristic exanthem and lymphadenopathy. Many infections are
  subclinical.
- **Congenital Rubella Syndrome.** Rubella virus infecting a pregnant female, although causing a
  benign illness in the mother, may result in a serious chronic fetal infection and malformation.
- Prophylaxis. Childhood immunization is highly effective at preventing infection.
- *Synonyms*: German measles, "3-day measles."

ETIOLOGY AND EPIDEMIOLOGY

ETIOLOGY *Rubella virus*, an RNA togavirus,
member of *Rubivirus* genus. Attenuated rubella
virus used in immunization can cause an illness
with rubella-like rash, lymphadenopathy, and
arthritis.
DEMOGRAPHY Before widespread immunization, most commonly occurred in children
<15 years. Currently young adults. *Risk fac-
tors:* Lack of active immunization and lack of
natural infection. After immunization began in
1969, incidence decreased by 99% in industrialized countries.
TRANSMISSION Inhalation of aerosolized respiratory droplets. Moderately contagious. 10 to
40% of cases asymptomatic. Period of infectiv-
ity from end of incubation period to disappearance of rash.

CLINICAL MANIFESTATION

PRODROME Prodrome usually absent, especially in young children. In adolescents and
young adults: Anorexia, malaise, conjunctivitis, headache, low-grade fever, and mild

upper respiratory tract symptoms. In women,
rubella-like illness frequently follows administration of attenuated live rubella virus with
arthralgias.
EXANTHEM Pink macules, papules (Fig. 27-22).
Initially on forehead, spreading inferiorly to
the face, trunk, and extremities during the first
day. By the second day, facial exanthem fades.
By the third day, exanthem fades completely
without residual pigmentary change or scaling.
Truncal lesions may become confluent, creating
a scarlatiniform eruption.
MUCOUS MEMBRANES Petechiae on soft palate
(Forchheimer sign) during prodrome (also
seen in infectious mononucleosis).
LYMPH NODES Enlarged during prodrome.
Postauricular, suboccipital, and posterior cervi-
cal lymph nodes enlarged and possibly tender.
Mild generalized lymphadenopathy may occur.
Enlargement usually persists for 1 week but
may last for months.
SPLEEN May be enlarged.
JOINTS Arthritis in adults; possible effusion.
Arthralgia, especially in adult women after
immunization.

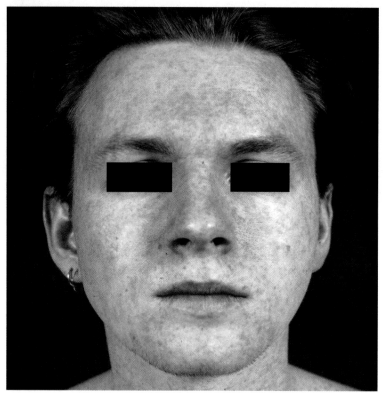

FIGURE 27-22 Rubella A 21-year-old male. Erythematous macules and papules appearing initially on the face and spreading inferiorly and centrifugally to the trunk and extremities, usually within the first 24 hours. Postauricular and posterior cervical lymph nodes were enlarged. Lesions becoming confluent on the cheeks while clearing on the forehead. Truncal lesions appear 24 hours after onset of facial lesions.

CONGENITAL RUBELLA SYNDROME Congenital heart defects; cataracts; microphthalmia, microcephaly, hydrocephaly, and deafness.

DIFFERENTIAL DIAGNOSIS

EXANTHEM Other viral exanthems, ACDE, and scarlet fever.
EXANTHEM WITH ARTHRITIS Acute rheumatic fever, rheumatoid arthritis, and erythema infectiosum.

DIAGNOSIS

Clinical diagnosis; can be confirmed by serology. Virus can be isolated from the throat, joint fluid aspirate.

COURSE

In most persons, rubella is a mild, inconsequential illness. However, when rubella occurs in a pregnant woman during the first trimester, the infection can be passed transplacentally to the developing fetus. Approximately half of infants who acquire rubella during the first trimester of intrauterine life will show clinical signs of damage from the virus.

TREATMENT

Rubella is preventable by immunization. Previous rubella should be documented in young women: If antirubella antibody titers are negative, rubella immunization should be given.

MEASLES ICD-10: B05

- A highly contagious childhood viral disease characterized by fever, coryza, and cough; an exanthema; conjunctivitis; pathognomonic enanthem (Koplik spots).
- Significant morbidity and mortality occur in acute and chronic course.
- Childhood immunization is highly effective at preventing infection.
- *Synonyms*: Morbilli and rubeola.

ETIOLOGY AND EPIDEMIOLOGY

ETIOLOGY Measles virus, member of RNA genus *Morbillivirus*, and family Paramyxoviridae.

DEMOGRAPHY Measles is no longer endemic in industrialized countries; cases result from importation of measles. Affects 30 million children yearly in developing countries.

RISK FACTORS Unvaccinated children are at the highest risk.

Transmission spread by respiratory droplets produced by sneezing and coughing. Infected persons contagious from several days before onset of rash up to 5 days after lesions appear. 90% of susceptible contacts will be infected.

PATHOGENESIS Virus enters cells of respiratory tract, replicates locally, spreads to regional lymph nodes, and disseminates hematogenously to skin and mucous membranes, where it replicates. Modified measles, a milder form of the illness, may occur in individuals with preexisting partial immunity induced by active or passive immunization. Persons deficient in cellular immunity are at high risk for severe measles.

CLINICAL MANIFESTATION

INCUBATION PERIOD 10 to 15 days.

PRODROME Fever. Malaise. Upper respiratory symptoms (coryza, hacking *bark-like cough*). Photophobia, conjunctivitis with lacrimation. Periorbital edema. As exanthem progresses, systemic symptoms subside.

EXANTHEM On the fourth febrile day, erythematous macules and papules appear on the forehead at hairline and behind the ears; it spreads centrifugally and inferiorly to involve the face, trunk (Fig. 27-23), extremities, and palms/soles, reaching the feet by third day. Initial discrete lesions may become confluent, especially on the face, neck, and shoulders. Lesions gradually fade in order of appearance, with subsequent residual yellow-tan stain or faint desquamation. Exanthem resolves in 4 to 6 days.

ENANTHEM Cluster of tiny bluish-white spots on red background, appearing on or after second day of febrile illness, are seen on buccal mucosa opposite premolar teeth, i.e., *Koplik spots* that are pathognomonic of measles. Appear before exanthem. Also: Entire buccal/inner labial mucosa may be inflamed.

BULBAR CONJUNCTIVAE Conjunctivitis, injected, and red.

GENERAL EXAMINATION Generalized lymphadenopathy. Diarrhea and vomiting. Splenomegaly.

MODIFIED MEASLES Milder clinical findings with preexisting partial immunity.

ATYPICAL MEASLES Occurs in individuals immunized with formalin-inactivated measles vaccine, subsequently exposed to measles virus. Exanthem begins peripherally and moves centrally; can be urticarial, maculopapular, hemorrhagic, and/or vesicular. Systemic symptoms can be severe.

MEASLES IN HOST WITH DEFENSE DEFECTS Rash may not occur. Pneumonitis and encephalitis more common.

DIFFERENTIAL DIAGNOSIS

DISSEMINATED MACULOPAPULAR ERUPTION Morbilliform drug eruption, scarlet fever. Kawasaki syndrome.

DIAGNOSIS

Clinical diagnosis confirmed by serology. Multinucleated giant cells in secretions. Isolate virus from blood, urine, and pharyngeal secretions. Detect measles antigen in respiratory secretions by immunofluorescent staining. Detects genomic sequences of measles virus RNA in serum, throat swabs, and cerebrospinal fluid (CSF).

COURSE

Self-limited infection in most patients, though there were 114,900 deaths globally in 2014.

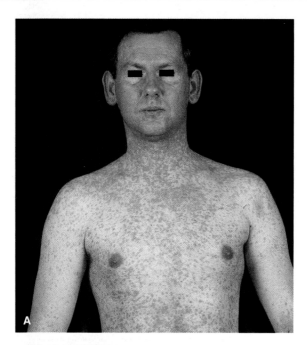

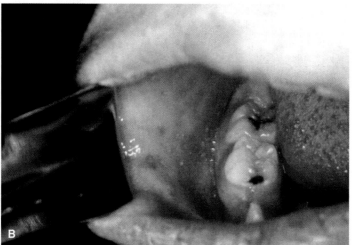

FIGURE 27-23 Measles with exanthem (A) Erythematous macules, first appearing on the face and neck where they become confluent, spreading to the trunk and arms in 2 to 3 days where they remain discrete. In contrast, rubella also first appears initially on the face but spreads to the trunk in one day. Koplik spots on the buccal mucosa were also present. Erythematous papules have become confluent on the face on the fourth day. **Measles with Koplik spots (B)** Red papules on buccal mucosa opposite premolars prior of appearance of exanthema. (From the Centers for Disease Control and Prevention.)

Children <5 years old are at the highest risk for death. Sites of complications: respiratory tract, central nervous system (CNS). Complications more common in malnourished children, the unimmunized, and those with congenital immunodeficiency and leukemia. Acute complications (10% of cases): otitis media, pneumonia (bacterial or measles), diarrhea, measles encephalitis, and thrombocytopenia. Chronic complication: subacute sclerosing panencephalitis (Dawson encephalitis).

TREATMENT

Prophylactic immunization. Supportive care.

ENTEROVIRAL INFECTIONS ICD-10: B34.1

- **Etiologic Agents.** Intestinal viruses echovirus 9 and 16, coxsackie A6 and A16 virus, and enterovirus 71 (EV71).
- **Enteroviral Infections with Rash:**
  - Echovirus 9 (E9): Discrete pink macules and papules resembling rubella ± fever.
  - Echovirus 16: Exanthem, roseola-like (confluent pink papules) ± fever.
  - Coxsackievirus A16, EV71: Hand foot and mouth disease.
  - Coxsackievirus A6: Eczema coxsackium.
  - A1–10, 16, 22, CB1–5; EV6, 9, 11, 16, 17, 25; EV71: Herpangina.
  - Other enteroviruses reported to cause erythema multiforme: vesicular, urticarial, petechial, and purpuric rashes.

HAND-FOOT-AND-MOUTH DISEASE ICD-10: 074.3

- Systemic viral infection characterized by ulcerative enanthem; vesicular exanthem on the distal extremities; mild constitutional symptoms.
- **Etiology.** Enterovirus (picornavirus group, single-stranded RNA, nonenveloped). Commonly: Coxsackievirus A16 and EV71. Coxsackie A6 associated with eczema coxsackium.
- **Demography.** Most common in first decade. Outbreaks during warmer months (late summer, or early fall) in temperate climates. Highly contagious, spread from person to person by oral–oral and fecal–oral routes.
- **Pathogenesis.** Enteroviral implantation in the GI tract (buccal mucosa and ileum) with extension into regional lymph nodes. Seventy-two hours later viremia occurs with seeding of the oral mucosa and skin of the hands and feet.

CLINICAL MANIFESTATION

SYMPTOMS Frequently 5 to 10 *painful* ulcerative oral lesions, leading to a refusal to eat in children. Few to 100 cutaneous lesions appear together or shortly after the oral lesions and may be asymptomatic or painful and tender.

Macules and papules that quickly evolve to *vesicles*. Characteristically, lesions occur on the palms and soles, especially on the sides of fingers, toes, and buttocks. Vesicles may have characteristic "linear" shape; tender, painful; usually do not rupture (Fig. 27-24). At other cutaneous sites, vesicles can rupture, with formation of *erosions* and *crusts*. Lesions heal without scarring.

Eczema coxsackium will also present with vesiculobullous lesions in the distribution of preexisting eczema.

ORAL LESIONS Macules → grayish vesicles, arising on the hard palate, tongue, and buccal mucosa (Fig. 27-25). Vesicles quickly erode to 5- to 10-mm, small, punched out painful ulcers.

GENERAL FINDINGS May be associated with high fever, severe malaise, diarrhea, and joint pains. EV17 infections may have associated CNS (aseptic meningitis, encephalitis, meningoencephalitis, or flaccid paralysis), and lung involvement.

DIFFERENTIAL DIAGNOSIS

A sudden outbreak of oral and distal extremity lesions is pathognomonic for hand foot and mouth disease. However, if only the oral lesions are present, the differential diagnosis would include HSV infection, aphthous stomatitis,

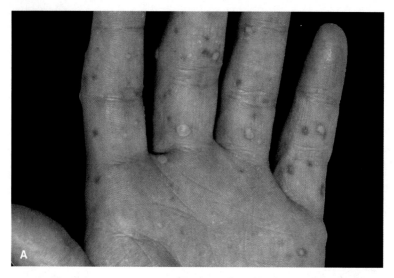

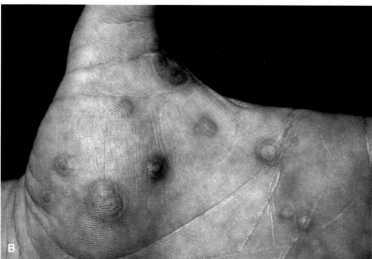

FIGURE 27-24 Hand-foot-and mouth disease (A) A 12-year-old male with classical oval vesicles on palms and fingers. **(B)** More extensive, almost bullous lesions on palm of another patient.

herpangina, erythema multiforme, and adverse drug reaction.

DIAGNOSIS

Usually made on clinical findings. Virus may be isolated from vesicles, throat washings, and stool specimens.

COURSE

Most commonly, hand foot and mouth disease is self-limited. Rise in serum antibodies eliminates the viremia in 7 to 10 days. Coxsackievirus has been implicated in cases of myocarditis, meningoencephalitis, aseptic meningitis, paralytic disease, and a systemic illness resembling measles. EV71 infections have higher morbidity/mortality rates resulting from CNS involvement and pulmonary edema.

TREATMENT

Symptomatic and supportive care.

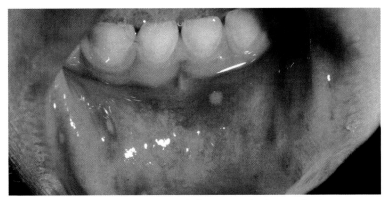

FIGURE 27-25 Hand-foot-and-mouth disease Multiple, superficial erosions with an erythematous halo on the lower labial mucosa; gingiva is normal. In primary herpetic gingivostomatitis, which presents with similar oral vesicular lesions, painful erosive gingivitis usually occurs as well.

HERPANGINA ICD-10: B08.5

- **Etiologic Agent.** Coxsackievirus A1–10; coxsackie B1–5; echoviruses; EV71.
- **Demography.** It usually affects children <5 year, prevalent in late summer and early fall in temperate climates.
- **Clinical Manifestation.** Sudden onset of fever, malaise, headache, anorexia, dysphagia, and sore throat.
- **Enanthem.** 1- to 2-mm gray-white papules/vesicles that evolve to ulcers with red halos, and diffuse pharyngeal hyperemia (Fig. 27-26). Distributed on the anterior tonsillar pillars, soft palate, uvula, and tonsils. Usually lasts 4 to 6 days, and its course is self-limited.

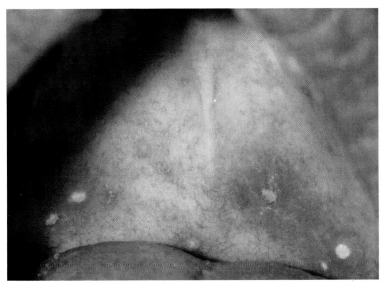

FIGURE 27-26 Herpangina Multiple, small vesicles and erosions with erythematous halos on the soft palate; some taste buds on the posterior tongue are inflamed and prominent.

ERYTHEMA INFECTIOSUM ICD-10: B08.3

- Childhood exanthem associated with primary human parvovirus B19 (HPVB19) infection.
- Characterized by edematous erythematous plaques on the cheeks ("slapped cheeks"); erythematous lacy eruption on the trunk and extremities.

ETIOLOGY AND EPIDEMIOLOGY

ETIOLOGY HPVB19 is a small single-stranded, nonenveloped virus. It is present in respiratory tract during the viremic stage of primary infection. Transmission by droplet aerosol.

DEMOGRAPHY More common in young. 60% of adolescents and adults are seropositive for antiparvovirus B19 IgG. Symptomatic rheumatic involvement is more common in adult women.

PATHOGENESIS Viremia develops 6 days after intranasal inoculation of HPVB19 into volunteers who lack serum antibodies to the virus. IgM and then IgG antibodies develop after a week and clear viremia. Significant bone marrow depression can occur at this time. The exanthem begins 17 to 18 days after inoculation and may be accompanied by arthralgia and/or arthritis; these findings are mediated by immune complexes. In compromised hosts, HPVB19 can destroy erythroid precursor cells,

causing severe aplastic crisis in adults and hydrops fetalis in the fetus.

CLINICAL MANIFESTATION

Constitutional symptoms are more severe in adults, with fever, and adenopathy. Arthritis/arthralgias involving the small joints of the hand, knees, wrists, ankles, and feet. Numbness and tingling of fingers.

CUTANEOUS LESIONS Edematous, confluent plaques on malar face ("slapped cheeks") (Fig. 27-27A) (nasal bridge, periorbital regions spared); lesions fade over 1 to 4 days. Usually absent in adults.

NONFACIAL LESIONS Appear after facial lesions. Erythematous macules and papules that become confluent, giving a lacy or reticulated appearance (Fig. 27-27B). Best seen on extensor arms; also trunk and neck. Fade in 5 to 9 days. Reticulated rash may recur. Adults: Reticulated macules on extremities.

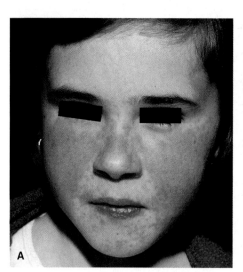 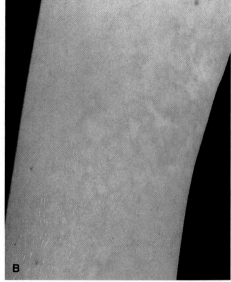

FIGURE 27-27 (A) Erythema infectiosum: slapped cheek A 10-year-old child. Diffuse erythema and edema of the cheeks with "slapped cheek" facies. **(B) Erythema infectiosum: reticulated erythema** A 10-year-old child. Discrete, erythematous macules with ring formation on the arm.

Less Commonly, morbilliform, confluent, circinate, and annular exanthems. Rarely, purpura, vesicles, pustules, and palmoplantar desquamation. HPVB19 also reported to cause papular purpuric "gloves and socks" *syndrome.*

MUCOSAL LESIONS Uncommonly, enanthem with glossal and pharyngeal erythema; red macules on buccal and palatal mucosa.

JOINTS Arthralgia and/or arthritis in 10% of children; typically involving large joints. Arthritis in adult women.

CNS AND PERIPHERAL NEUROPATHY Occur in persons with altered immunity.

DIFFERENTIAL DIAGNOSIS

CHILDREN WITH ERYTHEMA INFECTIOSUM Childhood exanthems, *Haemophilus influenzae* cellulitis, and adverse cutaneous drug reaction.

ADULTS WITH ARTHRITIS Lyme arthritis, rheumatoid arthritis, and rubella.

DIAGNOSIS

Usually made on clinical findings. Demonstration of IgM anti-HPVB19 antibodies or IgG seroconversion. Demonstration of HPVB19 in serum. During aplastic crisis: Absence of reticulocytes, falling hemoglobin, and hypoplasia or aplasia of erythroid series in bone marrow.

COURSE

CUTANEOUS "Slapped cheeks" are noted first, fading over 1 to 4 days. Then, reticulated rash appears on the trunk, neck, and extensor extremities. Eruption lasts 5 to 9 days but characteristically can recur for weeks or months.

ARTHRALGIAS Self-limited, lasting 3 weeks, but may persist for several months or years.

APLASTIC CRISIS In patients with chronic hemolytic anemias, transient aplastic crisis may occur, manifested by worsening anemia, fatigue, and pallor.

FETAL B19 INFECTION Intrauterine infection may be complicated by nonimmune fetal hydrops secondary to infection of RBC precursors, hemolysis, severe anemia, tissue anoxia, and high-output heart failure. Risk <10% after maternal infection.

IMMUNOCOMPROMISED HOST Prolonged chronic anemia associated with persistent lysis of RBC precursors. At risk: HIV disease, congenital immunodeficiencies, acute leukemia, organ transplants, systemic lupus erythematosus, and infants <1 year. Responds to intravenous immunoglobulin (IVIg).

TREATMENT

Symptomatic.

GIANOTTI–CROSTI SYNDROME ICD-10: L44.4

- Cutaneous reaction pattern associated with primary infection and immune response to viruses, bacteria, and vaccines.
- **Etiologic Agents.**
  - Viruses: EBV, CMV, hepatitis B virus (ayw strain), coxsackievirus, parainfluenza virus, respiratory syncytial virus, rotavirus, adenovirus, echovirus, pox virus, poliovirus, parvovirus, HIV, hepatitis A virus, and hepatitis C virus.
  - Bacteria: *Mycoplasma pneumoniae, Borrelia burgdorferi, Bartonella henselae,* and group A streptococcus.
  - Vaccines: Influenza, diphtheria, tetanus, pertussis, BCG, *H. influenzae* type b, and oral polio.
- **Epidemiology.** Occurs in children from 6 months to 12 years. Manifestation of immune response to transient viremia with immune complex deposition in the skin.

CLINICAL MANIFESTATION

Discrete, nonpruritic, erythematous, monomorphic papules (Fig. 27-28). Lesions become coalescent. Face, buttocks, and extensor surfaces of extremities; symmetric. Typically, the trunk is spared. Duration is 2 to 8 weeks. *Synonym*: Papular acrodermatitis of childhood (PAC).

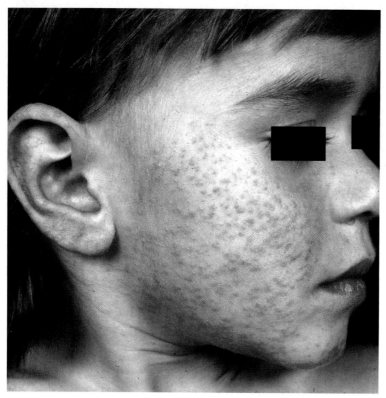

FIGURE 27-28 Gianotti–Crosti syndrome A 5-year-old girl with multiple red papules becoming confluent of the cheeks.

ARBOVIRUS ICD-10: A94

- Arbovirus (ARthropod-BOrne virus) is a group of RNA viruses transmitted to humans by arthropods.
- Vectors of Arbovirus. Mosquitoes, ticks, sandflies, and other arthropods feed on the blood of vertebrates and remain infective for life. The most important vector for human infection is the mosquito Aedes Aegypti, less commonly by A. albopictus. Mosquito acquires virus by feeding upon viremic human; remains infective for life.
- Dengue, chikungunya, and Zika virus are special among arboviruses, having dermatologic manifestations in addition to acute symptomatic illness with fever, malaise, and headache. Other arboviruses do not cause rash with the acute infection.
- Other arboviruses that do not cause rash include yellow fever, West Nile fever, Crimean-Congo hemorrhagic fever, and hundreds of others.

DENGUE ICD10: A90

- Self-limited systemic viral infection transmitted from mosquitoes to humans.
- **Incidence.** Globally, 390 million infections annually, of which 96 million present with clinical symptoms.

CLINICAL SYNDROMES

DENGUE FEVER Arthralgia–rash syndrome with abrupt onset of fever and muscle and joint pains, usually with retro-orbital pain, photophobia, and lymphadenopathy. *Rash:* Early flushing; later macules/papules; purpura.

DENGUE HEMORRHAGIC FEVER Increased vascular permeability and plasma leakage from blood vessels into tissues, thrombocytopenia, and bleeding manifestations (frank hemorrhage to spontaneous petechiae or elicited by tourniquet test). Plasma leakage causes a rise in hematocrit, effusions, and edema, especially in the chest and abdomen (Fig. 27-29).

DENGUE SHOCK SYNDROME Occurs when leakage or bleeding, or both, are sufficient to induce hypovolemic shock.

ETIOLOGY AND EPIDEMIOLOGY

ETIOLOGY Flavivirus, single-stranded RNA virus. Four distinct dengue serotypes (DEN-1, 2, 3, 4). Arthropod-borne virus (arbovirus). Infection confers lifelong protection against that serotype, but cross-protection between serotypes is of short duration. Infection with virus of a different serotype after the primary attack is more apt to result in severe disease, dengue hemorrhagic fever, or dengue shock syndrome.

VECTOR Transmitted by the bite of the *Aedes aegypti* mosquito; less commonly *A. albopictus*. Mosquito acquires virus by feeding upon viremic human; remains infective for life.

DEMOGRAPHY 2.5 billion people live in dengue endemic areas; 50 to 100 million cases of dengue occur annually worldwide. Most cases

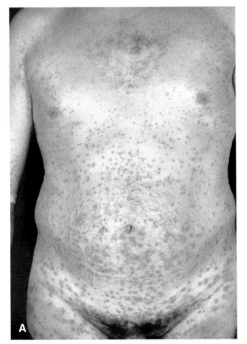
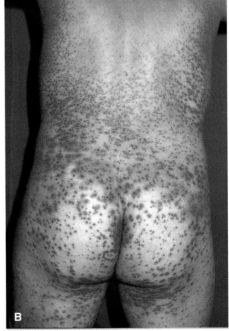

FIGURE 27-29 Dengue hemorrhagic fever A 39-year-old with fever and rash after a trip to Malaysia. Dermal hemorrhage and petechiae on normal tanned **(A)** and white skin are seen on the buttocks 48 hours later [white islands in a sea of red **(B)**]. (Courtesy of C Hafner et al. Hemorrhagic dengue fever after trip to Malaysia. *Hautarzt.* 2006;57(8):705–707. © Springer 2005.)

occurring in United States are imported in travelers returning from the tropics. Year-round transmission between latitudes 25°N and 25°S. Increased incidence associated with rapid urban population growth, overcrowding, lax mosquito control, and climate change.

PATHOGENESIS of severe syndrome involves preexisting dengue antibody. Virus–antibody complexes formed within a few days of second dengue infection; non-neutralizing enhancing antibodies promote infection of higher numbers of mononuclear cells, followed by release of cytokines, vasoactive mediators, and procoagulants, leading to the disseminated intravascular coagulation.

CLINICAL MANIFESTATION

INCUBATION PERIOD 3 to 7 days after bite of infected mosquito. Most dengue virus infections are asymptomatic.

FEBRILE PHASE High temperature ($\geq$38.5°C) accompanied by headache, vomiting, myalgia, and joint pain. In some cases, a *transient macular rash* (Fig. 27-29A). *Petechiae* and *bruising* may be noted at venipuncture sites (Fig. 27-29B). Lasts for 3 to 7 days after which most patients recover with complications.

CRITICAL PHASE Becomes apparent around the time of defervescence, evidenced by increasing hemoconcentration, hypoproteinemia, pleural effusions, and ascites. Hemorrhagic

manifestations occur, manifested by major skin bleeding, gastrointestinal (GI), or vaginal bleeding. Moderate-to-severe thrombocytopenia common, followed by rapid recovery during recovery phase.

RECOVERY PHASE Altered vascular permeability resolves after 48 to 72 hours. A second rash may be appearing during recovery phase, *mild macules/papules* to severe, pruritic *suggesting leukocytoclastic vasculitis*. Rash resolves with desquamation over 1 to 2 weeks. Profound fatigue persists for several weeks after recovery.

DIFFERENTIAL DIAGNOSIS

Other arboviral infection such as chikungunya and viral exanthems. Disease with local prevalence: Typhoid, malaria, leptospirosis, viral hepatitis, rickettsial diseases, and bacterial sepsis.

DIAGNOSIS

Consider diagnosis in travelers with febrile illness recently returned from endemic areas. During febrile phase, detection of viral nucleic acid in serum diagnostic. IgM seroconversion between paired samples is confirmatory finding.

TREATMENT

Symptomatic supportive therapy (http://www.cdc.gov/dengue/).

CHIKUNGUNYA ICD10: A92

CLINICAL MANIFESTATION

The majority of people infected with chikungunya virus become symptomatic. The incubation period is typically 3 to 7 days (range, 1 to 12 days). The disease is most often characterized by acute onset of fever (typically >39°C [102°F]) and polyarthralgia. Joint symptoms are usually bilateral and symmetric, and can be severe and debilitating. Other symptoms may include headache, myalgia, arthritis, conjunctivitis, nausea/vomiting, or maculopapular rash. Clinical laboratory findings can include lymphopenia, thrombocytopenia, elevated creatinine, and elevated hepatic transaminases.

RECOVERY PHASE Acute symptoms typically resolve within 7 to 10 days. Rare complications include uveitis, retinitis, myocarditis, hepatitis, nephritis, bullous skin lesions, hemorrhage, meningoencephalitis, myelitis, cranial nerve

palsies, and Guillain–Barré syndrome. Some patients might have relapse of rheumatologic symptoms (e.g., polyarthralgia, polyarthritis, tenosynovitis) in the months following acute illness. Variable proportions of patients with persistent joint pains for months to years. Mortality is rare and occurs mostly in older adults.

DIFFERENTIAL DIAGNOSIS Varies based on place of residence, travel history, and exposures. Dengue and chikungunya viruses are transmitted by the same mosquitoes and have similar clinical features. The two viruses can circulate in the same area and can cause occasional co-infections in the same patient.

MANAGEMENT There is no specific antiviral therapy for chikungunya virus infection. Treatment is for symptoms and can include rest, fluids, and use of non-steroidal anti-inflammatory drugs (NSAIDs) to relieve acute pain and fever.

ZIKA ICD10: A92

The explosive pandemic of Zika virus infection is occurring throughout South America, Central America, and the Caribbean.

ETIOLOGY AND EPIDEMIOLOGY

ETIOLOGY Zika virus is a single-stranded RNA virus of the Flaviviridae family, genus Flavivirus.

TRANSMISSION Anthroponotic (human-to-vector-to-human) occurs during outbreaks. Perinatal, in utero, and possible sexual and transfusion transmission events have also been reported.

CLINICAL MANIFESTATIONS

Most people infected with Zika virus are asymptomatic. Characteristic clinical findings are acute onset of fever with maculopapular rash, arthralgia, or conjunctivitis. Other commonly reported symptoms include myalgia and headache.

RECOVERY Illness is usually mild with symptoms lasting for several days to a week. Severe disease requiring hospitalization is uncommon and case fatality is low. Guillain–Barré syndrome reported in patients following suspected Zika virus infection. Fetal malformation with microcephaly has been reported with intrauterine Zika virus infection.

MANAGEMENT No specific antiviral treatment is available for Zika virus disease. Treatment is generally supportive.

HERPES SIMPLEX VIRUS DISEASE ICD-10: B00

- Classically with grouped vesicles arising on an erythematous base on keratinized skin (Fig. 27-30) or mucous membrane. Can also be "atypical," with patch(es) of erythema, small erosions, fissures, or subclinical lesions that shed HSV.
- Following primary infection, HSV persists in sensory ganglia for the life of the patient, recurring with lessening in immunity.
- **Clinical Manifestation:**
  - In healthy individuals, recurrent infections are asymptomatic or minor, resolving spontaneously or with antiviral therapy.
  - With host defense defects, mucocutaneous lesions can be extensive, chronic, or disseminate to skin or viscera.

FIGURE 27-30 Herpes simplex: Typical lesion A 39-year-old male with lesion on the abdomen above the waist. Grouped vesicles on an erythematous base/plaque are seen. The lesion is recurrent.

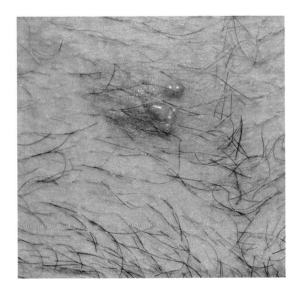

ETIOLOGY AND EPIDEMIOLOGY

ETIOLOGY HSV-1 and HSV-2.

- Labialis: HSV-1 (80), HSV-2 (20%).
- Urogenital: HSV-2 (80%), HSV-1 (20%).
- Herpetic whitlow: HSV-1 (60%), HSV-2 (40%).
- Neonatal: HSV-2 (80%), HSV-1 (20%).

TRANSMISSION Most transmission occurs when persons shed the virus but lack symptoms or lesions. Usually skin–skin, skin–mucosa, and mucosa–skin contact. Herpes gladiatorum is transmitted by skin-to-skin contact in wrestlers. Most commonly young adults; range, infancy to senescence.

FACTORS FOR RECURRENCE Approximately one-third of persons who develop herpes labialis will experience a recurrence; of these, one-half will experience at least two recurrences annually. Usual factors for herpes labialis: skin/mucosal irritation [ultraviolet (UV) radiation], menstruation, fever, common cold, altered immune states, and the site of infection (genital herpes recurs more frequently than labial). Host defense defections: HIV disease, malignancy (leukemia/lymphoma), transplantation (bone marrow, solid organ), chemotherapy, systemic glucocorticoids, other immunosuppressive drugs, and radiotherapy.

PATHOGENESIS Primary HSV infection occurs through close contact with a person shedding virus at a peripheral site, mucosal surface, or secretion. Transmission occurs via inoculation onto susceptible mucosal surface or break in skin (Fig. 27-31A). After exposure to HSV, the virus replicates in epithelial cells, causing lysis of infected cells, vesicle formation, and local inflammation. After primary infection at the inoculation site, HSV ascends peripheral sensory nerves and enters sensory (Fig. 27-31B) or autonomic nerve root (vagal) ganglia, where latency is established. Retrograde transport of HSV among nerves and establishment of latency are not dependent on viral replication in skin or neurons; neurons can be infected in the absence of symptoms (Fig. 27-31C).

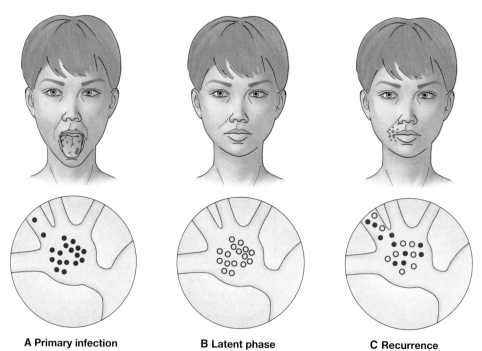

A Primary infection   **B Latent phase**   **C Recurrence**

FIGURE 27-31 Herpes labialis (A) With primary HSV infection, virus replicates in the oropharyngeal epithelium, ascends peripheral sensory nerves into the trigeminal ganglion. Herpes labialis **(B)** HSV persists in a latent phase within the trigeminal ganglion for the life of the individual. **(C)** Various stimuli initiate reactivation of latent virus, which then descends sensory nerves to the lips or perioral skin, resulting in recurrent herpes labialis.

Latency can occur after both symptomatic and asymptomatic primary infection. Periodically, HSV may reactivate from its latent state and virus particles then travel along sensory neurons to skin and mucosal sites to cause recurrent disease episodes. Recurrent mucocutaneous shedding can be associated with or without (asymptomatic shedding) lesions; the virus can be transmitted to a new host when shedding occurs.

Recurrences usually occur in the vicinity of the primary infection; may be clinically symptomatic or asymptomatic.

CLINICAL MANIFESTATION

See "Nongenital Herpes Simplex Virus Infection," p. 682.

LABORATORY EXAMINATIONS

TZANCK SMEAR (Fig. 27-32). Optimally, fluid from intact vesicle is smeared thinly on a microscope slide, dried, and stained with either Wright or Giemsa stain. Positive, if acantholytic keratinocytes or multinucleated giant acantholytic keratinocytes are detected. Positive in 75% of early cases, either primary or recurrent. *Antigen Detection Direct Fluorescent Antibody (DFA)*. Monoclonal antibodies, specific for HSV-1 and HSV-2 antigens, detect and differentiate HSV antigens on smear from lesion.

DIAGNOSIS

HSV infection confirmed by viral culture or antigen detection. Seroconversion diagnoses first-episode infections. Antibodies to (g)H1 or (g)G2 may take 2 to 6 weeks to develop. Recurring herpes can be ruled out if seronegative for HSV antibodies.

TREATMENT

PREVENTION Avoid skin-to-skin contact during outbreaks.

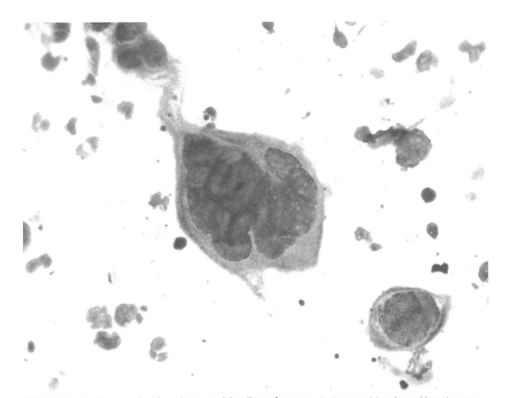

FIGURE 27-32 Herpes simplex virus: positive Tzanck smear A giant, multinucleated keratinocyte on a Giemsa-stained smear obtained from a vesicle base. Compare the size of the giant cell to that of the neutrophils also seen in this preparation. An isolated acantholytic keratinocyte is also seen. Identical findings are present in lesions caused by varicella zoster virus.

TOPICAL ANTIVIRAL THERAPY Minimal efficacy. Acyclovir 5% ointment, apply 6 times daily for 7 days. Penciclovir 1% cream every two hours while awake for recurrent orolabial infection.
ORAL ANTIVIRAL THERAPY DRUGS Acyclovir, valacyclovir, and famciclovir. Valacyclovir, the prodrug of acyclovir, has a better bioavailability and is nearly 85% absorbed after oral administration. Famciclovir is equally effective for cutaneous HSV infections.
Acyclovir: 400 mg 3 times daily or 200 mg 5 times daily for 7 to 10 days.
Valacyclovir: 1 g twice daily for 7 to 10 days for initial genital outbreak.

Famciclovir: 250 mg 3 times daily for 5 to 10 days.
RECURRENCES
Acyclovir: 400 mg three times daily for 5 days.
Valacyclovir: 1000 mg twice daily for 5 to 10 days for genital HSV recurrence, 2000 mg twice daily for 1 day for labialis recurrence.
Famciclovir: 1000 mg twice daily for 1 day for genital HSV recurrence, 1500 mg x 1 for labialis recurrence.
Continuous oral maintenance therapy (e.g. valaciclovir 500 mg/day) can be considered in patients with at least 6 episodes/year.

NONGENITAL HERPES SIMPLEX

- Nongenital HSV infection, whether primary or recurrent, is often asymptomatic.
- Lesions may present as group vesicles on an erythematous base (Fig. 27-30) or as recurrent erythematous plaque ± erosions.

For genital HSV infection, see Section 30.

CLINICAL MANIFESTATION

PRIMARY HSV INFECTION Asymptomatic primary infection is common. Symptomatic primary HSV is characterized by *vesicles at the site of inoculation* (Fig. 27-33), and may be associated with regional lymphadenopathy, and systemic symptoms (fever, headache, malaise, or myalgia). Primary herpetic gingivostomatitis is the most common symptom complex accompanying primary HSV infection in children (Fig. 27-34). Primary herpetic vulvovaginitis is seen most often in young women (see also Section 30).

Erythematous papules that quickly evolve to *grouped vesicles* and pustules occur at the site of inoculation (Fig. 27-33). Vesicles are often fragile, rupturing easily, to form *erosions* as the overlying epidermis sloughs. The most common sites of primary HSV infection are the mouth, anogenitalia, and hand/fingers. Erosions heal in 2 to 4 weeks, often with resultant postinflammatory hypo- or hyperpigmentation, uncommonly with scarring.
Regional Lymphadenopathy. May be tender.
PRIMARY HERPETIC GINGIVOSTOMATITIS Oral mucosa usually involved only in primary HSV infection with vesicles that quickly slough to form erosions (Fig. 27-34) at any site in the oropharynx: scanty to numerous. Gingival erythema, edema, and tenderness, edema. Severe

pain. Perioral facial involvement with vesicles and erosions common.
RECURRENT HERPES Prodrome of tingling, itching, or burning sensation usually precedes any visible skin changes by 24 hours. Systemic symptoms are usually absent. Grouped vesicles on erythematous base that evolve to erosions and crusts (Figs. 27-35A–D). Recurrent intraoral HSV is rare.
TRIGEMINAL NERVE HSV INFECTIONS

- *Perioral infection.* Recurrent facial herpes or cold sores are common (Fig. 27-35). Often preceded by prodromal symptoms (tingling, pain, burning sensation, or itching). Severe recurrences may complicate laser-resurfacing surgery.
- *Ocular infections.* Recurrent keratitis is a major cause of corneal scarring and visual loss. Continuous suppression therapy is recommended.
- *Herpetic facial paralysis.* Reactivation of geniculate ganglion infection implicated in pathogenesis of idiopathic facial palsy (Bell palsy). HSV-1 shedding detected in 40% of cases.
- *Herpes gladiatorum.* Transmission occurs during contact sports (wrestling, rugby, or football). Also occurs in cervical or lumbosacral dermatomes.

FIGURE 27-33 Herpes simplex: primary infection of the palm A 28-year-old female with a painful lesion on the palm for 3 days. A cluster of grouped pustules is seen on the palm. A red lymphangitis extends proximally on the wrist. The axillary lymph nodes were tender and enlarged. HSV-2 was detected on DFA. No antibodies to HSV-1 or 2 were detected, thus a primary infection.

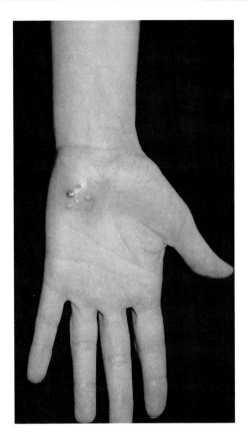

FIGURE 27-34 Herpes simplex: primary infection with gingivostomatitis A 6-year-old girl with history of atopic dermatitis. Multiple, very painful erosions on gingiva, labial mucosa and tongue (not shown). Tzanck smear was positive.

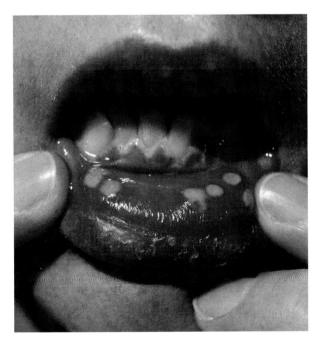

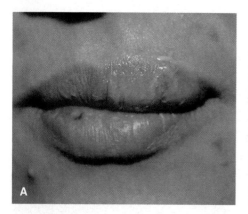
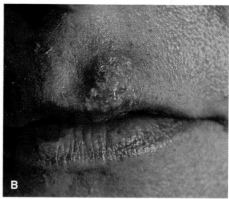
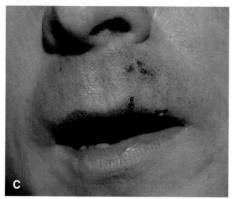
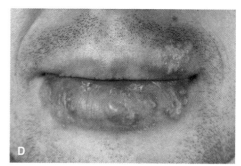

FIGURE 27-35 Herpes labialis: recurrent herpes labialis (A) Edematous lateral upper lip 24 hours after onset of tingling sensation. **(B)** Grouped vesicles on moustache area 48 hours after onset of symptoms. **(C)** Crusted erosion on upper lip and moustache area 7 days after onset of symptoms. **(D)** Painful vesicles, crusts and erosions on upper and lower lip in a 29-year-old male. The diagnosis was made on Tzanck smear.

HERPETIC FOLLICULITIS Occurs predominantly in the beard area (viral sycosis) in men. Characterized by follicular vesicles and later crusts (Fig. 27-36).

CERVICAL AND THORACIC SENSORY NERVE HSV INFECTIONS

- *Herpetic whitlow.* Infection of the tip of finger or thumb; uncommonly toe. Associated with painful neuritis in the affected finger (Fig. 27-37) and forearm.
- *HSV infection of the nipple.* Related to transmission of HSV from infant to mother during breast feeding.
- *HSV infections of the lumbosacral sensory nerves.* When lumbosacral ganglia become infected subsequent to anogenital herpes, recurrent lesions can occur on genitalia as well as the buttocks, thighs, and perianal mucosa. Perianal herpes does not necessarily imply direct anal inoculation of HSV. Herpes in the sacral dermatome may be accompanied by asymptomatic HSV reactivation/shedding from genital mucosa.

COMPLICATIONS OF HSV INFECTIONS OF PERIPHERAL SENSORY NERVOUS SYSTEM

- *Eczema herpeticum.* Usually follows autoinoculation of HSV (most commonly orolabial herpes) to atopic dermatitis (see "Herpes Simplex Virus: Widespread Cutaneous Infection Associated with Cutaneous Immunocompromise," p. 688).
- *S. aureus secondary infection.* Often occurs with eczema herpeticum.
- *Erythema multiforme.* In some individuals with recurrent HSV infections, erythema multiforme may occur with each recurrence (Fig. 27-38; see "Erythema Multiforme," Section 14).

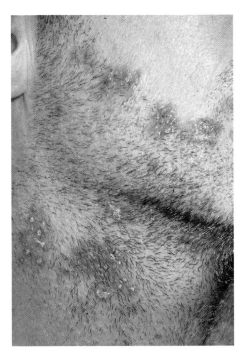

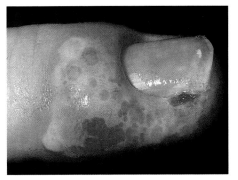

FIGURE 27-37 Herpes simplex virus infection: herpetic whitlow A 19-year-old male with painful finger lesions for 3 days. Painful, grouped, confluent vesicles on an erythematous edematous base of the distal finger were the first (and presumed primary) symptomatic infection.

FIGURE 27-36 Infectious folliculitis: herpes simplex virus A 40-year-old healthy male with discrete and grouped pustules and erosions in the beard area for 3 weeks. Lesions resolved with oral acyclovir.

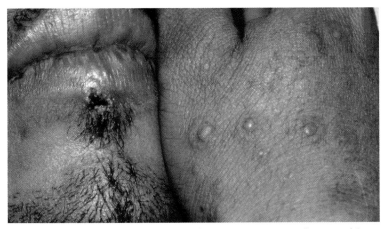

FIGURE 27-38 Herpes simplex virus infection: recurrent erythema multiforme A 31-year-old male with recurrent herpes labialis and disseminated lesions. Recurrent herpes labialis on the lower lip and IRIS-like edematous papules on the dorsum of the hand.

GENERAL FINDINGS Fever may be present during symptomatic primary herpetic gingivostomatitis.

REGIONAL LYMPHADENOPATHY Nonfluctuant, tender; usually unilateral.

CNS Signs of aseptic meningitis: Headache, fever, nuchal rigidity, CSF pleocytosis with normal sugar content, and positive HSV CSF culture.

DIFFERENTIAL DIAGNOSIS

PRIMARY INTRAORAL HSV INFECTION Aphthous stomatitis, hand foot and mouth disease, herpangina, and erythema multiforme.

RECURRENT LESION Fixed drug eruption.

LABORATORY EXAMINATIONS

See p. 681.

DIAGNOSIS

Clinical suspicion confirmed by Tzanck smear, viral culture, or antigen detection DFA.

COURSE

Recurrences of HSV tend to become less frequent in time. Eczema herpeticum may complicate various dermatoses. Patients with host defense defects may experience cutaneous dissemination of HSV, systemic dissemination of HSV, and chronic herpetic ulcers (see also Chronic Herpetic Ulcers). Erythema multiforme (see Section 14) may complicate each recurrence of herpes, occurring 1 to 2 weeks after an outbreak.

TREATMENT

See p. 682.

NEONATAL HERPES SIMPLEX ICD-10: P35.2

- **Risk factors** for neonatal HSV infection: Primary genital herpes in mother at time of delivery, absent maternal anti-HSV antibody, procedures on fetus, or father with HSV infection.
- **Etiology.** The majority of infections are caused by HSV-2; HSV-1 is more virulent in the newborn and associated with higher morbidity and mortality.
- **Transmission.** In utero (<5%); intrapartum (85%); postnatal acquisition. Mother is the most common source of infection. There is usually no clinical indication of shedding at the time of delivery. Shedding also occurs from uterine cervix. Incubation period in neonate: 4 to 21 days.
- **Demography.** Ninety-five percent of newborns with HSV infection contract it during labor and delivery (**Figs. 27-39** and **27-40**). Risk of transmission of HSV-2 from mother to newborn higher when primary infection occurs in the third trimester. Maternal antibodies transferred to fetus and protect against fetal infection.

CLINICAL MANIFESTATION

SKIN, EYES, MOUTH HERPES SIMPLEX Localized infection. Vesicles and erosions on skin, eyes, and mouth. Occurs at sites of trauma such as fetal scalp electrodes, extractors (vacuum and forceps), and circumcision. Margin of eyes and nasopharynx.

DISSEMINATED HERPES Disseminated infection. ±Vesicles, erosions. Hepatitis, pneumonitis, and disseminated intravascular coagulation. Difficult to diagnose in that up to 70% of infants have no mucocutaneous lesions.

CNS INFECTION ± Vesicles, erosions. Encephalitis. Presentation: Seizures, tremors, lethargy, unstable temperature, irritability, feeding problem, and bulging fontanelle.

TREATMENT

See p. 682.

FIGURE 27-39 Herpes simplex in neonate Fever and skin lesion. *Vesicles* and crusted erosions on the upper lip and large geographic ulcerations of the tongue, i.e., herpetic gingivostomatitis.

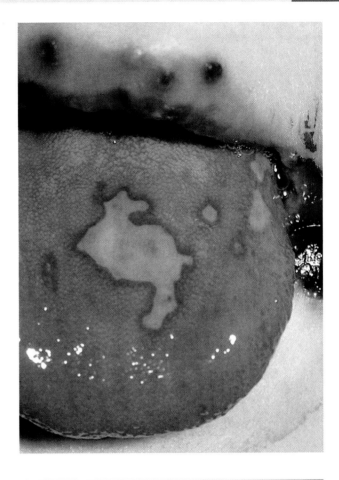

FIGURE 27-40 Herpes simplex virus infection: neonatal Neonate with skin lesion. Grouped and confluent vesicles with underlying erythema and edema on the shoulder, arising at the inoculation site.

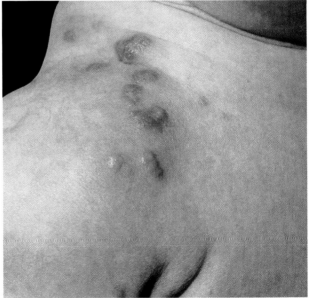

ECZEMA HERPETICUM

- HSV infects altered epidermis, most commonly the atopic dermatitis causing eczema herpeticum. Other dermatoses subject to HSV infection include Darier disease, thermal burns, Hailey–Hailey disease, immunobullous disease, ichthyosis vulgaris, and cutaneous T cell lymphoma.
- Epidemiology. HSV-1 > HSV-2. More common in children. May be transmitted from parental herpes labialis to child with atopic dermatitis, especially if erythrodermic.

CLINICAL MANIFESTATION

PRIMARY ECZEMA HERPETICUM May be associated with fever, malaise, and irritability. When recurrent, history of prior similar lesions; systemic symptoms less severe. Lesions begin in abnormal skin and may extend peripherally for several weeks during primary or recurrent HSV infections. Secondary infection with *S. aureus* is relatively common and may be painful. **CUTANEOUS LESIONS** Vesicles evolving into "punched-out" erosions (Figs. 27-41 and 27-42). Vesicles are first confined to eczematous skin. In contrast to primary or recurrent HSV eruptions, in eczema herpeticum, lesions are not grouped

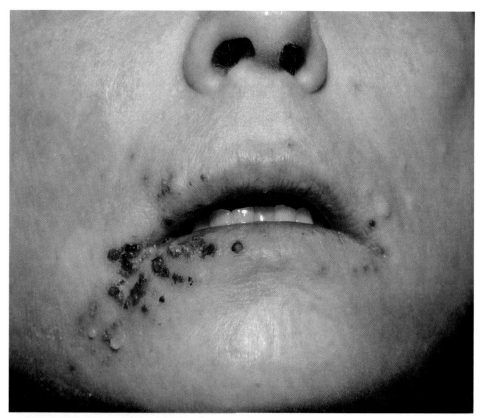

FIGURE 27-41 Herpes simplex: eczema herpeticum A 46-year-old female with painful crusted erosions and atopic dermatitis. DFA detected HSV-1.

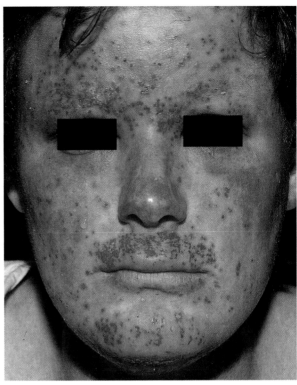

FIGURE 27-42 Herpes simplex: extensive eczema herpeticum Confluent and discrete crusted erosions associated with erythema and edema of the face of a 26-year-old male with atopic dermatitis.

but disseminated within the dermatosis. May later spread to normal-appearing skin. Erosions may become confluent, producing large denuded areas (Fig. 27-42). Successive crops of new vesiculation may occur. Common sites: face, neck, and trunk.

GENERAL EXAMINATION Primary infection may be associated with fever and lymphadenopathy.

DIFFERENTIAL DIAGNOSIS

WIDESPREAD VESICULOPUSTULES/EROSIONS
Varicella, disseminated VZV infection, and disseminated (systemic) HSV infection.

DIAGNOSIS

Clinical, confirmed by detection of HSV on culture or antigen detection. Rule out secondary infection by *S. aureus.*

COURSE AND TREATMENT

Untreated, primary episode of eczema herpeticum runs its course with resolution in 2 to 6 weeks. Recurrent episodes tend to be milder and not associated with systemic symptoms. Systemic dissemination can occur, especially with host defense defects. For treatment, see p. 682.

HERPES SIMPLEX WITH HOST DEFENSE DEFECTS

- In persons with host defense defects, herpes simplex may present as extensive local involvement, chronic herpetic ulcers, or skin disease associated with systemic HSV infection.
- **Host Defense Defects.** HIV disease, leukemia/lymphoma, bone marrow transplantation, chemotherapy for solid organ or BMT, autoimmune diseases, and malnutrition.
- **Pathogenesis.** After HSV viremia, disseminated cutaneous or visceral disease may occur. Factors determining whether severe localized disease, cutaneous dissemination, or visceral dissemination will occur are not well defined.

CLINICAL MANIFESTATION

PRIMARY HERPETIC INFECTION Local infection may be widespread on the face (Fig. 27-43),

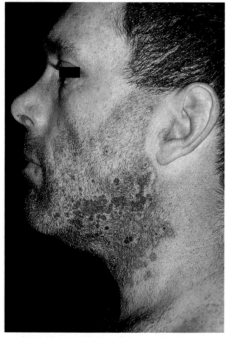

FIGURE 27-43 Herpes simplex: primary infection in HIV disease A 35-year-old male with HIV disease (CD4 cell count, 400/mL). Confluent vesicles and erosions with underlying erythema and edema (5–6-days duration) in the beard area. Gingivostomatitis and acute lymphadenopathy were also present, with onset of 5 days after orogenital sex.

oropharynx, and anogenital region with initial vesiculation followed by crusted erosions. Without antiviral therapy, lesions may persist to become chronic herpetic ulcers.

RECURRENT HERPES SIMPLEX With advanced HIV disease especially, mucocutaneous disease can be severe: Fingers with herpetic whitlow (Fig. 27-44A), oropharyngeal ulcers (Fig. 27-44B), esophageal ulcers, and anorectal ulcers. Systemic dissemination (see below) can occur from these sites, associated visceral HSV infection. Recurrent herpes simplex is manifested as persistent erosions and chronic ulcers. Chronic herpetic ulcers that persist in spite of adequate antiviral therapy (Fig. 27-45) (acyclovir, valacyclovir, and famciclovir) are usually caused by acyclovir-resistant HSV.

OROPHARYNGEAL ULCERS Large ulcerations occur on the tongue, hard palate, and gingivae. Linear ulcerations occur on the tongue (Fig. 27-44B).

ESOPHAGEAL ULCERS Usually associated with oropharyngeal herpetic ulcer. Esophagoscopy demonstrates mucosal erosions/ulceration.

ANOGENITAL ULCERS Acute ulceration of the vulva, penis, scrotum, and/or perineum may become chronic ulcers unless effectively treated. In individuals infected with acyclovir-resistant HSV, ulcerations do not respond to usual antiviral therapies. Anal ulcers usually occur via enlargement of perianal ulcers. Herpetic proctitis: Sigmoidoscopy shows friable mucosa and ulcerations.

MUCOCUTANEOUS DISSEMINATION Disseminated (nongrouped) vesicles and pustules often hemorrhagic with inflammatory halo; quickly rupture, resulting in "punched-out" erosions. Lesions may be necrotic and then ulcerate (Fig. 27-46).

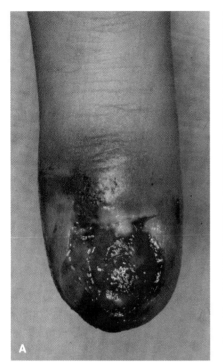
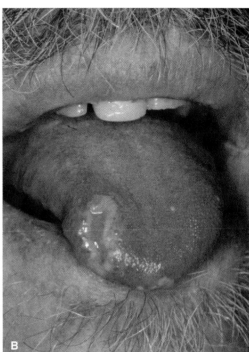

FIGURE 27-44 A 52-year-old male with advanced HIV disease had chronic herpetic ulcers on nares, finger, and tongue. **(A)** Herpetic whitlow with ulcer on the distal finger; nail had been avulsed by hand surgeon. **(B)** Chronic deep painful ulcer on the dorsolateral tongue.

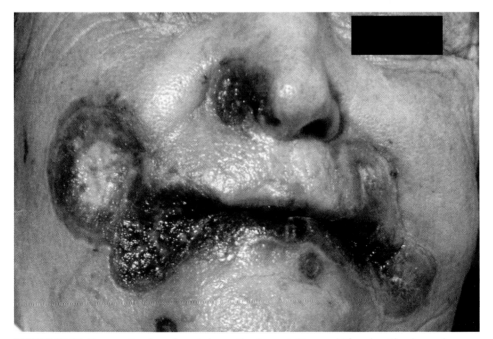

FIGURE 27-45 Herpes simplex: chronic herpetic ulcers A 65-year-old female with advanced myeloic leukemia. Ulcers did not respond to acyclovir but healed with foscarnet, but recurred.

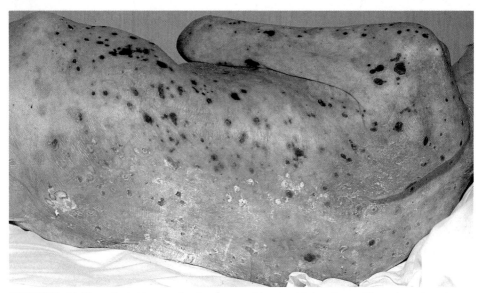

FIGURE 27-46 Disseminated herpes simplex 60-year old male with lymphoma. Disseminated erosions, ulcerations with hemorrhagic crusts on necrotic bases. Patients often have HSV visceral infection (lungs, liver, brain).

GENERAL EXAMINATION Widespread visceral involvement (liver, lungs, adrenals, GI tract, and CNS) can occur in persons with severe host defense defects.

DIFFERENTIAL DIAGNOSIS

CHRONIC HERPETIC ULCERS Chronic VZV infection, wound infection, and pressure ulcer.
ANORECTAL ULCERS HPV-induced SCC, Crohn disease
MUCOCUTANEOUS DISSEMINATION Varicella or disseminated herpes zoster (HZ), eczema herpeticum.

DIAGNOSIS

Clinical suspicion confirmed by Tzanck smear, positive HSV antigen detection DFA, or isolation of HSV on viral culture.

COURSE AND TREATMENT

For treatment, see p. 682. In HIV disease, persons successfully treated with ART experience reduction in frequency and severity of HSV recurrences. Infection with acyclovir-resistant strains results in chronic, progressive ulcerations that persist and/or continue to enlarge despite oral and IV acyclovir treatment.

VARICELLA ZOSTER VIRUS DISEASE ICD-10:B01

- **Varicella zoster virus** is a HHV that infects 98% of adults.
- **Primary VZV infection** *Varicella* **or** *chicken pox* is nearly always symptomatic and characterized by disseminated pruritic vesicles. During primary infection, VZV establishes lifelong infection in sensory ganglia.
- **When immunity to VZV declines**, VZV reactivates within the nerve cell, traveling down the neuron to the skin, where it erupts in a dermatomal pattern, i.e., HZ or *shingles*.
- **With host defense defects**, primary and reactivated VZV infections is often more severe, associated with higher morbidity rates and some mortality.
- **VZV vaccine** has reduced the incidence of varicella and HZ.

ETIOLOGY AND EPIDEMIOLOGY

ETIOLOGY VZV, a herpesvirus. Structurally similar to other herpesviruses.

AGE OF PRIMARY INFECTION Without immunization, 90% of cases occur in children <10 years, <5% in persons older than 15 years. With immunization (Varivax), the incidence is markedly reduced.

TRANSMISSION Airborne droplets and direct contact. Patients are contagious several days before varicella exanthem appears and until the last crop of vesicles. Crusts are not infectious. VZV can be aerosolized from the skin of persons with HZ, causing varicella in susceptible contacts.

PATHOGENESIS VZV enters through mucosa of the upper respiratory tract and oropharynx, followed by local replication, primary viremia, replication in cells of reticuloendothelial system, secondary viremia, and dissemination to skin and mucous membranes. During the course of varicella, VZV passes from skin lesions to the sensory nerves, travels to the sensory ganglia, and establishes latent infection. Immunity to VZV occurs with primary infection and with altered immunity, which results in VZV replication in sensory ganglia. VZV then travels down the sensory nerve, resulting in initial dermatomal symptoms, followed by skin lesions. Since the neuritis precedes the skin involvement, pain or itching appears before the skin lesions are visible. The locations of pain are varied and relate directly to the ganglion where VZV has emerged from latency to active infection. Prodromal symptoms may appear initially in the trigeminal, cervical, thoracic, lumbar, or sacral dermatome. *Postherpetic neuralgia* (PHN) is complex regional pain syndrome.

LABORATORY EXAMINATIONS

VZV ANTIGEN DETECTION DFA Smear of vesicle fluid or scraping from ulcer base/margin: DFA test detects VZV-specific antigen. Sensitive and specific method for identifying VZV-infected lesions. Higher yield than VZV cultures.

TZANCK SMEAR Cytology of fluid or scraping from base of vesicle or pustule shows both giant and multinucleated acantholytic epidermal cells (as does that of HSV infections) (Fig. 27-32).

SEROLOGY Seroconversion documents primary VZV infection.

DERMATOPATHOLOGY Lesional skin or visceral biopsy specimen shows multinucleated giant epithelial cells indicating HSV-1, HSV-2, or VZV infection. Immunoperoxidase stains specific for HSV-1, HSV-2, or VZV antigens can identify the specific herpesvirus.

VZV: VARICELLA

- The highly contagious primary infection caused by VZV. *Synonym*: Chicken pox.
- Characterized by successive crops of pruritic vesicles that evolve to pustules, crusts, and, at times, scars.
- Primary infection occurring in adulthood may be complicated by pneumonia and encephalitis.

EPIDEMIOLOGY

INCIDENCE Incidence of varicella has decreased as vaccination coverage has increased. Prior to 1995, there were 3 to 4 million cases in the United States annually.

CLINICAL MANIFESTATION

VESICULAR LESIONS occur in successive crops. Often single, discrete lesions: Scanty in number in children; more numerous in adults. Initial lesions are papules (often not observed) that may appear as *wheals* and quickly evolve to *vesicles*, superficial and thin-walled with surrounding erythema. Vesicles rapidly evolve to pustules and *crusted erosions* over an 8- to 12-hour period. With subsequent crops, all stages of evolution may be noted simultaneously, i.e., papules, vesicles, pustules, crusts, i.e., polymorphic (Figs. 27-47 and 27-48).

CRUSTED EROSIONS heal in 1 to 3 weeks, leaving a pink, somewhat depressed base. Characteristic *punched-out permanent scars* may persist.

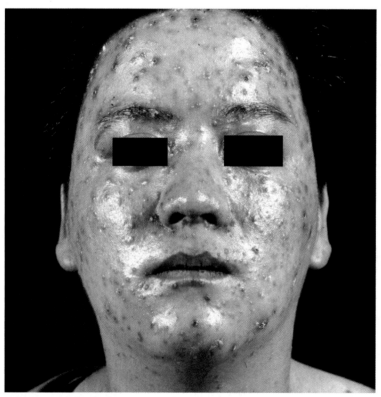

FIGURE 27-47 Varicella A 30-year-old female with pruritic eruption for 2 days. Multiple, pruritic, erythematous papules, vesicles and pustules on the face and neck. Several vesicles have evolved to crusted erosion. Note lesions are not in the same stage of evolution which contrasts small pox. **[compare this with** Fig. 27-8]

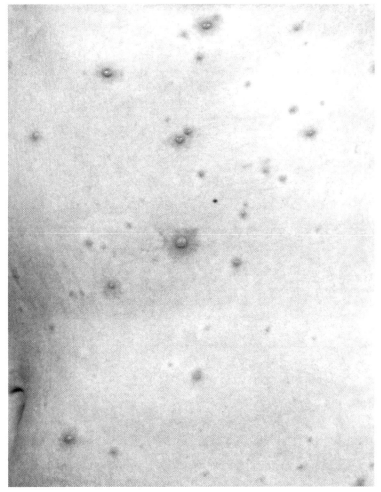

FIGURE 27-48 Varicella Lesions on the chest of a 23-year-old female. Vesicles, partly umbilicated, with an erythematous ring in different stages of development.

DISTRIBUTION First lesions begin on face (Fig. 27-47) and scalp, spreading inferiorly to trunk and extremities. Most profuse in areas least exposed to pressure, i.e., on the back between the shoulder blades, flanks, axillae, popliteal, and antecubital fossae. Density highest on the trunk (Fig. 27-48) and face, but less on the extremities. The palms and soles are usually spared.

MUCOUS MEMBRANES Vesicles (not often observed) and subsequent shallow erosions (2 to 3 mm). Most common on palate. Less common on other mucosal sites.

GENERAL EXAMINATION *VZV pneumonitis* occurs with increased frequency in adolescents and adults. *CNS* involvement with cerebellar ataxia and encephalitis can occur.

"MALIGNANT" VARICELLA occurs in persons with host defense defects. Pneumonitis, hepatitis, encephalitis, disseminated intravascular coagulation, and purpura fulminans may occur.

DIFFERENTIAL DIAGNOSIS

Disseminated HSV infection, cutaneous dissemination of zoster, eczema herpeticum, rickettsialpox, and enterovirus infections.

DIAGNOSIS

Usually made on clinical findings alone. Seroconversion, i.e., fourfold or greater rise in VZV titers.

COURSE

The most common complication in children <5 years is secondary bacterial infection. *Varicella encephalitis* and *Reye syndrome* occur in children 5 to 11 years of age. Two percent of fetal varicella are associated with maternal varicella in the first trimester of pregnancy. *Fetal varicella syndrome* is characterized by limb hypoplasia, eye and brain damage, and skin lesions. Varicella in immunocompromised may be complicated by hepatitis, encephalitis, and hemorrhagic complications.

TREATMENT

IMMUNIZATION Vaccination is 80% effective in preventing symptomatic VZV infection; 5 % of immunized children develop rash.

SYMPTOMATIC THERAPY Antihistamines lotions; avoid antipyretics because of the risk of Reye syndrome.

ANTIVIRAL AGENTS Decrease severity of course if given within 24 hours of onset.

Neonates: Acyclovir 10 mg/kg every 8h for 10 days.

Children: (2 to 18 yrs) Valaciclovir 20 mg/ kg every 8 h for 5 days or acyclovir 20 mg/kg every 6 h for 5 days.

Adolescents: Valaciclovir 1 g PO every 8 h for 7 days.

Immunocompromised: Valaciclovir 1 g PO for 7 to 10 days; acyclovir 800 mg by mouth 5 times a day; or famciclovir 500 mg by mouth every 8 h for 7 to 10 days.

Severely immunocompromised: Acyclovir 10 mg/kg IV every 8 h for 7 to 10 days.

Acyclovir resistant: Foscarnet 40 mg/kg IV every 8 h until resolution.

VZV: HERPES ZOSTER ICD-10: B02

- An acute dermatomal infection associated with reactivation of VZV. *Synonym*: Shingles.
- Characterized by unilateral dysesthesia. A vesicular or bullous eruption limited to a dermatome(s) innervated by a corresponding sensory ganglion.
- Postherpetic neuralgia is a major morbidity.

ETIOLOGY AND EPIDEMIOLOGY

The epidemiology of VZV infections is changing resulting from immunization with live (attenuated) virus vaccine for prevention of varicella in children and HZ in older adults. The cumulative lifetime incidence of HZ is 10 to 20% and higher in those with host defense defects.

PATHOGENESIS In varicella VZV passes from lesions in the skin and mucosa via sensory fibers centripetally to sensory ganglia. In the ganglia, the virus establishes lifelong latent infection. Reactivation occurs in those ganglia in which VZV has achieved the highest density and is triggered by immunosuppression, trauma, tumor, or irradiation (see risk factors). Virus multiplies and spreads centrifugally, down the sensory nerve to the skin/mucosa where it produces the characteristic vesicles (Fig. 27-49).

CLINICAL MANIFESTATION

Herpes zoster manifests in three distinct clinical stages: (1) prodrome, (2) active infection, and (3) PHN.

PRODROME *Pain*, *tenderness*, and *paresthesia* in the involved dermatome (Fig. 27-50) precedes the eruption. Pain can mimic angina or acute abdomen. *Allodynia*: Heightened sensitivity to mild stimuli. *Zoster sine herpete*: Nerve involvement can occur without cutaneous zoster. Flu-like constitutional symptoms can occur during prodrome and active infection.

DERMATOMAL LESIONS *Papules* (24 hours) → *vesicles*-bullae (48 hours) → pustules (96 hours) → *crusts* (7 to 10 days). New lesions continue to appear for up to 1 week. Erythematous, edematous base (Fig. 27-51) with superimposed clear vesicles, sometimes hemorrhagic. Vesicles erode forming crusted erosions.

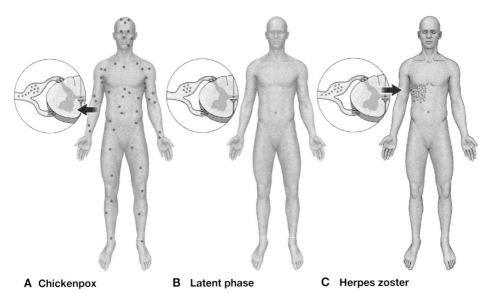

A Chickenpox   **B** Latent phase   **C** Herpes zoster

FIGURE 27-49 Varicella and herpes zoster (A) During primary VZV infection (varicella or chicken pox), virus infects sensory ganglia. **(B)** VZV persists in a latent phase within ganglia for the life of the individual. **(C)** With diminished immune function, VZV reactivates within sensory ganglia, descends sensory nerves, and replicates in skin.

Dermatomal crusting usually resolves in 2 to 4 weeks.

Distribution. Unilateral, dermatomal (Fig. 27-50). Two or more contiguous dermatomes may be involved. Noncontiguous dermatomal zoster is rare.

Hematogenous dissemination to other skin sites in 10% of healthy individuals (see herpes zoster with cutaneous dissemination, p. 701).

Site of Predilection. Thoracic (>50%) (Fig. 27-51), trigeminal (10 to 20%) (Fig. 27-52A), lumbosacral, and cervical (10 to 20%) (Fig. 27-53).

MUCOUS MEMBRANES Vesicles and erosions occur in mouth (Fig. 27-52B), vagina, and bladder, depending on dermatome involved.

LYMPHADENOPATHY Regional nodes draining the area are often enlarged and tender.

SENSORY OR MOTOR NERVE CHANGES Detectable by neurologic examination. Sensory defects (temperature, pain, or touch) and (mild) motor paralysis, e.g., facial palsy.

OPHTHALMIC ZOSTER Nasociliary involvement of V-1 (ophthalmic) branch of the trigeminal nerve occurs in about one-third of cases and is heralded by vesicles on the side and tip of the nose (Fig. 27-52A). Complications include uveitis, keratitis, conjunctivitis, retinitis, optic neuritis, glaucoma, proptosis, cicatricial lid retraction, and extraocular muscle palsies. Acute retinal necrosis is more common with immune deficiency.

DELAYED CONTRALATERAL HEMIPARESIS Typical presentation is headache and hemiplegia occurring in a patient with recent history of HZ ophthalmicus.

CONSTITUTIONAL SYMPTOMS Prodromal stage and active vesiculation: Flu-like symptoms. Chronic stages: Depression is very common in individuals with PHN.

POSTHERPETIC NEURALGIA Characterized by constant, severe, stabbing or burning, dysesthetic pain that may persist for months or years in a minority of patients, especially in the elderly.

SCARS Necrotic HZ lesions heal with disfiguring scars (Fig. 27-54).

DIFFERENTIAL DIAGNOSIS

PRODROMAL STAGE/LOCALIZED PAIN Can mimic migraine, cardiac or pleural disease, an acute abdomen, or vertebral disease.

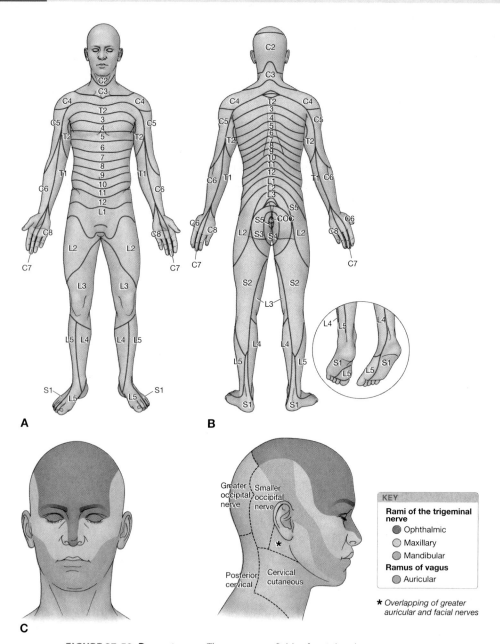

A

B

C

FIGURE 27-50 Dermatomes The cutaneous fields of peripheral sensory nerves.

FIGURE 27-51 Herpes zoster Close up of classical lesions. Grouped vesicles at different stages of development on an erythematous base in a dermatomal distribution on the abdomen.

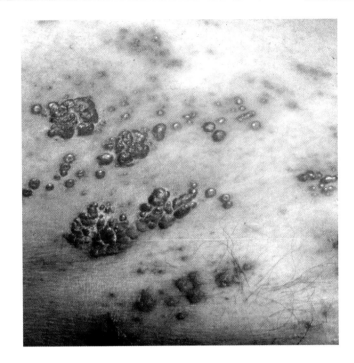

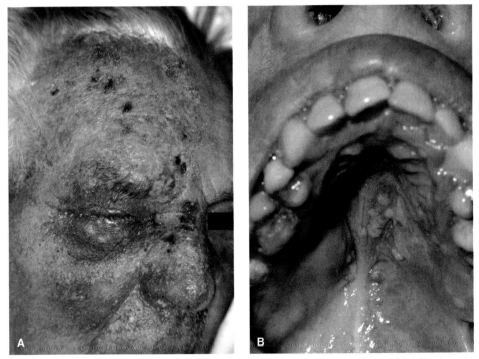

FIGURE 27-52 Herpes zoster (A) A 67-year old male with dermatomal zoster in the frontal and maxillary branch of the trigeminal nerve. Bullae, vesicle, and hemorrhagic crusts are seen. Note tremendous swelling of eye lids. **(B)** Mucosal lesions in another patient with involvement of the left maxillary branch of the trigeminal nerve. Unilateral erosions on the palate.

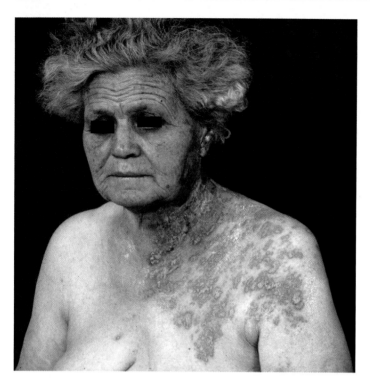

FIGURE 27-53 Herpes zoster cervical distribution (C 2 to C 5) A 65-year-old female being treated with prednisone for polymyalgia rheumatic has painful lesions for 5 days. Dermatomal grouped and confluent vesicles on the left neck, upper chest and shoulder.

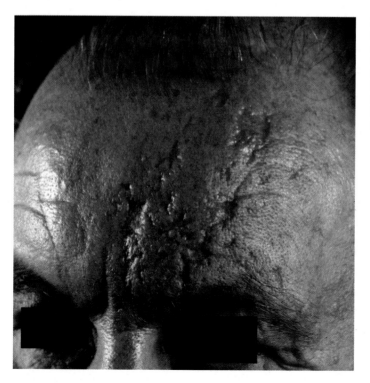

FIGURE 27-54 Herpes zoster: atrophic scars A 80-year-old male with a history of herpes zoster 1 year previously. Deep dermatomal (V1) scars are seen on the left forehead at the site of prior zoster.

DERMATOMAL ERUPTION HSV infection, photoallergic (poison ivy, poison oak) contact dermatitis, erysipelas, and necrotizing fasciitis.

DIAGNOSIS

PRODROMAL STAGE Suspect zoster in older or immunocompromised with unilateral pain.
ACTIVE VESICULATION Clinical findings usually adequate; may be confirmed by Tzanck test, DFA, or viral culture to rule out HSV infection.
POSTHERPETIC PAIN SYNDROME By history and clinical findings.

COURSE

Dissemination of Zoster. ≥20 lesions outside the affected or adjacent dermatomes; occurs in up to 10% of patients, usually with immune defects. VZV can disseminate hematogenously to skin and to viscera.
Neurological complications: Meningoencephalitis, cerebral vascular syndromes, cranial nerve syndromes [trigeminal (ophthalmic) branch (HZ ophthalmicus), facial and auditory nerves (Ramsay Hunt syndrome)], peripheral motor weakness, and transverse myelitis. *Visceral involvement*: Pneumonitis, hepatitis, pericarditis/myocarditis, pancreatitis, esophagitis, enterocolitis, cystitis, and synovitis.
Postherpetic Pain Syndrome. The risk of postherpetic neuralgia is 40% in patients >60 years with resolution in 87% at 6 months. The highest incidence is in ophthalmic zoster.

It does not appear to be more common in immune defects than in the general population.

Pain with HZ is associated with neural inflammation, nerve infection during the acute reactivation, and neural inflammation and scarring with PHN.
Zoster in Infants. Can occur albeit rarely. Usually not associated with neurological symptoms (Fig. 27-56).

TREATMENT

PREVENTION Vaccination against VZV with a live attenuated vaccine reduces the burden of illness by >60% and incidence of zoster by 51%.
ANTIVIRAL THERAPY Oral famciclovir 500 mg every 8 h for 7 days; valaciclovir 1 g every 8 h for 7 days; or acyclovir 800 mg 5 times a day for 7 days.
Mildly immunocompromised: As said previously, for up to 10 days. Severely immunocompromised: Acyclovir 10 mg/kg IV every 8 h for 7 to 10 days.
Acyclovir resistant: IV foscarnet 40 mg/kg IV every 8h until resolution.
SUPPORTIVE THERAPY Bed rest, sedation, pain management with narcotic analgesics; moist dressings.
POSTHERPETIC NEURALGIA Gabapentin, pregabalin, tricyclic antidepressants, i.e., doxepin, capsaicin cream topically. Nerve block.

VZV: HOST DEFENSE DEFECTS

■ **Host Defense Defects.** Immunosuppression, especially from lymphoproliferative disorders, cancer chemotherapy; HIV disease; immunosuppressive therapy.
■ **Primary and reactivation VZV disease** can be more severe with disseminated cutaneous and infection.

CLINICAL MANIFESTATION

NECROTIZING HERPES ZOSTER Severe dermatomal disease (Fig. 27-55).
HERPES ZOSTER WITH CUTANEOUS DISSEMINATION Variable numbers of vesicles or bullae are seen at any mucocutaneous site (Fig. 27-57). The condition thus appears clinically as zoster plus varicella.
HERPES ZOSTER WITH PERSISTENT DERMATOMAL INFECTION Chronic ulcers persist for months.

Papular or verrucous dermatomal lesions (Fig. 27-58).
EYE Acute retinal necrosis occurs in the absence of apparent conjunctival or cutaneous involvement with subsequent loss of vision.
VISCERAL DISSEMINATION Encephalitis, polyneuritis, myelitis, and vasculitis; pneumonitis; hepatitis; pericarditis/myocarditis; pancreatitis; enterocolitis.

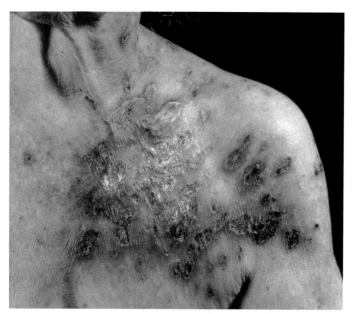

FIGURE 27-55 VZV: necrotizing herpes zoster Confluent, crusted ulcerations on an inflammatory base in several contiguous dermatomes in an elderly male with leukemia.

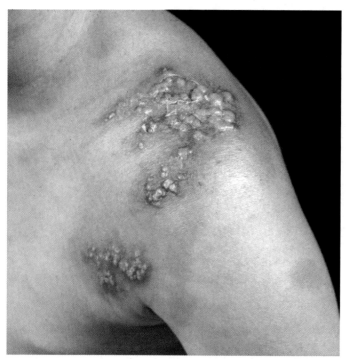

FIGURE 27-56 C-5-6 zoster on the shoulder of a 5-year-old boy The child had mild atopic dermatitis but was otherwise healthy and had only minimal pain. Diagnosis was verified by DFA. This image is shown to illustrate that herpes zoster can occur, albeit rarely, in infants and children.

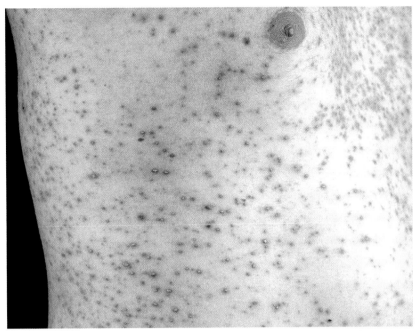

FIGURE 27-57 Varicella zoster virus infection: disseminated cutaneous, in an immunocompromised patient Hundreds of vesicles and pustules on erythematous bases of the trunk of a patient with lymphoma. Note the absence of grouping of lesions seen in herpes simplex or herpes zoster. The eruption is indistinguishable from varicella and must be differentiated from disseminated HSV infection.

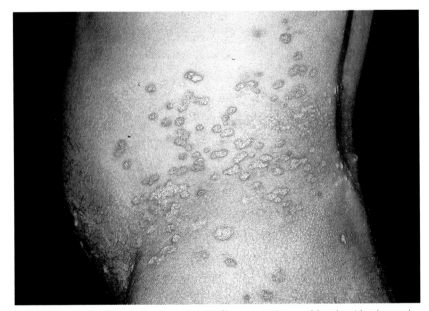

FIGURE 27-58 VZV: chronic zoster in HIV disease A 42-year-old male with advanced untreated HIV disease. Discrete and confluent hyperkeratotic papules/nodules in several contiguous dermatomes persistent for 2 years.

HUMAN HERPESVIRUS-6 AND 7 DISEASE ICD-10: B10

- Primary HHV-6 and HHV-7 infections cause exanthema subitum or roseola infantum, characterized by high fever in a healthy infant (9 to 12 months old), defervescence in 3 days followed by sudden appearance of exanthem.
- **Etiology.** HHV-6 (variants 6A and 6B) and HHV-7 share genetic, biologic, and immunologic features and are T cell tropic. At birth, most children have passively transferred anti-HHV-6 and anti-7 IgG. Primary infection is acquired via oropharyngeal secretions. HHV-6 antibodies reach a nadir at 4 to 7 months and increase throughout infancy. By 12 months, two-thirds of children become infected, with peak antibody levels reached at 2 to 3 years of age. Similarly, HHV-7 antibodies reach nadir at 6 months, with level peaking at 3 to 4 years of age. Latent infection may persist for the lifetime of the individual.
- **Pathogenesis.** HHV-6B causes exanthema subitum; pathogenesis of the exanthema is most likely immune response to viral antigens. HHV-6B reactivation occurs in transplant recipients and can cause encephalitis, bone marrow suppression, and pneumonitis.

CLINICAL MANIFESTATION

PRODROME High fever ranging from 38.9° to 40.6°C. Remains consistently high, with morning remission, until the fourth day, when it falls precipitously to normal, coincident with the appearance of rash. Infant remarkably well despite high fever. Asymptomatic primary HHV-6 and HHV-7 infection is common.

EXANTHEM SUBITUM OR ROSEOLA INFANTUM Small blanchable pink macules and papules, 1 to 5 mm in diameter (Fig. 27-59). Lesions may remain discrete or become confluent. Distribution: Trunk and neck.

GENERAL FINDINGS Absent in presence of high fever. Febrile seizures are common.

DIFFERENTIAL DIAGNOSIS

Other viral exanthems, ACDE, scarlet fever.

SEROLOGY Demonstration of IgM anti-HHV-6 or anti-HHV-7 antibodies or *IgG* seroconversion.

DIAGNOSIS

Usually made on clinical findings.

COURSE

Exanthem subitum is self-limited with rare sequelae. In some cases, high fever may be associated with seizures. Intussusception associated with hyperplasia of intestinal lymphoid tissue and hepatitis reported. As with other HHV infections, HHV-6 and HHV-7 persist throughout the life of the patient. The role of HHV-6 and HHV-7 in the pathogenesis of pityriasis rosea is being investigated.

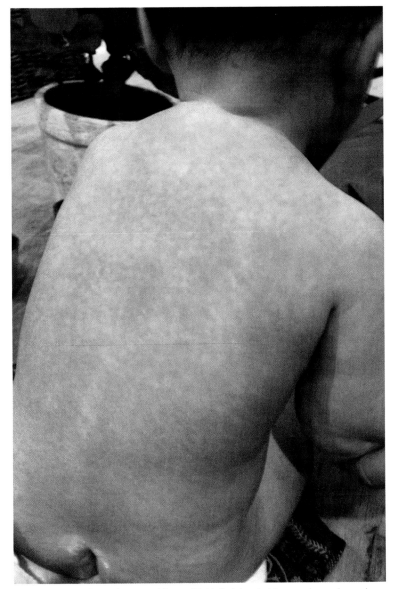

FIGURE 27-59 Exanthema subitum Multiple, blanchable macules and papules on the back of a febrile child, which appeared as the temperature fell.

HUMAN IMMUNODEFICIENCY VIRUS DISEASE ICD-10: B20-B24

- **HIV** originated in nonhuman primates in sub-Saharan Africa, evolving from simian immunodeficiency virus (SIV). Transmission to humans occurred in the early 20th century and has been linked to eating bush meats.
- **HIV disease** is characterized by a progressive quantitative and qualitative deficiency of *helper T cells* occurring in a setting of polyclonal immune activation.
- **Acquired immunodeficiency syndrome (AIDS),** the endstage of HIV disease, was first recognized in the United States (1981) and shortly after in Europe.
- **Transmission of HIV** occurs during sexual intercourse, exposure to blood or blood product, and perinatal exposure.
  - **Primary HIV infection** may be symptomatic with acute HIV seroconversion illness.
  - **Clinical manifestations** are of opportunistic infections and neoplasms. Clinical course is highly variable.
  - **Treatment.** When available, combination antiretroviral therapy (cART) is very effective in management of this chronic disease.

U.S. Department of Health and Human Services treatment guidelines for HIV disease: http://www.aidsinfo.nih.gov/

Updates on epidemiologic data from the Centers for Disease Control and Prevention (CDC): http://www.cdcnpin.org/

ETIOLOGY AND EPIDEMIOLOGY

ETIOLOGY HIV disease caused primarily by HIV-1 group of viruses. HIV-2 causes disease in western Africa and other foci.

TRANSMISSION Sexual intercourse, exposure to blood or blood product, perinatal or breast milk. Risk factors for acquisition: Genital ulcer disease, HIV-infected partner with high viral load (transmission more efficient), and receptive anal intercourse.

DEMOGRAPHY 36.9 million persons living with HIV infection in 2015. 25.8 million in sub-Saharan Africa. HIV disease has caused 39 million deaths since first recognized in 1981. In 2014, there were 2 million new cases of HIV globally.

PATHOGENESIS After primary HIV infection, billions of virions are produced and destroyed each day; a concomitant daily turnover of actively infected CD4+ cells is also in the billions. HIV infection is relatively unique among human viral infections in that, despite robust cellular and humoral immune responses that are mounted after primary infection, HIV is not cleared completely from the body. Chronic HIV disease follows primary infection with varying degrees of virus replication.

CLINICAL MANIFESTATION

Dermatologic disorders are nearly universal during the course of HIV disease. Some disorders are *highly associated with HIV disease*, and their diagnosis often warrants HIV serotesting: Acute retroviral syndrome, KS, oral hairy leukoplakia, proximal subungual onychomycosis, bacillary angiomatosis, eosinophilic folliculitis, chronic herpetic ulcers, any sexually transmitted disease, and skin findings of injecting drug use. *Moderate risk for HIV disease* is associated with HZ, molluscum contagiosum (multiple facial in adult), and candidiasis (oropharyngeal, esophageal, or recurrent vulvovaginal). *Possible risk for HIV disease*: Generalized lymphadenopathy, seborrheic dermatitis, and aphthous ulcers (recurrent, refractory to therapy).

ACUTE HIV INFECTION Acute viral illness with exanthem.

Unique to HIV disease acute HIV seroconversion illness (acute retroviral syndrome), oral hairy leukoplakia, eosinophilic folliculitis, pruritic popular eruption of HIV disease, and bacillary angiomatosis.

CUTANEOUS INFLAMMATORY DISORDERS Seborrheic dermatitis, atopic dermatitis, prurigo nodularis, psoriasis, xerosis, eosinophilic folliculitis, pruritus with secondary changes of excoriation, and adverse cutaneous drug reactions.

OPPORTUNISTIC INFECTIONS Molluscum contagiosum, VZV infection, herpes simplex, and HPV infections. *S. aureus* infections, bacillary angiomatosis, and mucosal candidiasis. Dermatophytoses. Systemic fungal infections with dissemination to skin.

OPPORTUNISTIC NEOPLASMS KS, HPV-induced dysplasia and invasive SCC (cervix, anus), Merkel cell carcinoma, non-Hodgkin and Hodgkin lymphoma, and primary CNS lymphoma.

IMMUNE RECONSTITUTION INFLAMMATORY SYNDROME (IRIS) IRIS occurs weeks or months after initiating cART, resulting from restored immunity to specific infectious or noninfectious antigens. Untreated mycobacterial and fungal coinfection predispose to IRIS. IRIS occurs most often in persons starting cART with CD4+ T cell count <50/μL who experience a precipitous drop in viral load; IRIS associated by an increase in CD4 cell count and/or a rapid decrease in HIV viral load. A paradoxical clinical worsening of a known condition or the appearance of a new condition after initiating therapy characterizes the syndrome. Potential mechanisms for the syndrome include a partial recovery of the immune system or exuberant host immunologic responses to antigenic stimuli. The infectious pathogens most frequently implicated in the syndrome are *Mycobacteria*, VZV, HSV, and CMV. Also, eosinophilic folliculitis and ACDE.

World Health Organization disease staging system for HIV infection and disease 2005:

- **Primary HIV infection:** May be either asymptomatic or associated with acute retroviral syndrome.
- **Stage I:** HIV infection is asymptomatic with a CD4 count of greater than 500/μL. May include generalized lymph node enlargement.
- **Stage II:** Mild symptoms that may include minor mucocutaneous manifestations and recurrent upper respiratory tract infections. A CD4 count of less than 500/μL.
- **Stage III:** Advanced symptoms that may include unexplained chronic diarrhea for longer than a month, severe bacterial infections including tuberculosis of the lung as well as a CD4 count of less than 350/μL.
- **Stage IV or AIDS:** Severe symptoms that include toxoplasmosis of the brain, candidiasis of the esophagus, trachea, bronchi or lungs, and KS. A CD4 count of less than 200/μL.

CDC 2008. In this system, HIV infections are classified based on CD4 counts and clinical symptoms.

- **Stage 1:** CD4 count ≥500 cells/μL and no AIDS defining conditions.
- **Stage 2:** CD4 count 200–500 cells/μL and no AIDS defining conditions.
- **Stage 3:** CD4 count ≤200 cells/μL or AIDS defining conditions.
- **Unknown:** If insufficient information is known to make one of the above classifications.

AIDS diagnosis remains even if, after treatment, the CD4+ T cell count rises to above 200 per μL of blood or other AIDS-defining illnesses are cured.

LABORATORY EXAMINATIONS

Diagnosis of HIV Infection HIV disease is diagnosed and monitored by measuring HIV RNA and antigens, CD4 cell counts, and serotesting (http://www.cdc.gov/std/treatment/2010/hiv.htm) (see Table 27-2).

TABLE 27-2 Laboratory Diagnosis of Human Immunodeficiency Virus (HIV) Infection

Test	Component Tested	Window Period	Role in Diagnosis
Enzyme-linked immunosorbent assay[a]	Antibodies (IgM and IgG)	3–6 weeks	Screening
Antigen capture[b]	HIV p24 antigen	2–3 weeks	Screening
Western blotting	Antibody (IgG)	3 weeks	Confirmatory
Immunofluorescence	Antibody (IgG)	3 weeks	Confirmatory
Nucleic acid testing	HIV RNA or DNA	2 weeks	Confirmatory
Viral culture	Virus, usually from peripheral blood mononuclear cells, not serum or plasma	—	Confirmatory, research

Ig = immunoglobulin
[a]Rapid tests as well as particle agglutination tests are also available.
[b]Detection can be increased with the use of immune complex dissociation techniques.

Modified from Maldarelli F. Diagnosis of human immunodeficiency virus infection. In: Mandell GL et al., eds. *Principles and Practice of Infectious Diseases*. Philadelphia, PA: Elsevier; 2005:1506, with permission. Copyright © Elsevier.

COURSE

The clinical course of HIV disease is highly variable in each person (Fig. 27-60). Symptomatic primary infection occurs often. A prolonged asymptomatic state following primary infection is common. Opportunistic infections and neoplasms occur in advanced disease. Early in the pandemic, prophylaxis for opportunistic infections and treatment of opportunistic infections improved morbidity and mortality. Currently, cART has been very effective in the majority of persons but may give rise to the metabolic syndrome and lipodystrophy.

TREATMENT

Guidelines for antiretroviral therapy (ART) evolve as new drugs become available as do local resources. Websites for updated guidelines of ART are as follows:

- United States: http://www.aidsinfo.nih.gov/guidelines.
- World Health Organization: http://www.who.int/hiv/topics/treatment/en/.

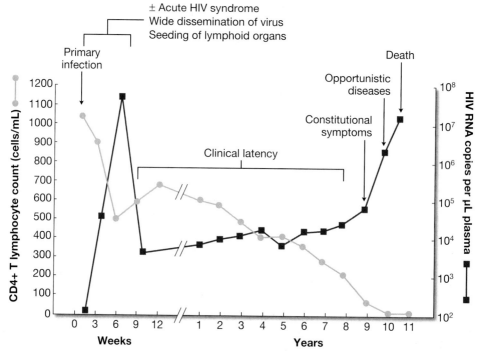

FIGURE 27-60 Typical disease course in an individual with HIV disease (Adapted from Fauci AS et al. Immunopathogenic mechanisms of HIV infection. *Ann Intern Med*. 1996;124(7):654–663.)

ACUTE HIV SYNDROME ICD-10: B23.0

- **Primary HIV Infection.** Up to 70% of primary infections are symptomatic, 3 to 4 weeks after exposure. Symptoms range from asymptomatic to severe.
- Infectious mononucleosis-like syndrome with fever, lymphadenopathy, and neurologic and GI symptoms.
- Infectious exanthema, enanthem, and mucocutaneous ulcerations.

CLINICAL MANIFESTATION

GENERAL FINDINGS Fever, pharyngitis, lymphadenopathy, headache/retro-orbital pain, arthralgias/myalgias, lethargy/malaise, anorexia/weight loss, and nausea/vomiting/diarrhea. Neurologic findings: Meningitis, encephalitis, peripheral neuropathy, and myelopathy.
EXANTHEM Appears 2 to 3 days after onset of fever, lasting 5 to 8 days. Morbilliform rash [infectious exanthem (Fig. 27-61)], with pink macules, papules up to 1 cm in diameter. Lesions remain discrete. Upper thorax and collar region, face, arms, scalp, and thighs.
OROPHARYNGEAL LESIONS Pharyngitis. *Enanthem*: Red macules, on hard and soft palate.

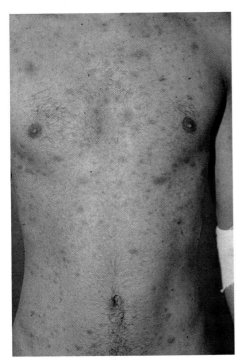

FIGURE 27-61 Acute HIV syndrome: exanthem Discrete, erythematous macules and papules on the anterior trunk; associated findings were fever and lymphadenopathy. (Used with permission from Armin Rieger, MD.)

Aphthous-like ulcers: Tonsils, palate, and buccal mucosa; esophageal ulcers. Uncommonly, *oral candidiasis.*
GENITAL LESIONS Aphthous-type painful ulcers. Prepuce of penis, scrotum, anus, and anal canal.

DIFFERENTIAL DIAGNOSIS

Infectious Exanthems. Adverse cutaneous drug reaction.

DIAGNOSIS

Demonstrated seroconversion of anti-HIV antibodies by ELISA, confirmed by Western blot, confirms diagnosis of primary HIV infection. Detection of HIV RNA and HIV antigens.

COURSE

The mean duration of symptomatic illness is 13 days. Prolonged symptomatic primary infection is associated with more rapid decline of immune function.
PRURITUS AND PRURITIC ERUPTIONS Pruritus is a common symptom in persons with advanced HIV disease. Primary or secondary dermatoses are usually the cause. *Eosinophilic folliculitis* and *popular pruritic eruption* of HIV disease are primary pruritic disorders occurring exclusively in HIV disease.

An atopic-like diathesis (atopic dermatitis, allergic rhinitis, or asthma) may become manifest. Findings secondary to chronic rubbing and scratching include excoriations, lichen simplex chronicus, prurigo nodularis, and hyperpigmentation (Figs. 27-62 and 27-64). Secondary *S. aureus* infection (impetiginization, furunculosis, or cellulitis) occur in traumatized lesions. Ichthyosis vulgaris and xerosis are common in advanced HIV disease and may be associated with mild pruritus. Protease inhibitors (particularly indinavir) may cause a retinoid dermatitis, which occurs soon after initiation of therapy. *Idiopathic pruritus* is associated with CD4+ T cell counts <200/μL and viral load >55,000 copies/μL, while cART has been associated with a decrease in idiopathic pruritus.

EOSINOPHILIC FOLLICULITIS

- **A chronic pruritic dermatosis** occurring in persons with advanced HIV disease. May occur before cART or flare with IRIS following initiation of cART.
- **Clinical Manifestation.** Extremely pruritic small pink to red, edematous, folliculocentric papules (Fig. 27-63), and less commonly pustules. Lesions tend to develop symmetrically above the nipple line on the chest, proximal arms, head, and neck. Secondary changes, *S. aureus* infections, and dyspigmentation are common (Fig. 27-64).
- **Laboratory Findings.** Lesional biopsy shows an inflammatory infiltrate of lymphocytes and eosinophils at the level of the isthmus and sebaceous gland. Peripheral eosinophilia.
- **Treatment.** A short tapered course of prednisone gives immediate relief of symptoms, e.g., 70 mg tapering by 5 or 10 mg daily. Lesions and symptoms often recur within a few weeks of completion of prednisone. Isotretinoin is also effective.

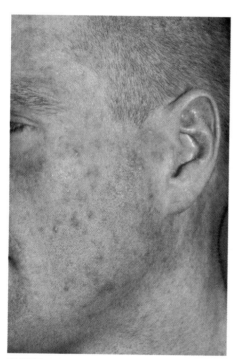

FIGURE 27-62 Eosinophilic folliculitis A 38-year-old male with HIV disease. Multiple pruritic red papules on the face and neck occurred shortly after reinstituting cART. This represents the immune reconstitution inflammatory syndrome (IRIS), occurring as immune parameters improve.

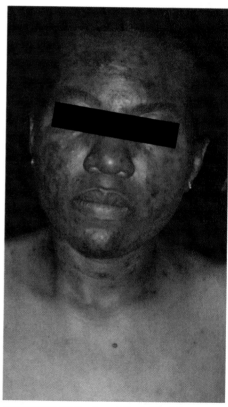

FIGURE 27-63 Eosinophilic folliculitis A 31-year-old African female with advanced HIV disease. Multiple pruritic edematous papules on the face and neck with marked postinflammatory hyperpigmentation. Note the absence of lesions and pigmentation on the adjacent chest.

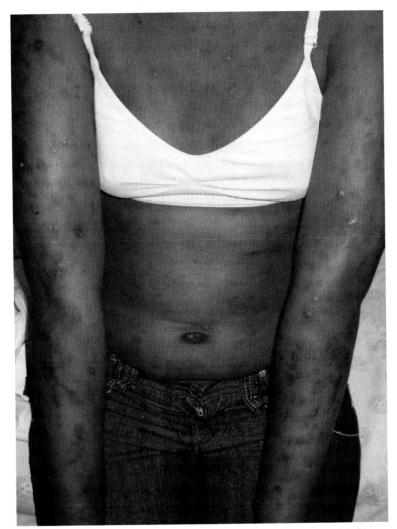

FIGURE 27-64 Papular pruritic eruption of HIV disease A 23-year-old African female with multiple excoriated papules on the arms and fewer lesions on the trunk. Primary lesions are thought to arise at sites of insect bites. (Used with permission from Adam Lipworth, MD.)

PAPULAR PRURITIC ERUPTION OF HIV

- **Epidemiology.** Prevalence high in developing nations, often the initial presenting manifestation of HIV disease. Rarely reported in Europe and North America. Papular pruritic eruption (PPE) appears to be a marker of advanced HIV disease; >80% of person with PPE have CD4+ T cell counts <100/μL (100). Etiopathogenesis is unclear; may represent a hypersensitivity reaction to arthropod bites.
- **Clinical Manifestation.** Urticarial papules and occasionally noninfectious pustules; occasionally folliculocentric. Usually symmetric and distributed primarily on the extremities, and less commonly on the trunk and face (Fig. 27-64). Because of intense pruritus, multiple excoriations, marked post-inflammatory hyperpigmentation, scarring is usually present.
- **Treatment.** Immune reconstitution with cART is an effective treatment for PPE, although several months of therapy may be required for lesions to resolve.

PHOTOSENSITIVITY IN HIV DISEASE (see Section 10)

Idiopathic photosensitivity may be the presenting complaint of advanced HIV disease. Photosensitive eruptions present with two distinct morphologies: photodistributed lichenoid eruptions (Fig. 27-65) and photodistributed eczematous eruptions. cART and other drugs cause photosensitive eruptions. Risk factors for photosensitivity include African ethnicity and cART. Photosensitivity occurs in association with other diseases such as porphyria cutanea tarda, chronic actinic dermatitis, lichenoid photo-eruption, and photosensitive granuloma.

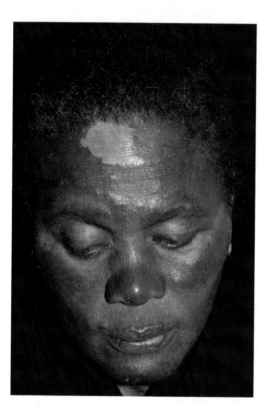

FIGURE 27-65 Lichenoid photosensitive eruption A 45-year-old African female with advanced HIV disease. Violaceous hyperpig-mented plaques in sun-exposed sites on the face. Depigmentation has occurred within a plaque on the forehead. Other than HIV dis-ease, neither underlying systemic disease nor drug exposure were identified.

ORAL HAIRY LEUKOPLAKIA ICD-10: K13.3

- **Etiology.** OHL emerges from latency in advanced HIV disease and causes benign mucosal hyperplasia. Occurs with CD4+ cell count <300/μL.
- **Clinical Manifestation.** Asymptomatic, but stigmatization of HIV disease. White or grayish-white, well-demarcated plaques (Fig. 27-66) with corrugated texture. Most commonly on the lateral and inferior surfaces of the tongue. Often present bilaterally. Oropharyngeal candidiasis often present as well.
- **Differential Diagnosis.** Pseudomembranous candidiasis (thrush), geographic or migratory glossitis, tobacco-associated leukoplakia, mucous patch of secondary syphilis, and SCCIS.
- **Diagnosis.** Clinical diagnosis. Lesions do not rub off; does not clear with adequate anticandidal therapy.
- **Course.** Usually resolves with cART and immune restoration. Recurs when cART failing.
- **Treatment.** Podophyllin 25% in tincture of benzoin applied to the lesion with a cotton-tipped applicator for 5 minutes. Effective cART results in regression and clearing of OHL.

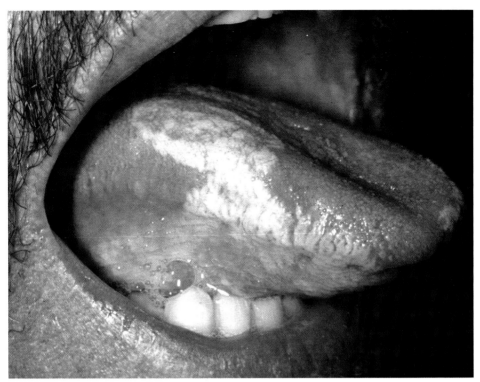

FIGURE 27-66 Hairy leukoplakia A 32-year-old male with advanced HIV disease. White plaques on the lateral tongue with corduroy-like pattern.

ADVERSE CUTANEOUS DRUG ERUPTIONS IN HIV DISEASE ICD-10: L27.0

- Incidence of ACDEs is estimated to be as much as 100 times more common in persons with HIV disease compared to that in the general population, becoming more frequent with advancing immunodeficiency.
- **Exanthematous or morbilliform eruptions** are the most common manifestation, accounting for up to 95% of cases.
- **Other morphologies** such as urticaria, erythema multiforme major, erythema multiforme minor, toxic epidermal necrolysis, lichenoid eruptions, vasculitis, and fixed drug eruptions also occur. Twenty percent of persons report systemic symptoms (fever, headache, myalgias, and arthralgias).
- **cART** can cause a wide spectrum of ACDE.

ETIOLOGY AND EPIDEMIOLOGY

Most common drugs causing adverse cutaneous drug eruptions (ACDE) in HIV disease are *aminopenicillins* and *sulfa drugs*. Factors associated with increased risk of drug eruptions include female gender, CD4+ T cell count <200/μL, CD8+ T cell count >460/μL, and history of prior drug eruptions. The incidence of toxic epidermal necrolysis is markedly increased in advanced HIV disease with a mortality rate 20%.

PATHOGENESIS Incidence increases with progressive HIV disease, and decline and dysregulation of immune function. After immune reconstitution by cART, some persons who previously tolerated a drug may develop allergic cutaneous drug reactions, a manifestation of IRIS.

CLASSIFICATION

Drug eruptions can mimic many dermatoses and must be first on the differential diagnosis in the appearance of a sudden symmetric eruption (see Section 23).

Exanthematous or morbilliform eruptions macules and papules. Account for 95% of ACDE in HIV disease as in the general population.

RETINOID DERMATITIS Indinavir has a retinoid effect on the skin and can cause eczematous dermatitis, chronic paronychia, cheilitis, and pyogenic granuloma.

Lipodystrophy syndrome: See below.

TREATMENT

In most cases, the implicated or suspected drug should be discontinued. In cases of urticaria/angioedema or early Stevens–Johnson syndrome, ACDE can be life threatening. Short-term oral corticosteroid therapy may be effective in reducing the risk of adverse drug eruptions.

Adverse Effects of Antiretroviral Therapy

Six classes of antiretroviral medications are currently in use:

- Non-nucleoside reverse transcriptase inhibitors (NNRTIs).
- Protease inhibitors.
- NRTIs.

- Integrase inhibitors.
- Chemokine receptor 5 antagonists.
- Entry inhibitors.

These medications are associated with a variety of cutaneous adverse effects, including hypersensitivity reactions, lipodystrophy, retinoid-like effects, hyperpigmentation, nail changes, and injection site reactions (Table 27-3).

Lipodystrophy and Metabolic Syndromes

HIV disease-related lipodystrophy is characterized by abnormal fat distribution with lipohypertrophy, lipoatrophy, or both. Abnormal fat distribution is often accompanied by metabolic abnormalities, i.e., elevation of fasting glucose and insulin levels, hypertriglyceridemia, hypercholesterolemia, and decreased high-density lipoprotein.

PATHOGENESIS Lipohypertrophy is most commonly associated with protease inhibitor therapy, while lipohypertrophy is frequently associated with NRTIs, particularly the thymidine analogues stavudine and zidovudine. HIV disease by itself may induce changes in fat distribution and metabolic anomalies such as insulin resistance.

CLINICAL MANIFESTATION Lipohypertrophy presents with central obesity, cushingoid habitus ("buffalo hump"), increased neck girth (Fig. 27-67), increased abdominal girth caused by intraabdominal fat ("protease pouch" or "crix belly"), and breast enlargement. Facial lipoatrophy, most pronounced on the cheeks and temples, is striking and stigmatizing for HIV disease (Fig. 27-68). Lipoatrophy of subcutaneous fat produces a pseudoathletic appearance with a prominent venous pattern and musculature on the extremities and buttocks. In cohort persons with HIV disease treated with ART, the overall prevalence of lipodystrophy was 38%, while the prevalence of lipoatrophy alone was 16% and lipohypertrophy alone was 12%. The prevalence of lipid anomalies was 49% and the prevalence of glucose disorders was 20%.

Treatment of lipodystrophy remains challenging. Substitution of regimens containing stavudine and zidovudine has been shown to be of partial benefit for lipoatrophy. Facial lipoatrophy has been treated with soft tissue fillers with varying degrees of success.

TABLE 27-3 Adverse Effects of Antiretroviral Drugs

Drug	Mechanism	Nonmucocutaneous Side Effects	Mucocutaneous Side Effects
Nucleoside Reverse Transcriptase Inhibitors			
Abacavir (ABC) Didanosine (ddI) Emtricitabine (FTC) Lamivudine (3TC) Stavudine (d4T) Tenofovir TDF) Zidovudine (AZT) Zalcitabine (ddC)	Nucleoside analogs that act by incorporating themselves into the growing viral DNA chain, which eventually induces termination of viral DNA elongation	▪ Pancreatitis, peripheral neuropathy, lactic acidosis, and hepatotoxicity with didanosine, stavudine, and zalcitabine ▪ Hepatotoxicity with emtricitabine and lamivudine ▪ Renal toxicity with tenofovir ▪ Anemia, granulocytopenia, myopathy, lactic acidosis, hepatotoxicity, and nausea with zidovudine	▪ Hypersensitivity, with rare instances of Stevens–Johnson syndrome/toxic epidermal necrolysis (SJS/TEN) ▪ Systemic hypersensitivity reactions in up to 5–8% with abacavir, associated with HLA-B5701/HLA-DR7/HLA-DQ3; incidence reduced by prescreening for HLA-B5701 ▪ Leukocytoclastic vasculitis, pancreatitis, and peripheral neuropathy with didanosine ▪ Hyperpigmentation of the nail bed, palms, and soles with emtricitabine ▪ Hyperpigmentation of the nails (including multiple longitudinal and transverse bands), diffuse hyperpigmentation of the skin and oral mucosa, leukocytoclastic vasculitis, and hypertrichosis with zidovudine ▪ Lipohypotrophy with stavudine and zidovudine ▪ Paronychia with nailfold pyogenic granuloma with lamivudine and zidovudine ▪ Oropharyngeal and esophageal ulcerations with zalcitabine
Non-Nucleoside Reverse Transcriptase Inhibitors			
Delavirdine Efavirenz Etravirine Nevirapine	Nonnucleosides that directly bind to reverse transcriptase to prevent conversion of viral RNA to DNA	▪ Hepatotoxicity ▪ Somnolence and depression with efavirenz	▪ Hypersensitivity reactions are common within the first 6 weeks of therapy, with rare progression to systemic hypersensitivity or SJS/TEN (highest incidence with nevirapine)
Protease Inhibitors			
Amprenavir Atazanavir Darunavir Fosamprenavir Indinavir Lopinavir Nelfinavir Ritonavir Saquinavir Tipranavir	Prevents cleavage of protein precursors essential for HIV maturation, infection of new cells, and replication	▪ Nausea, vomiting, diarrhea, headaches, lipid anomalies, and hyperglycemia ▪ Oral paresthesias with amprenavir ▪ PR prolongation and hyperbilirubinemia with atazanavir ▪ Hepatotoxicity and intracranial hemorrhage with tipranavir ▪ Nephrolithiasis and hyperbilirubinemia with indinavir ▪ Ritonavir may affect levels of many other medications, including saquinavir	▪ Hypersensitivity reactionswith rare progression to SJS, particularly with amprenavir, fosamprenavir, and tipranavir ▪ Acute exanthematous pustulosis ▪ Lipohypertrophy, most commonly with indinavir ▪ Dose-dependent retinoid-like effects (xerosis, cheilitis, alopecia, lateral nailfold pyogenic granuloma, curly hair, and recurrent paronychia), acute porphyria, "frozen shoulder," and venous thrombosis with indinavir ▪ Spontaneous bleeding and hematomas, particularly with ritonavir ▪ Rare cases of fixed drug eruptions with saquinavir ▪ Darunavir, tipranavir, fosamprenavir, and amprenavir contain sulfa moieties and should be used with caution in sulfa allergic patients

(continued)

TABLE 27-3 Adverse Effects of Antiretroviral Drugs (*Continued*)

Drug	Mechanism	Nonmucocutaneous Side Effects	Mucocutaneous Side Effects
Fusion Inhibitors			
Enfuvirtide	Inhibits binding of HIV to CD4 cells by binding to and inhibiting the action of gp40, a HIV protein that induces structural changes needed for fusion of HIV to host CD4 cells	■ Increased frequency of bacterial pneumonia	■ Systemic hypersensitivity reactions in <1%
Integrase Inhibitors			
Raltegravir	Inhibits HIV integrase, a viral enzyme that catalyzes the integration of HIV DNA into host chromosomal DNA	■ Nausea	■ Pruritus
Chemokine Receptor 5 (CCR5) Antagonists			
Maraviroc	Binds to the CCR5 receptor, a HIV co-receptor on CD4 cells, and thereby blocks attachment of HIV envelope proteins and HIV entry into host cells	■ Hepatotoxicity, nasopharyngitis, cough, abdominal pain, dizziness, musculoskeletal symptoms	■ Injection-site reactions in up to 98% of patients, requiring discontinuation in only 3%

Source: Reproduced with permission from Goldsmith LA, Katz SI, Gilchrest BA, et al., eds. *Fitzpatrick's Dermatology in General Medicine*. 8th ed. New York, NY: McGraw-Hill; 2012, p. 2447.

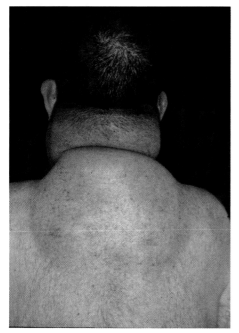

FIGURE 27-67 Lipohypertrophy A 51-year-old male with advanced HIV disease. Increase subcutaneous fatty tissue of neck with "buffalo hump on upper back." Gynecomastia was also present. Lipoatrophy was present on the face. His weight was normal.

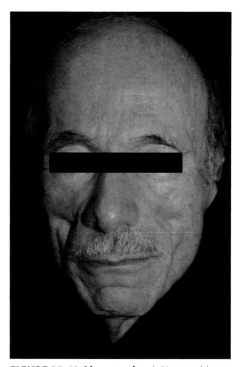

FIGURE 27-68 Lipoatrophy A 61-year-old male with advanced HIV disease. Striking loss of fat is seen on cheeks and temples. Lipohypertrophy of the neck and upper back were also present.

VARIATIONS IN COMMON MUCOCUTANEOUS DISORDERS IN HIV DISEASE

- Early in HIV disease when immune function is relatively intact, common dermatoses, ACDEs, and infections present as typical clinical manifestations have the usual course, and respond to standard therapies.
- With progressive decline in immune function, each of these characteristics of a disease can be strikingly altered.
- With effective management with cART and immune reconstitution, diseases either do not occur, resolve without specific therapy, or respond more readily to therapy.

Kaposi Sarcoma

Early in the HIV epidemic in the United States and Europe, 50% of men who have sex with men (MSM) had KS at the time of initial AIDS diagnosis. In persons with HIV disease, the risk for KS is 20,000 times that of the general population and 300 times that of other immunosuppressed individuals. In untreated HIV disease, KS may progress rapidly with extensive mucocutaneous and systemic involvement. KS in persons successfully treated with cART does not occur, resolves without specific therapy other than immune reconstitution, or responds better to chemotherapies (see also "Kaposi Sarcoma," Section 21).

Nonmelanoma Skin Cancers

The incidence of a SCC is increased in advanced HIV disease. Infection with oncogenic types of HPV is the more common cause of SCC. Cervix, external genitalia, and the anorectal areas are the most common involved sites for SCC in situ and invasive SCC. The incidence of UV light-induced invasive SCC is increased in advanced HIV disease in persons with skin phototypes I to III with much UVL exposure during early decades of life. These SCCs can be quite aggressive, invading locally, growing rapidly, and metastasizing by lymphatics and blood, with increased morbidity and mortality.

Aphthous Ulcers

Recurrent aphthous ulcers occur more frequently, become larger (often >1 cm), and/or become chronic with advanced HIV disease. Ulcers may extensive and/or multiple; commonly involving the tongue, gingiva, lips, and esophagus, causing severe odynophagia with rapid weight loss. Intralesional triamcinolone. Prednisone 70 mg tapered by 10 or 5 mg per day over 7 or 14 days. In resistant cases, thalidomide is an effective agent (see also "Aphthous Ulcers," Section 33).

Staphylococcus aureus Infection

S. aureus is the most common cutaneous bacterial pathogen in the general population and in HIV disease. The nasal carriage rate of *S. aureus* is up to 50%, which is twice that of HIV-seronegative control groups. In most instances, *S. aureus* infections are typical, presenting as primary infections (folliculitis, furuncles, or carbuncles), secondarily infections (excoriations, eczema, scabies, herpetic ulcer, or KS), cellulitis, or venous access device infections, all of which can be complicated by bacteremia and disseminated infection. Methicillin-resistant *S. aureus* (MRSA) infections, if not identified, may be more severe because of delay in initiation of effective anti-MRSA therapy (see also Section 25).

Dermatophytoses

Epidermal dermatophytosis can be extensive, recurrent, and difficult to eradicate. Proximal subungual onychomycosis occurs in advanced HIV disease, presents as a chalky-white discoloration of the undersurface of the proximal nail plate, and is an indication for HIV serotesting (see also "Dermatophytoses," Section 26, and "Fungal Infections: Onychomycosis," Section 32).

Mucosal Candidiasis

Mucosal candidiasis affecting the upper aerodigestive tracts and/or vulvovagina is common in HIV disease. Oropharyngeal candidiasis, the most common presentation, is often the initial manifestation of HIV disease and is a marker for disease progression. Esophageal and tracheobronchial candidiasis occur in advanced HIV disease and are AIDS-defining conditions. The incidence of cutaneous candidiasis may be increased; with insulin resistance associated with cART, balanoposthitis can be seen. In young children, chronic candidal paronychia and nail dystrophy occur (see also "Candidiasis," Section 26).

Disseminated Fungal Infection

Latent pulmonary fungal infections with *Cryptococcus neoformans, Coccidioides immitis, Histoplasma capsulatum,* and *Penicillium marneffei* can be reactivated in HIV disease and disseminated to the skin and other organs. The most common cutaneous presentation of disseminated infection is molluscum contagiosum-like lesions on the face; other lesions such as nodules, pustules, ulcers, abscesses, or a papulosquamous eruption resembling guttate psoriasis (seen with histoplasmosis) also occur (see also "Disseminated Cryptococcosis," "Histoplasmosis," and "Disseminated Coccidioidomycosis," Section 26).

Herpes Simplex

HSV-1 or 2 infection is common opportunistic infections of HIV disease. Most reactivation is subclinical. Anogenital reactivation is particularly frequent. With advancing HIV disease, early lesions present with erosions or ulcerations associated with epidermal necrosis without vesicle formation. Untreated, these lesions may evolve to large, painful ulcers with rolled margins in the oropharynx, esophagus, and anogenitalia. Treatment of HSV reduces genital and plasma HIV RNA levels (see also "Herpes Simplex with Host Defense Defects," p. 690).

Varicella-Zoster Virus (VZV) Infection

Primary VZV infection (varicella or chicken pox) in HIV disease can be severe, prolonged, and complicated by visceral VZV infection, bacterial secondary infection, and death. HZ occurs in 25% of persons during the course of HIV disease, associated with modest decline in immune function. Cutaneous dissemination of HZ is relatively common. However, visceral involvement is rare. With increasing immuno-deficiency, VZV infection can present clinically as chronic dermatomal verrucous lesions; one or more chronic painful ulcers or ecthymatous lesions within a dermatome; crusted erosions, ulcer, or nodule. Untreated, these lesions persist for months. HZ can recur within the same dermatome(s) or in other dermatomes. VZV can infect the CNS causing a rapidly progressive chorioretinitis with acute retinal necrosis, chronic encephalitis, myelitis, radiculitis, or meningitis. Extensive HZ may heal with hypertrophic or keloidal scar (see also "VZV: Host Defense Defects," p. 701").

Molluscum Contagiosum

In advanced HIV disease, molluscum contagiosum has up to 18% prevalence; the severity of molluscum contagiosum is a marker for advanced immunodeficiency. Patients may have multiple small papules or nodules or large tumors, >1 cm in diameter, most commonly arising on the face, especially the beard area, the neck, and intertriginous sites. Cyst-like mollusca occur on the ears. Occasionally, mollusca can arise on the non-hair-bearing skin of the palms/soles (see also "Molluscum Contagiosum," p. 649").

Human Papillomavirus Infection

With advancing immunodeficiency, cutaneous and/or mucosal warts can become extensive and refractory to treatment. Of more concern, however, HPV-induced intraepithelial neoplasia, termed *squamous intraepithelial lesion* (SIL), is a precursor to invasive SCC, arising most often on the cervix, vulva, penis, perineum, and anus (Fig. 27-69). In females with HIV disease, the incidence of cervical SIL is six to eight times that of controls. The current trend toward longer median survival of patients with advanced HIV may lead to an increased incidence of HPV-associated neoplasia and invasive SCC in the future. SIL on the external genitalia, perineum, or anus is best managed

with local therapies such as imiquimod cream, cryosurgery, electrosurgery, or laser surgery rather than with aggressive surgical excision (see also "Human Papillomavirus: Mucosal Infections," Section 30).

Syphilis

The clinical course of syphilis in persons with HIV disease is most often the same as in the normal host. However, an accelerated course with the development of neurosyphilis or tertiary syphilis has been reported within months of initial syphilitic infection (see also "Syphilis," Section 30).

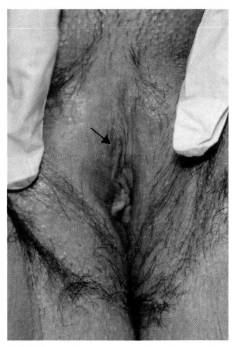

FIGURE 27-69 Squamous cell carcinoma in situ A 32-year-old female with HIV disease and cervical dysplasia. A subtle velvety plaque is seen on the vulva superior to the clitoris.

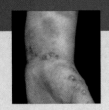

ARTHROPOD BITES, STINGS, AND CUTANEOUS INFESTATIONS

CUTANEOUS REACTIONS TO ARTHROPOD BITES

- Arthropods are defined by an exoskeleton, segmented body, and jointed appendages. Arthropods causing local and systemic reactions associated with their bites: Arachnida, Chilopoda, Diplopoda, and Insecta.
- Cutaneous reactions to arthropod bites are inflammatory and/or allergic reactions.
- Characterized by an intensely pruritic eruption at the bite sites, whether immediately or minutes to hours to days after the bite, persisting for days to weeks, manifested by solitary or grouped: Urticarial papules; papulovesicles; bullae. Persons are often unaware of having been bitten.
- Systemic symptoms may occur, ranging from mild to severe, with death occurring from anaphylactic shock.
- Arthropods are vectors of many systemic infections.

ARTHROPODS THAT BITE, STING, OR INFEST

Four of nine classes of arthropods cause local or systemic reactions.

1. **Arachnida** (four pairs of legs): Mites, ticks, spiders, and scorpions.
   a. **Acarina.** (mites and ticks) *Sarcoptes scabiei* (scabies). *Demodex folliculorum* and *D. brevis* (demodicidosis). Environmental mites. *Ticks* (Fig. 28-1) that feed on humans and are vectors for disease include blacklegged or *Ixodes* tick, *Amblyomma americanum* (lone star) tick, and *Dermacentor* (American dog or Wood) tick.
   b. **Araneae.** (spiders) *Loxosceles reclusa* or brown recluse spider. *Latrodectus* or black widow spiders. *Tegenaria or hobo spiders* cause necrotic arachnidism in the Pacific Northwest of United States. *Tarantula*: Mild inflammatory response to bite and to shed hairs.
   c. **Scorpionida.** Venom contains a neurotoxin that can cause severe local and systemic reactions.
2. **Chilopoda** or centipedes.
3. **Diplopoda** or millipedes.
4. **Insecta** (three pairs of legs).
   a. **Anoplura.** *Phthirius pubis* or crab lice. *Pediculus capitis* or head lice. *Pediculus corporis* or body lice.
   b. **Coleoptera.** Beetles. Blister beetles contain the chemical cantharidin, which produces a blister when the beetle is crushed on the skin.
   c. **Diptera.** Mosquitoes, black flies (bites produce local reactions as well as black fly fever with fever, headache, nausea, generalized lymphadenitis), midges (punkies, no-see-ums, sand flies), Tabanidae (horseflies, deerflies, clegs, breeze flies, greenheads, mango flies); botflies, *Callitroga americana, Dermatobia hominis, Phlebotomid* sand flies, and tsetse flies.
   d. **Hemiptera.** Bedbugs and kissing bugs.
   e. **Hymenoptera.** Ants, bees, wasps, and hornets.
   f. **Lepidoptera.** Caterpillars, butterflies, and moths.
   g. **Siphonaptera.** Fleas, chigoe, or sand flea.

ARTHROPOD-BORNE INFECTIONS

- Lyme borreliosis, tularemia, and bubonic plague.
- Scrub typhus, endemic (murine) typhus, spotted fever groups, and Q fever.
- Human granulocytic anaplasmosis.
- Tick-borne meningoencephalitis.
- Leishmaniasis and trypanosomiasis (sleeping sickness or Chagas disease).
- Malaria and babesiosis.

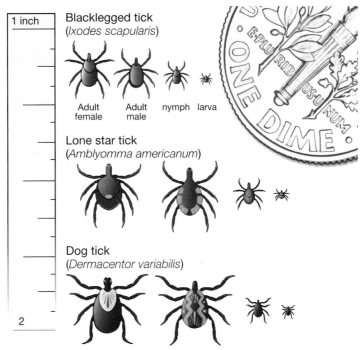

FIGURE 28-1 Comparison of blacklegged, lone star, and dog ticks Black-legged or *Ixodes* nymphal ticks transmit *Borrelia burgdorferi* (Lyme disease) and other infections. Lone star ticks or *Amblyomma americanum* is the vector for ana-plasmosis, tularemia, and Southern tick-associated rash illness. Dog or wood ticks, *Dermacentor variabilis*, transmit Rocky Mountain spotted fever and tularemia.

- Filariasis, onchocerciasis (river blindness), and loiasis.

CLINICAL MANIFESTATION

ERYTHEMATOUS MACULES Occur at bite sites and are usually transient.

PAPULAR URTICARIA or urticarial papules persistent for >48 h (Figs. 28-2 and 28-3); usually <1 cm; vesicle may for on papule. Large urticarial plaques may occur.

BULLOUS LESIONS Tense bullae with clear fluid on a slightly inflamed base (Fig. 28-4); excoriation results in erosion.

SECONDARY LESIONS Excoriations of urticarial, papular, and vesicular lesions common. Painful erosion may be secondarily infected with *Staphylococcus aureus*. Excoriated or secondarily infected lesions may heal with hyper- or hypopigmentation and/or raised or depressed scars, especially in more darkly pigmented individuals.

SYSTEMIC FINDINGS May occur associated with toxin or allergy to the substance injected during the bite. Many varied systemic infections can be injected during the bite.

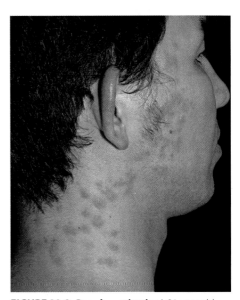

FIGURE 28-2 Papular urticaria A 21-year-old male awoke with multiple pruritic erythematous papules on his exposed face, neck, forearms, and hands. Bedding was heavily colonized with bedbugs.

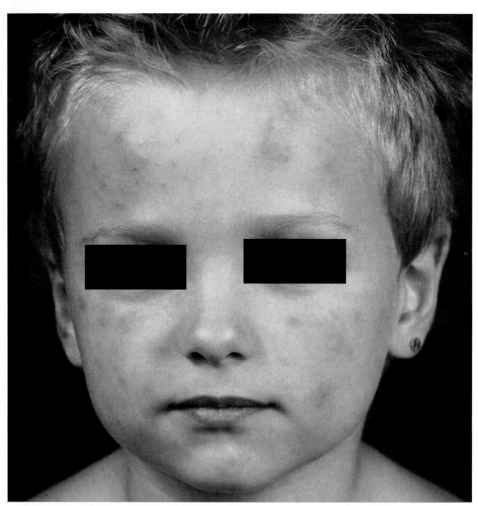

FIGURE 28-3 Papular urticaria A 6-year-old girl with multiple mosquito bites on face.

CLINICAL VARIATIONS BY ARTHROPOD

MITES *Sarcoptes scabiei* causes infestation *scabies* (see Scabies). *Demodex folliculorum* and *D. brevis* live in human hair follicles and sebaceous glands, causing *demodicidosis* (see Demodicidosis, p. 731).

Food, fowl, grain, straw, harvest, and animal mite bites cause papular urticaria.

FOOD MITES Cheese, grain, or mold mites can cause mild contact dermatitis: Baker's or grocer's itch. *Straw mites.* Bites occur during harvest season causing dermatitis; straw itch. *Harvest mite:* Chiggers. Bites can cause dermatitis. One species transmits *Rickettsia tsutsugamushi*, the cause of scrub typhus.

Dermatophagoides species of house dust mites are implicated in the pathogenesis of asthma and atopic dermatitis. Feed on desquamated human skin and other organic detritus, living in bedding, carpets, and furniture. Bodies and excreta may have a role in asthma and other allergies. Affected persons respond with production of IgE antibodies. *Fowl mites.* Chicken, pigeons, etc. Bites cause papular urticaria on exposed sites. *Rat mites* cause painful bites and dermatitis and transmit endemic/murine typhus. *House mouse mite* is the vector for rickettsialpox. *Cheyletiella* spp. (dog and cat mites) bite pet owners causing pruritic lesions on forearms, chest, and abdomen. Canine sarcoptic mange (*S. scabiei* var. *canis*) and feline

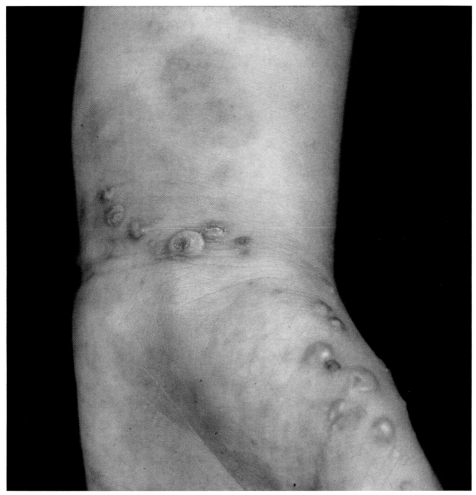

FIGURE 28-4 Bullous insect bite A 10-year-old child with bullous lesions on the ventral wrist and popular urticarial on the forearm.

mange (*Notoedres cati*) cause a pruritic dermatosis in pet owners.

TICKS Ticks attach and feed painlessly. Secretions can produce local bite reactions (erythema), febrile illness, and paralysis. Black-legged or *Ixodes* tick, lone star tick, and dog tick are vectors for diseases. Erythema migrans (see Fig. 25-81), characteristic of primary Lyme disease or borreliosis, occurs at the bite site of an infected *Ixodes* tick that transmits *Borrelia burgdorferi*, *B. mayonii* (Midwestern US).

Lymphocytoma cutis (see Fig. 25-82) also occurs at the site of bite of an infected *Ixodes* tick. **SPIDERS** *Brown recluse spider* bites can result in mild local urticarial reactions to full-thickness

skin necrosis. Associated with a maculopapular exanthem, fever, headache, malaise, arthralgia, and nausea/vomiting. Most lesions diagnosed as brown recluse spider bites are bite reactions to other arthropods. *Widow spiders* inject a neurotoxin (α-latrotoxin) that produces bite site reactions as well as varying degrees of systemic toxicity.

INSECTS *Pubic lice, head lice, body lice* papular urticaria, excoriations, and secondary infections (see pages 726–731).

Mosquitoes. Bites usually present as papular urticaria (Fig. 28-3) on exposed sites; reactions can be urticaria, eczematous, or granulomatous.

Black Flies. Anesthetic is injected, resulting in a painless initial bite; may subsequently become painful with itching, erythema, and edema. Black fly fever is characterized by fever, nausea, and generalized lymphadenitis.

Midges. Bites produce immediate pain with erythema at bite site with 2- to 3-mm papule and vesicles, followed by indurated nodules (up to 1 cm) persisting for many months.

Tabanidae or horse flies. Bites painful with papular urticaria; rarely associated with anaphylaxis.

Dermatobia hominis (human botfly) in tropical regions causes furuncular myiasis, painful lesions that resemble pyogenic granuloma or abscess. Female botfly captures a mosquito, attaches its eggs to the mosquito body, and then releases the mosquito. Eggs hatch on the mosquito becoming larvae and are deposited on human skin. Larvae use bite site as portal of entry into skin. A pruritic papule develops at the site, slowly enlarging over several weeks into a domed nodule (resembles a furuncle) with a central pore (Fig. 28-5). Larvae drop out after 8 weeks to pupate in soil.

House Flies. Larvae deposited into any exposed skin site (ear, nose, paranasal sinuses, mouth, eye, anus, and vagina) or at any wound site (leg ulcers, ulcerated squamous and basal cell carcinomas, hematomas, or umbilical stump)

and grow into maggots, which can be seen on the surface of wound causing wound myiasis (Fig. 28-6). Maggot debridement therapy is used to selectively debride necrotic wound tissue.

Cimex lectularius or bedbugs bite exposed skin (face, neck, arms, or hands) of sleeping humans. Feeding takes 5 to 10 minutes. Grouped papular urticaria (Fig. 28-2) occur at bite sites, usually, but now always, in groups of three ("breakfast, lunch, and dinner"). Bedbug hides in crevices of walls, mattresses, and furniture. Reddish brown streaks may be seen on mattress; bedbugs defecate old blood meal while ingesting a new meal.

Reduviid or kissing bugs bite usually present as papular urticaria; severe reactions can produce necrosis and ulceration. Subfamily of reduviid bugs transmits *Trypanosoma cruzi,* the agent of Chagas disease.

Fleas. Papular urticaria at bite site. Dog fleas often live in carpeting and bite exposed lower legs. Secondary changes of excoriation, prurigo nodularis, and *S. aureus* infection occur.

Tunga Penetrans or Chigoe Flea. Papule, nodule, or vesicle (6 to 8 mm in diameter) with a central black dot (tungiasis) produced by posterior part of the flea's abdominal segments. As eggs mature, papule becomes a black, pea-sized nodule (Fig. 28-7). With severe infestation, nodules and plaques appear with a

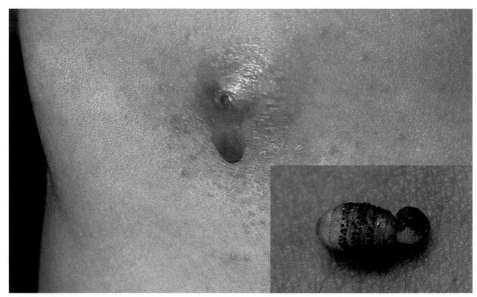

FIGURE 28-5 Furuncular myiasis A pruritic papule at the site of deposition of a botfly larva, slowly enlarging over several weeks into a domed nodule (resembles a furuncle). The lesion has a central pore through which the posterior end of the larva (inset) intermittently protrudes and thus respires.

FIGURE 28-6 Wound myiasis
Multiple housefly larvae in a chronic stasis ulcer on the ankle after castellani paint and Unna boot treatment for 1 week. Upon removal, the maggots were visible; and the base of the ulcer was red and clean, having been debrided by maggots.

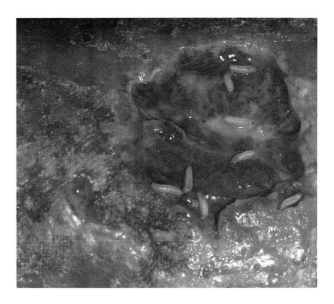

honeycombed appearance. Ulceration, inflammation, and secondary infection can occur. Most common on feet, especially under the toenails, webspaces, plantar aspect of the feet, and sparing weight-bearing areas; in sunbathers, any area of exposed skin.

Female bee, hornet, or wasp sting producing immediate burning/pain, followed by intense, local, erythematous reaction with swelling and urticaria. Severe systemic reactions occur in individuals who are sensitized, with angioedema/generalized urticaria and/or respiratory insufficiency from laryngeal edema or bronchospasm and/or shock.

Fire and *harvester ants* produce local skin necrosis and systemic reactions to sting; bite reaction begins as an intense local inflammatory reaction that evolves to a sterile pustule.

Caterpillar/moth contact can produce burning/itching sensation, papular urticaria, irritation caused by histamine release, allergic contact dermatitis (Fig. 28-8), and/or systemic reactions. Wind-borne hairs can cause keratoconjunctivitis.

DIFFERENTIAL DIAGNOSIS

Papular urticaria. Allergic contact dermatitis, especially to plants such as poison ivy or poison oak.

DIAGNOSIS

Clinical diagnosis, at times, confirmed by lesional biopsy.

TREATMENT

PREVENTION Apply insect repellent such as diethyltoluamide (DEET) to skin and permethrin spray to clothing. Use screens, nets, and clothing. Treat flea-infested cats and dogs; spray household with insecticides (e.g., malathion, 1 to 4% dust).

LARVAE IN SKIN *Tungiasis.* Remove flea with needle, scalpel, or curette; topical petrolatum to suffocate fleas; topical ivermectin; oral thiabendazole or metrifonate for heavy infestations.

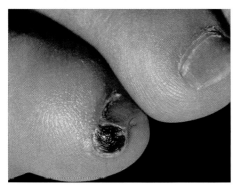

FIGURE 28-7 Tungiasis Periungual papule with surrounding erythema on the lateral margin of the fifth toe; the larva is visualized by removing the overlying crust.

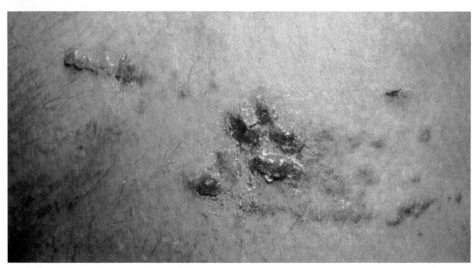

FIGURE 28-8 Immunologic IgE-mediated contact urticaria: pine processionary caterpillar Linear edematous papules and vesicles occurred on the exposed arm shortly after exposure to *Thaumeto-poea pityocampa* in a pine forest.

FURUNCULAR MYIASIS Suffocate larvae by covering with petrolatum and removing the following day.

GLUCOCORTICOIDS Give potent topical glucocorticoids for a short duration for intense pruritus.

Oral glucocorticoids can be given for persistent pruritus.

ANTIMICROBIAL AGENTS Secondary infection antibiotic treatment with topical agents.

SYSTEMIC INFECTION/INFESTATION Treat with appropriate antimicrobial agent.

PEDICULOSIS CAPITIS ICD-10: B85.0

- Infestation of the scalp by the head louse.
- Feeds on scalp and neck and deposits its eggs on hair.
- Presence of head lice is associated with few symptoms but much consternation.

ETIOLOGY AND EPIDEMIOLOGY

SUBSPECIES *Pediculus Humanus Capitis.* Sesame seed size, 1 to 2 mm. Feed every 4 to 6 h. Move by grasping hairs close to scalp; can crawl up to 23 cm/day. Lice lay nits within 1 to 2 mm of scalp. Nits are ova within chitinous case. Young lice hatch within 1 week, passing through nymphal stages and maturing to adults over a period of 1 week. One female can lay 50 to 150 ova during a 16-day lifetime. Survive only for a few hours off scalp. Transmission: Head-to-head contact; shared hats, caps, brushes, combs; theater seats; pillows. Head louse is not a vector of infectious disease.

DEMOGRAPHY In the United States, more common in whites than blacks; claws have adapted to grip cylindrical hair; hair pomade may inhibit infestation. In Africa, pediculosis capitis is relatively uncommon. Estimated that 6 to 12 million persons in the United States are infested annually.

CLINICAL MANIFESTATION

SYMPTOMS Pruritus of the back and sides of scalp. Scratching and secondary infection associated with occipital and/or cervical lymphadenopathy. Some individuals exhibit obsessive-compulsive disorder or delusions of parasitosis after eradications of lice and nits.

INFESTATION *Head lice* are identified by eye or by microscopy (hand lens or dermatoscope) but are difficult to find. Most patients have a population of <10 head lice. *Nits* are the oval grayish-white egg capsules (1 mm long) firmly cemented to the hairs (Fig. 28-9); vary in number from only a few to thousands. Nits are deposited by head

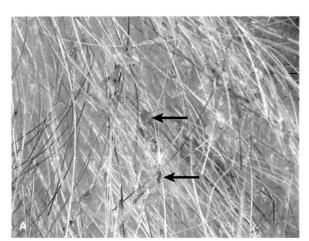
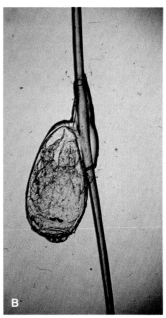

FIGURE 28-9 Pediculosis capitis: nits (A) *Arrows:* Grayish-white egg capsules (nits) are firmly attached to the hair shafts, visualized with a lens. **(B)** Magnified, an egg with a developing head louse nymph attached to a hair shaft is seen.

lice on the hair shaft as it emerges from the follicle. With current infestation, nits are near the scalp; with infestation of long standing, nits may be 10 to 15 cm from the scalp. In that scalp hair grows 0.5 mm daily, the presence of nits 15 cm from the scalp indicates that the infestation is approximately 9 months old. New viable eggs have a creamy-yellow color; empty eggshells are white. *Sites of predilection*: Head lice nearly always confined to the scalp, especially occipital and postauricular regions. Rarely, head lice infest the beard or other hairy sites. Although more common with crab lice, head lice can also infest the eyelashes (*pediculosis palpebrarum*). **SKIN LESIONS** *Bite reactions*: Papular urticaria on the neck. Reactions related to immune sensitivity/tolerance. *Secondary lesions: Eczema, excoriation, or lichen simplex chronicus* on the occipital scalp and neck secondary to chronic scratching/rubbing. *Secondary infection* with *S. aureus* of eczema or excoriations; may extend onto the neck, forehead, face, or ears. Posterior occipital lymphadenopathy.

DIFFERENTIAL DIAGNOSIS

Small White Hair "Beads" Hair casts (inner root sheath remnants), hair lacquer, hair gels, dandruff (epidermal scales), and piedra.

SCALP PRURITUS Atopic dermatitis, impetigo, and lichen simplex chronicus.
NO INFESTATION Delusions of parasitosis.

LABORATORY EXAMINATIONS

MICROSCOPY *Nits* 0.5-mm oval, whitish eggs (Fig. 28-9B). Nonviable nits show an absence of an embryo or operculum. *Louse.* Insect with six legs, 1 to 2 mm in length, wingless, translucent grayish-white body that is red when engorged with blood.

DIAGNOSIS

Clinical findings, confirmed by detection of lice. Louse comb increases chances of finding lice. Nits alone are not diagnostic of active infestation. Nits within 4 mm of scalp suggest active infestation.

TREATMENT

TOPICALLY APPLIED INSECTICIDES Permethrin, malathion, pyrethrin, ivermectin, and spinosad.
SYSTEMIC Oral ivermectin, levamisole, and albendazole.

PEDICULOSIS CORPORIS ICD-10:B85.1

- Body lice reside and lay eggs in clothing. They occur in poor socioeconomic conditions.
- Lice leave clothing to feed on a human host. Body louse survives more than a few hours away from the human host.
- Body lice are vectors of many systemic infections.

EPIDEMIOLOGY AND ETIOLOGY

ETIOLOGIC AGENT *Pediculus Humanus Humanus.* Larger than head louse: 2 to 4 mm; otherwise indistinguishable. Life span 18 days. Female lays 270 to 300 ova. Nits: Ova within chitinous case. Nits incubate for 8 to 10 days; nymphs mature to adults in 14 days.

HABITAT Live in seams of clothing; can survive without blood meal for up to 3 days. Attaches to body hairs to feed. Risk factors for infestation include poverty, war, natural disasters, indigence, homelessness, and refugee-camp populations.

BODY LICE AS VECTORS OF DISEASE Body lice transmit many infectious agents while feeding. *Bartonella quintana* causes trench fever and endocarditis. *Rickettsia prowazekii* causes epidemic typhus. *Brill–Zinsser disease (louse-borne relapsing fever)* is recrudescence of epidemic typhus fever.

CLINICAL MANIFESTATION

INFESTATION Lice and nits are found in clothing seams (Fig. 28-10). Lice grab on to body hairs to feed.

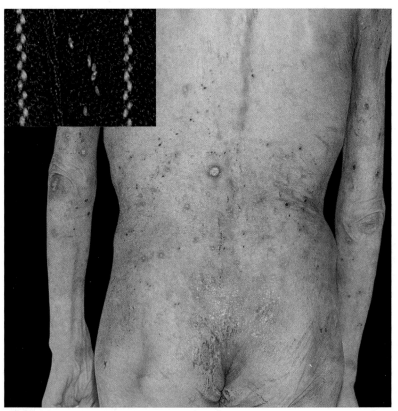

FIGURE 28-10 Pediculosis corporis A 60-year-old homeless male. Multiple lesions secondary to excoriations, prurigo nodularis, and lichen simplex chronicus. Lice and nits are seen in the seams of clothing (inset).

REACTIONS TO BITES Bite reactions such as papular urticarial (Fig. 28-10) are similar to those of head lice. Changes secondary to rubbing and scratching include excoriations, eczema, lichen simplex, infection with *S. aureus*, and postinflammatory hyperpigmentation (Fig. 28-10). Scabies, pediculosis capitis, and *Pulex irritans* (the human flea) can coexist.

DIFFERENTIAL DIAGNOSIS

Atopic dermatitis, contact dermatitis, scabies, or adverse cutaneous drug reaction.

DIAGNOSIS

Lice and eggs are found in clothing seams.

TREATMENT

DECONTAMINATION OF CLOTHING AND BEDDING Hygiene measures.
DELOUSING Pyrethrin, permethrin.

PEDICULOSIS PUBIS ICD-10: B85.2

- In infestation of hair-bearing regions by the crab or pubic lice.
- Most commonly inhabit the pubic area; hairy parts of the chest and axillae; upper eyelashes.
- Manifested clinically by mild-to-moderate pruritus, papular urticaria, and excoriations.

ETIOLOGY AND EPIDEMIOLOGY

Phthirius pubis, the crab or pubic louse. Size 0.8 to 1.2 mm. First pair of legs vestigial; other two clawed (Fig. 28-11). Life span 14 days. Female lays 25 ova. Nits incubate for 7 days; nymphs mature over 14 days. Mobility: Adults can crawl 10 cm/day. Prefer a humid environment; tend not to wander. Infestation most common in young males. Transmission during close physical contact: Sharing bed. May coexist with other sexually transmitted diseases.

CLINICAL MANIFESTATION

OFTEN ASYMPTOMATIC Mild-to-moderate pruritus for months. With excoriation and secondary infection, lesions may become tender and be associated with enlarged regional.
INFESTATION *Lice* appear as 1- to 2-mm, brownish-gray specks (Figs. 28-12 and 28-13) in hairy areas involved. Remain stationary for days; mouth parts embedded in skin; claws grasping a hair on either side. Usually few in number. *Nits* attached to hair appear as tiny white-gray specks

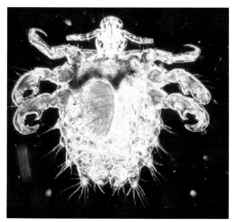

FIGURE 28-11 Crab louse Adult female with an egg developing within her body.

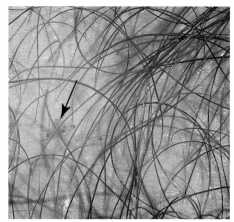

FIGURE 28-12 Crab louse Crab louse (*arrow*) on the skin in the pubic region.

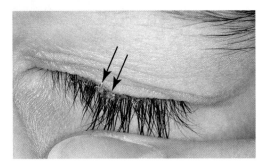

FIGURE 28-13 Crab lice in eyelashes A 10-year-old child. Crab lice (*arrows*) and nits on the upper eyelashes of a child; this was the only site of infestation.

(Fig. 28-13). Few to numerous. Eggs at hair–skin junction indicate active infestation. *Infestation* most common in pubic and axillary areas; also, perineum, thighs, lower legs, trunk, and periumbilical. In children, eyelashes (Fig. 28-13) and eyebrows may be infested without pubic involvement. Maculae coeruleae (see below)

most common on lower abdominal wall, buttocks, and upper thighs.

SKIN LESIONS *Papular urticaria* (small erythematous papules) at sites of feeding, especially periumbilical (Fig. 28-14). *Changes secondary to rubbing lichenification and excoriations.* Secondary *S. aureus* infection. *Maculae coeruleae*

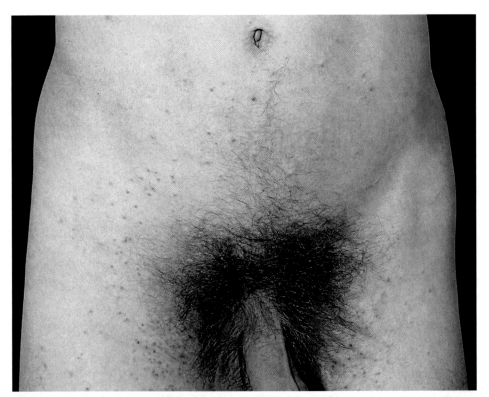

FIGURE 28-14 Crab lice infestation: papular urticaria A 25-year-old with pruritus. Multiple inflammatory papules at sites of crab lice bites on the abdomen and the inner aspects of the thighs.

(*taches bleues*) are slate-gray or bluish-gray macules around 0.5 to 1 cm in diameter, non-blanching. Result from crab louse bites. With eyelid infestation, serous crusts may be present along with lice and nits; occasionally, edema of eyelids with severe infestation.

With secondary impetiginization, regional lymphadenopathy.

DIFFERENTIAL DIAGNOSIS

Atopic dermatitis, seborrheic dermatitis, tinea cruris, molluscum contagiosum, and scabies. These disorders may coexist with crab louse infestation.

DIAGNOSIS

Demonstration of live adult lice, nymphs, or nits in the pubic area to diagnose active infestation.

COURSE

Treatment is usually effective. Reinfestation can occur. Retreatment may be necessary if lice are found or if eggs are observed at the hair–skin junction.

TREATMENT

PEDICULOSIS See p. 727. Decontaminate bedding and clothing. Treat sex partners.

DEMODICIDOSIS ICD-10: B88.0

Demodex species are human face mites, part of the human cutaneous microbiome. *D. folliculorum* resides in hair follicles; *D. brevis*, infundibulum of sebaceous glands. Mites do not invade tissue. Site of habitation usually symptomatic. In some cases, this causes an inflammatory reaction (demodicidosis) that occurs with lesions resembling rosacea, suppurative folliculitis, or perioral dermatitis (Fig. 28-15).

■ **Treatment.** Topical ivermectin, permethrin; in severe cases oral ivermectin 200 μg/kg.

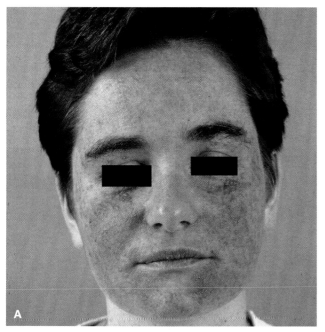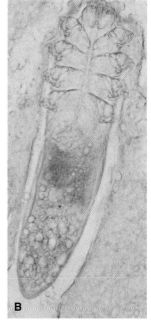

FIGURE 28-15 Demodicidosis A 25-year-old female noted facial rash the day after a heavy workout. **(A)** Tender red papules on the face. Lesions look like papular rosacea. **(B)** Microscopic examination of curetting of papule demonstrates *Demodex* mite. Lesions resolved with oral ivermectin.

SCABIES ICD-10: B86

- **Superficial epidermal infestation** by the mite *Sarcoptes scabiei* var. *hominis*. ***Transmission:*** Usually spread by skin-to-skin contact and fomites.
- **Clinical Manifestation.** *Pruritus* often with minimal cutaneous findings. *Burrows* under stratum corneum.
- **Scabetic Nodules.** *Eczematous dermatitis. Hyperinfestation* (crusted or hyperkeratotic or Norwegian scabies).
- **Diagnosis.** Easily missed and should be considered in a patient of any age with persistent generalized severe pruritus.

ETIOLOGY AND EPIDEMIOLOGY

ETIOLOGIC AGENT *S. scabiei* var. *hominis*. Obligate human parasite. Mites of all developmental stages burrow into epidermis shortly after contact, no deeper than stratum granulosum; deposit feces in tunnels (Fig. 28-16). Female life span 4 to 6 weeks; lays 40 to 50 eggs. Lays 3 eggs per day in burrows; eggs hatch in 4 days. Leave burrow, usually at night, and lay eggs during the day. Hatched larvae migrate to skin surface and mature into adults. Males and females copulate. Gravid female burrows back under stratum corneum; male falls off. In classic scabies, approximately 10 females per patient are present. With hyperinfestation, >1 million mites may be present. Estimated at 300 million cases/year worldwide.

DEMOGRAPHY Major public health problem in many less-developed countries. In some areas of South and Central America, prevalence is about 100%. In Bangladesh, the number of children with scabies exceeds that of children with diarrheal and upper-respiratory disease. In countries where human T cell leukemia/lymphoma virus (HTLV-I) disease is common, hyperinfestation scabies is a marker of this infection. Transmission by skin-to-skin contact and fomites. Mites can remain alive for >2 days on clothing or in bedding. Persons with hyperinfestation shed many mites into their environment daily and pose a high risk of infecting those around them.

PATHOGENESIS

Hypersensitivity of both immediate and delayed types occurs in the development of lesions other than burrows. During *first infestation*, pruritus occurs after sensitization to *S. scabiei* has occurred, usually within 4 to 6 weeks. After *reinfestation*, pruritus may occur within 24 h. With *hyperinfestation*, persons are often *immunocompromised* or have *neurologic disorders*.

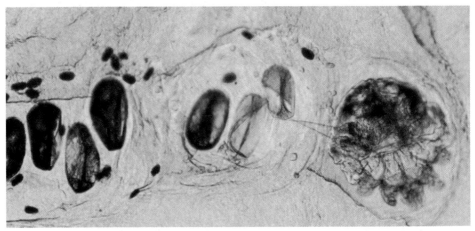

FIGURE 28-16 Burrow with Sarcoptes scabiei (female), eggs, and feces Female mite at the end of a burrow with seven eggs and smaller fecal particles obtained from a papule on the webspace of the hand.

CLINICAL MANIFESTATION

Symptoms

Patients are often aware of similar symptoms in family members or sexual partners. *Pruritus* is intense, widespread, but usually spares the head and neck. Itching often interferes with or prevents sleep. Pruritus may be absent with hyperinfestation. *Rash* ranges from no rash to generalized erythroderma. Patients with atopic diathesis scratch, producing eczematous dermatitis. Some individuals experience pruritus for many months with no rash. Tenderness of lesions suggests secondary bacterial infection.

Cutaneous Findings

(1) Lesions occurring at the sites of mite infestation, (2) cutaneous manifestations of hypersensitivity to mites, (3) lesions secondary to chronic rubbing and scratching, (4) secondary infection, (5) hyperinfestation, and (6) variants of scabies in special hosts: those with an atopic diathesis, nodular scabies, scabies in infants/small children, and scabies in the elderly.

INTRAEPIDERMAL BURROWS Skin-colored ridges, 0.5 to 1 cm in length (Figs. 28-17 to 28-19), either linear or serpiginous, with minute vesicle or papule at end of tunnel. Each infesting female mite produces one burrow. Mites are about 0.5 mm in length. Burrows average 5 mm in length but may be up to 10 cm. *Distribution*: Areas with few or no hair follicles, usually where stratum corneum is thin and soft, i.e., the interdigital webs of the hands (Fig. 28-17), wrists, palms and soles in infants (Fig. 28-18), shaft of penis, elbows, feet, buttocks, or axillae (Figs. 28-19 and 28-20). In infants, infestation may also occur on head and neck.

Scabies with nodules 5 to 20 mm in diameter, red, pink, tan, or brown in color, smooth (Fig. 28-21); burrow sometimes seen on the surface of a very early lesion. *Distribution*: Scrotum, penis (Fig. 28-21), axillae, waist, buttocks (Fig. 28-22), or areolae. Resolve with postinflammatory hyperpigmentation. May be more apparent after treatment, as eczematous eruption resolves.

SCABIES WITH HYPERINFESTATION (FORMERLY CALLED NORWEGIAN SCABIES) May begin as ordinary scabies. In others, clinical appearance is of chronic eczema, psoriasiform dermatitis, seborrheic dermatitis, or erythroderma. Lesions often markedly hyperkeratotic and/or crusted (Figs. 28-23 and 28-24). Warty dermatosis of the hands/feet with nail bed hyperkeratosis. Erythematous scaling eruptions occur on the face, neck, scalp, and trunk. Affected persons have a characteristic odor. *Distribution*:

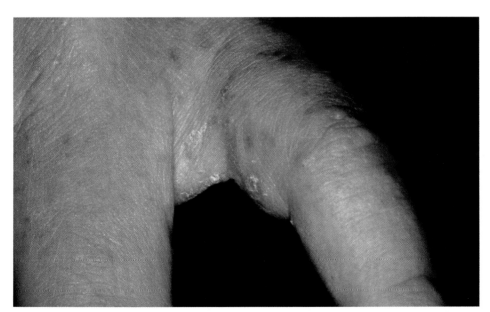

FIGURE 28-17 Scabies with burrows Papules and burrows in typical location on the finger web. Burrows are tan or skin-colored ridges with linear configuration with a minute vesicle or papule at the end of the burrow; they are often difficult to define.

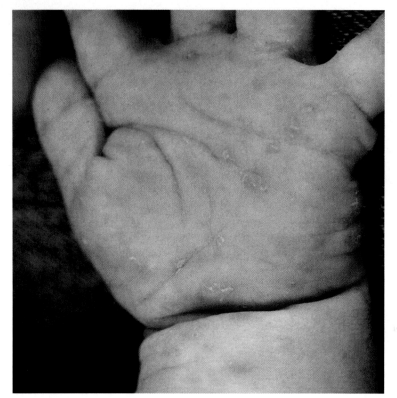

FIGURE 28-18 Burrows of scabies on the palm of a 3-year-old infant. There are many linear and even semi-circular lesions. The whole family was affected.

Generalized (even involving head and neck in adults) or localized. In patients with neurologic deficit, hyperinfestation may occur only in an affected limb. May be localized only to the scalp, face, finger, toenail bed, or sole.

"Id" or autosensitization-type reactions characterized by widespread small urticarial edematous papules mainly on the anterior trunk, thighs, buttocks, and forearms. **SECONDARY CHANGES** Excoriations, lichen simplex chronicus, and prurigo nodules. Postinflammatory hyper- and hypopigmentation in more deeply pigmented individuals. Bullous scabies can mimic bullous pemphigoid. Secondary infection by *S. aureus*.

DIFFERENTIAL DIAGNOSIS

Pruritus, localized or generalized, rash delusions of parasitosis, adverse cutaneous drug reaction, atopic dermatitis, allergic contact dermatitis, and metabolic pruritus.

Nodular scabies. urticaria pigmentosa (in young child), papular urticaria (insect bites), prurigo nodularis, and pseudolymphoma. **SCABETIC HYPERINFESTATION** Psoriasis, eczematous dermatitis, seborrheic dermatitis, and erythroderma.

LABORATORY EXAMINATIONS

MICROSCOPY Highest yield in identifying a mite is in typical burrows on the finger webs, flexor aspects of wrists, and penis. A drop of mineral oil is placed over a burrow, and the burrow is scraped off with a curette or no. 15 scalpel blade and placed on a microscope slide. Three findings are diagnostic of scabies: *S. scabiei* mites, eggs, and fecal pellets (scybala) (Fig. 28-24). **DERMATOPATHOLOGY** *Scabietic burrow*: Located within stratum corneum; female mite with eggs situated in blind end of burrow. Spongiosis (epidermal edema) near mite with vesicle formation common. Dermis shows infiltrate

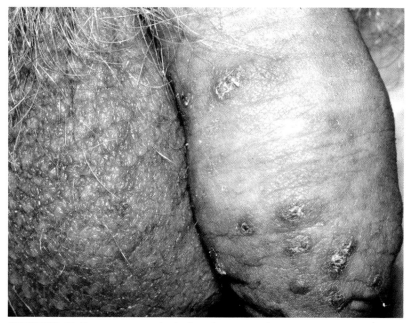

FIGURE 28-19 Burrows on penis shaft and scrotum If you suspect scabies in a male, always look at the penis.

FIGURE 28-20 Scabies: Predilection sites Burrows are most easy to identify on the webspace of the hands, wrists, and lateral aspects of the palms. Scabietic nodules occur uncommonly, arising on the genitalia, especially the penis and scrotum, waist, axillae, and areolae.

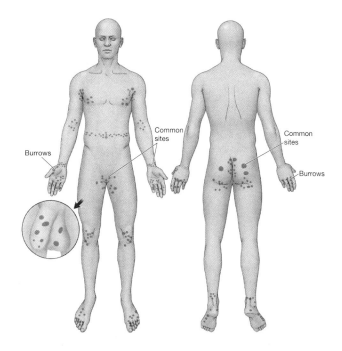

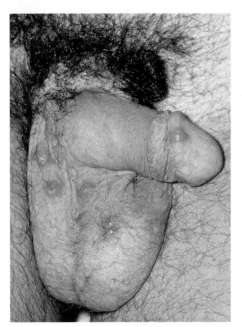

FIGURE 28-21 Scabies with nodules Red-brown papules and nodules on the penis and scrotum; these lesions are pathognomonic for scabies, occurring at sites of infestation in some individuals.

with eosinophils. Nodules: Dense chronic inflammatory infiltrate with eosinophils. In some cases, persistent arthropod reaction resembling lymphoma with atypical mononuclear cells. Hyperinfestation: Thickened stratum corneum riddled with innumerable mites.

DIAGNOSIS

Clinical findings, confirmed by microscopy (identification of mites, eggs, or mite feces).

COURSE

Pruritus often persists up to several weeks after successful eradication of mite infestation, understandable in that the pruritus is a hypersensitivity phenomenon to mite antigen(s). If reinfestation occurs, pruritus becomes symptomatic within a few days. Delusions of parasitosis can occur in individuals who have been successfully treated for scabies or have never had scabies. Hyperinfestation: May be impossible to eradicate; recurrence more likely to relapse than reinfestation. Nodules: In treated patients, 80% resolve in 3 months but may persist up to 1 year.

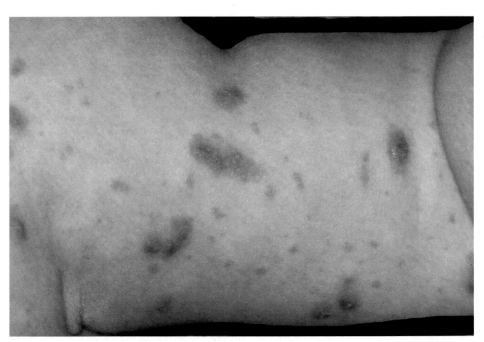

FIGURE 28-22 Scabies with nodules A 4-year-old infant with reddish brown nodules on thigh and buttocks persisting after treatment with permethrin.

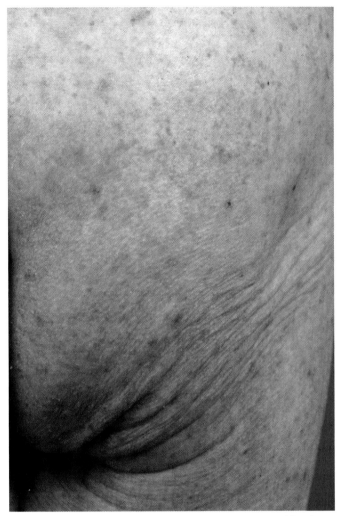

FIGURE 28-23 Scabies with hyperinfestation A 60-year-old mal-nourished female with hundreds of papular lesions and burrows on the back and buttocks. Pruritus was excruciating.

MANAGEMENT

PRINCIPLES OF TREATMENT Treat infested individuals and close physical contacts (including sexual partners) at the same time, whether or not symptoms are present. Application should be to all skin sites.

RECOMMENDED REGIMENS Permethrin 5%. Cream applied to all areas of the body. Lindane (g-Benzene Hexachloride) 1% lotion or cream applied thinly to all areas of the body from the neck down; wash off thoroughly after 8 h. Note: Lindane should not be used after a bath or shower, or by patients with extensive dermatitis, pregnant or lactating women, or children younger than 2 years. Mite resistance to lindane exists. Low cost makes lindane a key alternative in many countries.

ALTERNATIVE REGIMENS *Topical.* Crotamiton 10%, sulfur 2 to 10% in petrolatum, benzyl benzoate 10% and 25%, benzyl benzoate with sulfiram, malathion 0.5%, sulfram 25%, and ivermectin 0.8%.

Systemic. Oral ivermectin, 200 mg/kg; single dose reported very effective in 15 to 30 days. Two to three doses, separated by 1 to 2 weeks,

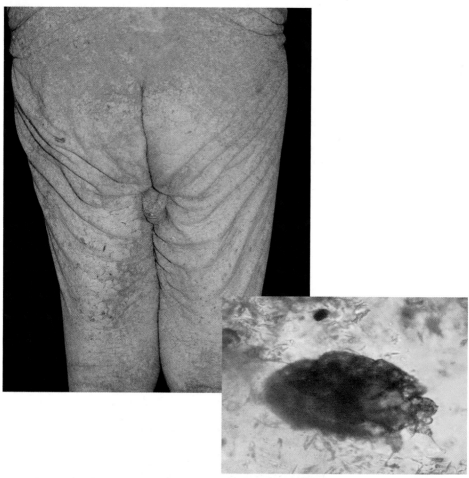

FIGURE 28-24 Scabies with hyperinfestation A 79-year-old male with hyperkeratotic scabies for 4 years. The patient had been treated in his home with topical antiscabetic agents and oral ivermectin as well as extensive decontamination of his home on multiple occasions. Confluent hyperkeratotic plaques are seen on the back, buttocks, and legs. As many as five scabetic mites were seen on one microscope field (see inset).

usually required for heavy infestation or in immunocompromised individuals. May effectively eradicate epidemic or endemic scabies in institutions such as nursing homes, hospitals, and refugee camps. Not approved by U.S. Food and Drug Administration or European Drug Agency. Do not use in infants, young children, or pregnant/lactating women.

CRUSTED SCABIES Oral ivermectin combined with topical scalicides (not ivermectin). Decontamination of the environment.

NODULES of scabies resolve after intralesional injection of triamcinolone acetonide.

POSTSCABIETIC ITCHING Generalized itching that persists a week or more is probably caused by hypersensitivity to remaining dead mites and mite products. Antihistamines, topical steroids can be used. For severe, persistent pruritus, especially in individuals with a history of atopic disorders, a 14-day tapered course of prednisone is indicated.

SECONDARY BACTERIAL INFECTION Treat with mupirocin ointment or systemic antimicrobial agent.

CUTANEOUS LARVA MIGRANS ICD-10: B76

- **Creeping Eruption.** Cutaneous infestation following percutaneous penetration and epidermal migration of hookworm larvae.
- **Etiologic Agents.** *Cutaneous larva migrans*: Hookworms larvae of *Ancylostoma braziliense* in the United States. Ova of hookworms are deposited in sand and soil in warm shady areas, hatching into larvae that penetrate human skin. Humans are aberrant, dead-end hosts who acquire the parasite from an environment contaminated with animal feces. Larvae penetrate human skin, migrating within the epidermis up to several centimeters a day. Most larvae are unable to develop further or invade deeper tissues and die after days or months. *Larva currens*: *Strongyloides stercoralis; filariform* larvae can penetrate skin (usually on buttocks), producing lesions similar to larva migrans.

CLINICAL MANIFESTATION

CUTANEOUS LARVA MIGRANS Serpiginous, thin, linear, raised, and tunnel-like lesion 2 to 3 mm wide containing serous fluid (Fig. 28-25). Several or many lesions may be present, depending on the number of penetrating larvae (Fig. 28-26). Larvae move a few to many millimeters daily, confined to an area of several centimeters in diameter. Infestation most commonly occurs on the feet, lower legs, and buttocks.

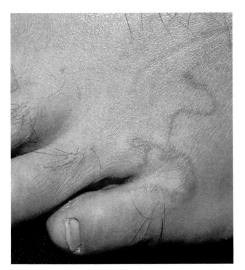

FIGURE 28-25 Cutaneous larva migrans A serpiginous, linear, raised, tunnel-like erythematous lesion outlining the path of migration of the larva.

LARVA CURRENS (CUTANEOUS STRONGYLOIDIASIS) A distinctive form of larva migrans. Papules, urticaria, papulovesicles at the site of larval penetration (Fig. 28-27). Associated with intense pruritus. Occurs on buttocks, thighs, back, shoulders, and abdomen. Pruritus and eruption disappear when larvae enter blood vessels and migrate to intestinal mucosa.

DIFFERENTIAL DIAGNOSIS

Migratory lesions from other parasites, photoallergic contact dermatitis, jellyfish sting, and epidermal dermatophytosis.

LABORATORY FINDINGS

DERMATOPATHOLOGY Parasites seen on biopsy specimens from advancing point of the lesion.

DIAGNOSIS

Clinical findings.

COURSE

Self-limited; humans are "dead-end" hosts. Most larvae die and the lesions resolve within 2 to 8 weeks.

TREATMENT

TOPICAL AGENTS Thiabendazole, ivermectin, and albendazole are effective.
SYSTEMIC AGENTS Thiabendazole, orally 50 mg/kg per day in two doses (maximum 3 g/d) for 2 to 5 days; ivermectin, 6 mg twice daily, albendazole, 400 mg/d for 3 days; highly effective.
REMOVAL OF PARASITE Do not attempt; parasite not in visible lesions.

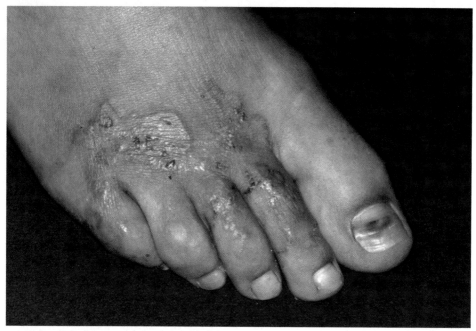

FIGURE 28-26 Cutaneous larva migrans   Multiple raised, tunnel-like, partially crusted and scaly lesions on forefoot.

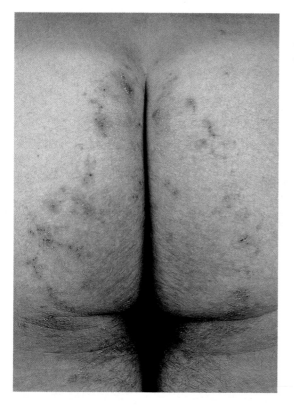

FIGURE 28-27 Larva currens   Multiple, pruritic, serpiginous, inflammatory lines on the buttocks at sites of penetration of *S. stercoralis* larvae.

WATER-ASSOCIATED DISEASES

- Various aquatic microorganisms can cause soft-tissue infections after exposure.
- Bacteria. *Aeromonas hydrophila*, *Edwardsiella tarda*, *Erysipelothrix rhusiopathiae*, *Mycobacterium marinum*, *Pfiesteria piscicida*, *Pseudomonas* species, *Streptococcus* iniae, *Vibrio vulnificus*, and other *Vibrio* species.
- Alga. *Prototheca wickerhamii*.
- Localized Cutaneous Infestations. Cercarial dermatitis and seabather's eruption can occur after exposure to microscopic marine animals.
- Cnidaria (jellyfish) and echinoderms (sea urchins, starfish) can cause envenomation.

SCHISTOSOME CERCARIAL DERMATITIS ICD-10: B65.3

- Swimmer's itch, clam digger's itch, schistosome dermatitis, and sedge pool itch.
- Acute pruritic papular eruption at the sites of cutaneous penetration by *Schistosoma cercariae* larvae of schistosomes whose usual hosts are birds and small mammals.
- Schistosomes implicated: *Trichobilharzia, Gigantobilharzia, Ornithobilharzia, Microbilharzia*, and *Schistosomatium*.
- Exposure can be to fresh, brackish, or saltwater. Eggs produced by adult schistosomes living in animals are shed with animal feces into the environment; on reaching water, schistosome eggs hatch, releasing fully developed larvae (miracidia). Snails are the appropriate hosts for miracidia, from which they emerge as cercariae. These must penetrate the skin of a vertebrate host to continue development.
- **Transmission.** Humans are dead-end hosts. Cercariae penetrate human skin, elicit an inflammatory response, and die without invading other tissues. Occurs worldwide in areas with fresh and saltwater inhabited by appropriate molluscan hosts. Acquired by skin exposure to fresh/saltwater infested by cercariae.

CLINICAL MANIFESTATION

Pruritus and rash begin within hours after exposure. A pruritic macular, papular, papulovesicular, and/or urticarial eruption develops at exposed sites with marked pruritus (Fig. 28-28), sparing parts of the body covered by clothing. (In contrast, seabather's eruption occurs on areas of the body covered by swimsuits.) *Papular urticaria* occurs at each site of penetration in previously sensitized individuals. In highly sensitized persons, lesions may progress to eczematous plaques, urticarial wheals, and/or vesicles, reaching a peak 2 to 3 days after exposure. Schistosomes capable of causing invasive disease in humans (*Schistosoma mansoni, S. haematobium,* and *S. japonicum*) may cause a similar skin eruption shortly after penetration as well as late *visceral complications*.

COURSE

Lesions usually resolve within a week.

TREATMENT

Topical and/or systemic glucocorticoids may be indicated in more severe cases.

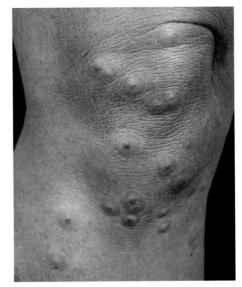

FIGURE 28-28 Schistosome cercarial dermatitis A highly pruritic papulovesicular eruption on the knees acquired after the patient waded through a slow-flowing creek.

SEABATHER'S ERUPTION ICD-10: B65.3

- **Etiology.** Caused by exposure to two marine animals: Larvae of the thimble jellyfish, *Linuche unguiculata,* in waters off the coast of Florida, Caribbean, Mexico, and Brazil. Planula larvae of the sea anemone, *Edwardsiella lineata,* Long Island, NY.
- Pathogenesis nematocysts of coelenterate larvae sting the skin of hairy areas or under swimwear, presumably causing an allergic reaction. Some affected individuals recall a stinging or prickling sensation while in the water.

CLINICAL MANIFESTATION

Lesions present clinically as inflammatory papules 4 to 24 h after exposure (Fig. 28-29). A monomorphous eruption of erythematous papules or papulovesicles is seen most commonly: vesicles, pustules, and papular urticaria, which may progress to crusted erosions. In comparison with cercarial dermatitis, which occurs on exposed sites, seabather's eruption occurs at sites covered by bathing apparel while bathing in saltwater.

COURSE

On average, lesions persist for 1 to 2 weeks. In sensitized individuals, the eruption can become progressively more severe with repeated exposures and may be associated with systemic symptoms.

TREATMENT

Topical or systemic glucocorticoids provide symptomatic relief.

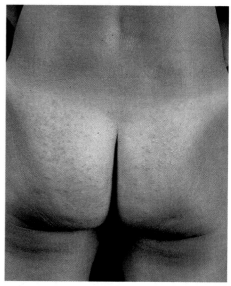

FIGURE 28-29 Seabather's eruption This papulovesicular rash appeared on a swimmer while on vacation in the Caribbean. During swimming, the patient experienced slight stinging in the regions covered by her bikini; later that evening she noticed the eruption. The rash is characteristically confined to the areas covered by the swimwear.

CNIDARIA ENVENOMATIONS ICD-10: T63.6

- **Etiology.** There are >10,000 Cnideria spp. that are swimming medusa or sessile polyps which inject toxin/venom that has local and systemic effects. Members of the Cnidaria phylum that can affect humans are jellyfish, Portuguese man-of-war, sea anemones, and fire "coral."
- **Pathogenesis.** Cnidarian stings elicit toxic rather than allergic reactions. Ranging from mild, self-limited irritations to extremely painful and serious injuries.

CLINICAL MANIFESTATION

Pruritic, burning, and painful papules in linear arrangement (Figs. 28-30 and 28-31).

COURSE

Stings from box jellyfish can be fatal.

TREATMENT

Wet dressings, topical corticosteroids.

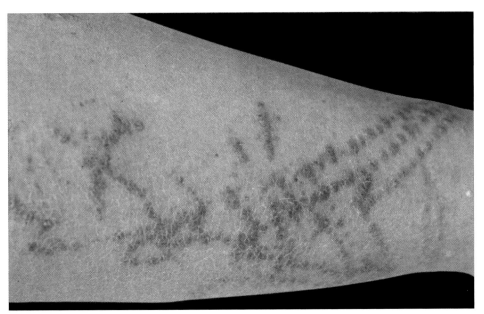

FIGURE 28-30 Jellyfish envenomation Pruritic and painful papules in a linear arrangement on the leg, appearing after contact with jellyfish.

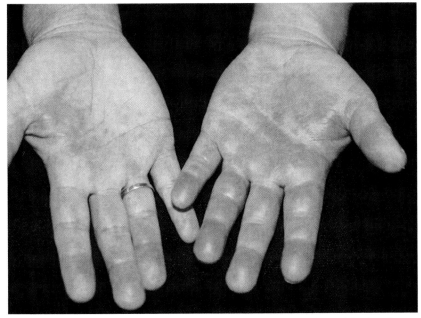

FIGURE 28-31 Fire coral envenomation A 47-year-old female with painful palms that occurred after contact with fire coral. The palms and palmar fingers are red and edematous at sites of envenomation.

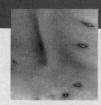

SYSTEMIC PARASITIC INFECTIONS

LEISHMANIASIS ICD-10: B55

- **Etiology.** Many species of obligate intracellular protozoa *Leishmania*; predominant species are:
  - **New World:** *Leishmania mexicana* complex, *Viannia* subgenus.
  - **Old World:** *L. tropica, L. major,* and *L. aethiopica.*
- **Vector.** Sandflies. Old World: *Phlebotomus.* New World: *Lutzomyia.*
- **Pathogenesis.** Infection of macrophages in skin, naso-oropharyngeal mucosa, and the reticuloendothelial system (viscera). Diversity of clinical syndromes resulting from a particular parasite, vector, and host species.

CLINICAL SYNDROMES

Cutaneous leishmaniasis (CL) characterized by development of single or multiple cutaneous papules at the site of a sandfly bite, often evolving into nodules and ulcers, which heal spontaneously with a depressed scar.

- New World cutaneous leishmaniasis (NWCL).
- Old World cutaneous leishmaniasis (OWCL).

Diffuse (anergic) cutaneous leishmaniasis (DCL).

Mucosal leishmaniasis (ML).

Visceral leishmaniasis (VL); kala-azar; post–kala-azar dermal leishmaniasis (PKDL).

Synonyms: NWCL: chiclero ulcer, pian bois (bush yaws), uta. OWCL: Baghdad/Delhi boil or button, oriental/Aleppo sore/evil, *bouton d'Orient.* ML: Espundia. VL: Kala-azar (Hindu for black fever).

EPIDEMIOLOGY AND ETIOLOGY

Infection in humans is caused by 20 *Leishmania* species (*Leishmania* and *Viannia* subgenera). Stages of parasite: Promastigote: Flagellated form found in sandflies and culture; amastigote: nonflagellated tissue form (2 to 4 μm in diameter); replicates in macrophage phagosomes in mammalian hosts.

TRANSMISSION Vector-borne by bite of infected female phlebotomine sandflies, which become infected by taking blood meal from infected mammalian host. About 30 species of sandflies have been identified as vectors. They rest in dark, moist places, and are typically most active in evening and nighttime hours. Other modes: Congenital and parenteral (i.e., by blood transfusion, needle sharing, or laboratory accident).

RESERVOIRS Varies with geography and leishmanial species. Zoonosis involves rodents/canines.

VECTORS Transmitted by 30 species of female sandflies of genera *Lutzomyia* (New World) and *Phlebotomus* (Old World).

PREVALENCE An estimated 12 million people infected worldwide. 1.5 to 2 million new cases annually; 350 million individuals are at risk of infection. 50% of new cases are in children. 75,000 individuals die annually of ML.

GEOGRAPHY All inhabited continents except Australia; endemic in focal areas of 90 countries. Tropics, subtropics, and southern Europe. More than 90% of cases of CL occur in Afghanistan, Algeria, Iran, Iraq, Saudi Arabia, Syria, Brazil, and Peru. Climates: Range from deserts to rain forests, and from rural to urban.

HOST DEFENSE DEFECTS *Leishmania*-specific anergy: Patients develop DCL. Poor immune response or immunosuppression (HIV disease): VL. Hyperergic variant: Leishmaniasis recidivans caused by *L. tropica.*

PATHOGENESIS

The clinical and immunologic spectrum of leishmaniasis parallels that of leprosy. CL occurs in a host with good protective immunity. MCL occurs in those with an intense inflammatory reaction. DCL occurs with extensive and widespread proliferation of the organism in the skin but without much inflammation or tendency for visceralization. VL

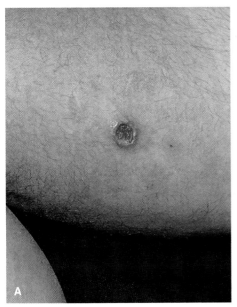 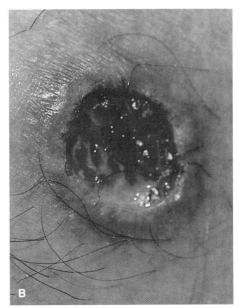

FIGURE 29-1 A and B New World cutaneous leishmaniasis: ulcer on thigh A 42-year-old with HIV disease noted a painless lesion on the medial thigh 6 weeks after returning from Mexico. Ulcer with rolled borders and base with granulation tissue. Leishmania were seen on lesional biopsy. *L. mexicana* was isolated on the tissue culture of lesional biopsy.

occurs in the host with little immune response and/or in immunosuppression. Unlike leprosy, extent and pattern are strongly influenced by the specific species of *Leishmania* involved. Additional factors that affect the clinical picture: Number of parasites inoculated, site of inoculation, nutritional status of host, and nature of the last nonblood meal of vector. Infection and recovery are followed by lifelong immunity to reinfection by the same species of *Leishmania*. In some cases, interspecies immunity occurs.

CLINICAL MANIFESTATION

Primary lesions occur at site of sandfly bite, usually on the exposed site.

INCUBATION PERIOD Inversely proportional to size of inoculum: Shorter in visitors to endemic area. OWCL: *L. tropica major*, 1 to 4 weeks; *L. tropica*, 2 to 8 months; acute CL: 2 to 8 weeks or more.

SYMPTOMS Noduloulcerative lesions usually asymptomatic. With secondary bacterial infection, may become painful.

NWCL *L. mexicana* complex. Small erythematous papule develops at sandfly bite site, evolving into ulcerated nodule (Fig. 29-1). Enlarges to 3 to 12 cm with raised border. Nonulcerating nodules may become verrucous. Lymphangitis, regional lymphadenopathy. Isolated lesions on the hand or head usually do not ulcerate. Eventually lesion heals with a depressed scar. Ear lesions may persist for years, destroying cartilage (chiclero ulcers) (Fig. 29-2).

ML Characterized by naso-oropharyngeal mucosal involvement, a metastatic complication of CL. Mucosal disease usually becomes evident several years after healing of original cutaneous lesions; cutaneous and mucosal lesions can coexist or appear decades apart. Edema and inflammatory changes lead to epistaxis and coryzal symptoms. In time, the nasal septum, floor of the mouth, and tonsillar areas are destroyed (Fig. 29-3). Results in marked disfigurement (referred to as *espundia* in South America). Death may be caused by superimposed bacterial infection, pharyngeal obstruction, or malnutrition.

OWCL Begins as small erythematous papule, which may appear immediately after sandfly bite but usually 2 to 4 weeks later. Papule slowly enlarges to 2 cm over a period of several weeks and assumes a dusky violaceous hue (Figs. 29-4 and 29-5). Eventually, lesion becomes crusted

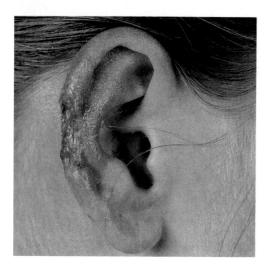

FIGURE 29-2 New World cutaneous leishmaniasis: chiclero ulcer A deep ulcer on the helix at the site of a sandfly bite. This variant typically occurs in leishmaniasis acquired in Central and South America.

in center with a shallow ulcer and raised indurated border = volcano sign. In some cases, the center of the nodule becomes hyperkeratotic, forming a cutaneous horn. Small satellite papules may develop at periphery of lesion, and occasionally subcutaneous nodules along the course of proximal lymphatics. Peripheral extension usually stops after 2 months, and an ulcerated nodule persists for another 3 to 6 months, or longer. The lesion then heals with a slightly depressed scar. In some cases, CL remains active with positive smears for 24 months (nonhealing chronic CL). The number of lesions depends on the circumstances of the exposure and extent of infection within the sandfly vector. May result in multiple lesions, up to 100 or more (Figs. 29-4 and 29-5).

DCL Resembles lepromatous leprosy; large number of parasites in macrophages in dermis; no visceral involvement. In the Old

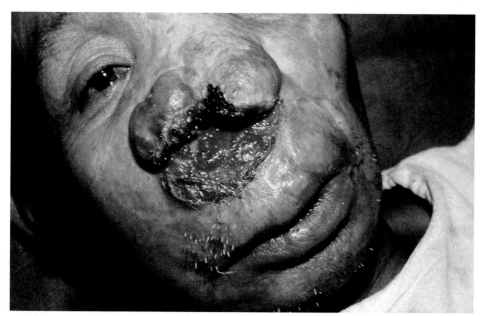

FIGURE 29-3 Mucocutaneous leishmaniasis: espundia Painful, mutilating ulceration with destruction of portions of the nose. (Used with permission from Eric Kraus, MD.)

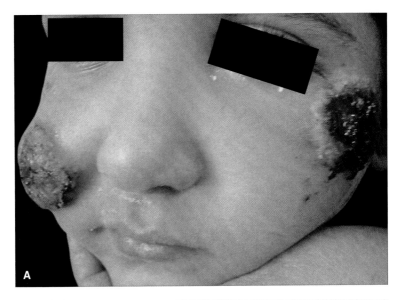

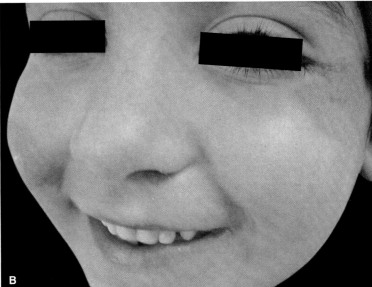

FIGURE 29-4 Old World cutaneous leishmaniasis: face A 7-year-old Jorda-
nian girl with painful lesions on the cheeks for 6 weeks. **(A)** Large crusted nodules
with surrounding edema on both cheeks. **(B)** Three weeks after successful therapy
(sodium stibogluconate pentostam injections; 15 mg/kg per day IM injection for
21 days), lesions have healed with minimal residual erythema and no scarring.
(Used with permission from Mohammad Tawara, MD.)

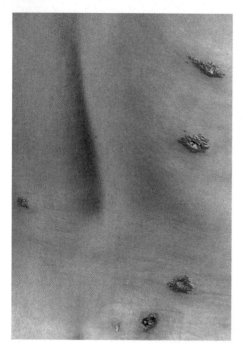

FIGURE 29-5 Old World cutaneous leishmaniasis Multiple, crusted nodules on the exposed back, arising at sites of sandfly bites. Many of the lesions resemble a volcano with a central depressed center, i.e., volcano sign.

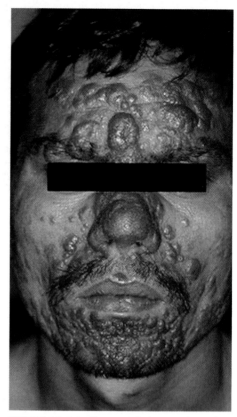

FIGURE 29-6 Indian post-kala-azar dermal leishmaniasis Coalescent erythematous dermal papules and nodules over the face in a picture similar to leonine facies. (Used with permission from Raj Kubba, MD.)

World, occurs in 20% of individuals with leishmaniasis in Ethiopia and Sudan. In South America, attributed to a member of *L. braziliensis* complex. Presents as a single nodule, which then spreads locally, often through extension from satellite lesions, and eventually by metastasis. In time, lesions become widespread with nonulcerating nodules appearing diffusely over the face and trunk. Responds poorly to treatment.

LEISHMANIASIS RECIDIVANS (LR) Complication of *L. tropica* infection. Dusky-red plaques with active, spreading borders and healing centers, giving rise to gyrate and annular lesions. Most commonly affects the face; can cause tissue destruction and severe deformity.

PKDL Sequel to VL that has resolved spontaneously or during/after adequate treatment. Lesions appear ≥1 year after course of therapy with macular, papular, nodular lesions, and hypopigmented macules/plaques on face (Fig. 29-6), trunk, and extremities. Resembles lepromatous leprosy when lesions are numerous. Develops in 20% of Indian patients treated for VL caused by *L. donovani* and in a small percentage of Ethiopian patients with VL caused by *L. aethiopica*.

VL Can remain subclinical or become symptomatic, with acute, subacute, or chronic course. Inapparent VL cases outnumber clinically apparent cases. Malnutrition is risk factor for clinically apparent VL. Bone marrow, liver, and the spleen are involved. Term *kala-azar* (Hindi for "black fever," some patients had gray color) refers to profoundly cachectic febrile patients with life-threatening disease. Patients present with fever, splenomegaly, pancytopenia, and wasting.

DIFFERENTIAL DIAGNOSIS

ACUTE CL Insect bite reaction, impetigo, ecthyma, furuncle, *Mycobacterium marinum* infection, furuncular myiasis, and chancre.

DIAGNOSIS

Clinical suspicion, confirmed by demonstrating:
- Intracellular nonflagellated amastigote in a biopsy of skin, mucosa, liver, lymph nodes or aspirate of spleen, bone marrow, and lymph node.
- Flagellated promastigote in culture of tissues (requires up to 21 days).

COURSE

In general, NWCL tends to be more severe and progressive than OWCL.

TREATMENT

Antimony-containing compounds meglumine antimoniate and sodium stilbogluconate (see Fig. 29-4) are given systemically. Other drugs used to treat leishmaniasis: amphotericin B, miltefosine, paromomycin, and pentamidine.

HUMAN AMERICAN TRYPANOSOMIASIS ICD-10: B57.2

- *Synonym.* Chagas disease.
- **Etiology.** *Trypanosoma cruzi.*
- **Demography.** Central and South America. 16 to 18 million persons infected.
- **Transmission.** *T. cruzi* deposited in feces of reduviid bugs onto the skin; enters host via breaks in skin (excoriations), mucous membranes, or conjunctivae. Can also be transmitted by transfusion of blood from infected persons, by organ transplantation, and from mother to fetus.
- **Dissemination.** Via lymphatics and bloodstream to muscles.

CLINICAL MANIFESTATION

INOCULATION SITE CHAGOMA An indurated area of erythema and swelling, at the portal of entry, occurring 7 to 14 days after inoculation. May be accompanied by local lymphadenopathy. Parasites located within leukocytes and cells of subcutaneous tissues. These initial local signs are followed by malaise, fever, anorexia, and edema of the face and lower extremities.

ROMAÑA SIGN Unilateral painless edema of palpebrae and periocular tissues. Occurs when conjunctiva is the portal of entry. Classic finding in acute AT.

Edema of face and lower extremities.

TRYPANOSOMIDES Morbilliform, urticariform, or erythematopolymorphic eruptions.

HEMATOGENIC OR METASTATIC CHAGOMAS Nodule(s) caused by dissemination of infection. Hard, painful, wine-colored nodules; rarely soften or ulcerate.

SYSTEMIC FINDINGS Generalized lymphadenopathy. Hepatosplenomegaly. Severe myocarditis may occur; most deaths result from heart failure.

INDETERMINATE/ASYMPTOMATIC PHASE Characterized by subpatent parasitemia, detectable antibodies to *T. cruzi*, absence of associated signs and symptoms.

SYMPTOMATIC CHRONIC INFECTION May take several decades to develop. Symptomatic disease: Heart (rhythm disturbances, cardiomyopathy, and thromboembolism), megaesophagus, megacolon, and peripheral nervous system disease.

COURSE Most infected persons remain so for life. Heart and GI involvement associated with serious morbidity and mortality.

HUMAN AFRICAN TRYPANOSOMIASIS ICD-10: B56

- *Synonym.* Sleeping sickness.
- **Etiology.** *Trypanosoma brucei gambiense* causes West African sleeping sickness; accounts for 95% of reported cases. *Trypanosoma brucei rhodesiense* causes East African sleeping sickness.
- **Epidemiology.** Vector: tse-tse flies.
- **Primary reservoir.** West African sleeping sickness: humans. East African sleeping sickness: antelope and cattle.
- **Demography.** >66 million persons infected. West Africa: Ivory Coast, Chad, Central African Republic; rural populations. East Africa: Sudan; workers in wild areas, rural populations, and tourists in game parks.

CLINICAL MANIFESTATION

ACUTE INFECTION Stage I disease. *Trypanosomal chancre* appears in some patients at inoculation site (Fig. 29-7); painful; 7 to 14 days after tse-tse fly bite. Typically 2 to 5 cm indurated; may ulcerate; resolved in few weeks. Parasites can be seen in fluid expressed from chancre and buffy coat. *Systemic findings.* Fever, arthralgias, malaise, localized facial edema, and moderate splenomegaly. Lymphadenopathy is prominent in *T. b. gambiense* trypanosomiasis. Course is more rapid in East African type. Tourist with *T. b. rhodesiense* disease may develop systemic signs of infection near the end of the trip.

CHRONIC INFECTION Stage II disease. Characterized by insidious development of protean neurologic symptoms. Progressive indifference and daytime somnolence develops. East African type may develop arrhythmias and congestive heart failure before CNS disease develops.

TREATMENT

Pentamidine, melarsoprol, and eflornithine. For late-stage disease, difluoromethylornithine.

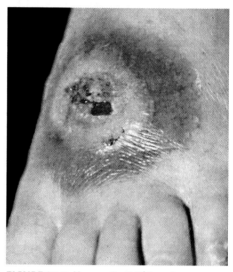

FIGURE 29-7 Human East African trypanosomiasis: trypanosomal chancre Ulcerated plaque at bite site on dorsal foot. A macular exanthem was present on the trunk. (Reprinted with permission from Moore AC et al. Case 20-2002. A 37-year-old man with fever, hepatosplenomegaly, and a cutaneous foot lesion after a trip to Africa. *N Engl J Med.* 2002;346:2069. © 2002 Massachusetts Medical Society.)

CUTANEOUS AMEBIASIS ICD-10 : A06.7

Amebiasis is caused by *Entamoeba histolytica,* which infects the GI tract and rarely the skin.

- **Incidence.** 10% of world population infected with *Entamoeba*. Majority of infections caused by non-invasive *E. dispar*. 10% of those colonized with *E. histolytica* develop amebic colitis. More prevalent in tropics and in rural areas; inadequate sanitation and crowding. Skin involvement is associated with malnutrition and immunocompromise (HIV/AIDS and solid organ transplantation).

CLINICAL MANIFESTATIONS

Cutaneous amebiasis begins as an indurated pustule that evolves to a painful ragged ulcer, foul smelling, and covered with pus or necrotic debris (Fig. 29-8). Usually, a consequence of underlying amebic abscess invading skin. Typical sites are perianal area (extension of sigmorectal involvement) (Fig. 29-8) or abdominal wall (draining sinus from liver or colon). Penis or vulva may become infected during intercourse. Surgical wound infections may follow removal of hepatic or abdominal abscess. Remote ulcers (e.g., face) may result from autoinoculation.

COURSE AND TREATMENT

Without treatment lesion progressively enlarges. Treat with sulfadiazine and pyrimethamine, clindamycin.

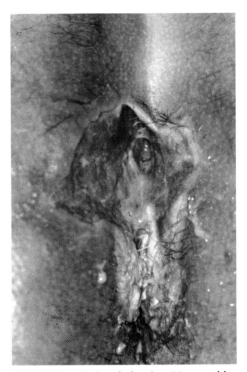

FIGURE 29-8 Perianal ulcer in a 35-year-old man, 4 weeks after removal of condylomata acuminata by electrodesiccation The ulcer showed no tendency to heal and a biopsy of its base revealed an inflammatory infiltrate with oval protozoa with phagocytosed red blood cells. Real time PCR was positive for entameba histolytica. (Reproduced with permission from Posch C et al. *J Dtsch Dermatol Ges.* 2011;9:649–50. © The authors. Journal compilation © Blackwell Verlag GmbH, Berlin.)

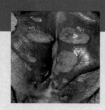

SEXUALLY TRANSMITTED DISEASES

HUMAN PAPILLOMAVIRUS: ANOGENITAL INFECTIONS ICD-10: B97.7

- Mucosal human papilloma virus (HPV) infections are the most common sexually transmitted infection (STIs) seen by the dermatologist. Only 1 to 2% of HPV-infected young, sexually active persons have any visibly detectable clinical lesion.
- HPV present in the birth canal can be transmitted to a newborn during vaginal delivery and can cause external genital warts (EGW) and respiratory papillomatosis.
- **Warts.** Barely visible papules to nodules to confluent masses occurring on anogenital skin or mucosa and oral mucosa. EGW: External genitalia, perineum. Cervix. Oropharynx.
- **Dysplasia** of anogenital and oral skin and mucosa ranging from mild to severe to squamous cell carcinoma (SCC) in situ (SCCIS). Invasive SCC can arise within SCCIS. Most commonly in the cervix and anal canal.

ETIOLOGY AND EPIDEMIOLOGY

ETIOLOGY HPV is DNA papovirus that multiplies in the nuclei of infected epithelial cells (see Section 27). More than 20 types of HPV can infect the genital tract: types 6, 11 most commonly. Types 16, 18, 31, 33, and 35 are strongly associated with anogenital dysplasia and carcinoma. In persons with multiple sexual partners, subclinical infection with multiple HPV types is common.

RISK FACTORS FOR ACQUIRING HPV INFECTION Number of sexual partners/frequency of sexual intercourse. Sexual partner with HPV anogenital infection. Infection with other STIs.

TRANSMISSION Through sexual contact: genital–genital, oral–genital, and genital–anal. Microabrasions occur on the epithelial surface allowing virions from the infected partner to gain access to the basal cell layer of the noninfected partner.

- During delivery, mothers with anogenital warts can transmit HPV to the neonate, resulting in EGW and laryngeal papillomatosis in children.

INCIDENCE Most sexually active individuals are subclinically infected with HPV; most HPV infections are asymptomatic, subclinical, or unrecognized. 1% of sexually active adults (15 to 19 years of age) develop clinical lesions.

PATHOGENESIS "Low-risk" and "high-risk" HPV types both cause anogenital infections. HPV infection may persist for years in a dormant state and becomes infectious intermittently. Exophytic warts are probably more infectious than subclinical infection. *Immunosuppression* may result in new extensive HPV lesions, poor response to treatment, increased multifocal intraepithelial neoplasia. All HPV types replicate exclusively in the host's cell nucleus. In benign HPV-associated lesions, HPV exists as a plasmid in cellular cytoplasm, replicating extrachromosomally. In malignant HPV-associated lesions, HPV integrates into the host's chromosome, following a break in the viral genome (around E1/E2 region). E1 and E2 function is deregulated, resulting in cellular transformation.

GENITAL WARTS

CLINICAL MANIFESTATION

Usually asymptomatic, except for cosmetic appearance. Anxiety of having STI. Obstruction if large mass.

MUCOCUTANEOUS LESIONS Four clinical types of genital warts occur:

Small papular (Fig. 30-1).

   Condyloma acuminatum. Cauliflower-floret (acuminate or pointed) lesions (Figs. 30-2 to 30-4).

   Keratotic warts (Figs. 30-5 and 30-6).

   Flat-topped papules/plaques (most common on cervix) (Fig. 30-7).

   Skin-colored, pink, red, tan, and brown. Solitary, scattered, and isolated, or they form voluminous confluent masses. In immunocompromised individuals, lesions may be huge (Fig. 30-5).

   Sites of predilection. Male: Frenulum, corona, glans penis, prepuce, shaft (Figs. 30-1 and 30-3), and scrotum. *Female*: Labia, clitoris, periurethral area, perineum, vagina, and cervix (flat lesions) (Fig. 30-7). *Both sexes*: Perineal, perianal (Fig. 30-5), anal canal, rectal; urethral meatus, urethra, and bladder; oropharynx.

Laryngeal Papillomas

- Relatively uncommon; associated with HPV-6 and 11.
- Arise most commonly on true vocal cords of the larynx.
- Age: Children <5 years of age, adults >20 years of age.
- Risk of SCCIS and invasive SCC.

DIFFERENTIAL DIAGNOSIS

PAPULAR/NODULAR EXTERNAL GENITAL LESIONS
Normal anatomy (e.g., sebaceous glands, pearly penile papules, and vestibular papillae), squamous intraepithelial lesions (SILs), SCCIS, invasive SCC, benign neoplasms (moles, seborrheic keratoses, skin tags, pilar cyst, and angiokeratoma), inflammatory dermatoses (lichen nitidus, lichen planus), molluscum contagiosum, condylomata lata, folliculitis, and scabetic nodules.

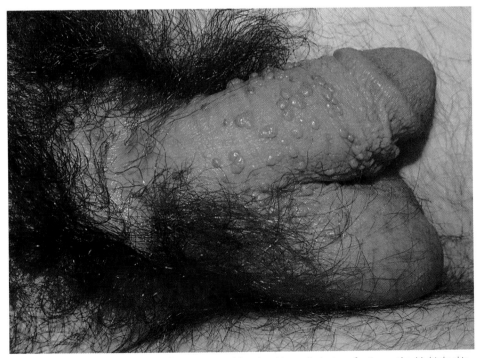

FIGURE 30-1 Papular warts: penis A 23-year-old male with penile lesions for 6 months. Multiple skin-colored papules on the penis and scrotum.

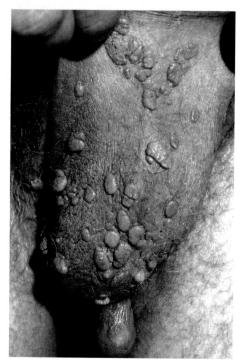

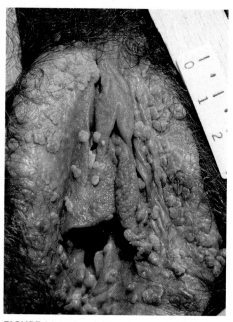

FIGURE 30-4 Condylomata acuminata: vulva Multiple, pink-brown, soft papules on the labia.

FIGURE 30-2 Condyloma acuminata A 35-year-old male with cluster of warts on the scrotum for 2 months.

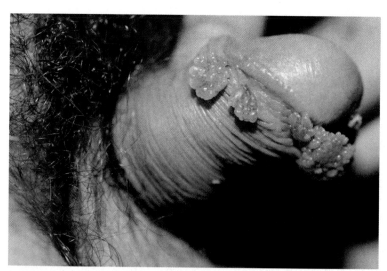

FIGURE 30-3 Condylomata acuminata: penis A 20-year-old male with Crohn disease treated with infliximab infusion. Condylomata on the distal foreskin resemble cauliflower floret-like papules.

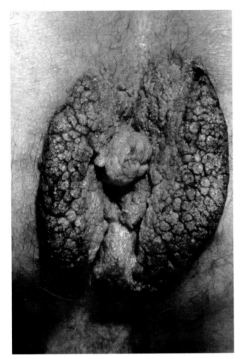

FIGURE 30-5 Genital warts A 45-year-old male with HIV disease and hyperkeratotic condylomata acuminata seen on the anal and perineal area.

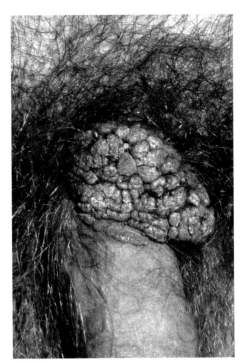

FIGURE 30-6 Keratotic external genital warts (EGW): male A 51-year-old male with lesions at the base of penis for several years. Lesional biopsy reported EGW ruling out verrucous carcinoma.

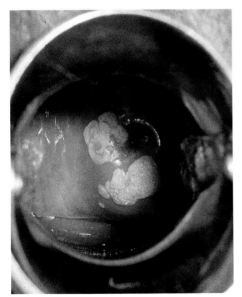

FIGURE 30-7 Condylomata acuminata: uterine cervix Sharply demarcated, whitish, and flat plaques becoming confluent around the cervix.

LABORATORY EXAMINATIONS

PAP SMEAR Encourage all women to have an annual Pap smear since HPV is the major etiologic agent for cancer of the cervix. Anal Pap test with a cervical brush and fixative solution helps detect anal dysplasia.

DERMATOPATHOLOGY Biopsy is indicated if diagnosis is uncertain; lesions do not respond to standard therapy and worsen during therapy; the patient is immunocompromised; warts are pigmented, indurated, fixed, and/or ulcerated. Indicated in some cases to confirm diagnosis and/or rule out SCCIS or invasive SCC.

DETECTION OF HPV DNA Presence of HPV DNA and specific HPV types determined on smears and lesional biopsy by in situ hybridization.

Serology. Genital warts are markers of unsafe sexual practices, and patients should be screened for other STDs.

DIAGNOSIS

Clinical diagnosis, occasionally confirmed by biopsy.

COURSE

HPV is highly infectious, with an incubation period of 3 weeks to 8 months. Most HPV-infected individuals who develop genital warts do so 2 to 3 months after becoming infected. If left untreated, genital warts may resolve on their own, remain unchanged, or grow. After regression, *subclinical infection may persist for life.* Recurrence may occur with normal immune function as well as in immunocompromised. Recurrences more commonly are reactivation of subclinical infection than reinfection. In pregnancy, genital warts may increase in size and number, show increased vaginal involvement, and have an increased rate of secondary bacterial infection. Children delivered vaginally of mothers with genital HPV infection are at risk for developing recurrent respiratory papillomatosis in later life.

HPV types 16, 18, 31, and 33 are the major etiologic factors for in situ and invasive SCC: Cervix; external genitalia (vulva and penis); anus and perineum.

MANAGEMENT

PREVENTION Use of condoms reduce transmission. HPV vaccine protects against four strains of HPV and cervical cancer later in life.

GOAL OF TREATMENT Removal of exophytic warts and reduction of signs and symptoms. No therapy has been shown to eradicate HPV or prevent cervical or anogenital cancer. Treatment is more successful if warts are small and present for <1 year. Risk of transmission might be reduced by "debulking" genital warts.

SELECTION OF TREATMENT Guided by preference of patient—avoid expensive therapies, toxic therapies, and procedures that result in scarring. See Section 27.

PATIENT APPLIED AGENTS Imiquimod 5% cream, podophylox 0.5% solution.

CLINICIAN ADMINISTERED THERAPY Cryosurgery, podophyllin 10 to 25%, trichloroacetic acid 80 to 90%, surgical removal, and electrodesication.

HPV: SQUAMOUS CELL CARCINOMA IN SITU (SCCIS) AND INVASIVE SCC OF ANOGENITAL SKIN

- HPV infection of the anogenital epithelium can result in a spectrum of changes referred to as SILs, ranging from mild dysplasia to SCCIS.
- Over time, these lesions can regress, persist, progress, or recur, in some cases to invasive SCC.
- Clinically, lesions appear as multifocal macules, papules, and plaques on the external anogenital region.
- Lesions involving the cervix and anus have the highest risk for transformation to invasive SCC; however, lesions can transform at any site.
- *Synonyms*: Vulvar intraepithelial neoplasia, penile intraepithelial neoplasm, bowenoid papulosis.

ETIOLOGY AND EPIDEMIOLOGY

The Bethesda System (National Cancer Institute) is currently used as terminology for "dysplastic" lesions caused by HPV on anogenital sites. The terminology applies to both cytologic (Pap test) and histologic assessments. Intraepithelial neoplasia are designated as cervical (CIN), vulvar (VIN), penile (PIN), and anal (AIN). VIN is classified as VIN1 (mild dysplasia), VIN2 (moderate dysplasia), VIN3 (severe dysplasia or carcinoma in situ), and VIN3 differentiated type.

ETIOLOGY HPV types 16, 18, 31, and 33.

TRANSMISSION HPV transmitted sexually. Autoinoculation. Rarely, HPV-16 is transmitted from mother to newborn.

DEMOGRAPHY Cervical SCC is the second most common female malignancy worldwide, second only to breast cancer. It is the most frequent malignancy in developing countries, with 500,000 new cases and 200,000 deaths worldwide attributed to it annually.

RISK FACTORS Host defense defects and cigarette smoking are risk factors for more dysplastic lesions and invasive SCC.

PATHOGENESIS HPV-16- and 18-infected cells may not be able to differentiate fully as a result of either: (1) functional interference of cell cycle–regulating proteins, caused by viral gene expression or (2) overproduction of E5, E6, and E7. When this occurs, the host DNA synthesis continues unchecked and leads to rapidly dividing undifferentiated cells with

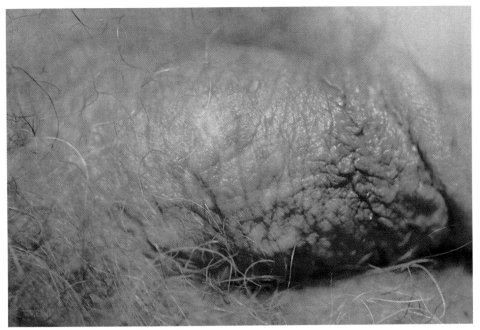

FIGURE 30-8 HPV squamous cell carcinoma in situ A 48-year-old male with penile lesion for 2 years. Pink papules forming a 1-cm plaque on the shaft of the penis. Lesional biopsy reported SCCIS with HPV changes (koilocytosis).

morphologic characteristics of intraepithelial neoplasia. Accumulated chromosomal breakages, rearrangements, deletions, and other genomic mutations can lead to invasive capability and malignancy.

CLINICAL MANIFESTATION

Prior history of condylomata acuminata. Female partners of males may have CIN.

Mucocutaneous Lesions

- Erythematous flat-topped papules.
- Lichenoid (flat-topped) or pigmented papules (called *bowenoid papulosis*) (Figs. 30-8 and 30-9).
- May show confluence or form plaque(s).
- Leukoplakia-like plaque (Fig. 30-10). Surface usually smooth and velvety.

COLORS Tan, brown, pink, red, violaceous, and white. Nodule or ulceration in field of SIL suggests invasive SCC (Figs. 30-11 and 30-12).

ARRANGEMENT Characteristically clusters, i.e., commonly multifocal. May be solitary.

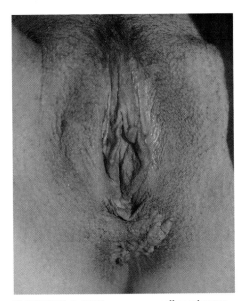

FIGURE 30-9 HPV squamous cell carcinoma in situ A 33-year-old heart transplant recipient with anogenital lesions for several years. Lesional biopsy was reported to show SCCIS with HPV changes (koilocytosis).

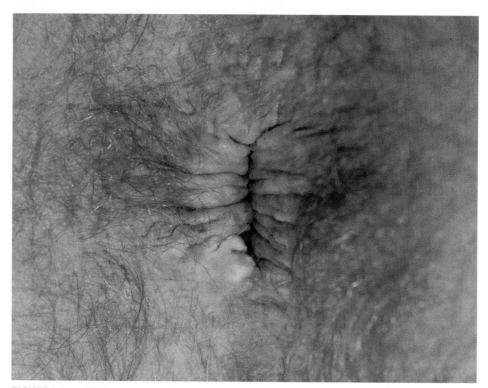

FIGURE 30-10 HPV squamous cell carcinoma in situ A 49-year-old male with HIV disease noted to have anal lesions for 1 month. A white firm nodule on the rim of the anus. Biopsy reported SCCIS with HPV changes. No lesions were detected on anal colposcopy.

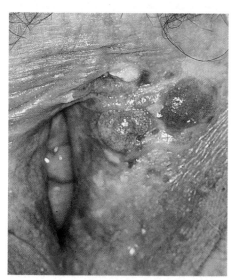

FIGURE 30-11 HPV-induced in situ and invasive squamous cell carcinoma: vulva Several red nodules (invasive SCC) arising within a white plaque (SCCIS) on the left labium.

DISTRIBUTION Males: Glans penis, prepuce (75%) (flat lichenoid papules or erythematous macules); penile shaft (25%) (pigmented papules). Females: Labia majora and minora, clitoris. Multicentric involvement of the cervix, vulva, perineum, and/or anus occurs not infrequently. Both sexes: Inguinal folds, perineal/perianal skin. Oropharyngeal mucosa. Sites other than external genitalia may be associated with cervical dysplasia, CIN, cervical SCC; rarely, SCCIS of other sites, i.e., nail unit (periungual, nail bed); intraurethral (Fig. 30-13).

DIFFERENTIAL DIAGNOSIS

MULTIPLE SKIN-COLORED PAPULES ± HYPERKERATOSIS Genital warts, psoriasis vulgaris; lichen planus. **PIGMENTED ANOGENITAL MACULE(S)/PAPULE(S)** Genital lentiginosis, melanoma (in situ or invasive), pigmented basal cell carcinoma, and angiokeratomas.

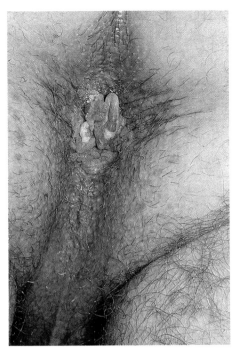

FIGURE 30-12 HPV-induced in situ and invasive squamous cell carcinoma: perineal/perianal A 38-year-old male with HIV disease aware of perianal lesions for several months; he had a prior history of EGW. Brown perineal and perianal macules and papules (SCCIS) with a pink nodule arising at the anal verge. Excisional biopsy of the nodule reported invasive SCC arising within SCCIS.

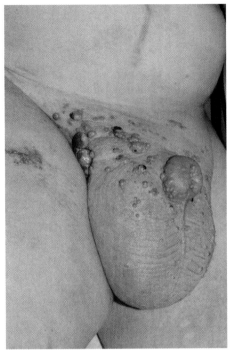

FIGURE 30-13 Metastatic SCC of urethra A 38-year-old male with primary urethral squamous cell carcinoma metastatic to inguinal lymph nodes with lymphedema. Red nodules and plaques are cutaneous metastases. PCR of thigh metastasis detected HPV-16.

LABORATORY EXAMINATIONS

DERMATOPATHOLOGY Epidermal proliferation with vacuolated keratinocytes (koilocytes). Recent application of podophyllin to condyloma acuminatum may cause changes similar to SCCIS.
SOUTHERN BLOT ANALYSIS Identifies HPV type.
PAP SMEAR Koilocytotic atypia.
EXFOLIATIVE CYTOLOGY Cervical Pap smears have been recommended for women 21 -to 65 years. Cytology of the anal canal may also be helpful in management of individuals with a history of anal HPV infection, especially if immunocompromised (HIV disease, transplant recipients). By the Bethesda System, these cytologic findings are reported as atypical squamous cells of undetermined significance (ASCUS), low-grade squamous intraepithelial lesion (LSIL), high-grade (HSIL), and SCC.

DIAGNOSIS

Clinical suspicion, confirmed by biopsy of the lesion.

COURSE

Invasive SCC develops only through well-defined precursor lesions (Figs. 30-11 and 30-12). Over time, these lesions can regress, persist, recur, or progress, in some cases to invasive SCC. Natural history of CIN is best studied: Progression to invasive SCC occurs in 36% of cases over a 20-year period. Patients with intraepithelial neoplasias, which often occur in immunocompromised individuals, should be followed indefinitely, with monitoring by exfoliative cytology and lesional biopsy specimens.

LABORATORY FINDINGS

Colposcopy

The most common indication for colposcopy is abnormal exfoliative cytology. Acetic acid, 3 to 5%, is applied to the cervix, which causes columnar and abnormal epithelium to become edematous. Abnormal (atypical) epithelium adopts a white or opaque appearance that can be distinguished from the normal pink epithelium. Abnormal epithelium is then biopsied. Colposcopy can also be performed on individuals with abnormal anal exfoliative cytology, and biopsy specimens obtained from abnormal site(s).

Biopsy

In cases of documented SIL or SCCIS, biopsy specimens should be obtained from rapidly enlarging lesions, areas of ulceration or bleeding, exuberant tissue with abnormal vascularity.

TREATMENT

The only way of possibly reducing the potential risk of invasive SCC is diagnosis and eradication of intraepithelial disease. Because lesions are relatively uncommon, cases are often best managed by a dermatologist with clinical experience in the care of these patients, an oncologic gynecologist, or a colorectal surgeon. If lesion biopsy specimens do not show early invasion, lesions can be treated medically or surgically.

Medical Management

5-Fluorouracil cream has been used but is difficult to use because of erosions. Imiquimod cream 5% is also effective.

Surgical Management

Surgical excision, Mohs surgery, electrosurgery, laser vaporization, and cryosurgery.

HERPES SIMPLEX VIRUS: GENITAL DISEASE ICD-10: A60

■ Genital herpes (GH) is a chronic sexually transmitted viral disease, characterized by symptomatic and asymptomatic viral shedding.

ETIOLOGY AND EPIDEMIOLOGY

ETIOLOGY HSV-2 > HSV-1. See also Section 27.
PREVALENCE Highly variable. Depends on many factors: country, region of residence, population subgroup, gender, and age. Greater among higher risk sexual behavior groups. Prevalence of HSV-2 seropositivity in general population: United States: 16.2%; Europe: 4 to 18%; Ssub-Saharan Africa: up to 70%.
TRANSMISSION Usually skin-to-skin contact. Seventy percent of transmission occurs during times of asymptomatic HSV shedding. Transmission rate in discordant couples (one partner infected, the other not) approximately 10% per year; 25% of females become infected, compared with only 4 to 6% of males. Prior HSV-1 infection is protective; in females with anti-HSV-1 antibodies, 15% become infected with HSV-2, but in those without anti-HSV-1 antibodies, 30% become infected with HSV-2.

CLINICAL MANIFESTATION

Only 10% of HSV-2 seropositive individuals are aware that symptoms are those of GH.

Ninety percent do not recognize symptoms of GH. Most clinical lesions are minor breaks in the mucocutaneous epithelium, presenting as erosion, "abrasions," fissures. The "classically" described findings are *uncommon*. Symptoms of aseptic HSV-2 meningitis can occur with primary or recurrent GH.
PRIMARY GENITAL HERPES Most individuals with primary infection are asymptomatic. Those with symptoms report fever, headache, malaise, myalgia, peaking within the first 3 to 4 days after onset of lesions, resolving during the subsequent 3 to 4 days. *Erythematous papules* initially evolve to *vesicles or pustules*, which become *eroded* as the overlying epidermis sloughs (Figs. 30-14 and 30-15). Primary infection occurs anywhere on the anogenital skin, cervix, and anorectal mucosa. Epithelial defects heal in 2 to 4 weeks, often with resulting postinflammatory hypo- or hyperpigmentation, uncommonly with scarring.

With host defense defects, lesions tend to be more extensive and delayed in healing.
RECURRENT GENITAL HERPES New symptoms may result from old infections. Most individuals do

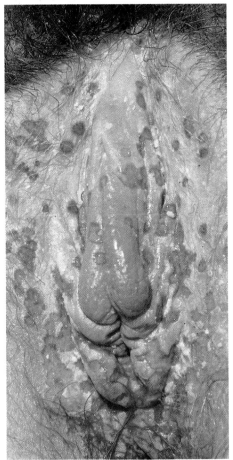

FIGURE 30-14 Genital herpes, primary
Multiple, extremely painful, punched-out, confluent, and shallow ulcers on the edematous vulva
and perineum. Micturition is often very painful.
Associated inguinal lymphadenopathy is common.

not experience "classic" findings of grouped
vesicles on erythematous base. Common symptoms are itching, burning, fissure, redness, and
irritation prior to eruption of vesicles. Dysuria,
sciatica, and rectal discomfort. Lesions may be
similar to primary infection but on a reduced
scale. Often a 1- to 2-cm erythematous plaque
with vesicles (Figs. 30-16 to 30-20), which
rupture with of erosions.
DISTRIBUTION *Males.* Primary infection: Glans,
prepuce, shaft, sulcus, scrotum, thighs, and

buttocks. Recurrences: Penile shaft, glans,
and buttocks. *Females.* Primary infection:
Labia majora/minora, perineum, and inner
thighs. Recurrences: Labia majora/minora and
buttocks.
ANORECTAL INFECTION Occurs following anal
intercourse; characterized by tenesmus, anal
pain, proctitis, discharge, and ulcerations
(Figs. 30-18 and 30-19) as far as 10 cm into
anal canal.
GENERAL FINDINGS *Inguinal/femoral lymph
nodes* may be enlarged, tender with primary
infection. *Signs of aseptic meningitis.* Fever,
nuchal rigidity; can occur in the absence of
GH. Pain along sciatic nerve.

DIFFERENTIAL DIAGNOSIS

Trauma, candidiasis, syphilitic chancre, fixed-
drug eruption, chancroid, and gonococcal
erosion.

LABORATORY STUDIES

See Section 27 "Herpes Simplex Virus Disease."

DIAGNOSIS

Diagnosis can be made on clinical finding. Confirmation by viral culture or direct
fluorescent antibody (DFA) or serology may
be indicated. Coinfection with another STD
should be ruled out.

COURSE

GH is a lifetime infection and recurrences are
the rule. Seventy percent are asymptomatic.
Recurrence rates are high in those with an
extended first episode of infection, regardless of whether antiviral therapy is given.
Chronic suppressive therapy reduces shedding.
Treatment of first-episode infection prevents
complications such as meningitis and radiculitis. Erythema multiforme may complicate
recurrences, occurring 1 to 2 weeks after an
outbreak.

TREATMENT

PREVENTION Advise patients to abstain from
sexual activity while lesions are present and
encourage use of condoms during all sexual
activity.

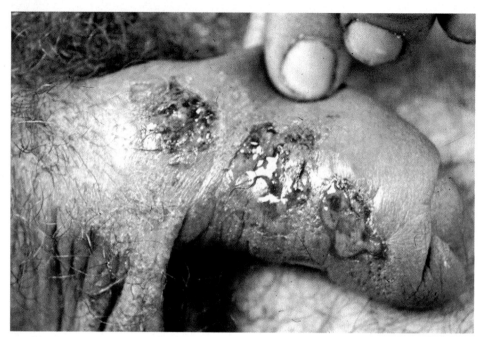

FIGURE 30-15 Genital herpes, primary A 18-year-old male, homeless with painful genital lesions for 7 days. Multiple erosions on the penis and scrotum.

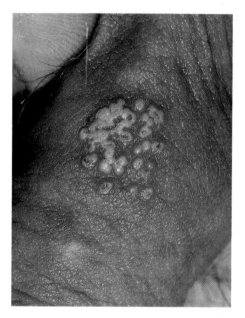

FIGURE 30-16 Genital herpes, recurrent Group of vesicles with early central crusting on a red base arising on the shaft of the penis. This "textbook" presentation, however, is much less common than small asymptomatic erosions or fissures.

FIGURE 30-17 Genital herpes, recurrent: vulva Large, painful erosions on the labia. Extensive lesions such as these are uncommon in recurrent genital herpes in an otherwise healthy individual.

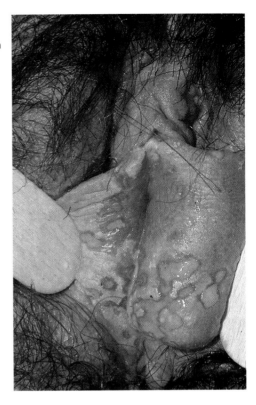

FIGURE 30-18 Genital herpes, recurrent A 30-year-old male with HIV disease. Multiple, painful, sharply demarcated ulcers are seen on the anus and perineum.

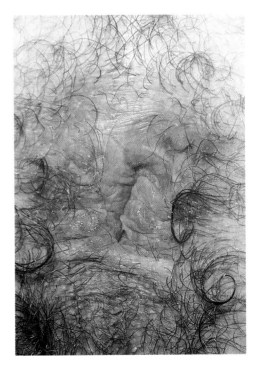

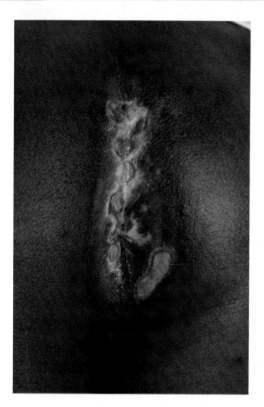

FIGURE 30-19 Chronic herpetic ulcers A 32-year-old male with extensive painful erosions of perineum and anus. This was the presenting complaint that led to HIV serotesting and diagnosis of HIV disease.

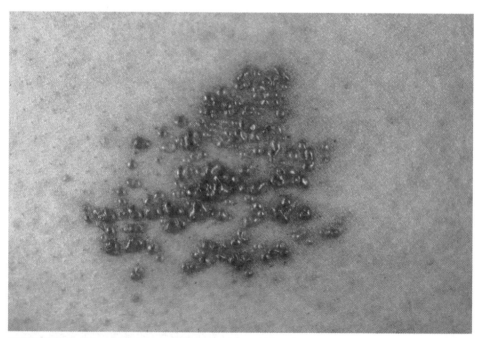

FIGURE 30-20 Genital herpes, recurrent A 55-year-old female with recurring lesions on buttock. She is otherwise healthy.

FIRST EPISODE Oral antivirals. Acyclovir 400 mg 3 times daily for 10 days or until lesions resolve. Valacyclovir 1000 mg twice daily for 7 to -10 days.

RECURRENCES Oral antivirals. Acyclovir 400 mg 3 times daily for 5 days or 800 mg twice daily for 5 days, or 800 mg 3 times daily for 2 days. Valacyclovir 500 mg twice daily for three days or 1 mg twice daily for 3 days. Famciclovir 125 mg twice daily for 5 days or 1 g once a day for 5 days.

MAINTENANCE THERAPY Oral antivirals: Daily suppressive therapy. Acyclovir 400 mg twice daily. Valcyclovir 500 to 1000 mg once daily. Famciclovir 250 mg once daily.

SEVERELY IMMUNOCOMPROMISED IV acyclovir 5 mg/kg every 8h for 5 to 7 days or oral acyclovir 400 mg 5 times a day for 7 to 14 days.

ACYCLOVIR RESISTANT IV foscarnet 40 mg/kg every 8h for 14 to 21 days.

NEONATES See Section 27.

NEISSERIA GONORRHOEAE DISEASE

- **Etiology.** *N. gonorrhoeae*, the gonococcus.
- **Colonize Mucosa.** Oropharynx, anogenital sites.
- **Epidemiology.** STI. Shares clinical spectrum of *Chlamydia trachomatis*; symptoms are usually more severe with gonococcal infections.

CLINICAL MANIFESTATION

LOCAL INFECTION Gonorrhea or "clap." Gonococcus infects mucocutaneous surfaces of the lower genitourinary tract, the anus and rectum, and the oropharynx.

INVASIVE INFECTION Pelvic inflammatory disease (PID).

DISSEMINATED INFECTION If untreated, disseminated gonococcal infection (DGI) may occur spreading to deeper structures with abscess formation. Colonizes oropharyngeal or anogenital mucosa from which gonococcus seeds blood.

ETIOLOGY AND EPIDEMIOLOGY

ETIOLOGY *N. gonorrhoeae*, the gonococcus (Fig. 30-21). Humans are the only natural reservoir of the organism. Strains that cause disseminated infection tend to cause minimal genital inflammation. In the United States, these strains have occurred infrequently during the past decade. Up to 40% of persons coinfected with *C. trachomatis*. Gonorrhea enhances transmission as well as acquisition of HIV/AIDS.

INCIDENCE Gonorrhea is the second most commonly reported notifiable disease in the United States: in 2010, 310,000 cases reported having it in the United States. Higher in developing countries.

DEMOGRAPHY Young, sexually active. Symptomatic infection more common in males. In the United States, highest incidence of gonorrhea is in blacks, lowest in those of Asian/Pacific Island descent. In Africa, median prevalence of gonorrhea in pregnant women is 10%.

TRANSMISSION *Sexually*, from partner who either is asymptomatic or has minimal symptoms. *Neonate* exposed to infected secretions in birth canal. About 1% of patients with untreated mucosal gonococcal infection develop disseminated infection (see the following). Gonorrhea may enhance HIV transmission.

PATHOGENESIS Gonococcus has an affinity for columnar epithelium; stratified and squamous

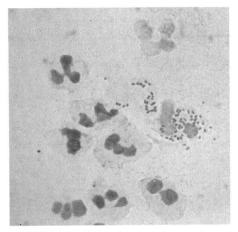

FIGURE 30-21 *Neisseria gonorrhoeae:* **Gram stain** Multiple, gram-negative diplococci within polymorphonuclear leukocytes as well as in the extracellular areas of a smear from a urethral discharge.

epithelia are more resistant to attack. Gonococcus penetrates between epithelial cells, causing a submucosal inflammation with polymorphonuclear (PMN) leukocyte reaction with resultant purulent discharge. Strains of gonococcus that cause disseminated infection tend to cause little genital inflammation and thereby escape detection. Most signs and symptoms of disseminated infection are manifestations of immune complex formation and deposition. Multiple episodes of disseminated infection may be associated with abnormality of terminal complement component factors.

NEISSERIA GONORRHOEAE: GONORRHEA ICD-10: A54

- In men, the most common presentation is purulent urethral discharge.
- Most infected women are asymptomatic and cervical infection is most common.
- Most men (90%) develop symptoms of urethritis within 5 days.
- Most women are asymptomatic; when symptoms occur, it is usually > 14 days since exposure.
- If untreated, infection can spread to deeper structures with abscess formation and disseminated gonococcal infection (DGI).

CLINICAL MANIFESTATIONS

GENITALIA *Men:* Urethral discharge ranging from scanty and clear to purulent and copious (Fig. 30-22).
Women: Periurethral edema, urethritis. Purulent discharge from cervix but no vaginitis. In prepubescent females, vulvovaginitis. Bartholin abscess.
ANORECTUM Proctitis with pain and purulent discharge.
PHARYNX Pharyngitis with erythema occurs secondary to oral-genital sexual exposure. Always coexists with genital infection.
DISSEMINATED INFECTIONS Hemorrhagic, painful pustules on erythematous base on palms and fingers (Fig. 30-23) often associated with fever.
GONOCOCCAL ARTHRITIS Usually monoarticular knees, ankles.
GONOCOCCAL VESICULITIS AND PROSTATITIS in males, **pelvic disease** in females leads to obliteration of the tubes and thus infertility.
NEONATE Conjunctivitis, swollen eyelid, severe hyperemia, chemosis, and profuse purulent discharge; rarely, corneal ulcer and perforation. Usually in absence of genital infection. Infections occur intrapartum.

DIFFERENTIAL DIAGNOSIS

URETHRITIS GH with urethritis, *C. trachomatis* urethritis, *Ureaplasma urealyticum* urethritis, *Trichomonas vaginalis* urethritis, and reactive arthritis.
CERVICITIS *C. trachomatis* or HSV cervicitis.

LABORATORY EXAMINATIONS

GRAM STAIN Gram-negative diplococci intracellularly in PMN leukocytes in exudate (Fig. 30-21).
CULTURE *Men:* Urethra, rectum, oropharynx. *Women:* Cervix, rectum, oropharynx. *DGI:* Blood. Isolation on gonococcal-selective media, i.e., chocolatized blood agar, Martin–Lewis medium, and Thayer–Martin medium. Antimicrobial susceptibility testing important caused by resistant strains.

DIAGNOSIS

Clinical suspicion, confirmed by laboratory findings, and culture. Coinfection with other sexually pathogens should be ruled out.

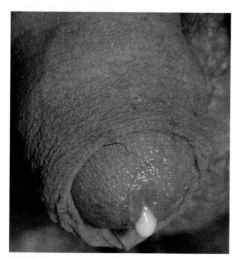

FIGURE 30-22 Gonorrhea Purulent, creamy urethral discharge from the distal urethra.

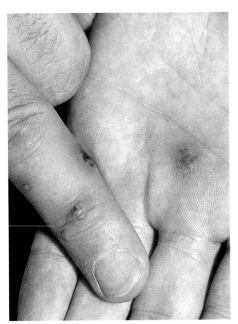

FIGURE 30-23 Disseminated gonococcal infection Hemorrhagic, painful pustules on erythematous bases on the palms and the fingers. These lesions occur at acral sites and are few in number.

COURSE

Most infected men seek treatment resulting from symptoms early enough to prevent serious sequelae, but not to prevent transmission to others. Most infected women have no recognizable symptoms until complications such as PID, tubal scarring, infertility, or ectopic pregnancy occur. DGI more common in women with asymptomatic cervical, endometrial, or tubal infection, and homosexual men with asymptomatic rectal or pharyngeal gonorrhea.

TREATMENT

LOCALIZED UNCOMPLICATED GONORRHEA Single dose intramuscular ceftriaxone 125 mg or oral cefixime 400 mg. *Alternatives:* Intramuscular ceftizoxime 500 mg, or intramuscular cefotaxime 500 mg, or intramuscular cefoxitin 2 g with oral probenecid 1 g.
PENICILLIN ALLERGY intramuscular spectinomycin 2 mg.
DISSEMINATED GONOCOCAL INFECTION Intramuscular or intravenous ceftriaxone 1 g every 24 hours. *Alternatives:* Intravenous cefotaxime or ceftizoxime 1 g every 8 hours or intramuscular spectinomycin 2 g every 12 hours.

SYPHILIS ICD-10: A50-53

- Chronic systemic infection caused by the spirochete *T. pallidum,* transmitted through skin and mucosa, with manifestations in nearly every organ system.
- Incidence is greater than 10 million cases annually worldwide, and almost 20,000 cases annually in the United States.
- Primary infection: A painless ulcer or chancre on the mucocutaneous site of inoculation. Associated with regional lymphadenopathy (chancriform syndrome: distal ulcer associated with proximal lymphadenopathy).
- Systemic infection: Shortly after inoculation, syphilis becomes a systemic infection with characteristic secondary and tertiary stages.
- Course: Clinical course and response to standard therapy may be altered in HIV/AIDS.

ETIOLOGY AND EPIDEMIOLOGY

ETIOLOGY Venereal syphilis caused by *T. pallidum*. *T. pallidum* is a thin delicate spirochete with 6 to 14 spirals. Only natural host for *T. pallidum* is the human. Subspecies of *T. pallidum* cause the nonvenereal diseases endemic syphilis (bejel), yaws, and pinta.
TRANSMISSION *Sexual contact*: Contact with infectious lesion (chancre, mucous patch, condyloma latum, and cutaneous lesions of secondary syphilis). Sixty percent of those in contact with persons having primary and secondary syphilis become infected. *Congenital infection*: In utero or perinatal transmission.
PATHOGENESIS The spirochetes pass through an intact mucous membrane and microscopic abrasion in skin, enter lymphatics and blood within a few hours, and produce systemic infection and metastatic foci before development of a primary lesion. Spirochetes divide locally, with resulting host inflammatory

response and chancre formation, either a single lesion or, less commonly, multiple lesions. Cellular immunity is of major importance in healing of early lesions and control of infection (T_H1 type). Primary syphilis is the most contagious stage of the disease. Later syphilis is essentially a vascular disease, lesions occurring secondary to obliterative endarteritis of terminal arterioles and small arteries, and by the resulting inflammatory and necrotic changes.

LABORATORY EXAMINATIONS

DARK-FIELD MICROSCOPY Positive in primary chancre and papular lesions of secondary syphilis such as condylomata lata. Unreliable in oral cavity because of the presence of saprophytic spirochetes, and negative in patients treated systemically or topically with antibiotics. Regional lymph node aspirated and aspirate examined in the dark-field microscope.

Direct Fluorescent Antibody T. pallidum (DFA-TP) Test. Fluorescent antibodies are used to detect *T. pallidum* in exudate from lesion, lymph node aspirate, or tissue.

SEROLOGIC TESTS FOR SYPHILIS (STS) Positive in persons with any treponemal infection. Tests always positive in secondary syphilis.
Nontreponemal STS. Measures IgG and IgM directed against cardiolipin–lecithin–cholesterol antigen complex. Rapid plasma reagin (RPR) test (automated RPR: ART). VDRL slide test; nonreactive in 25% of patients with primary syphilis. In early syphilis: Either do the fluorescent treponemal antibody-absorbed (FTA-ABS) test or repeat VDRL in 1 to 2 weeks if the initial VDRL is negative. *Prozone phenomenon*: If antibody titer high, test may be negative; must dilute serum; becomes nonreactive or reactive in lower titers following therapy for early syphilis.
Treponemal STS FTA-ABS Test. Agglutination assays for antibodies to *T. pallidum*:

Microhemagglutination assay (MHA-TP; Serodia TPPA test); *T. pallidum hemagglutination* test (TPHA). Often remain reactive after therapy; not helpful in determining infectious status of patient with past syphilis.

DERMATOPATHOLOGY In primary and secondary syphilis, lesional skin biopsy shows central thinning or ulceration of epidermis. Lymphocytic and plasmacytic dermal infiltrate. Proliferation of capillaries and lymphatics with endarteritis; may have thrombosis and small areas of necrosis. Dieterle stain demonstrates spirochetes.

COURSE

Even without treatment, chancre heals completely in 4 to 6 weeks. The infection either becomes latent or clinical manifestations of secondary syphilis appear. Secondary syphilis usually manifests as macular exanthem initially; after weeks, lesions resolve spontaneously and recur as *maculopapular* or *papular eruptions*. In 20% of untreated cases, up to three to four such recurrences followed by periods of clinical remission may occur over a period of 1 year. Infection then enters a latent stage, in which there are no clinical signs or symptoms of the disease. After untreated syphilis has persisted for >4 years, it is rarely communicable, except in the case of pregnant women, who, if untreated, may transmit syphilis to their fetuses, regardless of the duration of their disease. One-third of patients with untreated latent syphilis developed clinically apparent tertiary disease. Gummas hardly ever heal spontaneously. Noduloulcerative syphilides undergo spontaneous partial healing, but new lesions appear at the periphery.

TREATMENT

Antibiotics (see p. 769 for specific doses). Educate patients and treat sex partners. In the United States, report cases to the Department of Health.

PRIMARY SYPHILIS ICD-10: A51

CLINICAL MANIFESTATION

Genital or extragenital lesions occur at sites of inoculation. Ulcers are usually painless unless secondarily infected. Incubation period: 21 days (average); range, 10 to 90 days.

Chancre Button-like papule develops at the site of inoculation into a painless erosion and then ulcerates with raised border and scanty serous exudate (Figs. 30-24 and 30-25). Surface may be crusted. Lesions few millimeters to 1 or 2 cm in diameter. Usually single lesions; less commonly, few, multiple, or kissing lesions. Extragenital chancres occur at any site of inoculation; lesions on the fingers are painful.

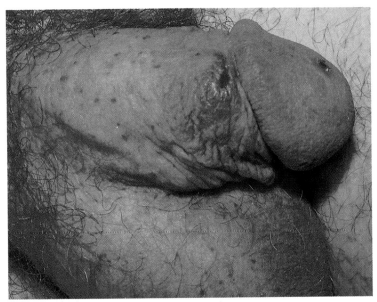

FIGURE 30-24 Primary syphilis: penile chancre A 28-year-old male with penile lesion for 7 days. Painless ulcer on distal penile shaft with smaller erosion on the glans. The ulcer is quite firm on palpation.

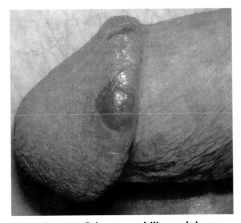

FIGURE 30-25 Primary syphilis: nodule on glans A 58-year-old male with penile lesion for 10 days. Red firm nodule on the glans; the lesion resolved without therapy and did not ulcerate. Biopsy reported inflammatory changes. The diagnosis was made in retrospect when STS obtained before marriage was positive.

SITES OF PREDILECTION Genital sites are most common. Male: Inner prepuce, coronal sulcus of the glans penis, shaft, base. Female: Cervix, vagina, vulva, clitoris, breast; chancres observed less frequently in women. Extragenital chancres: Anus or rectum, mouth, lips, tongue (Fig. 30-26), tonsils, fingers (painful!), toes, breast, and nipple.

LYMPHADENOPATHY Appears within 7 days. Nodes are discrete, firm, rubbery, nontender, and more commonly unilateral; may persist for months.

DIFFERENTIAL DIAGNOSIS

GENITAL EROSION/ULCER GH, traumatic ulcer, fixed drug eruption, chancroid, and lymphogranuloma venereum (LGV).

DIAGNOSIS

Clinical suspicion, confirmed by dark-field microscopy or serologically.

TREATMENT

Intramuscular benzathine penicillin G 2.4 million units in single dose or oral doxycycline 100 mg twice daily for 14 days.

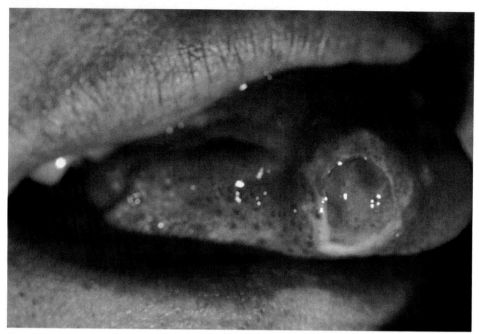

FIGURE 30-26 Primary syphilis: chancre on tip of the tongue A 24-year-old male with painful lesion on the tongue for 10 days.

SECONDARY SYPHILIS ICD-10: A51.3

CLINICAL MANIFESTATION

Appears 2 to 6 months after primary infection; 2 to 10 weeks after appearance of the primary chancre; 6 to 8 weeks after healing of the chancre. Chancre may still be present when secondary lesions appear (15% of cases). Concomitant HIV infection may alter the course of secondary syphilis.

Fever, sore throat, weight loss, malaise, anorexia, headache, and meningismus. Mucocutaneous lesions are asymptomatic.

SKIN LESIONS OF SECONDARY SYPHILIS Macules and papules 0.5 to 1 cm, round to oval; pink brownish-red. *First exanthem* always macular and faint (Fig. 30-27). Later eruptions may be papulosquamous (Figs. 30-28 and 30-29), pustular, or acneiform. Vesiculobullous lesions occur only in neonatal congenital syphilis (palms and soles). On the palms and soles lesions are psoriasiform (Figs. 30-30 and 30-31). On palpation, papules are firm (Figs. 30-30 and 30-31); condylomata lata, soft.

In the face, they look like seborrheic dermatitis and occur on the forehead and the nasolabial folds (Fig. 30-29). Lesions may also be annular or polycyclic, especially on the face in dark-skinned persons (Fig. 30-32). In relapsing secondary syphilis, arciform lesions. Always sharply defined except for macular exanthem. Lesions are scattered, tend to remain discrete, and are usually symmetric.

Condylomata lata (Fig. 30-33). Most commonly in the anogenital region and mouth; can be seen on any body surface where moisture can accumulate between intertriginous surfaces, i.e., axillae or toe webs.

HAIR Diffuse hair loss, including temples and parietal scalp. Patchy, *moth-eaten alopecia* on the scalp and beard area. Loss of eyelashes or lateral third of eyebrows.

MUCOUS MEMBRANES Small, asymptomatic, round or oval, slightly elevated, flat-topped macules and papules 0.5 to 1 cm in diameter, covered by hyperkeratotic white to gray membrane,

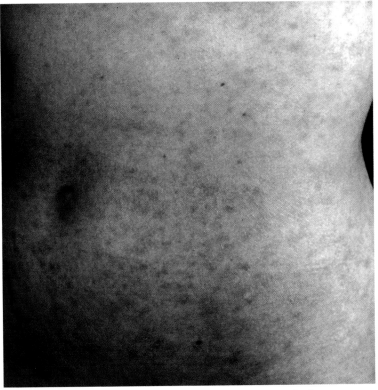

FIGURE 30-27 Secondary syphilis A 21-year-old female with the first exanthem of secondary syphilis (roseola syphilitica). These are barely visible, relatively ill-defined macules of salmon color, disseminated over chest, abdomen and back. Similar to pityriasis rosea but without or very little scale.

occurring on the oral or genital mucosa. Split papules at the angles of the mouth.

GENERALIZED LYMPHADENOPATHY Cervical, suboccipital, inguinal, epitrochlear, or axillary. Splenomegaly.

ASSOCIATED FINDINGS *Musculoskeletal involvement*: Periostitis of long bones, particularly tibia (nocturnal pain); arthralgia; hydrarthrosis of knees or ankles without X-ray changes. *Eyes*: Acute bacterial iritis, optic neuritis, and uveitis. *Meningovascular reaction*: CSF positive for inflammatory markers. *Gastrointestinal (GI) involvement*: Diffuse pharyngitis, hypertrophic gastritis, hepatitis, patchy proctitis, ulcerative colitis, and rectosigmoid mass. *Genitourinary involvement*: Glomerulonephritis and nephrotic syndrome, cystitis, and prostatitis.

LABORATORY EXAMINATIONS

DERMATOPATHOLOGY Epidermal hyperkeratosis; capillary proliferation with endothelial swelling; perivascular infiltration by monocytes, plasma cells, and lymphocytes. Spirochete is present in many tissues including the skin, eye, and CSF.

CSF Abnormal in 40% of patients. Spirochetes in CSF in 30% of cases.

LIVER FUNCTION Elevated enzymes.

RENAL FUNCTION Immune complex-induced membranous glomerulonephritis.

COURSE

Recurrent eruptions appear after month-long asymptomatic intervals. Initially a relatively

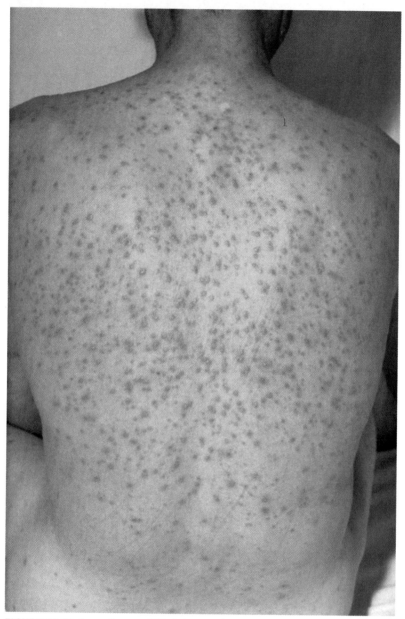

FIGURE 30-28 Secondary syphilis Later exanthema, papulosquamous and of more tan or copper-like color.

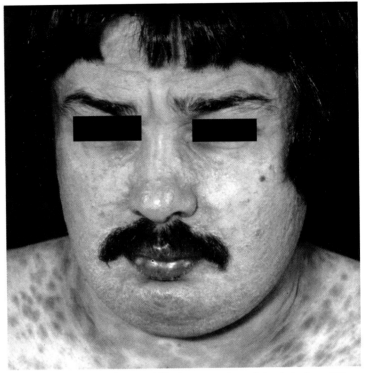

FIGURE 30-29 Secondary syphilis Later exanthem. Seborrheic dermatitis like papulosquamous lesions on the face and a copper tone papular rash on the neck and trunk.

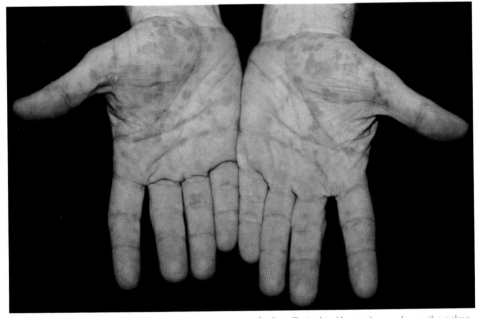

FIGURE 30-30 Secondary syphilis: papulosquamous lesion Typical red keratotic papules on the palms.

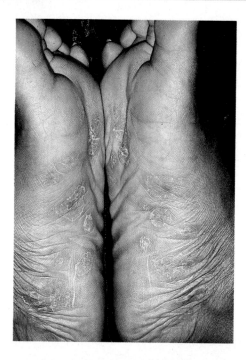

FIGURE 30-31 Secondary syphilis: papulosquamous lesions A 20-year-old female with hyperkeratotic, scaling plaques on the plantar aspects of both feet. Similar lesions were present on the palms.

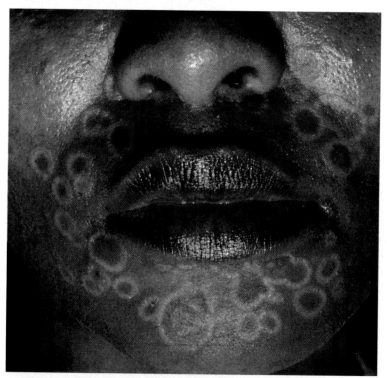

FIGURE 30-32 Secondary syphilis: annular facial lesions Annular plaques merging on the face of a South African woman. (Used with permission from Jeffrey S. Dover, MD.)

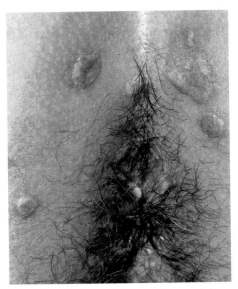

FIGURE 30-33 Secondary syphilis: condylomata lata Soft, flat-topped, moist, pink-tan papules and nodules on the perineum and perianal area. The lesions are teeming with *T. pallidum.*

faint *exanthem*, always macular, pink; lesions are ill defined. Later lesions of early syphilis are papular, brownish, and tend to be more localized. Symptoms may last 2 to 6 weeks (4 weeks average) and may recur in untreated or inadequately treated patients. Secondary lesions subside within 2 to 6 weeks, with the infection entering the latent stage.

DIFFERENTIAL DIAGNOSIS

EXANTHEM Adverse cutaneous drug eruption, pityriasis rosea, viral exanthem, infectious mononucleosis, tinea corporis, tinea versicolor, scabies, "id" reaction, condylomata acuminata, acute guttate psoriasis, and lichen planus.

DIAGNOSIS

Clinical suspicion confirmed by lab tests. Darkfield is positive in all secondary syphilis lesions except for macular exanthem.

TREATMENT

As for primary syphilis (see p. 769).

LATENT SYPHILIS ICD-10: A53.0

- Suspected on the basis of a history of primary or secondary lesions, history of exposure to syphilis, or delivery of an infant with congenital syphilis; can occur without prior recognized primary or secondary lesions.
- **Treatment:** As for primary syphilis (see p. 769).

CLINICAL MANIFESTATION

No clinical signs or symptoms of infection; STS positive; CSF is normal.
COURSE A previous negative STS defines the duration of latency. Early latent syphilis (<1 year) is distinguished from late latent disease (≥1 year). Latent disease does not preclude infectiousness or the development of gummatous skin lesions, cardiovascular lesions, or neurosyphilis. Maternal-fetal transmission can occur. Seventy percent of untreated patients never develop clinically evident tertiary syphilis. The more sensitive treponemal antibody test rarely becomes negative without treatment.

TERTIARY/LATE SYPHILIS ICD-10: 52.9

CLINICAL MANIFESTATION

GUMMA Nodular or papulosquamous plaques that may ulcerate and form circles/arc (Fig. 30-34). May expand rapidly causing destruction. May be indolent and heal with scarring. Solitary. Skin: Any site, especially on the scalp, face, chest (sternoclavicular), or calf.

Internal: Skeletal system (long bones of legs), oropharynx, upper respiratory tract (perforation of nasal septum, palate), larynx, liver, and stomach.
NODULAR ULCERATIVE SYPHILIDES Like gumma but flatter. Undergo spontaneous partial healing but recur at periphery. May be circular or serpiginous.

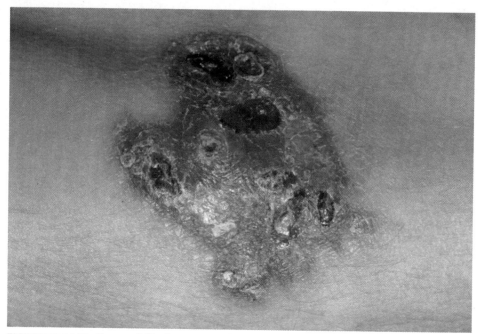

FIGURE 30-34 Tertiary syphilis. Gumma Tan, firm, well-defined plaque with multiple ulcerations in the scapular region.

ASYMPTOMATIC NEUROSYPHILIS Occurs in 25% of patients with untreated late latent syphilis. Lack neurologic symptoms/signs and CSF abnormalities. Twenty percent of patients with asymptomatic neurosyphilis progress to clinical neurosyphilis in the first 10 years; risk increases with time.

MENINGEAL SYPHILIS Onset of symptoms <1 year after infection; headache, nausea/vomiting, stiff neck, cranial nerve palsies, seizures, and changes in mental status. Meningovascular syphilis. Onset of symptoms 5 to 10 years after infection; subacute encephalitis prodrome followed by stroke syndrome, progressive vascular syndrome.

GENERAL PARESIS Onset of symptoms 20 years after infection. PARESIS: Paresis, Affect, Reflexes (*hyperactive*), Eye (*Argyll Robertson pupils*), Sensorium (illusions, delusions, hallucinations), Intellect (decrease in recent memory, orientation, calculations, judgment, insight), and Speech.

TABES DORSALIS Onset of symptoms 25 to 30 years after infection; ataxic wide-based gait and foot slap, paresthesia, bladder disturbances, impotence, areflexia, loss of position, deep pain, temperature sensations (Charcot or neuropathic joints, foot ulcers), and optic atrophy.

CARDIOVASCULAR SYPHILIS Results from endarteritis obliterans of vasa vasorum. Occurs in 10% of late untreated syphilis, 10 to 40 years after infection. Uncomplicated aortitis, aortic regurgitation, saccular aneurysm, and coronary ostial stenosis.

DIFFERENTIAL DIAGNOSIS

Plaque(s) ± ulceration ± granulomas: Cutaneous tuberculosis, cutaneous atypical mycobacterial infection, lymphoma, and invasive fungal infections.

DIAGNOSIS

Clinical findings, confirmed by STS and lesional skin biopsy; dark-field examination always negative.

COURSE

In *untreated* syphilis, 15% of patients develop late benign syphilis, mostly skin lesions. Tertiary syphilis is now rare. Previously, patients presenting with tertiary syphilis gave a history of lesions of 3 to 7 years' duration (range, 2 to 60 years); gumma developing by the 15th year. As noted, there are neurologic and cardiovascular complications of tertiary syphilis if left untreated. Consider neurosyphilis in differential diagnosis of neurologic disease in HIV disease.

TREATMENT

Intramuscular benzathine penicillin 2.4 million units once a week for three weeks. Patients allergic to penicillin should be treated by an infectious disease specialist.

NEUROSYPHILIS consult CDC guidelines.

CONGENITAL SYPHILIS ICD-10: A50.9

- **Transmission.** During gestation or intrapartum. Risk of transmission: Early maternal syphilis, 75 to 95%; >2 years' duration, 35%.
- **Pathogenesis.** Lesions usually develop after the fourth month of gestation, associated with fetal immunologic competence. Pathogenesis depends on the immune response of fetus. Adequate treatment of mother before the 16th week of pregnancy prevents fetal damage. Untreated: Fetal loss up to 40%.

CLINICAL MANIFESTATION

EARLY MANIFESTATIONS Appear before 2 years of age, often at 2 to 10 weeks of age. Infectious. Resembles severe secondary syphilis in adult. Bullae, vesicles on palms and soles, superficial desquamation, petechiae, and papulosquamous lesions. *Rhinitis or snuffles* (23%); *mucous patches*, condylomata latum. Bone changes: Osteochondritis, osteitis, and periostitis. Hepatosplenomegaly, jaundice, and lymphadenopathy. Anemia, thrombocytopenia, ad leukocytosis.

LATE MANIFESTATIONS Appear after 2 years of age. Noninfectious. Similar to late acquired syphilis in adults. Cardiovascular syphilis. Interstitial keratitis. Eighth nerve deafness. Recurrent arthropathy; bilateral knee effusions (Clutton joints). Gummatous periostitis results in destructive lesions of nasal septum/palate. Asymptomatic neurosyphilis in 33% of patients; clinical syphilis in 25%.

RESIDUAL STIGMATA *Hutchinson teeth* [centrally notched, widely spaced, peg-shaped upper central incisors; "mulberry" molars (multiple poorly developed cusps)]. *Abnormal facies*: Frontal bossing, saddle nose, poorly developed maxillae, and rhagades (linear scars at angles of mouth, caused by bacterial secondary infection of early facial eruption). Saber shins. Nerve deafness. Old chorioretinitis, optic atrophy, and corneal opacities caused by interstitial keratitis.

TREATMENT

Consult CDC guidelines.

LYMPHOGRANULOMA VENEREUM ICD-10: A55

■ Clinical manifestations depend on the site of entry of *C. trachomatis* (the sex contact site) and the stage of disease progression: Inguinal syndrome, rectal syndrome, and pharyngeal syndrome.

ETIOLOGY AND EPIDEMIOLOGY

ETIOLOGY *C. trachomatis*, obligate intracellular bacterium. Major outer-membrane protein delineates >20 serovars (immunotypes): *Trachoma*: Serovars A, B, Ba, and C. *Mucosal STDs*: Serovars D-K (most common bacterial STD). *Invasive STD*: Serovars L_1, L_2, L_3 (in United States, L_2 most commonly).

TRANSMISSION *Sexual: C. trachomatis* in purulent exudate is inoculated onto skin or mucosa of sexual partner and gains entry through minute lacerations and abrasions. *Perinatal. Heterosexual men*: Acute infection presents as inguinal syndrome. *Women/homosexual men*: Anogenitorectal syndrome most common.

PREVALENCE Chlamydial urethritis more common in heterosexual men and high socioeconomic status. Prevalence of cervical infection in the United States: 5% for asymptomatic college students; >10% in family planning clinics: >20% in STD clinics.

PATHOGENESIS Primarily an infection of lymphatics and lymph nodes. Lymphangitis and lymphadenitis occur in the drainage field of the inoculation site with subsequent perilymphangitis and periadenitis. Necrosis occurs; loculated abscesses, fistulas, and sinus tracts develop. As the infection subsides, fibrosis replaces acute inflammation with resulting obliteration of lymphatic drainage, chronic edema, and stricture.

CLINICAL MANIFESTATION

ACUTE LYMPHOGRANULOMA VENEREUM Primary genital lesion noticed in less than one-third of men and rarely in women. *In heterosexual men and women*: Small painless vesicle or nonindurated ulcer/papule on the penis or labia/posterior vagina/fourchette; heals in a few days. With receptive anal intercourse, primary anal or rectal infection develops after receptive anal intercourse. Infection can spread from the primary site of infection to regional lymphatics.

Papule, shallow erosion or ulcer, grouped small erosions or ulcers (herpetiform), or nonspecific urethritis. *Cordlike lymphangitis* of dorsal penis may follow. Lymphangial nodule (bubonulus) may rupture, resulting in sinuses and fistulas of the urethra and deforming scars of the penis. Multilocular suppurative lymphadenopathy. Cervicitis, perimetritis, salpingitis may occur. Receptive anal intercourse: Primary anal rectal infection (hemorrhagic proctitis with regional lymphadenitis).

Erythema nodosum in 10% of cases (see Section 7).

INGUINAL SYNDROME Characterized by painful inguinal lymphadenopathy beginning 2 to 6 weeks after presumed exposure. Unilateral in two-thirds of cases; palpable iliac/femoral nodes often present on same side (Fig. 30-35). Initially, nodes are discrete, but progressive periadenitis results in a matted mass of nodes that may become fluctuant and suppurative. Overlying skin becomes fixed, inflamed, thin, and eventually develops multiple draining fistulas. *Groove sign*: Extensive enlargement of chains of inguinal nodes above and below the inguinal ligament (Fig. 30-35).

Unilateral bubo in two-thirds of cases (most common presentation) (Fig. 30-35). Marked edema and erythema of skin overlying node. One-third of inguinal buboes rupture; two-thirds slowly involute. Seventy-five percent of cases have deep iliac node involvement with a pelvic mass that seldom suppurates.

Anogenitorectal syndrome associated with receptive anal intercourse, proctocolitis, hyperplasia of intestinal and perirectal lymphatic tissue. Resultant abscesses, fistulas, and rectal stricture. Overgrowth of lymphatic tissue results in lymphorrhoids (resembling hemorrhoids) or perianal condylomata.

ESTHIOMENE Elephantiasis of genitalia, usually females, which may ulcerate, occurring 1 to 20 years after primary infection.

DIFFERENTIAL DIAGNOSIS

PRIMARY STAGE GH, primary syphilis, and chancroid.

INGUINAL SYNDROME Incarcerated inguinal hernia, plague, tularemia, tuberculosis, GH, syphilis, chancroid, and lymphoma.

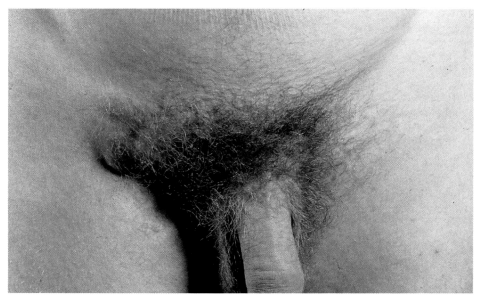

FIGURE 30-35 Lymphogranuloma venereum: Groove sign Striking tender lymphadenopathy occurring at the left femoral and inguinal lymph nodes separated by a groove made by Poupart ligament (groove sign).

DIAGNOSIS

Diagnosis is based on clinical findings. Exclude other causes of inguinal lymphadenopathy or genital ulcers.

COURSE

Highly variable. Bacterial secondary infections may contribute to complications. Rectal stricture is late complication. Spontaneous remission is common.

TREATMENT

Oral doxycycline 100 mg twice daily for 21 days or oral erythromycin base 500 mg four times daily for 21 days.

CHANCROID ICD-10: A57

- Etiology: *Haemophilus ducreyi,* a gram-negative streptobacillus.

EPIDEMIOLOGY AND ETIOLOGY

ETIOLOGY *H. ducreyi,* a gram-negative streptobacillus.

DEMOGRAPHY Uncommon in industrialized nations. Endemic in tropical and subtropical developing countries, especially in poor, urban, and seaport populations. Much more common in young males. Lymphadenitis more common in males.

TRANSMISSION Most likely during sexual intercourse with partner who has *H. ducreyi* genital ulcer. Chancroid is a cofactor for HIV/AIDS transmission; high rates of HIV/AIDS infection among those who have chancroid. Ten percent of individuals with chancroid acquired in the United States are coinfected with *T. pallidum* and HSV.

PATHOGENESIS Primary infection develops at the site of inoculation (break in epithelium), followed by lymphadenitis. The genital ulcer is characterized by perivascular and interstitial infiltrates of macrophages and of CD4+ and CD8+ lymphocytes, consistent with a delayed-type hypersensitivity, cell-mediated immune response. CD4+ cells and macrophages in the ulcer may explain the facilitation of transmission of HIV/AIDS in patients with chancroid ulcers.

CLINICAL MANIFESTATION

Incubation period is 4 to 7 days.

PRIMARY LESION Tender papule with erythematous halo that evolves to pustule, erosion, and ulcer. *Ulcer* is usually quite *tender* or *painful*. Its borders are sharp, undermined, and not indurated (Figs. 30-36 and 30-37). Base is friable with granulation tissue and covered with gray to yellow exudate. *Edema* of prepuce common. Ulcer may be singular or multiple, merging to form large or giant ulcers (>2 cm) with serpiginous shape.

DISTRIBUTION Male: Prepuce, frenulum, coronal sulcus, glans penis, and shaft. Female: External genitalia, vaginal wall by direct extension from introitus, cervix, perianal. Extragenital lesions: Breast, fingers, thighs, oral mucosa. Bacterial superinfection of ulcers can occur. Multiple ulcers (Fig. 30-37) develop by autoinoculation.

PAINFUL INGUINAL LYMPHADENITIS Usually unilateral, occurs in 50% of patients 7 to 21 days after primary lesion. Ulcer may heal before buboes occur. Buboes occur with overlying erythema and may drain spontaneously.

Painful ulcer at the site of inoculation, usually on the external genitalia.

REGIONAL LYMPH NODES Tender adenopathy. Suppurative adenopathy.

STI most strongly associated with increased risk for HIV/AIDS transmission.

Synonyms. Soft chancre, ulcus molle, and chancre mou.

DIFFERENTIAL DIAGNOSIS

GENITAL ULCER GH, primary syphilis, LGV, and traumatic lesions.

TENDER INGUINAL MASS GH, secondary syphilis, LGV, incarcerated hernia, plague, and tularemia.

DIAGNOSIS

Combination of a painful ulcer with tender lymphadenopathy (one-third of patients) is suggestive of chancroid. Smear: Short gram-negative rods in linear arrangement. A definitive diagnosis of chancroid requires the identification of *H. ducreyi* on special culture media. Rule out HIV, *T. pallidum*, and HSV coinfection.

COURSE

The time required for complete healing is related to the size of the ulcer; large ulcers may require 14 days. Complete resolution of fluctuant lymphadenopathy is slower than that of ulcers

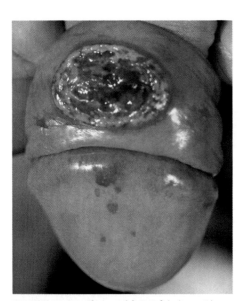

FIGURE 30-36 Chancroid Painful ulcer with marked surrounding erythema and edema. (Used with permission from Prof. Alfred Eichmann, MD.)

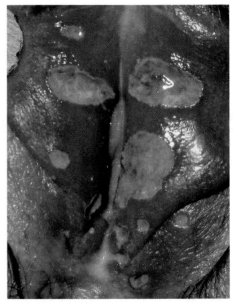

FIGURE 30-37 Chancroid Multiple, painful, punched-out ulcers with undermined borders on the vulva occurring after autoinoculation.

and may require needle aspiration through adjacent intact skin, even during successful therapy.

TREATMENT

Azithromycin 1 g in single dose. Ciprofloxacin 500 mg twice daily for 3 days (contraindicated in pregnancy). Erythromycin base 500 mg three times daily for 7 days. Intramuscular ceftriaxone in single dose. Resistance to ciprofloxacin and erythromycin has been reported.

DONOVANOSIS ICD-10: A58

- STI caused by *Klebsiella granulomatis*, an encapsulated intracellular gram-negative rod. Rare in industrialized nations. Endemic foci in tropical and subtropical environments.

CLINICAL MANIFESTATION

Painless, progressive, ulcerative lesions of anogenital areas. Highly vascular (i.e., a beefy red appearance) (Fig. 30-38) and bleed easily on contact. Spreads by continuity or by autoinoculation of approximated skin surfaces. Distribution. *Males*: Prepuce or glans, penile shaft, and scrotum. *Females*: Labia minora, mons veneris, and fourchette. Ulcerations then spread by direct extension or autoinoculation to inguinal and perineal skin. Extragenital lesions occur in mouth, lips, throat, face, GI tract, and bone.
REGIONAL LYMPH NODES Not enlarged. Large subcutaneous nodule may mimic a lymph node, i.e., pseudobubo.
VARIANT TYPES Ulcerovegetative (Fig. 30-38); nodular; hypertrophic; sclerotic/cicatricial.
COMPLICATIONS Deep ulcerations, chronic cicatricial lesions, phimosis, lymphedema (elephantiasis of penis, scrotum, vulva), and exuberant epithelial proliferation that grossly resembles carcinoma.

DIFFERENTIAL DIAGNOSIS

Differential diagnosis in endemic areas, syphilitic chancre, chancroid, chronic herpetic ulcer, LGV, cutaneous tuberculosis, and invasive SCC.

DIAGNOSIS

Visualize Donovan bodies (rod-shaped organisms seen in cytoplasm of mononuclear phagocytes) in tissue samples or touch or crush preparation or in lesional biopsy specimen. Rule out other or concurrent cause of genital ulcer disease.

COURSE

Little tendency toward spontaneous healing. Heals with antibiotic treatment. Relapse may occur.

TREATMENT

All antibiotic treatments should be given for at least three weeks or until all lesions have healed.
RECOMMENDED REGIMEN Oral doxycycline twice daily.
ALTERNATIVE REGIMEN Oral azithromycin 1 g once a week. Ciprofloxacin 750 mg twice daily. Erythromycin base 500 mg four times daily. Trimethoprim-sulfamethoxazole double strength tablet (160 mg/800 mg) twice daily.

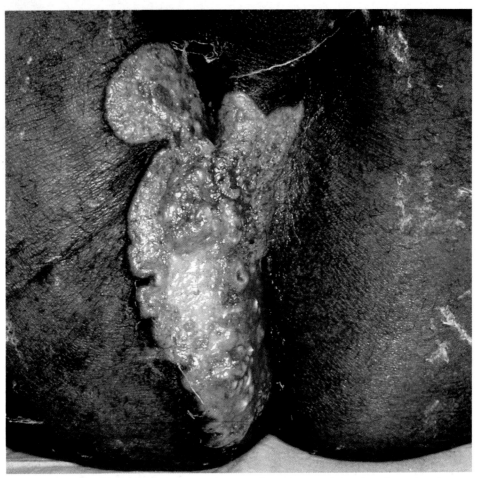

FIGURE 30-38 Donovanosis: ulcerovegetative type Extensive granulation tissue formation, ulceration, and scarring of the perineum, scrotum, and penis.

PART IV

Skin Signs of Hair, Nail, and Mucosal Disorders

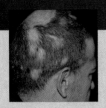

DISORDERS OF HAIR FOLLICLES AND RELATED DISORDERS

BIOLOGY OF HAIR GROWTH CYCLES

GLOSSARY OF TERMS

Hair Follicle Cycle

The hair follicle undergoes life-long cyclic transformations into three primary phases: anagen, catagen, and telogen (Fig. 31-1).

ANAGEN Growth phase; determines the ultimate length of hair at a site. Anagen hair matrix has rapidly proliferating epithelial cells and is exquisitely sensitive to drugs, growth factors, hormones, stress, and immunologic and physical injury. Destruction of epithelial stem cells results in permanent hair loss.

Anagen hairs have pigmented malleable proximal ends (Fig. 31-2A). About 85 to 99% of hairs will be in this phase, with some individual variation.

TELOGEN Period of relative quiescence, prior to shedding. *Telogen hairs* are club hairs with depigmented rounded proximal ends (Fig. 31-2B). About 1 to 15% of hairs are in this phase at any given time.

CATAGEN Apoptosis-driven phase between telogen and anagen phase. Only about 1% of hairs are seen in this phase.

EXOGEN Active process of hair shaft shedding.

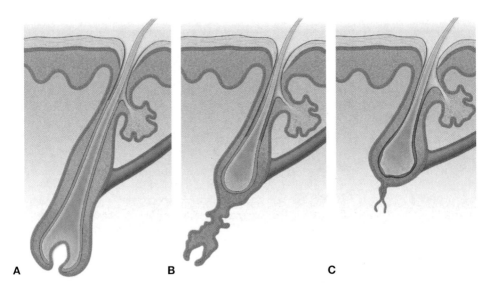

A   B   C

FIGURE 31-1 Hair growth cycle Diagrammatic representation of the changes that occur to the follicle and hair shaft during the hair growth cycle. **(A)** Anagen (growth stage); **(B)** Catagen (degenerative stage); **(C)** Telogen (resting stage). (Used with permission from Lynn M. Klein, MD.)

FIGURE 31-2 Hair mount (A) Anagen: Note the malleable proximal ends and **(B)** Telogen: club hairs. (Reproduced with permission from Goldsmith LA, Katz SI, Gilchrest BA, et al, eds. *Fitzpatrick's Dermatology in General Medicine.* 8th ed. New York, NY: McGraw-Hill; 2012.)

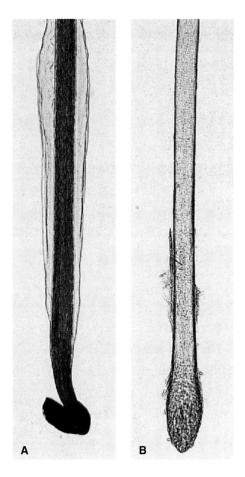

A   B

Types of Hair

LANUGO HAIR Soft fine pigmented hair that covers much of fetus; usually shed before birth.

VELLUS HAIR Fine, nonpigmented hair; growth not affected by hormones.

TERMINAL HAIR Thick, pigmented hair found on scalp, eyebrow/eyelashes, beard, axillae, pubic area; growth is influenced by hormones.

LABORATORY EXAMINATIONS

HAIR PULL Scalp is gently pulled. Normally, three to five hairs are dislodged; shedding more hair suggests pathology.

TRICHOGRAM Determines the number of anagen and telogen hairs and is made by epilating (plucking) 50 hairs or more and counting the number of anagen and telogen hairs.

SCALP BIOPSY Offers insight into pathogenesis of alopecia.

HAIR LOSS: ALOPECIA ICD-10: L63-L66

- Shedding of hair is termed *effluvium* or *defluvium*, and the resulting condition is called *alopecia* (Greek alópekia, "baldness").
- Alopecia classified into:
- *Noncicatricial alopecia*: No clinical sign of tissue inflammation, scarring, or atrophy of skin.
- *Cicatricial alopecia*: Evidence of tissue destruction such as inflammation, atrophy, and scarring may be apparent.

NONSCARRING ALOPECIA (Table 31-1)

TABLE 31-1 Etiology of Hair Loss

Diffuse (global) hair loss (nonscarring)	Focal (patchy, localized) hair loss
Failure of follicle production	Nonscarring
Hair shaft abnormality	Production decline
Abnormality of cycling (shedding)	Triangular alopecia
Telogen effluvium	Pattern hair loss (androgenetic alopecia)
	Hair breakage
Anagen effluvium	Trichotillomania
	Traction alopecia
Loose anagen syndrome	Infection (tinea capitis)
	Primary or acquired hair shaft abnormality
Alopecia areata	Unruly hair
	Abnormality of cycling
	Alopecia areata
	Syphilis
	Scarring (cicatricial) alopecia (see "Scarring Alopecia" p. 798)

PATTERN HAIR LOSS ICD-10: L64.9

- Pattern hair loss is the most common type of progressive balding.
- Occurs through the combined effect of:
  - Genetic predisposition.
  - Action of androgen on scalp hair follicles.
- In males, pattern/extent of hair loss varies from bitemporal recession, to frontal and/or vertex thinning, to loss of all hair except that along the occipital and temporal margins ("Hippocratic wreath").
- *Synonyms*: Males: Androgenetic alopecia (AGA), male-pattern baldness, common baldness. Females: Hereditary thinning, female-pattern baldness.

ETIOLOGY AND EPIDEMIOLOGY

ETIOLOGY Combined effects of androgen on genetically predisposed hair follicles. Genetics: (1) autosomal dominant and/or polygenic; (2) inherited from either or both parents.

AGE OF ONSET

- *Men*: May begin any time after puberty, as early as the second decade; often fully expressed in 40s.

- *Women*: Later, in about 40% occurs in the sixth decade.

SEX Men >> women.

CLASSIFICATION

Hamilton classified male-pattern hair loss into stages (Fig. 31-3A).

Ludwig classified hair loss in women (Fig. 31-3B).

A. Male (Hamilton classification)

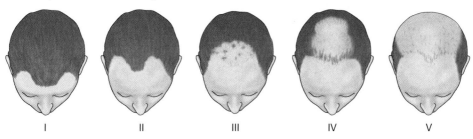

I　　　　II　　　　III　　　　IV　　　　V

B. Female (Ludwig classification)

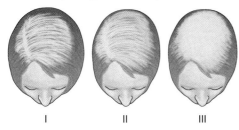

I　　　　II　　　　III

FIGURE 31-3 Androgenetic alopecia: patterns in men and women (A) Hamilton classified the severity and pattern of hair loss in men into types I to V. **(B)** Ludwig classified hair loss in women into types I to III.

PATHOGENESIS

- *Dihydrotestosterone* causes growth of the prostate, growth of terminal hair, AGA, and acne.
- Testosterone causes growth of axillary hair and lower pubic hair, as well as sex drive, growth of the phallus and scrotum, and spermatogenesis.
- Testosterone is converted to (DHT) by 5α-reductase (5α-R). Two isozymes of 5α-R occur: type I and type II.
- Type I 5α-R is localized to sebaceous glands (face, scalp), chest/back skin/liver, adrenal gland, kidney.
- Type II 5α-R is localized to the scalp hair follicle, beard, chest skin, liver, seminal vesicle, prostate, epididymis, and foreskin/scrotum.
- Finasteride inhibits conversion of testosterone to DHT by type II 5α-R.

CLINICAL MANIFESTATION

SKIN FINDINGS Scalp skin is normal.

- In young women, look for signs of virilization (acne, excess facial or body hair, male-pattern or escutcheon).

HAIR (Figs. 31-4 to 31-7) Hair in areas of pattern hair loss becomes finer in texture (shorter in length and reduced diameter). In time, hair becomes vellus and eventually atrophies completely.

DISTRIBUTION

- Men usually exhibit patterned loss in the frontotemporal and vertex areas (Figs. 31-4 and 31-5). Paradoxically, men with extensive pattern hair loss may have excess growth of secondary sexual hair, i.e., axillae, pubic area, chest, and beard.
- Women, including those who are endocrinologically normal, also lose scalp hair according to the male pattern, but hair loss is far less pronounced. Often, hair loss is more diffuse in women, following the pattern described by Ludwig (Fig. 31-3B).

SYSTEMIC FINDINGS In young women with AGA, look for signs of virilization (clitoral hypertrophy, acne, and facial hirsutism).However, most women with pattern hair loss are endocrinologically normal.

DIFFERENTIAL DIAGNOSIS

DIFFUSE NONSCARRING SCALP ALOPECIA Diffuse pattern of hair loss with alopecia areata, telogen

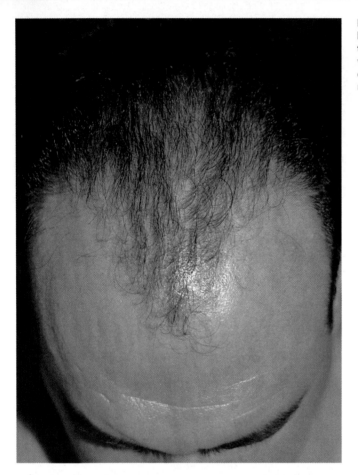

FIGURE 31-4 Pattern hair loss: male, Hamilton type III A 46-year-old male with bitemporal recession of hairline and frontal thinning of hair.

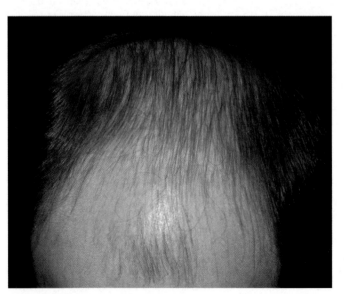

FIGURE 31-5 Pattern hair loss: male, Hamilton types IV to V A 37-year-old male with loss of hair in the frontotemporal and vertex areas in a male corresponding to Hamilton types IV and V.

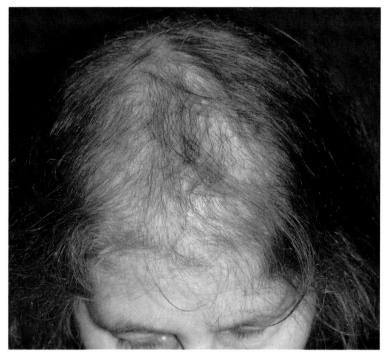

FIGURE 31-6 Pattern hair loss: female, Ludwig type II A 66-year-old female with diffuse thinning of hair on the crown.

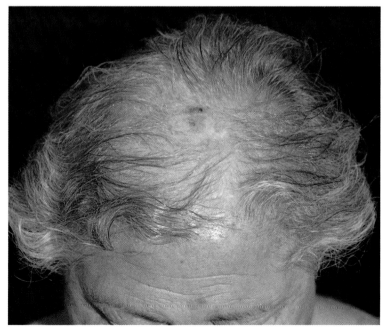

FIGURE 31-7 Pattern hair loss: female, Lugwig type III with basal cell carcinoma (BCC) A 67-year-old Greek female with advanced alopecia of the crown with BCC arising within it.

defluvium, secondary syphilis, systemic lupus erythematosus (SLE), iron deficiency, hypothyroidism, hyperthyroidism, trichotillomania (pulling of one's own hair, compulsive), and seborrheic dermatitis. The so-called alopecia, senescent due to age, was described initially in patientns with diffuse thinning, no family history of pattern balding, and no evidence of increased minituarization on scalp biopsy (see below). This diagnosis remains controversial and some authorities believe that most causes of significant hair loss in the elderly are also androgen-driven.

LABORATORY EXAMINATIONS

TRICHOGRAM In pattern hair loss, the earliest changes are an increase in the percentage of telogen hairs.

DERMATOPATHOLOGY Abundance of telogen-stage follicles is noted, associated with hair follicles of decreasing size and eventually nearly complete atrophy.

HORMONE STUDIES In women with hair loss and evidence of increased androgens (menstrual irregularities, infertility, hirsutism, severe cystic acne, or virilization), determine the following:

- Testosterone: total and free.
- Dehydroepiandrosterone sulfate (DHEAS).
- Prolactin.

OTHER STUDIES Other causes of thinning hair should be excluded with measurement of thyroid-stimulating hormone (TSH), T_4, serum iron, serum ferritin, and/or total iron-binding capacity, complete blood count, and antinuclear antibodies (ANA).

DIAGNOSIS

Clinical diagnosis is made on the history, pattern of alopecia, and family incidence of AGA. Skin biopsy may be necessary in some cases.

COURSE

The progression of alopecia is usually very gradual, over years to decades.

MANAGEMENT

ORAL FINASTERIDE 1 mg/day. Finasteride has no affinity for androgen receptors and therefore does not block other actions of testosterone (growth of the phallus and scrotum, spermatogenesis, or libido). Two percent of men taking finasteride report decrease in libido and erectile function; these effects were reversible when the drug was stopped and disappeared in two-thirds of those who continued taking finasteride. Dutasteride (2.5 mg) inhibits both type I and II reductase enzymes, perhaps more potently than finasteride.

TOPICAL MINOXIDIL Topically applied minoxidil, 2% and 5% solution, may be helpful in reducing the rate of hair loss or in partially restoring lost hair in both men and women.

ANTIANDROGENS In women with AGA who have elevated adrenal androgens, spironolactone, cyproterone acetate, flutamide, and cimetidine bind to androgen receptors and block the action of DHT. These must not be used in men.

TOPICAL LATANOPROST 0.1%, a prostaglandin analogue, may stimulate hair follicle growth.

HAIRPIECE Wigs, toupees, prosthetics; hair weaves.

Surgical Treatment

Hair transplantation: Grafts of one or two follicles are taken from androgen-insensitive hair sites (peripheral occipital and parietal hairy areas) to bald androgen-sensitive scalp areas. *Scalp reduction/rotation flaps.*

ALOPECIA AREATA ICD-10: L63.9

- A localized loss of hair in round or oval areas with no apparent inflammation of the skin.
- Nonscarring; hair follicle intact; hair can regrow.
- Clinical findings: Hair loss ranging from solitary patch to complete loss of all terminal hair.
- Prognosis: good for limited involvement. Poor for extensive hair loss.
- Management: intralesional triamcinolone effective for limited number of lesions.

ETIOLOGY AND EPIDEMIOLOGY

ETIOLOGY Unknown. Association with other autoimmune diseases; 10 to 20% of persons with alopecia areata (AA) have a familial history of AA.
AGE OF ONSET Young adults (<25 years); children are affected more frequently. Can occur at any age.
PREVALENCE 1.7% of the US population experiences at least one episode of AA in a lifetime.

PATHOGENESIS

- Follicular damage occurs in anagen followed by rapid transformation to catagen and telogen; then to dystrophic anagen status. While the disease is active, follicles are unable to progress beyond early anagen.
- Follicular stem cell is spared; hair follicles are not destroyed (there is no scarring).

CLINICAL MANIFESTATIONS

DURATION OF HAIR LOSS Patches of AA can be stable and often show spontaneous regrowth over a period of several months; new patches may appear while others resolve.
ASSOCIATED FINDINGS Autoimmune thyroiditis. Down syndrome. Autoimmune polyendocrinopathy-candidiasis–ectodermal dysplasia syndrome.

Hair

- Alopecia often sharply defined with normal-appearing skin with follicular openings present (Figs. 31-8 to 31-10).

- "Exclamation mark" hairs. Diagnostic broken-off stubby hairs (distal ends are broader than proximal ends) (Fig. 31-8); seen at margins of hair loss areas.
- Scattered, discrete areas of alopecia (Fig. 31-9) or confluent with total loss of scalp hair (Fig. 31-10), or generalized loss of body hair (including vellus hair).
- Diffuse AA of scalp (noncircumscribed) gives the appearance of thinned hair; can be difficult to differentiate from telogen effluvium (TE) or hair loss with thyroid disease.

Sites of Predilection. Scalp most commonly. Any hair-bearing area. Beard, eyebrows, eyelashes, pubic hair.

- *Alopecia areata (AA)*: Solitary or multiple areas of hair loss (Figs. 31-8 and 31-9).
- *AA totalis (AAT)*: Total loss of terminal scalp hair.
- *AA universalis (AAU)*: Total loss of all terminal body and scalp hair (Fig. 31-10).
- *Ophiasis*: Bandlike pattern of hair loss over periphery of scalp.

NAILS Fine pitting ("hammered brass") of dorsal nail plate. (see also Section 32, Fig. 32-10).

DIFFERENTIAL DIAGNOSIS

NONSCARRING ALOPECIA White-patch tinea capitis, trichotillomania, early scarring alopecia, pattern hair loss, secondary syphilis (alopecia areolaris) ("moth-eaten" appearance in beard or scalp).

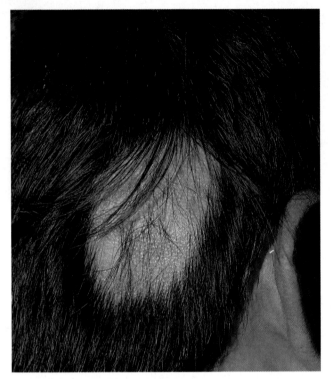

FIGURE 31-8 Alopecia areata (AA) of scalp: solitary lesion An area of alopecia without scaling, erythema, atrophy, or scarring on the occipital scalp. The short, broken-off hair shafts (so-called exclamation mark hair) appear as very short stubs emerging from the bald scalp.

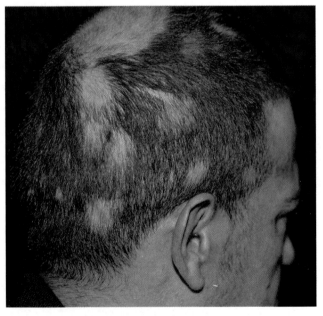

FIGURE 31-9 Alopecia areata of scalp: multiple, extensive lesions A 46-year-old male with multiple, confluent patches of alopecia areata.

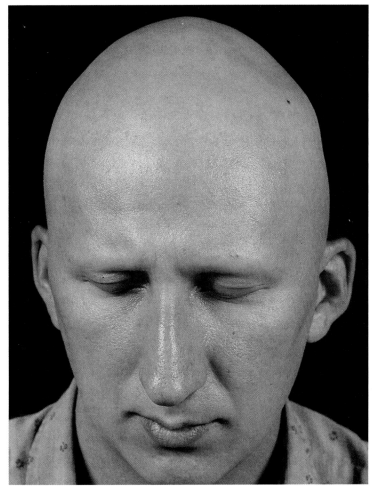

FIGURE 31-10 Alopecia areata universalis (AAU) This patient has lost all scalp hair (alopecia totalis), eyebrows, eyelashes, beard, and all body hair (alopecia universalis) and has dystrophic ("hammered brass") nails.

LABORATORY EXAMINATIONS

SEROLOGY ANA (to rule out SLE); rapid plasma reagin (RPR) test (to rule out secondary syphilis).
KOH PREPARATION Rule out tinea capitis.
DERMATOPATHOLOGY Acute lesions show peribulbar, perivascular, and outer root sheath mononuclear cell infiltrate of T cells and macrophages; follicular dystrophy with abnormal pigmentation and matrix degeneration. May show increased number of catagen/telogen follicles.

COURSE

- Spontaneous remission is common in patchy AA but is less so with AAT or AAU.

- Poor prognosis associated with onset in childhood, loss of body hair, nail involvement, atopy, and family history of AA.
- Recurrences of AA, however, are frequent.

MANAGEMENT

- Treatment directed at inflammatory infiltrate. No curative treatment is currently available.
- In many cases, the most important factor in management of the patient is psychological support from the dermatologist, family, and support groups (The National Alopecia Areata Foundation, http://-www.naaf.org/).

- Persons with extensive scalp involvement such as AAT may prefer to wear a wig or hairpiece.
- Makeup applied to eyebrows is helpful. Eyebrows can be tattooed.

GLUCOCORTICOIDS *Topical.* Superpotent agents not usually effective.

Intralesional Injection. Few and small lesions of AA can be treated with intralesional triamcinolone acetonide, 3 to 7 mg/mL.

Systemic Glucocorticoids. May induce regrowth, but AA recurs on discontinuation.

SYSTEMIC CYCLOSPORINE Induces regrowth, but AA recurs when drug is discontinued.

INDUCTION OF ALLERGIC CONTACT DERMATITIS Dinitrochlorobenzene, squaric acid dibutylester, or diphencyprone reported to be successful, but local discomfort resulting from allergic contact dermatitis and swelling of regional lymph nodes poses a problem.

ORAL PUVA (PHOTOCHEMOTHERAPY) Variably effective, as high as 30%, and worth a trial in patients who are highly distressed about the problem. Entire body must be exposed.

JANUS KINASE INHIBITORS ("JAK inhibitors:" ruxolitinib and tofacitinib) are FDA approved for moderate to severe (greater than 30% loss) disease and are effective. It has yet to be determined how long such agents have to be administered.

TELOGEN EFFLUVIUM ICD-10: L65.0

- Telogen effluvium is the transient increased shedding of normal club (telogen) hairs from resting scalp follicles.
- Secondary to accelerated shift of anagen (growth phase) into catagen and telogen (resting phase).
- Results in increased daily hair loss and, if severe, diffuse thinning of scalp hair.

ETIOLOGY AND EPIDEMIOLOGY

ETIOLOGY A reaction pattern to a variety of physical or mental stressors.

Endocrine: Hypo- or hyperthyroidism; postpartum; discontinuation or changing type of estrogen containing drugs.

Nutritional deficiency: Biotin, zinc, iron, and essential fatty acid.

Rapid weight loss, caloric or protein deprivation, chronic iron deficiency, and excessive vitamin A ingestion.

Physical stress: Febrile illnesses, catabolic illnesses (e.g., malignancy, chronic infection), major surgery, major trauma, acute, or chronic psychological stress.

Psychological stress: Anxiety, depression, and bipolar disorder.

Intoxication: Thallium, mercury, and arsenic.

Drugs: See Table 31-2.

Idiopathic: No obvious cause is apparent in a significant number of cases.

AGE OF ONSET Any age.

SEX More common in women, caused by parturition, cessation of an oral contraceptive, and "crash" dieting.

INCIDENCE Second most common cause of alopecia after AGA.

PATHOGENESIS

- TE: Many more hairs than normal are shed daily. The precipitating stimulus results in a premature shift of anagen follicles into the telogen phase. TE occurs in 3 to 4 months after the inciting event occurred.
- Can become chronic but rarely goes beyond 50% loss.

CLINICAL MANIFESTATION

SKIN LESIONS No abnormalities of the scalp are detected.

HAIR (Fig. 31-11) Diffuse shedding of the scalp hair. Gentle hair pull gathers several to many club or telogen hairs.

Distribution. Hair loss occurs diffusely throughout the scalp. Hairs are finer than older hairs and have tapered ends.

NAILS The precipitating stimulus for TE may also affect the growth of nails, resulting in Beau lines (see Transverse or Beau Lines, see Section 32), which appear as transverse lines or grooves on the fingernail and toenail plates.

TABLE 31-2 Drug-Induced Alopecia

Drugs	Features of Alopecia
ACE inhibitors Enalapril	Probable telogen effluvium
Anticoagulants Heparin Warfarin	Probable telogen effluvium
Antimitotic agents Colchicine	Anagen effluvium
Antineoplastic agents Bleomycin, cyclophosphamide, cytarabine, dacarbazine, dactinomycin, daunorubicin, doxorubicin, etoposide, fluorouracil, hydroxyurea, ifosfamide, mechlorethamine, melphalan, methotrexate, mitomycin, mitoxantrone, nitrosourea, procarbazine, thiotepa, vinblastine, vincristine	Anagen effluvium
Antiparkinsonian agents Levodopa	Probable telogen effluvium
Antiseizure agents Trimethadione	Probable telogen effluvium
Beta-blockers Metoprolol Propranolol	Probable telogen effluvium
Birth control agents Oral contraceptives	Diffuse hair loss (telogen effluvium) 2–3 months after cessation of oral contraceptive
Drugs used in treatment of bipolar disorders Lithium	Probable telogen effluvium
Ergot derivatives (used in treatment of prolactinemia) Bromocriptine	Probable telogen effluvium
H$_2$ blockers Cimetidine	Probable telogen effluvium
Heavy metals (poisoning) Thallium Mercury and lead	Diffuse shedding of abnormal anagen hair 10 days after ingestion; complete hair loss in 1 month; characteristic is pronounced hair loss on sides of head, also of lateral eyebrows Diffuse hair loss with acute and chronic exposure
Cholesterol-lowering drugs Clofibrate	Occasionally associated with hair loss
Pesticides Boric acid	Total scalp alopecia reported after acute intoxication; with chronic exposure, hair becomes dry and falls out
Retinoids Etretinate Isotretinoin	Increased hair shedding and plucked telogen count; decreased duration of anagen phase Diffuse loss; probably same mechanism as above

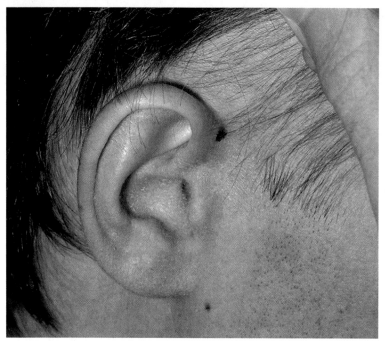

FIGURE 31-11 Telogen effluvium A clump of hair in the hand, associated with striking thinning of scalp hair. Using the fingers as shown, 30 to 40 hairs could be removed with each "hair pull."

DIFFERENTIAL DIAGNOSIS

INCREASED SHEDDING OF SCALP HAIR ± NONSCARRING ALOPECIA Pattern hair loss, diffuse-pattern alopecia areata, loose anagen syndrome, hyperthyroidism, hypothyroidism, SLE, secondary syphilis, and drug-induced alopecia (Table 31-2).

LABORATORY EXAMINATIONS

HAIR PULL Compared with the normal hair pull, in which 80 to 90% of hair is in the anagen phase, TE is characterized by a reduced percentage of anagen hairs.
CBC Rule out iron-deficiency anemia.
CHEMISTRY Serum iron, iron-binding capacity.
TSH Rule out thyroid disease.
SEROLOGY ANA and RPR.

HISTOPATHOLOGY Increase in the proportion of follicles in telogen.

DIAGNOSIS

Made on history, clinical findings, hair pull, and possible biopsy, excluding other causes.

COURSE AND PROGNOSIS

Complete regrowth of hair is the rule. In postpartum TE, if hair loss is severe and recurs after successive pregnancies, regrowth may never be complete. TE may continue for up to a year after the precipitating cause.

MANAGEMENT

No intervention is needed or required. The patient should be reassured that the process is part of a normal cycle of hair growth.

ANAGEN EFFLUVIUM ICD-10: L65.1

- Etiology: Radiation therapy to head; chemotherapy with alkylating agents; intoxications; protein malnutrition.
- Onset is usually rapid and extensive (see **Fig. 31-12**).
- Pathogenesis: Occurs after any insult to the hair follicle that impairs its mitotic/metabolic activity.
- More common and severe with combination chemotherapy than with the use of a single drug. Severity is generally dose dependent.
- Regrowth is usually rapid after discontinuation of chemotherapy.

ETIOLOGY

Anagen cycle disrupted causing varying degrees of hair follicle dystrophy:

- *Radiation therapy* to head.
- *Alkylating agents*: See Table 31-2.
- *Intoxications*: Mercury, boric acid, and thallium.
- Severe protein malnutrition.

PATHOGENESIS

- Occurs after any insult to hair follicle that impairs its mitotic/metabolic activity.

CLINICAL MANIFESTATIONS

HAIR Scalp hair loss is diffuse and extensive (Fig. 31-12). Hair breaks off at the level of the scalp. Eyebrows/lashes, beard, and body hair may also be lost.

NAILS Show transverse banding or ridging.

COURSE

- Hair regrows after discontinuation of chemotherapy.
- Regrowth after radiation depends on type, depth, dose fractionation; may result in irreversible hair follicle stem cell damage.

MANAGEMENT

No effective preventive measures are available.

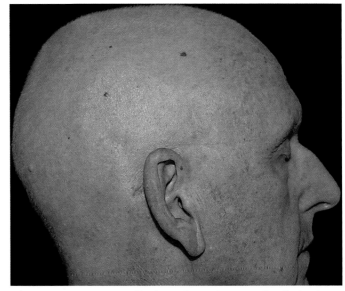

FIGURE 31-12 Anagen effluvium: chemotherapy All scalp, facial, and bodily hair have fallen out. Close inspection reveals that scalp hair has begun to regrow.

CICATRICIAL OR SCARRING ALOPECIA ICD-10: L66.0-L66.9

- Primary cicatricial (scarring) alopecia results from damage or destruction of the hair follicles stem cells by:
- Inflammatory (usually noninfectious) processes.
- Infection: e.g., "kerion" tinea capitis and necrotizing herpes zoster.
- Other pathologic processes: Surgical scar, primary or metastatic neoplasm.
- Manifestations: Effacement of follicular orifices in a patchy or focal distribution, usually in scalp or beard.
- The end result is effacement of follicular orifices and replacement of the follicular structure by fibrous tissue (Table 31-3).
- Scarring is irreversible. Therapies are ineffective.

Chronic Cutaneous (Discoid) Lupus Erythematosus (CCLE): See Section 14.

- May occur without other manifestations or serologic evidence of lupus erythematosus.
- Manifestations:
- CCLE: erythematous plaques (Figs. 31-13 to 31-15). Keratotic follicular plugs ("carpet tacks"). Scattered. Variable in number. May become confluent. Postinflammatory hypopigmentation, and/or follicular plugging.
- SLE: Diffuse scalp erythema with diffuse hair thinning (Fig. 31-14).
- Tumid LE: Violaceous dermal inflammatory plaque with overlying hair loss.
- Dermatopathology: See "Lupus Erythermatosus" in Section 14.

LICHEN PLANOPILARIS (LPP) See "Lichen Planus" in Section 14.

TABLE 31-3 Classification of Primary Cicatricial Alopecias

Lymphocytic
Chronic cutaneous (discoid) lupus erythematosus
Lichen planopilaris (LPP)
  Classic LPP
  Frontal fibrosing alopecia
  Graham-Little syndrome
Classic pseudopelade of Brocq
Central centrifugal cicatricial alopecia
Alopecia mucinosa
Keratosis follicularis spinulosa decalvans

Neutrophilic
Folliculitis decalvans
Dissecting folliculitis (cellulitis)

Mixed
Folliculitis keloidalis
Folliculitis necrotica
Erosive pustular dermatosis

- Follicular lichen planus (LP) is associated with cicatricial scalp alopecia, resulting in permanent hair loss (Fig. 31-16).
- LPP may or may not be associated with lichen planus of the skin or mucosa.
- Most commonly affects middle-aged women.
- Manifestations in scalp: Perifollicular erythema ± hyperkeratosis. Violaceous discoloration of scalp. Prolonged inflammation results in scarring alopecia. In some cases, follicular inflammation and scale are absent, with only areas of scarring alopecia, so-called footprints in the snow or pseudopelade. Distribution: Most common on parietal scalp; also affects other hair-bearing sites such as the groin and axilla.
- Symptoms: Scalp pain.
- Variants:
  - *Graham-Little syndrome*: LP-like lesions + follicular "spines"/keratosis pilaris– like lesions in areas of alopecia on scalp, eyebrows, axillary, and pubic areas.
  - *Frontal fibrosing alopecia*: Frontotemporal hairline recession and eyebrow loss in postmenopausal women with perifollicular erythema (Fig. 31-17); histology shows LPP.

Pseudopelade of Brocq

- End stage of all noninflammatory scarring alopecias and a variety of initially inflammatory disorders.
- Manifestations:
  - Early lesions: Discrete, smooth, skin- or pink-colored irregularly shaped areas of alopecia without follicular hyperkeratosis or perifollicular inflammation (Fig. 31-18).
  - Pattern of alopecia: Early moth-eaten pattern with eventual coalescence into larger patches of hair loss ("footprints-in-the-snow").
  - Dermatopathology: Similar to lichen planopilaris.

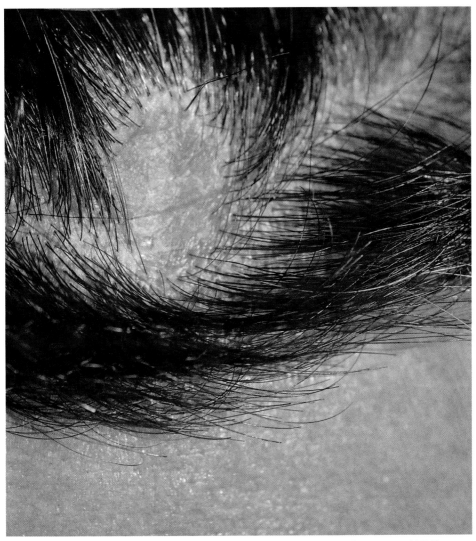

FIGURE 31-13 Scarring alopecia of scalp: chronic cutaneous lupus erythematosus (CCLE)
A 41-year-old white male with multiple red discoid keratotic patches on the scalp for 1 year. A red scaling lesion with scarring alopecia is seen on the frontal scalp.

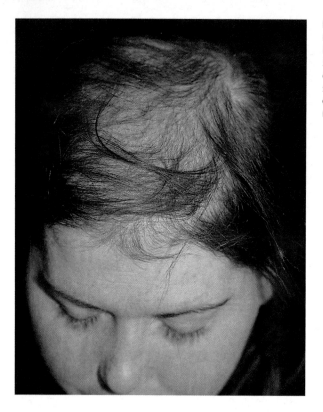

FIGURE 31-14 Diffuse and scarring alopecia of scalp: Systemic LE (SLE) and CCLE lesions A 36-year-old female with poorly controlled SLE for 3 years. Diffuse scalp alopecia is seen associated discrete discoid lesions with scarring alopecia.

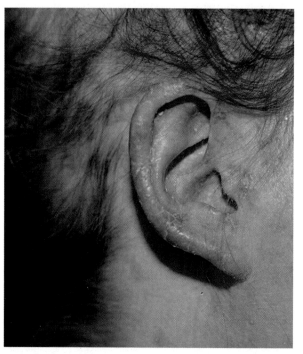

FIGURE 31-15 This is the same patient as in **Figure 31-14**. She has erythema of the ears and red areas of scarring alopecia on the scalp.

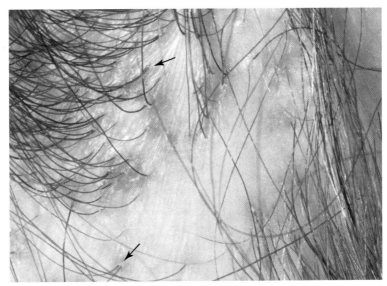

FIGURE 31-16 Scarring alopecia of scalp: pseudopelade of Brocq caused by lichen planus The scalp is smooth, shiny, and devoid of hair and hair follicles in many areas; some of the remaining follicles are inflamed with perifollicular erythema and scale. Several hairs are seen emerging from a single site within the area of alopecia (*arrows*). The term pseudopelade implies that the lesions resemble alopecia areata.

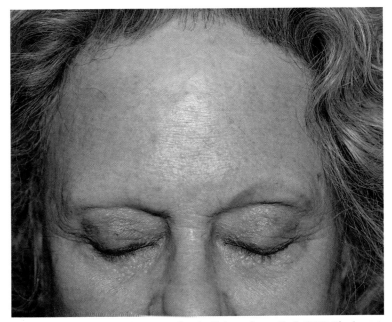

FIGURE 31-17 Scarring alopecia of scalp: lichen planopilaris (LPP) The frontal hairline has gradually receded; the area of alopecia lacks the pigmentation of forehead skin, which has had lifelong sun exposure. Both eyebrows have no hair; the eyebrow on the left is penciled in. The eyelashes appear normal. No other clinical findings of LP were detected. This clinical variant of LPP is called frontal fibrosing alopecia.

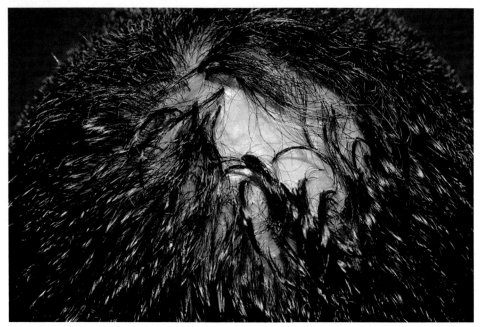

FIGURE 31-18 Scarring alopecia of scalp: pseudopelade of Brocq Extensive scarring alopecia with residual islands of hair follicles and hair on the vertex. Note follicular tufting (several hair follicles emerging the scalp in groups) and the absence of erythema, scale, or crust.

Central Centrifugal Scarring Alopecia (CCSA)

- *Synonyms*: Follicular degeneration syndrome, hot comb alopecia, and pseudopelade.
- Most commonly occurs in black women. Relation to chemical processing, heat, or chronic tension on the hair is uncertain, but they are best avoided.
- Slowly progressive alopecia begins in the crown/midvertex and advances centrifugally to surrounding areas.
- Dermatopathology: Earliest most distinctive change is premature desquamation of the inner root sheath with later changes through the outer root sheath, loss of the follicular epithelium, and replacement with fibrous tissue.

Alopecia Mucinosa (Follicular Mucinosis)

- Erythematous lesions (papules, plaques, or flat patches) of alopecia, occurring mainly on the scalp and/or face.
- Dermatopathology: Prominent follicular, epithelial/sebaceous gland mucin, and perifollicular lymphohistiocytic infiltrate without concentric lamellar fibrosis.

- May be symptom of cutaneous T-cell lymphoma (see Section 21).

Folliculitis Decalvans

- Pustular folliculitis leading to hair loss. Surviving hairs clustered, emerging from a single follicular orifice (tufted folliculitis).
- Bogginess or induration of scalp/beard with pustules, erosions, crusts (Fig. 31-19), and scale.
- *Staphylococcus aureus* infection is common. Whether *S. aureus* infection is the primary process or secondary is uncertain.
- Dermatopathology: Acute suppurative folliculitis, early.
- Scarring alopecia is irreversible. Systemic antibiotics, rifampin, systemic and/or topical and/or intralesional glucocorticoids, and systemic retinoid have been used. *S. aureus* infection should be documented and treated with appropriate antimicrobial agent.

Dissecting Folliculitis

- *Synonyms*: Dissecting cellulitis, perifolliculitis abscedens et suffodiens.
- Race: Most common in black men.
- Initial deep inflammatory nodules, primarily over the occiput, that progress to coalescing

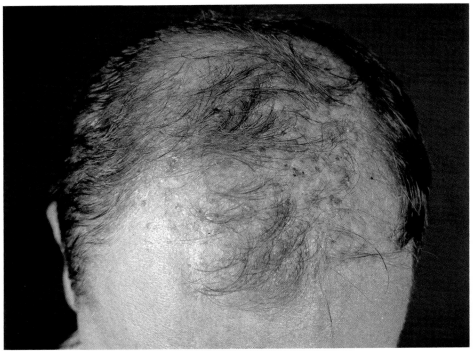

FIGURE 31-19 Scarring alopecia of scalp: folliculitis decalvans Erythema, inflammatory papules, crusts, and scarring of the scalp. Male pattern hair loss is also present.

regions of boggy scalp (Fig. 31-20). Sinus tracts may form; purulent exudates can be expressed. *S. aureus* secondary infection is common.

- Dermatopathology: Early follicular plugging and suppurative follicular/perifollicular abscesses with mixed inflammatory infiltrate; later, foreign-body giant cells, granulation tissue, scarring with sinus tracts.
- Scarring alopecia is irreversible. *S. aureus* infection should be documented and treated with appropriate antimicrobial agent.

Follicultis Keloidalis Nuchae

- *Synonym*: Acne keloidalis (nuchae).
- Occurs most commonly in black men.
- Usually occurs on the occipital scalp and nape of the neck, starting with a chronic papular or pustular eruption (Fig. 31-21). Keloidal scar formation may occur.
- Early mild involvement may respond to intralesional triamcinolone. If *S. aureus* is isolated on culture, treat with appropriate antimicrobial agent.

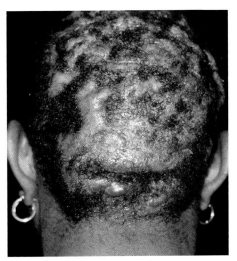

FIGURE 31-20 Scarring alopecia of scalp: dissecting folliculitis A 46-year-old black female with longstanding abscess formation of the scalp has resulted in very severe hypertrophic scarring. There was associated cystic acne and hidradenitis suppurativa.

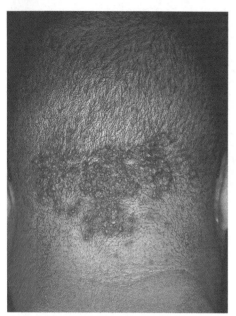

FIGURE 31-21 Scarring alopecia of scalp: folliculitis keloidalis A 31-year-old black male with papular scars of 3 years' duration, and follicular pustules becoming confluent on the occipital scalp and neck.

Pseudofolliculitis Barbae

- *Synonym*: "razor bumps."
- Occurs commonly in black men who shave.
- Related to curved hair follicles. Cut hair retracts beneath skin surface, grows, and penetrates follicular wall (transfollicular type) or surrounding skin (extrafollicular type), causing a foreign-body reaction.
- Distribution: Any shaved area, i.e., beard (Fig. 31-22), scalp, or pubic.
- Keloidal scarring in varying degrees occurs at involved sites.
- *S. aureus* secondary infection is common.

Acne Necrotica

- Pruritic or painful erythematous follicular-based papule with central necrosis, crusting, and healing with depressed scar.
- Lesions occur on anterior scalp, forehead, and nose; at times, the trunk.
- Dermatopathology: Lymphocytic necrotizing folliculitis.
- Poor response to treatment. Systemic antimicrobial agents and isotretinoin reported to be effective.

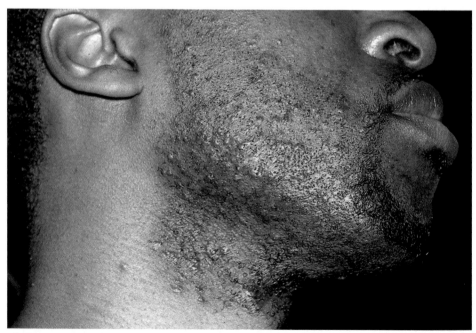

FIGURE 31-22 Pseudofolliculitis barbae A 29-year-old black male with multiple follicular papular scars in the beard; the presence of follicular pustules usually indicates secondary *Staphylococcus aureus* folliculitis.

Erosive Pustular Dermatosis of Scalp

- A disease of the elderly, mainly women, although pediatric cases do occur.
- Manifestations: Chronic, boggy, crusted plaque(s) on the scalp overlying exudative erosions and pustules, eventually leading to scarring alopecia.
- May follow trauma or treatment of actinic keratoses.
- Dermatopathology: Lymphoplasmacytic infiltrate with or without foreign-body giant cells and pilosebaceous atrophy.
- Poor response to therapy. Treat documented *S. aureus* infection.

LABORATORY EXAMINATION

SCALP BIOPSY 4-mm punch biopsy including subcutaneous tissue, prepared for horizontal section. A second 4-mm punch biopsy specimen for vertical sections and direct immunofluorescence, particularly if lupus is suspected.

MANAGEMENT

GLUCOCORTICOIDS Topical high-potency and intralesional glucocorticoids (e.g., triamcinolone) are the mainstay of treatment, improving symptoms and hair growth.

ANTIBIOTICS May be effective, especially if *S. aureus* infection is documented. Anti-inflammatory properties of plaquenil and doxycycline have also been used, even in the absence of documented infection, particularly for lymphocytic scarring alopecias in early clinical presentation (LPP and, CCSA).

EXCESS HAIR GROWTH ICD-10: L68

- Excess hair growth occurs in two patterns.
  - *Hirsutism*: Occurs in women at sites where hair is under androgen control.
  - *Hypertrichosis*: Hair density or length beyond accepted limits of normal for age, race, and sex (generalized, localized; lanugo, vellus, and terminal hair).

HIRSUTISM

- Excessive hair growth (women) in androgen-dependent hair patterns, secondary to increased androgenic activity.
- Normally only postpubescent males have terminal hair in these sites.

ETIOLOGY AND EPIDEMIOLOGY

DEFINITION Secondary to increased androgenic activity.

ETIOLOGY See Table 31-4.

RISK FACTORS Familial, ethnic, and racial influences. Hirsuteness: white > black > Asian.

PREVALENCE IN THE UNITED STATES Survey of college-aged women: 25% had easily noticeable facial hair and17% had periareolar hair.

PATHOGENESIS

- Dihydrotestosterone, derived from conversion of testosterone by 5α-R at the hair follicle, is the hormonal stimulus for hair growth; 50 to 70% of circulating testosterone in normal women is derived from precursors, androstenedione, and DHEA; the rest is secreted directly, mostly by the ovaries. In hyperandrogenic women, a greater percentage of androgens may be secreted directly.
- In women, adrenal glands secrete androstenedione, DHEA, DHEA sulfate, and testosterone; ovaries secrete mainly androstenedione and testosterone.

CLINICAL MANIFESTATION

HISTORY

- Virilization symptoms: Female pattern hair loss to male pattern balding, acne, deepened voice, increased muscle mass, clitoromegaly, increased libido, and personality change. Relatively recent or rapid onset of symptoms and signs *not* associated with puberty.
- Other: Amenorrhea or changes in menstruation. New-onset hypertension.

TABLE 31-4 Etiology of Hirsutism

Androgen-secreting tumors: Usually associated with irregular menses/amenorrhea	
Adrenal	Ovarian
Adenoma	Gonadal stromal tumor
Adenocarcinoma	Thecoma
Ectopic ACTH-secreting tumor	Lipoid tumor
Functional androgen excess	
Adrenal enzyme deficiencies (congenital adrenal hyperplasia)	Cushing syndrome
Early onset 21-hydroxylase deficiency	Polycystic ovarian disease
Late onset 21-hydroxylase deficiency	With and without adrenal
11β-hydroxylase deficiency	contribution
3β-dehydroxylase deficiency	Hyperthecosis
"Idiopathic" hirsutism	
Medication/drug induced	

Hirsutism. (1) Note the amount of excess hair, (2) note all sites of hair, and (3) evaluate progression and therapy.

■ New growth of terminal hair (Fig. 31-23), especially on the face (Fig. 31-23A), chest, abdomen, upper back, and shoulders.

CUSHING SYNDROME Centripetal obesity, muscle wasting (especially peripheral muscle weakness), and violaceous striae.

PELVIC EXAMINATION If polycystic ovary syndrome is suspected.

LABORATORY EVALUATION OF HIRSUTISM

SERUM TESTOSTERONE If >200 ng/mL, exclude androgen-secreting tumor.

SERUM-FREE TESTOSTERONE AND DEHYDROEPI-ANDROSTERONE More sensitive; most women with moderately elevated androgen levels have polycystic ovarian syndrome. If >800 μg/d, suggestive of adrenal tumor.

17-HYDROXYPROGESTERONE Raised level suggests CAH; confirm diagnosis by repeat measurement after ACTH stimulation.

SERUM PROLACTIN Hyperprolactinemia resulting from macro- or microprolactinoma or treatment with neuroleptic drugs; may have

associated menstrual abnormalities, infertility, or galactorrhea.

URINARY 17-KETOSTEROID Helpful in evaluating the overall amount of androgen secretion. Results checked against age-appropriate normal levels; peak levels occur at 30 years (significant decline with age thereafter).

OLIGOMENORRHEA/AMENORRHEA Prolactin, follicle-stimulating hormone, total testosterone.

MANAGEMENT

COSMETIC TREATMENT Bleaching: Hydrogen peroxide. Temporary removal: Shaving, waxing, and chemical (Nair). Eflornithine (Vaniqa) cream. LASER epilation. Electrolysis.

WEIGHT LOSS Obesity increases free testosterone levels by reducing sex hormone–biding hormone.

ENDOCRINOLOGY CONSULTATION For suspected late-onset CAH, Cushing syndrome, tumor.

SYSTEMIC ANTIANDROGEN THERAPY Oral Antiandrogens. Spironolactone (100 to 200 mg daily). Cyproterone acetate. Finasteride.

ORAL CONTRACEPTIVES Inhibit androgen synthesis by inhibiting output of gonadotropins; most effective if combined with antiandrogens.

BROMOCRIPTINE For treatment of prolactinoma.

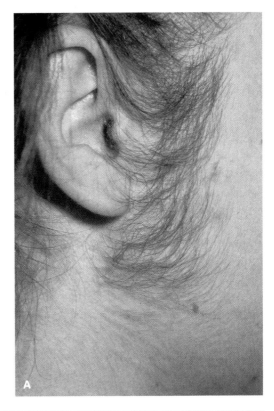

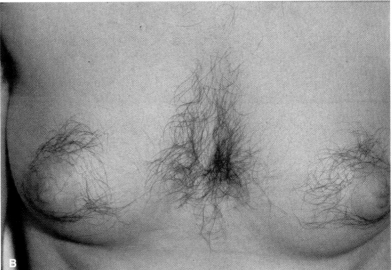

FIGURE 31-23 Hirsutism: face and chest (A) Increased hair growth in androgen-dependent hair follicles of the sideburn area, associated with androgen excess. **(B)** Increased hair growth in androgen-dependent hair follicles of the presternal and periareolar regions.

HYPERTRICHOSIS

- Hypertrichosis is excessive hair growth (density, length) beyond accepted limits of normal for age, race, sex in areas that are not androgen sensitive (see **Fig. 31-24**).
- May be generalized/universal or localized.
- May consist of lanugo, vellus, or terminal hair.

ETIOLOGY

Congenital or hereditary; acquired (see "Acquired Hypertrichosis Lanuginosa" see below), drugs (minoxidil, phenytoin, cyclosporine, glucocorticoids, streptomycin, and PUVA), porphyria, POEMS syndrome, and hypothyroidism.

CLINICAL MANIFESTATION

LOCALIZED HYPERTRICHOSIS Trauma/scar/occupation-related sites of irritation. Drug-induced: topical minoxidil. Becker nevus.
ACQUIRED HYPERTRICHOSIS LANUGINOSA Production of lanugo (wasp) hair in follicles previously producing vellus hair ("malignant down"). Hair may be >10 cm in length in nonscalp areas. Can involve entire body, except for palms and soles. In mild types, downy hair is limited to the face; hair on previously hairless areas such as the nose and eyelids is usually noticed first.
UNIVERSAL HYPERTRICHOSIS (Fig. 31-24) Increase of lanugo, vellus, or terminal hair.

MANAGEMENT

- Find and remove the inciting cause.
- Similar to "Cosmetic Treatment" of hirsutism (see the preceding).

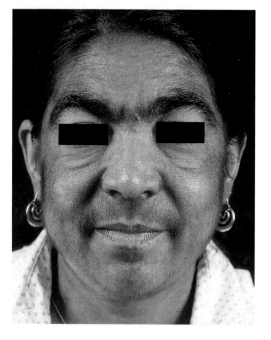

FIGURE 31-24 Hypertrichosis of face Excessive hair growth in nonandrogen-sensitive areas of the face in a female treated with cyclosporine.

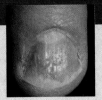

DISORDERS OF THE NAIL APPARATUS

NORMAL NAIL APPARATUS

- The nail apparatus is made up of:
  - Nail plate, the horny "dead" product.
  - Four specialized epithelia: Proximal nail fold, nail matrix, nail bed, and hyponychium.

COMPONENTS OF THE NORMAL NAIL APPARATUS (See Fig. 32-1)

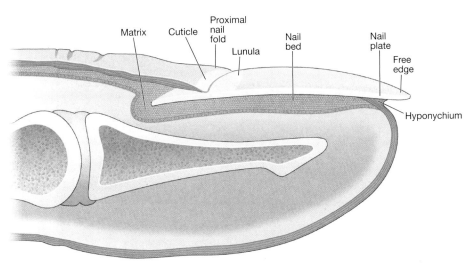

FIGURE 32-1 Schematic drawing of normal nail.

LOCAL DISORDERS OF NAIL APPARATUS

CHRONIC PARONYCHIA ICD-10: L03.0

- Associated with damage to the cuticle, mechanical or chemical.
- At risk: Adult women, food handlers, and house cleaners.
- Chronic dermatitis of proximal nail fold and matrix: chronic inflammation (eczema, psoriasis) with loss of cuticle, separation of nail plate from proximal nail fold (Fig. 32-2).
- Predisposing factors:
  - Dermatosis: Psoriasis, dermatitis [atopic, irritant (occupational), allergic contact], and lichen planus.
  - Drugs: oral retinoids (isotretinoin, acitretin), indinavir.
  - Foreign body: Hair, bristle, and wood splinters.
- Manifestations: First, second, and third fingers of the dominant hand; proximal and lateral nail folds erythematous and swollen; cuticle absent.
- Secondary infection/colonization: *Candida* spp., *Pseudomonas aeruginosa*, or *Staphylococcus aureus*. Nail plate may become discolored; green undersurface with *Pseudomonas*. Infection associated with painful acute inflammation.
- *Management:*
  - Protection.
  - Treat the dermatitis with glucocorticoid: topical, intralesional triamcinolone, or a short course of prednisone.
  - Treat secondary infection.

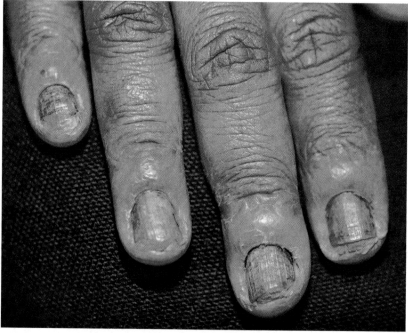

FIGURE 32-2 Chronic paronychia The distal fingers and periungual skin are red and scaling. The cuticle is absent; a pocket is present, formed as the proximal nail folds separate from the nail plate. The nail plates show trachonychia (rough surface with longitudinal ridging) and onychauxis (apparent nail plate thickening caused by subungual hyperkeratosis of nail bed). The underlying problem is psoriasis. *Candida albicans* or *Staphylococcus aureus* can cause space infection in the "pocket" with intermittent erythema and tenderness of the nail fold.

ONYCHOLYSIS ICD-10: L60.1

- Detachment of the nail from its bed at distal and/or lateral attachments (Fig. 32-3).
- Etiology
  - Primary: Idiopathic (fingernails in women; mechanical or chemical damage); trauma (fingernails, occupational injury; toenails, podiatric abnormalities, poorly fitting shoes).
  - Secondary: Vesiculobullous disorders (contact dermatitis, dyshidrotic eczema, herpes simplex); nail bed hyperkeratosis (onychomycosis, psoriasis, or chronic contact dermatitis); nail bed tumors; drugs.
  - In psoriasis, the yellowish-brown margin is visible between the pink normal nail and white separated areas (Fig. 32-3). In "oil spot" or "salmon-patch" variety, nail plate–nail bed separation may start in the middle of nail.
- Colonization with *P. aeruginosa* results in a biofilm on the undersurface of the onycholytic nail plate, causing a brown or greenish discoloration (Fig. 32-4).
- Other secondary pathogens that can colonize/infect the space are *Candida* spp., dermatophytes, and numerous environmental fungi.
- Underlying disorders in fingernail onycholysis: trauma (e.g., splinter), psoriasis, photoonycholysis (e.g., doxycycline), dermatosis adjacent to nail bed (e.g., psoriasis, dermatitis, and chemical exposure), and congenital/hereditary.
- Underlying toenail onycholysis: Additional factors of onychomycosis (*Trichophyton rubrum*), shoe trauma.
- *Management:* Debride all nails separated from nail bed (patient should continue weekly debridement); remove debris on nail bed; treat underlying disorders.

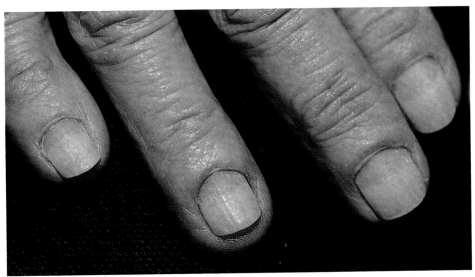

FIGURE 32-3 Onycholysis A 60-year-old female with distal onycholysis of fingernails, mild chronic paronychia, and loss of cuticle. Psoriasis is the likely underlying problem.

GREEN NAIL SYNDROME

- Usually associated with onycholysis (as previously mentioned). *P. aeruginosa*, the most common cause, produces the green pigment pyocyanin (Fig. 32-4).
- *Management*: debride "lytic" nail. See the preceding.

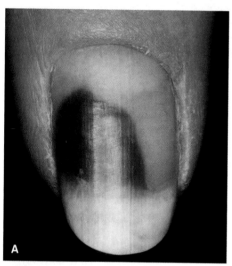 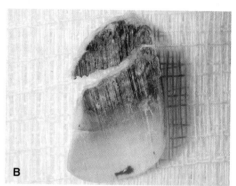

FIGURE 32-4 Onycholysis with *Pseudomonas* colonization (A) Psoriasis has resulted in distal onycholysis of the thumbnail. **(B)** A biofilm of *Pseudomonas aeruginosa* has produced the green-black discoloration of the undersurface of the onycholytic nail, which resolved following the debridement and treatment of the nail bed with glucocorticoid cream.

ONYCHAUXIS AND ONYCHOGRYPHOSIS

- *Onychauxis*: Thickening of entire nail plate, seen in elderly.
- *Onychogryphosis*: Onychauxis with ram's hornlike deformity, most commonly of the great toe (Fig. 32-5).
- *Etiology*: Pressure from footwear in elderly; also, inherited autosomal dominant.

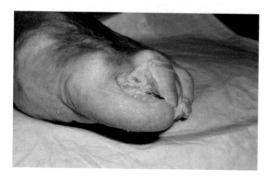

FIGURE 32-5 Onychauxis and onychogryphosis The great toenails appear grossly thickened with transverse ridging (onychauxis) with some medial deviation (onychogryphosis or ram's horn deformity). (Used with permission from Dr. Nathaniel Jellinek.)

PSYCHIATRIC DISORDERS

Repeated manipulation of the nail apparatus can result in changes of the paronychial skin and the nail plate.

Habit-tic Deformity. Caused by chronic, mechanical injury (Fig. 32-6). The cuticle is pushed back with inflammation and thickening of the proximal nail fold. Occurs most commonly on thumbnail(s), as compulsive disorders (tic habit), caused by the index finger repeatedly picking at the cuticle of the thumbnail.

Obsessive Compulsive Disorder. Repeat picking at the paronychia skin can result in lichen simplex chronicus. *S. aureus* secondary infection is a common complication. In extreme cases, the nail plate can be destroyed (Fig. 32-7); nail biting.

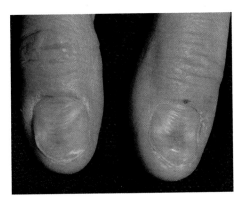

FIGURE 32-6 Habit-tic deformity The nail plates of both thumbs are dystrophic with transverse ridging and discoloration. The cuticle is absent and the proximal nail folds excoriated. When the proximal nails and nail fold were covered with tape continually, normal nails regrew in 5 months.

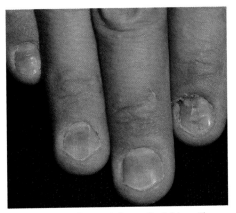

FIGURE 32-7 Compulsive nail picking The cuticles are not formed, the proximal nail folds are inflamed and excoriated. The breaks in the integrity provide a portal of entry for *S. aureus* and acute paronychia.

NAIL APPARATUS INVOLVEMENT OF CUTANEOUS DISEASES

PSORIASIS

- Most common dermatosis affecting the nail apparatus.
- >50% of persons with psoriasis have nail involvement at one point in time, with lifetime involvement up to 80 to 90%.

LABORATORY EXAMINATION

KOH preparation and/or nail clipping to pathology for PAS stain to rule out fungal colonization/infection. Onychomycosis is more common in nails with onycholysis.

CLINICAL FINDINGS

SKIN Typical psoriatic lesion on nail folds (Fig. 32-8).

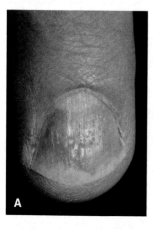
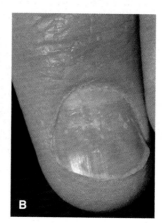
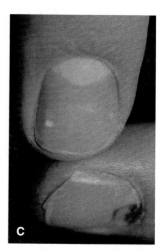

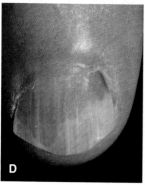

FIGURE 32-8 Psoriasis vulgaris (A) Multiple nail pits on the dorsal nail plate, "oil staining" of the nail bed, and distal onycholysis. **(B)** Trachonychia (rough surface) with oil staining and distal onycholysis. **(C)** Punctate leukonychia is pathognomonic for psoriasis and may be seen in only one finger. As can be seen in the nail below with traumatic subungual hemorrhage, punctate leukonychia did not occur at this site of trauma. **(D)** Oil staining, distal onycholysis, longitudinal ridging, adherence of the cuticle to the distal nail plate.

Matrix

- *Pitting or elkonyxis*: Punctate depressions; small, shallow; vary in size, depth, shape (Fig. 32-8A). May occur as regular lines (transverse; long axis) or in a grid-like pattern. Uncommon on toenails. Also seen in atopic dermatitis. Geometric and superficial pits seen in alopecia areata (hammered brass nails).
- *Trachyonychia*: Nail dull, rough, and fragile (Fig. 32-8B). Twenty-nail dystrophy or sandpaper nails associated with proximal nail matrix damage: nonspecific and can also be seen in alopecia areata (see Alopecia areata: trachyonychia, p. 791), lichen planus, atopic dermatitis. May regress spontaneously.

- *Serial transverse depressions*: May mimic "washboard" nails of tic habit (pushing back cuticle).
- *Longitudinal ridging*: Resembles melted wax.
- *Punctate leukonychia*: 1- to 2-mm white spots in nail plate (mistakenly attributed to trauma) (Fig. 32-8C).
- *Leukonychia*: Proximal matrix involvement: Surface rough and nail coarse (Fig. 32-8C).

Nail Bed

- *"Oil" spots*: Oval, salmon-colored nail beds (Figs. 32-8A and D).
- *Onycholysis*: Secondary to "oil" spots affecting hyponychium medially or laterally (Fig. 32-8A). May become colonized

with *Candida*, environmental fungi (e.g., *Aspergillus*), *Pseudomonas*. Predisposes to distal/lateral onychomycosis in toenail. Up to 20% of psoriatic nails have secondary onychomycosis.
- *Subungual hyperkeratosis*: Nail plate becomes raised off hyponychium.
- *Splinter hemorrhages.*

DIFFERENTIAL DIAGNOSIS

Onycholysis, onychomycosis, trauma (toenails), eczema, and alopecia areata.

MANAGEMENT

- Often unsatisfactory. See "Psoriasis" in Section 3.
- For matrix involvement, intralesional triamcinolone 3 to 5 mg/mL may be effective.
- For nail bed psoriasis, topical steroid (occluded) reduces hyperkeratosis.
- Systemic therapy such as methotrexate, acitretin, or "biologics" often improves nail apparatus psoriasis but may lag a few months after completion of therapy.

LICHEN PLANUS (LP)

- Nail involvement occurs in 10% of individuals with disseminated LP.
- Nail apparatus involvement may be the only manifestation.
- One, several, or all 20 nails may be involved ("twenty-nail syndrome," where there is loss of all 20 nails without any other evidence of lichen planus elsewhere on the body). **Onychorrhexis is seen** (longitudinal ridging and fissuring of the nail plate with brittleness and breakage.), though this is not a specific feature and can be seen with aging.

CLINICAL MANIFESTATIONS

Skin swelling with blue/red discoloration of proximal nail fold.

MATRIX
- *Small focus in matrix*: Bulge under proximal nail fold (Fig. 32-9A).
- *Subsequent longitudinal red line*: Thinned nail plate evolving into distal split nail (onychorrhexis) (Fig. 32-9B).
- *Diffuse matrix involvement*: Selective atrophy of nail plate with onychorrhexis and/or transverse splitting.
- *Red lunula*: Focal or disseminated.
- *Melanonychia, longitudinal*: Transitory.
- *Complete nail split.*
- *Pterygium formation (scar, matrix destroyed)*: Partial loss of the central nail plate presents as a V-shaped extension of skin of proximal nail fold adherent to the nail bed (Figs. 32-9A and B).

- *"Idiopathic atrophy of nails"*: Acute progressive nail destruction leading to diffuse nail atrophy with and without pterygium; complete loss of nail (anonychia) (Figs. 32-9B–D).

NAIL BED Onycholysis, distal subungual hyperkeratosis, bulla formation, and permanent anonychia.
VARIANTS
- *20-nail dystrophy of childhood*: Resolves spontaneously.
- *LP-like eruptions following bone marrow transplant*: Graft-versus-host disease.
- *Drug-induced LP-like reaction.*

MANAGEMENT
- See "Lichen Planus," Section 14.
- Intralesional triamcinolone.
- Systemic glucocorticoids.
- Urea may help hydrate and smooth out the nail plate.

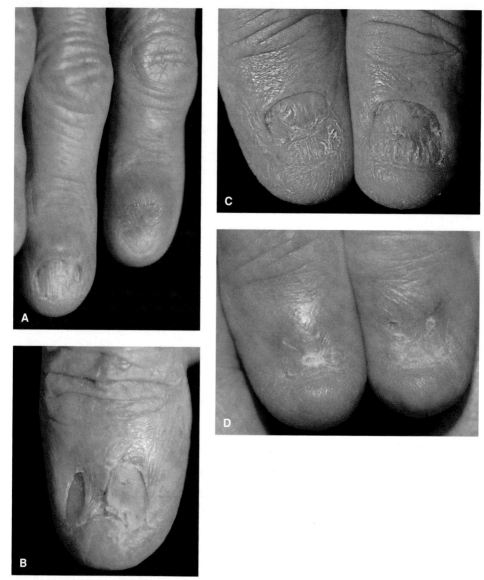

FIGURE 32-9 Lichen planus (A) Middle finger: Involvement of the proximal fold and matrix has caused trachonychia, longitudinal ridging, and pterygium formation. Index finger: Destruction of the matrix and nail plate is complete with anonychia. Seven of ten fingernails are involved; the others are normal. **(B)** Involvement of the nail matrix with scarring or pterygium formation proximally dividing the nail plate in two. **(C)** Early involvement of the matrix with thinning of the thumbnail plates. **(D)** Same patient as Figure 32-8C, two years later, the nail plate is completely destroyed, i.e., anonychia.

ALOPECIA AREATA (AA)

- Manifestations:
  - Geometric pitting (Fig. 32-10) (small, superficial, and regularly distributed).
  - Hammered brass appearance.
  - Mottled erythema of lunulae.
  - Trachonychia (roughness caused by excessive longitudinal striations).

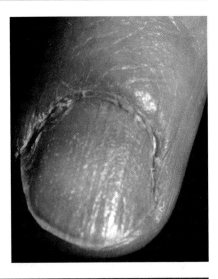

FIGURE 32-10 Alopecia areata: trachonychia The nail plate is rough with a "hammered brass" appearance.

DARIER DISEASE (DARIER–WHITE DISEASE, KERATOSIS FOLLICULARIS)

Nail changes are pathognomonic: Longitudinal streaks (red and white); distal subungual hyperkeratotic papules with distal V- or wedge-shaped fissuring of nail plate (Fig. 32-11).

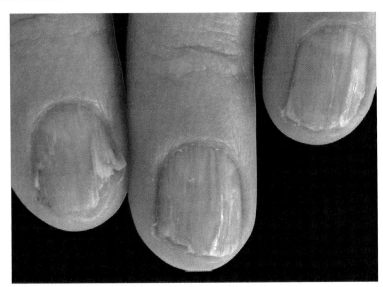

FIGURE 32-11 Darier disease Red and white longitudinal streaks on the fingernails with V-nicking in distal portion of plate. (Reproduced with permission from Goldsmith LA, Katz SI, Gilchrest BA, et al, eds. *Fitzpatrick's Dermatology in General Medicine.* 8th ed. New York, NY: McGraw-Hill; 2012.)

CHEMICAL IRRITANT OR ALLERGIC DAMAGE OR DERMATITIS

Chemicals in nail polish and adhesive for paste-on nails can cause damage to the nail plate, i.e., discoloration, onychoschizia (splitting or lamination of the nail plate, usually in the horizontal plane at free edge; Fig. 32-12). Irritant or allergic contact dermatitis can also occur on the paronychial skin.

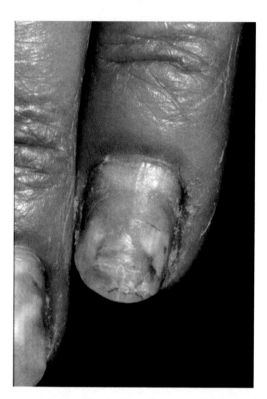

FIGURE 32-12 Chemically damaged nail
False nail glued to the fingernail has chemically damaged the nail plate with leukonychia and onychoschizia (splitting and lamination of nail plate).

NEOPLASMS OF THE NAIL APPARATUS ICD-10: L60

- Benign tumors: Fibroma/fibrokeratoma, subungual exostosis, myxoid cyst, glomus tumor (painful red nail bed patch), onychomatricoma, or nail matrix nevi.
- Malignant tumors: Squamous cell carcinoma, melanoma, or Merkel cell tumor.

MYXOID CYSTS OF DIGITS (See "Digital Myxoid Cyst" in Section 9)

- Pseudocyst or ganglion originates in distal interphalangeal joint, associated with osteoarthritis (Heberden nodes).
- Lesions can present on the proximal nail fold (Fig. 32-13), above and compressing the matrix, resulting in a longitudinal depressed groove in the nail plate.
- When cysts expand between the periosteum and matrix, the nail becomes dystrophic with a dusky red lunula.

LONGITUDINAL MELANONYCHIA

- *Manifestations:* Tan, brown, or black longitudinal streak within the nail plate (Fig. 32-14).
- *Pathogenesis:* (1) Increased melanin synthesis in normally nonfunctional matrix melanocytes, (2) increase in total number of melanocytes synthesizing melanin, and (3) nevomelanocytic nevus (junctional, Fig. 32-14).
- *Onset:* Congenital or acquired. Most originate in distal matrix.
- *Differential diagnosis:* Focal activation of nail matrix (e.g., trauma), hyperplasia of nail matrix melanocytes, nevomelanocytic nevus (junctional), drug-induced [e.g., zidovudine (AZT)] hydroxychloroquine, or melanoma of nail matrix.

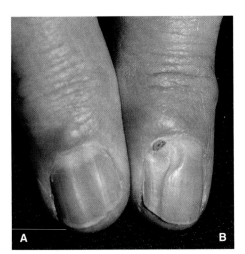

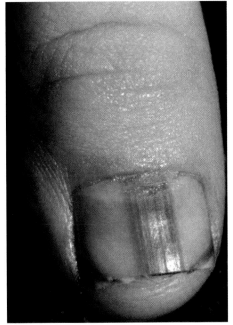

FIGURE 32-13 Myxoid cysts (A) Dermal erythema and swelling of the proximal nail folds with associated longitudinal groove of the nail plate. **(B)** Clear gelatinous fluid has drained from the index finger on the right (crusted site). Degenerative joint disease is present in both distal interphalangeal joints.

FIGURE 32-14 Junctional nevomelanocytic nevus of the nail matrix A junctional nevus is present in the nail matrix resulting in a longitudinal brown stripe in the nail bed. The proximal nail fold/cuticle is not pigmented.

ACROLENTIGINOUS MELANOMA (ALM) (See Section 12)

- *Mean age*: 55 to 60 years. *Incidence*: 2 to 3% of melanomas in whites; 15 to 20% in blacks, Asian, Native Americans. Usually asymptomatic; most patients notice pigmented lesion, usually after trauma.
- *Dermatopathology*: In situ or invasive proliferation of atypical melanocytes.
- *Findings*: Arises subungually or periungually, presenting with longitudinal melanonychia and/or nail plate dystrophy (**Fig. 32-15**).
- *Hutchinson sign*: Periungual extension of brown-black pigmentation onto proximal and lateral nail folds (**Fig. 32-15A**).
- 25% of ALM may be amelanotic (pigmentation not obvious or prominent).
- *Distribution*: Thumbs, great toes (hallux).
- *Differential diagnosis*: Subungual hemorrhage (**Fig. 32-15B**). Dermoscopy is helpful.
- *Indications for biopsy*: Periungual pigmentation, adult age, change in color/width of band, hyperpigmented lines within the band, proximal portion of band wider than distal; thumb, index finger, or toe involvement; blurred margins and history of trauma.
- *Prognosis*: 5-year survival rates from 35% to 50%.

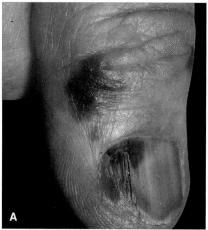 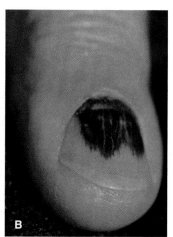

FIGURE 32-15 Acrolentiginous melanoma versus subungual hemorrhage
(A) Melanoma arose in the nail matrix of the thumb with resultant nail plate dystrophy, subungual melanosis, and extension into the proximal nail fold and beyond it (Hutchinson sign). **(B)** Trauma to the proximal nail resulted in hemorrhage and a transverse depression across the nail plate. Hemorrhage extends to the longitudinal dermal ridges. Dermoscopy helps in distinguishing this from ALM.

SQUAMOUS CELL CARCINOMA (See Section 11)

- SCC in situ (SCCIS) occurring periungually is usually caused by the oncogenic human papillomavirus types 16 and 18.
  - *Findings*: Skin-colored or hyperpigmented, keratotic, hyperkeratotic, or warty papules/plaques; onycholysis; failure of nail formation.
  - *Distribution*: Proximal and lateral nails, matrix, and hyponychium (**Fig. 32-16**).
- *Invasive* SCC arises within SCCIS.
  - *Symptoms*: Pain if periosteal invasion has occurred.
  - *Findings*: Solitary nodule is most common, often destroying the nail.
  - *Distribution*: Much more common on the fingers (thumb and index finger most often) than toes; multiple fingers may be involved in the immunocompromised host.
  - *Management*: Mohs surgery or amputation of digit for more deeply invasive lesions involving periosteum.

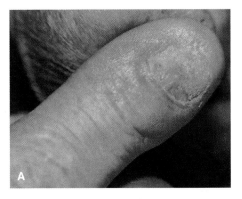

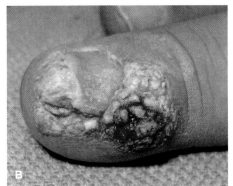

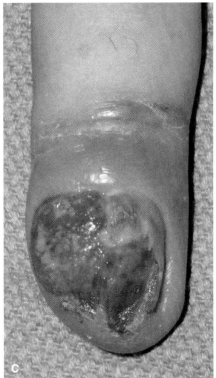

FIGURE 32-16 HPV-induced in situ and invasive squamous cell carcinoma (A) The right index fingernail bed shows hyperkeratotic failure of nail plate formation. Biopsy of the nail bed reported SCCIS with HPV-induced changes (koilocytosis). **(B)** Progression into invasive squamous cell carcinoma may present as hyperkeratotic papules or **(C)** complete obliteration of the nail unit. (Parts B and C used with permission from Dr. Nathaniel Jellinek.)

INFECTIONS OF THE NAIL APPARATUS ICD-10: L03.019

- Dermatophytes are the most common pathogens infecting the nail apparatus.
- *S. aureus* and group A streptococcus cause acute soft-tissue infection of the nail fold.
- *Candida* and *S. aureus* can cause secondary infection of chronic paronychia.
- Recurrent herpes simplex virus infection.

BACTERIAL INFECTIONS

- *S. aureus* is the most common cause of acute paronychia.

- Felon is an acute infection of the finger tip.
- *Management*: See "Antimicrobial Therapy" in Section 25.

ACUTE PARONYCHIA ICD-10 ∘ L03.01

- Acute infection of lateral or proximal nail fold.
- Usually associated with a break in integrity of the epidermis (e.g., hang nail) or trauma.
- *Findings*: Throbbing pain, erythema, swelling, pain, and ± abscess formation (Fig. 32-17).
- Infection may extend deeper, forming a felon (Fig. 32-18).

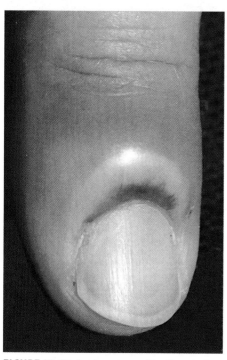

FIGURE 32-17 Acute paronychia The proximal nail fold is red and edematous (cellulitis) with pus formation.

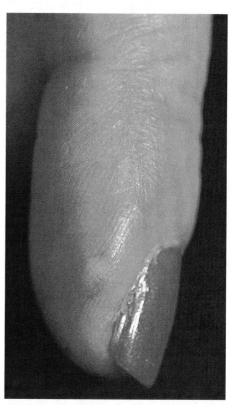

FIGURE 32-18 Felon An abscess is seen on the fingertip with surrounding erythema and swelling. Methicillin-sensitive *S. aureus* (MSSA) was isolated on culture of the pus.

FELON ICD-10: L03.0

- Soft-tissue infection of pulp space of distal phalanx (Fig. 32-18); closed space infection of multiple compartments created by fibrous septa passing between the skin and periosteum.
- *History*: Penetrating injury, splint, and paronychia.
- *Findings*: Pain, erythema, swelling, and abscess (Fig. 32-18).
- *Distribution*: Thumb and index finger.
- *Complications*: Osteitis, osteomyelitis of distal phalanx, joint with septic arthritis; extension into distal end of flexor tendon sheath, and producing tenosynovitis.
- *Course*: May be rapid and severe.

FUNGAL INFECTIONS AND ONYCHOMYCOSIS

- *Candida* spp. usually cause "space" infections of chronic paronychia or onycholytic nail and can cause destruction of the nail in the immunocompromised host.
- Dermatophytes infect the skin around the nail apparatus and cause superficial destruction of the nail.

- *Onychomycosis*: Chronic progressive fungal infection of nail apparatus, most commonly caused by dermatophytes, less often by *Candida* spp.; molds and environmental fungi can be cultured from diseased nails but are not usually primary pathogens.

CANDIDA ONYCHIA

- *Candida albicans* infections of the nail apparatus occur most often on the fingers, commonly as a secondary infection of chronic paronychia. Onychia describes inflammation of the matrix of the nail resulting in shedding of nail.
- Invasion of nail plate usually occurs only in the immunocompromised host, i.e., chronic mucocutaneous candidiasis (CMC) or HIV/AIDS disease.

ETIOLOGY AND EPIDEMIOLOGY

ETIOLOGY *C. albicans* and other species.
Chronic CMC. See "Candidiasis," Section 26.

CLINICAL FINDINGS

HIV/AIDS Candidal onychia and paronychia are common in children with HIV/AIDS, often associated with mucosal candidiasis.
Nail Apparatus. Chronic Paronychia with Acute Candidal Flare. *Candida* spp. can cause painful chronic infection with pain, tenderness, erythema, ± pus. Nail may become dystrophic with areas of opacification; white, yellow, green, or black discoloration; with transverse furrowing.
Colonization in Tinea Unguium. Secondary pathogen in distal/lateral onychomycosis.
Total Nail Dystrophy. Proximal/lateral nail folds are inflamed and thickened. Fingertips appear bulbous. Nail is invaded and may eventually become totally dystrophic (Fig. 32-19). HIV/AIDS: One nail may be involved. CMC: 20 nails may be involved in time.

DIFFERENTIAL DIAGNOSIS

Tinea unguium, psoriasis, eczema, chronic paronychia, lichen planus.

MANAGEMENT

See "Candidiasis," Section 26.

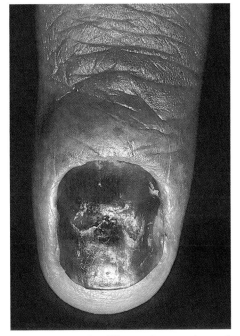

FIGURE 32-19 *Candida* onychomycosis: total dystrophic type The entire fingernail plate is thickened and dystrophic and is associated with a paronychial infection; both findings were caused by *C. albicans* in an individual with advanced HIV/AIDS disease.

TINEA UNGUIUM/ONYCHOMYCOSIS

- Symptoms: Nails lose protective and manipulative function.
- Complications:
  - Pain in toenail with pressure from shoes.
  - Predispose to secondary bacterial infections.
  - Ulcerations of the underling nail bed.
- Complications occur more commonly in the growing population of immunocompromised individuals and diabetic patients.

CLASSIFICATION BY ANATOMIC SITE INVOLVED

DISTAL AND LATERAL SUBUNGUAL ONYCHOMYCOSIS (DLSO) (Fig. 32-20) Infection begins in hyponychial area or nail fold, extending subungually. May be either primary, i.e., involving a healthy nail apparatus, or secondary (e.g., psoriasis) associated with onycholysis. Always associated with tinea pedis.

SUPERFICIAL WHITE ONYCHOMYCOSIS (SWO) Pathogen invades surface of dorsal nail (Fig. 32-21). Etiology: *Trichophyton mentagrophytes* or *T. rubrum* (children). Much less commonly, mold: *Acremonium, Fusarium*, and *Aspergillus terreus.*

PROXIMAL SUBUNGUAL ONYCHOMYCOSIS (PSO) Pathogen enters by way of the posterior nail fold–cuticle area and then migrates along the proximal nail groove to involve the underlying matrix, proximal to the nail bed, and finally the underlying nail (Fig. 32-22). Etiology: *T. rubrum.* Findings: Leukonychia that extends distally from under proximal nail fold. Usually one or two nails involved. Always associated with immunocompromised states.

ETIOLOGY AND EPIDEMIOLOGY

AGE OF ONSET Children or adults. Once acquired, usually does not remit spontaneously. Therefore, the incidence increases with advancing age;.

SEX Somewhat more common in men.

ETIOLOGIC AGENTS Between 95% and 97% caused by *T. rubrum* and *T. mentagrophytes.*

Molds. *Acremonium, Fusarium*, and *Aspergillus* spp. can rarely cause SWO. Dermatosis such as psoriasis, which results in onycholysis and subungual hyperkeratosis, or dermatophytic onychomycosis can be secondarily colonized/infected by molds.

GEOGRAPHIC DISTRIBUTION Worldwide.

PREVALENCE Incidence varies in different geographic regions. In the United States and Europe, up to 10% of adult population affected (related to occlusive footwear).

TRANSMISSION Dermatophytes. Anthropophilic dermatophyte infections are transmitted from one individual to another, by fomite or direct contact, commonly among family members. Some spore forms (arthroconidia) remain viable and infective in the environment for up to 5 years.

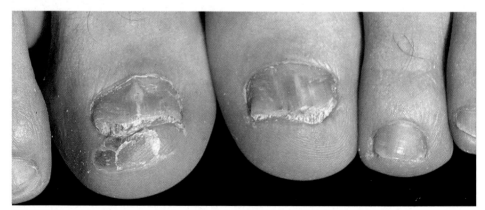

FIGURE 32-20 Onychomycosis of toenails: distal and lateral subungual type (DLSO) The toenails are white, caused by onycholysis and subungual hyperkeratosis. The dorsum of the feet shows erythema and scaling, i.e., tinea pedis. *T. rubrum* was detected on culture.

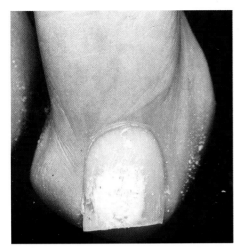

FIGURE 32-21 Onychomycosis of toenails: superficial white type (SWO) The dorsal nail plate is chalky white. White nail dystrophy can easily be treated by curettage; KOH preparation of the curetting shows hyphae.

Molds. Ubiquitous in environment; not transmitted between humans.

RISK FACTORS Atopics are at increased risk for *T. rubrum* infections. Diabetes mellitus, treatment with immunosuppressive drugs, and HIV/AIDS. For toenail onychomycosis, most important factor is wearing of occlusive footwear.

PATHOGENESIS

PRIMARY ONYCHOMYCOSIS/TINEA UNGUIUM The probability of nail invasion by fungi increases with defective vascular supply in posttraumatic states or disturbance of innervation.

SECONDARY ONYCHOMYCOSIS Infection occurs in already altered nail apparatus, such as psoriatic or traumatized nail.

DLSO (Fig. 32-20) Nail bed produces soft keratin stimulated by fungal infection that accumulates under the nail plate, thereby raising it. Matrix is usually not invaded, and production of normal nail plate remains unimpaired despite fungal infection.

CLINICAL MANIFESTATION

Approximately 80% of onychomycosis occurs on the feet; simultaneous occurrence on toe- and fingernails is not common.

DLSO White patch is noted on the distal or lateral undersurface of the nail and nail bed. With progressive infection, the nail becomes

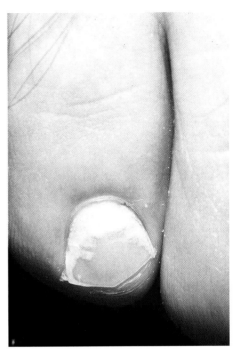

FIGURE 32-22 *Tinea unguium:* **proximal subungual onychomycosis type (PSO)** The proximal nail plate is a chalky white color caused by invasion from the undersurface of the nail matrix. The patient had advanced HIV/AIDS disease.

opaque, thickened, cracked, friable, raised by underlying hyperkeratotic debris in hyponychium (Fig. 32-20). When fingernails are involved, pattern is usually two feet and one hand.

SWO A white chalky plaque is seen on the proximal nail plate, which may become eroded with loss of the nail plate (Fig. 32-21). SWO may coexist with DLSO. Occurs almost exclusively on the toenails, rarely on the fingernails.

PSO (Fig. 32-22) A white spot appears from beneath proximal nail fold. In time, white discoloration fills lunula, eventually moving distally to involve much of undersurface of the nail. Occurs more commonly on toenails.

DIFFERENTIAL DIAGNOSIS

DLSO Psoriatic nails ("oil drop" staining of the distal nail bed and nail pits is seen in psoriasis but not onychomycosis), eczema, Reiter syndrome, keratoderma blennorrhagicum, onychogryphosis, pincer nails, and congenital nail dystrophies.

SWO Traumatic or chemical injury to nail, psoriasis with leukonychia.

LABORATORY EXAMINATIONS

All clinical diagnoses of onychomycosis should be confirmed by laboratory testing (see "Dermatophytoses," Section 26).

NAIL SAMPLES For DLSO: Distal portion of involved nail bed; SWO: Involved nail surface; PSO: Punch biopsy through nail plate to involved nail bed.

DIRECT MICROSCOPY Specific identification of pathogen is usually not possible by microscopy, but, in most cases, yeasts can be differentiated from dermatophytes by morphology.

FUNGAL CULTURE Isolation of the pathogen permits better use of oral antifungal agents.

HISTOLOGY OF NAIL CLIPPING Indicated if clinical findings suggest onychomycosis after negative KOH wet mounts. PAS stain is used to detect fungal elements in the nail. *Most reliable technique for diagnosing onychomycosis.*

COURSE AND PROGNOSIS

Without effective therapy, onychomycosis does not resolve spontaneously; progressive involvement of multiple toenails is the rule. Prevalence in diabetic patients estimated to be 32%; *Diabetic patients need early intervention and should be screened regularly by a dermatologist and/or podiatrist.* Untreated HIV/AIDS is associated with increased prevalence of dermatophytoses. Long-term relapse rate with newer oral agents such as terbinafine or itraconazole reported to be 15 to 21% 2 years after successful therapy; mycologic cultures may be positive without any clinically apparent disease.

MANAGEMENT

See Section 26 and Table 32-1.

New topical drugs in development include azoles (eficonazole), allylamines (TDT-067), benzoxaboroles (tavaborole), and nanoemulsions. They are reportedly improved

TABLE 32-1 Management of Tinea Unguium

Debridement	Debride dystrophic nails; patients should debride weekly.
Topical agents	Available as lotions and lacquer. *Usually not effective* except for SWO. *Ciclopirox (Penlac) nail lacquer:* monthly professional nail debridement recommended.
Systemic agents	*Note:* In systemic treatment of onychomycosis, nails usually do not appear normal after the treatment times recommended because of slow growth of nail. If cultures and KOH preparations are negative after these time periods, medication can nonetheless be stopped and nails will usually regrow normally.
Terbinafine (Allylamine)	250 mg/d for 6 weeks for fingernails and 12–16 weeks for toenails; most effective against dermatophyte infections.
Itraconazole: approved (USA) for onychomycosis. Effective in dermatophytes and *Candida* only	200 mg/d for 6 weeks (fingernails), 12 weeks (toenails) (continuous therapy). Although not approved for toenail onychomycosis, pulse dosing is used, given for 3–4 months at 200 mg twice daily for first 7 days of every month (continue treatment for 12 weeks for toenail involvement).
Fluconazole: not approved (USA) for onychomycosis. Effective in dermatophytes and *Candida*	Reported effective at dosing of 150–400 mg 1 day per week or 100–200 mg/d until the nails grow back normally. Effective in yeasts and less so in dermatophytes.
Ketoconazole: not approved for onychomycosis.	Effective at 200 mg/d; more effective for *Candida* than dermatophytes; however, infrequently hepatotoxicity and antiandrogen effect have limited its long-term use for onychomycosis.
Secondary prophylaxis	Antifungal cream, lotion, or powder daily. Antiseptic gels: ethanol or isopropyl alcohol. Pedicures/manicures: make sure instruments are sterilized or individuals have their own.

at permeating the nail plate. Photodynamic therapy and laser therapy such as long pulse, short pulse and also Q-switched have also been used recently, though effectivity has been a source of controversy.

INDICATIONS FOR SYSTEMIC THERAPY Fingernail involvement, limitation of function, pain

physical disability, potential for secondary bacterial infection, source of recurrent epidermal dermatophytosis, and quality-of-life issues. Early onychomycosis is easier to cure in younger, healthier individuals than in older individuals with more extensive involvement and associated medical conditions.

NAIL SIGNS OF MULTISYSTEM DISEASES ICD-10: L60.0

TRANSVERSE OR BEAU LINES

Systemic disease is implicated if all 20 nails involved. Single nail involvement is usually traumatic, compulsive picking, or tearing at the nails (onychotillomania). *Etiology*: High fever, postnatal, cytotoxic drugs, severe adverse cutaneous drug reaction, dermatologic disease (eczema, erythroderma, paronychia), viral infection (hand-foot-and-mouth disease, measles), Kawasaki syndrome, and peripheral ischemia. *Findings*: Transverse, bandlike depressions in nail, extending from one lateral edge to the other, affecting all nails at corresponding levels (Fig. 32-23). If duration of disease completely inhibits matrix activity for 7 to 14 days, transverse depression results in total division of nail plate (onychomadesis). Multiple parallel lines with chemotherapy. *Duration*: Thumbnails (lines present for 6 to 9 months) and large nails (lines present for up to 2 years) are most reliable markers.

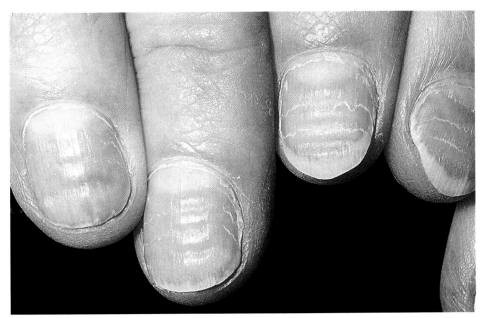

FIGURE 32-23 Cancer chemotherapy: Beau lines Multiple transverse ridging of multiple fingernails was associated with chemotherapy for breast cancer.

LEUKONYCHIA

True Leukonychia. Attributable to matrix dysfunction:

- *Total leukonychia*: Usually inherited.
- *Transverse leukonychia*: 1- to 2-mm wide arcuate bands.
- *Punctate leukonychia*: Psoriasis and trauma.
- *Longitudinal leukonychia*: Darier disease (see **Fig. 32-11**).

Pseudoleukonychia. SWO (**Fig. 32-21**), chemical damage to nail keratin.

Apparent Leukonychia. Caused by alteration of matrix and/or nail bed (e.g., apparent macrolunula); may involve all fingernails:

- *Terry-type leukonychia*.
  - *Association*: Hepatic disorders.
  - *Findings*: Opaque white plate obscuring lunula and extending to within 1 to 2 mm from distal edge of nail (**Fig. 32-24**). Involves all nails evenly.
- *Uremic Half-and-Half Nail of Lindsay*
  - *Association*: Renal disorders.
  - *Findings*: Proximal nail dull white obscuring lunula (20–60% of nail); distal nail pink/reddish.
- *Banded nails (Muehrcke lines)* (see **Fig. 32-34**).
  - Paired, narrow, and white transverse bands.
  - *Association*: Cancer antineoplastic chemotherapy, hypoalbuminemia; unilateral following trauma.
  - *Findings*: Bands are parallel to lunula, separated from one another, and from lunula, by strips of pink nail.

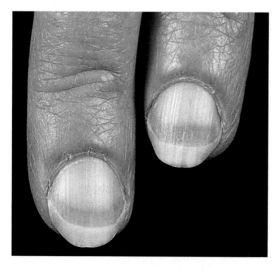

FIGURE 32-24 Apparent leukonychia: Terry-type nails The proximal two-thirds of the nail plate is white, whereas the distal third shows the red color of the nail bed.

YELLOW NAIL SYNDROME

Symptoms: Nails stop growing. *Association*: Lymphedema, respiratory tract disease (bronchiectasis, chronic bronchitis, malignant neoplasms), rheumatoid arthritis, and internal malignancies. *Findings*: Nails hard, excessively curved from side to side; diffuse pale yellow to dark yellow-green discoloration (**Fig. 32-25**). Cuticles absent. Secondary onycholysis common. *Distribution*: 20 nails.

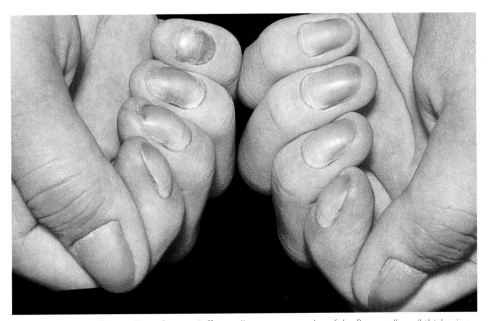

FIGURE 32-25 Yellow nail syndrome Diffuse yellow-to-green color of the fingernails, nail thickening, slowed growth, and excessive curvature from side to side of all 10 fingernails.

PERIUNGUAL FIBROMA

Synonym: Koenen tumors. *Association*: Tuberous sclerosis (see "Tuberous Sclerosis," Section 16); occur in 50% of individuals. *Onset*: Puberty. *Findings*: Usually multiple, small to large, elongated to nodular tumors; produce a longitudinal groove in nail plate caused by matrix compression (Fig. 32-26).

SPLINTER HEMORRHAGES

Distal splinter hemorrhages seen with minor trauma (most common cause, occurring in up to 20% of normal population); psoriasis and atopic dermatitis. *Proximal splinter hemorrhages*: trauma (Fig. 32-15B), sideropenic anemia, bacterial endocarditis (Fig. 32-27), trichinosis, antiphospholipid antibody syndrome, and altitude sickness. *Findings*: Tiny linear structures, usually 2 to 3 mm long, arranged in the long axis of nail; they subsequently move superficially and distally with nail growth.

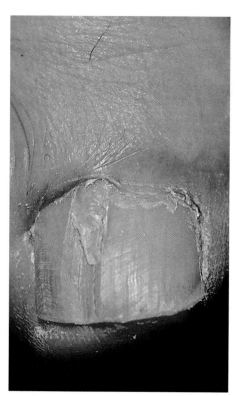

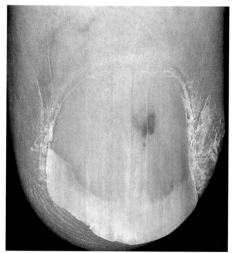

FIGURE 32-26 Tuberous sclerosis: periungual fibroma A skin-colored tumor is seen emerging from beneath the proximal nail fold associated with a longitudinal groove in the nail plate.

FIGURE 32-27 Infective endocarditis: splinter hemorrhage Subungual hemorrhage in the mid-portion of the fingernail bed in a 60-year-old female with enterococcal endocarditis; subconjunctival hemorrhage was also present.

NAIL FOLD/PERIUNGUAL ERYTHEMA AND TELANGIECTASIA

Associated with connective tissue (collagen-vascular) disease.

Periungual Erythema. *Association*: Systemic lupus erythematosus (SLE), dermatomyositis (DM). HIV/AIDS or hepatitis C virus infection, scleroderma, hypertrophic pulmonary osteodystrophy, Kawasaki disease, hand and foot syndrome, and microvasculitis. *Findings*: Periungual erythema, edema, alterations of cuticle, and secondary nail changes.

Telangiectasia. *Association*: Scleroderma, SLE, DM; rheumatoid arthritis. *Findings*: Linear wiry vessels perpendicular to nail base overlie proximal nail folds (**Fig. 32-28**); usually bright red; may be black if thrombosed. SLE and DM: arise within erythema. Scleroderma and DM: Enlarged capillary loops with *reduced* capillary density and avascular areas.

Cuticle Hyperkeratosis and Hemorrhages. SLE and DM.

Discoid LE. See **Figure 32-29**.

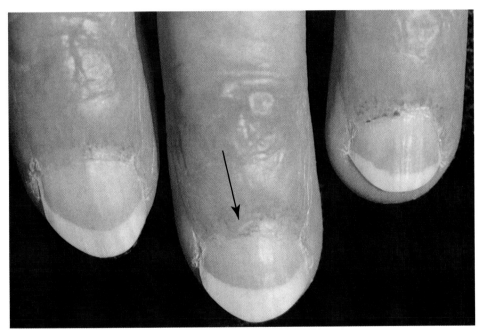

FIGURE 32-28 Systemic lupus erythematosus: Nail fold erythema and telangiectasia A 64-year-old female with systemic LE with arthritis, fatigue, and photosensitivity for decades. Proximal nail folds are enlarged with erythema, teleangiectasia (*arrow*), and thromboses. The cuticle is elongated.

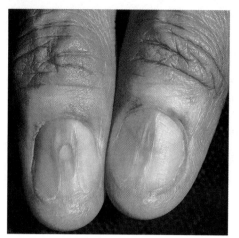

FIGURE 32-29 Discoid lupus erythematosus: Nail fold and matrix involvement and nail dystrophy Proximal nail folds show erythema, scarring, and depigmentation associated with nail matrix inflammation.

PTERYGIUM INVERSUM UNGUIUM

Nail plate adheres to fingertip skin in scleroderma.

SYSTEMIC AMYLOIDOSIS

Nail dystrophy resembling lichen planus with severe onychodystrophy (nail plate thinned, longitudinally fissured with subungual hemorrhages) can precede diagnosis of primary systemic amyloidosis. Biopsy of nail apparatus confirms the diagnosis of amyloidosis with amyloid deposits in the superficial dermis of the nail matrix (Fig. 32-30).

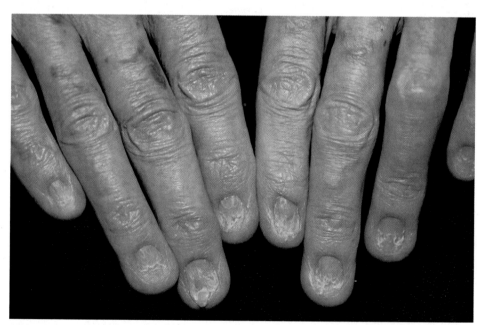

FIGURE 32-30 Systemic amyloidosis Nail findings preceded the diagnosis of systemic amyloidosis. The matrix is inflamed with resultant thinning of the proximal nail plate and disintegration distally.

KOILONYCHIA

Spoon-shaped nails (Fig. 32-31). *Etiology* (more often resulting from local rather than systemic factors): hereditary and congenital; Plummer–Vinson syndrome (iron-deficiency anemia, dysphagia, and glossitis). *Findings:* In early stages, nail plate becomes flattened; later, edges become everted upward and nail appears concave.

FIGURE 32-31 Koilonychia The fingernail plate is concave; no other nails were involved. There were no associated systemic factors.

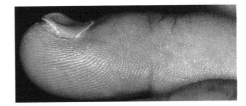

CLUBBED NAILS

Angle between proximal nail fold and nail plate is >180°. May occur with or without cyanosis. *Pathogenesis*: Hypertrophy of soft-tissue components of digital pulp; hyperplasia of fibrovascular tissue at base of nail (nail can be "rocked"); local cyanosis. *Etiology*:

- Cardiovascular disorders: Aortic aneurysm, congenital, and acquired cardiovascular disease.
- Bronchopulmonary disorders: Intrathoracic neoplasms, chronic intrathoracic, and suppurative disorders.
- Gastrointestinal disorders: Inflammatory bowel disease, GI neoplasms, hepatic disorders, multiple polyposis, bacillary dysentery, and amoebic dysentery.
- Chronic methemoglobinemia.

Findings: Digit is bulbous; nail plate enlarged and excessively curved (Fig. 32-32). Increased curvature usually affects all 20 nails.

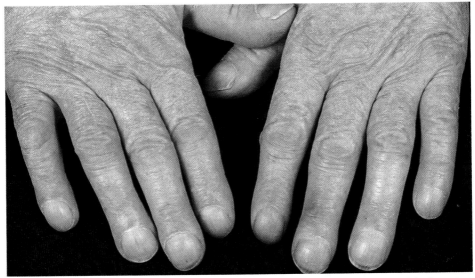

FIGURE 32-32 Lung cancer: clubbed fingers Bulbous enlargement and broadening of the fingertips in a smoker with lung cancer. The tissue between the nail and underlying bone has a spongy quality giving a "floating" sensation when pressure is applied downward and forward at the junction between the plate and proximal fold. Cigarette smoke has stained the left index and middle finger.

DRUG-INDUCED NAIL CHANGES

Drugs causing adverse nail changes are similar to those causing adverse changes in cutaneous and mucosal sites.

- Antimalarials: Discoloration (Fig. 32-33).
- Chemotherapy: Beau lines (Fig. 32-23), onychomadesis, Muehrcke lines (Fig. 32-34), hemorrhagic onycholysis, pyogenic granulomas, and melanonychia.
- Antiretrovirals: Melanonychia [zidovudine (AZT)]; pyogenic granuloma (indinavir).
- Beta-blockers: Digital ischemia.
- Bleomycin: Digital ischemia.
- PUVA: Photo-onycholysis, melanonychia.
- Retinoids: Nail fragility, pyogenic granuloma, and paronychia.
- Silver-containing compounds: Blue–grey discoloration of the lunula (Fig. 32-35).

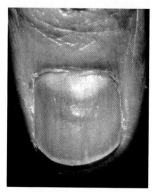

FIGURE 32-33 Nail discoloration: quinacrine Bluish discoloration of the nail in a patient with SLE treated with quinacrine.

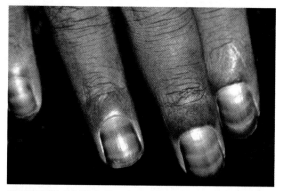

FIGURE 32-34 Nail discoloration and transverse bands (Muehrcke lines): Period transverse bands on the fingernail in a patient with breast cancer being treated with chemotherapy (5-fluorouracil).

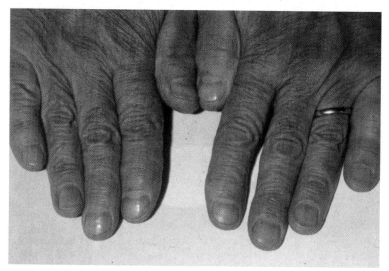

FIGURE 32-35 Nail discoloration: argyria The lunula shows blue-grey discoloration. Such changes have been reported in exposure to silver salts (medication and environmental) but are also noted in Wilson's disease, hemoglobin M disease and hereditary acrolabial telangiectases. This patient had taken silver nitrate for gastritis for many years.

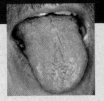

DISORDERS OF THE MOUTH

DISEASES OF THE LIPS ICD-10: K13.0

ANGULAR CHEILITIS (PERLÈCHE)

- Associated with increased moisture at commissures, salivation (at sleep).
- *Predisposing factors*: Thumb sucking in children; sagging face and loss of teeth in older persons; candidiasis in immunocompromised persons; *Staphylococcus aureus* in atopic dermatitis and isotretinoin treatment.
- *Findings*: Erythema and maceration at commissures (see Fig. 33-1).
- *Diagnosis*: KOH for candidiasis; culture for *S. aureus, Candida*.
- *Management*: Identify and treat causes.

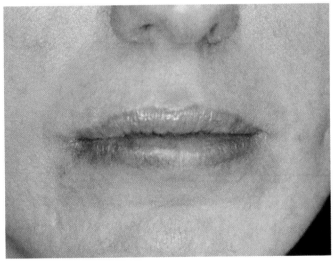

FIGURE 33-1 Angular cheilitis Mild erythema and scaling in bilateral commissures. (Used with permission from Dr. Nathaniel Treister.)

ACTINIC CHEILITIS

Actinic/solar keratoses, usually of the lower lip. Rule out squamous cell carcinoma in situ (SCCIS) or invasive if papule or nodule or ulcer occurs (see Section 11).

CONDITIONS OF THE TONGUE, PALATE, AND MANDIBLE ICD-10: K14

FISSURED TONGUE

- Normal variant in up to 11% of population. Asymptomatic.
- *Findings*: Multiple folds with anterior-posterior orientation on the dorsal surface of the tongue (Fig. 33-2).
- *Associated disorders*: Psoriasis, Down syndrome, acromegaly, and Sjögren syndrome.
- *Synonyms*: Lingua fissurata, lingua plicata, scrotal tongue, grooved tongue, furrowed tongue.

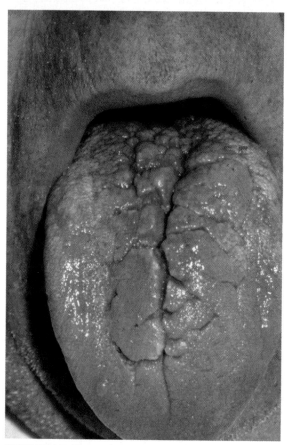

FIGURE 33-2 Fissured tongue Deep furrows on the dorsum of the tongue are asymptomatic.

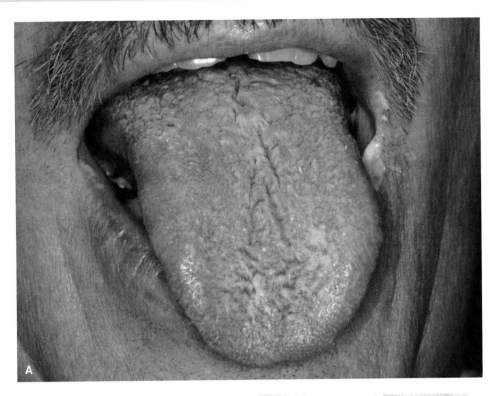

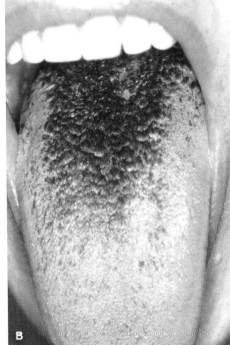

FIGURE 33-3 (A) Hairy tongue Defective desquamation of filiform papilla noted in posterior aspect of tongue. Tongue has a white surface caused by retained keratin. (Used with permission from Dr. Nathaniel Treister.) **(B) Black hairy tongue** In this example, chrormogenic bacteria have stained the tongue black.

BLACK OR WHITE HAIRY TONGUE

- *Pathogenesis*: Defective desquamation of filiform papillae resulting in hair-like projections on the dorsum of the tongue.
- *Associations*: Heavy tobacco use, mouth breathing, systemic antibiotic therapy, poor oral hygiene, general debilitation, radiation therapy, chronic use of bismuth-containing antacids, or lack of dietary roughage.
- *Findings*: Furry plaques on dorsal tongue (**Fig. 33-3**). Candidiasis may occur secondarily.
- *Management*: Eliminate predisposing factors; good oral hygiene.
- *Synonym*: Lingua villosa (nigra).

ORAL HAIRY LEUKOPLAKIA (See Section 27)

- *Pathogenesis*: Epstein–Barr virus infection; low CD4 cell counts.
- *Findings*: White corrugated plaques on lateral aspects of tongue (see **Fig. 27-66**). Does not occur in successfully treated HIV/AIDS.

MIGRATORY GLOSSITIS ICD-10: K14.1

- Irregular areas of dekeratinized and desquamated filiform papillae (red in color) are surrounded by elevated whitish or yellow margins (**Fig. 33-4**).
- *Etiology*: Unknown; possible link with psoriasis. Incidence: Common; usually asymptomatic.
- *Synonym*: Geographic tongue.

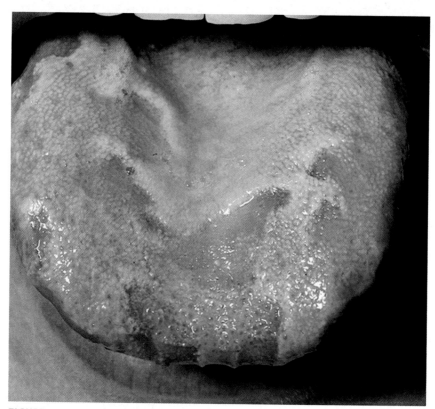

FIGURE 33-4 Migratory glossitis Areas of hyperkeratosis alternate with areas of normal pink epithelium, creating a geographic pattern in a female with psoriasis.

PALATE AND MANDIBULAR TORUS

- *Pathogenesis*: Genetic predisposition, autosomal dominant in some series, more common in females, Native Americans, Eskimos (torus palatini); local stressors (mandibular and palatal tori).
- *Associations*: Bruxism
- *Symptoms*: May be complicated by ulceration; usually asymptomatic.
- *Findings*: Palatal tori are usually in midline of palate and less than 2 cm, but can vary in size through life; mandibular tori found usually near premolars; rarely bilateral. They are smooth, nodular protrusions (**Figure 33-5**).
- *Management*: Not needed; if it creates ulcerations or complicate dental prosthesis, surgery can be done.

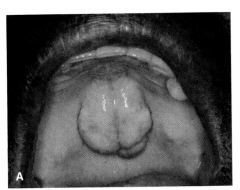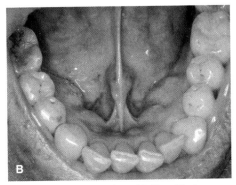

FIGURE 33-5 (A) Torus palatinus Bony protrusion in the midline, upper palate. **(B) Mandibular torus** Unilateral protrusion near premolars, above the mylohyoid muscle insertion into the mandible. (Used with permission from Dr. Nathaniel Treister.)

DISEASES OF THE GINGIVA, PERIODONTIUM, AND MUCOUS MEMBRANES ICD-10: K06

GINGIVITIS AND PERIODONTITIS

- *Gingivitis*: Erythema, edema, and blunting of interdental papillae without bone loss. Predisposing factors: poor oral hygiene, tobacco use, and diabetes.
- *Periodontitis*: Chronic infection of connective tissue, periodontal ligament, and alveolar bone; most common cause of tooth loss in adults.
- *Course*: Accumulation of subgingival calculus (calcified plaque) and Actinobacillus actinomycetemcomitans infection results in painless soft tissue edema, insidious alveolar bone resorption, deepening periodontal pockets, and tooth loss.

EROSIVE GINGIVOSTOMATITIS

Reaction pattern associated with viral infection, autoimmunity, lichen planus (LP), erythema multiforme, pemphigus, and cicatricial pemphigoid.
Findings: Erythema, desquamation, and edema of gingivae. Other mucocutaneous sites may be affected.

LICHENOID MUCOSITIS

Findings: Reticulated white plaques and painful erosions on mucosal surfaces.
Etiology: LP, drugs (NSAIDs, antihypertensive agents), allergic contact dermatitis, and graft-versus-host disease.

LICHEN PLANUS (See Section 14)

- *Incidence*: 40 to 60% of individuals with LP have oropharyngeal involvement.
- *Findings*:
  - Milky-white papules.
  - Wickham striae: Reticulate (netlike) patterns of lacy-white hyperkeratosis [buccal mucosa (Fig. 33-6), lips, tongue, and gingivae].
  - Hypertrophic LP: Leukoplakia with Wickham striae usually on the buccal mucosa.
  - Atrophic LP: Shiny plaque often with Wickham striae in surrounding mucosa.
  - Erosive/ulcerative LP: Superficial erosions with overlying fibrin clots that are seen on the tongue and buccal mucosa; can be painful (Fig. 33-6). Should follow carefully for development of squamous cell carcinoma (1 to 3% of cases), particularly in drinkers, smokers, the immunosuppressed or those infected with HPV.
  - Bullous LP: Intact blisters (rupture and result in erosive LP).
  - Desquamative gingivitis: Bright red gingiva (Fig. 33-7).

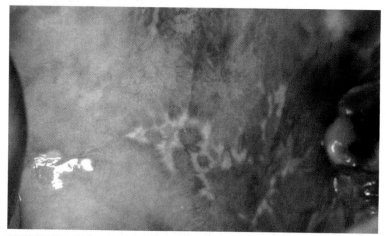

FIGURE 33-6 Lichen planus: Wickham striae Poorly defined violaceous plaque with lacy, white pattern on the buccal mucosa.

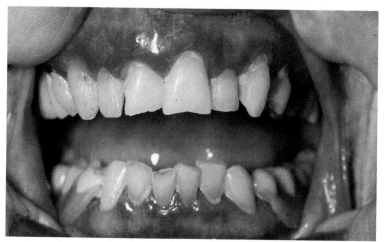

FIGURE 33-7 Lichen planus: desquamative gingivitis The gingival margins are erythematous, edematous, and retracted. The lesions were painful, making dental hygiene difficult, resulting in plaque formation on the teeth.

ACUTE NECROTIZING ULCERATIVE GINGIVITIS

- *Precipitating factors*: Poor oral hygiene, HIV/AIDS, immunosuppression, alcohol and tobacco use, and nutritional deficiency.
- *Findings* (Fig. 33-8): Punched-out ulcers of the interdental papillae. Gingival hemorrhage, severe pain, foul odor/halitosis, fever, and lymphadenopathy; alveolar bone destruction.
- *Etiologic agents*: *Bacteroides fusiformis, Prevotella intermedia, Borrelia vincentii, and Treponema*.
- *Management*: Systemic antibiotics such as clindamycin, metronidazole, and amoxicillin. Dental hygiene.
- *Synonyms*: Trench mouth, Vincent disease.

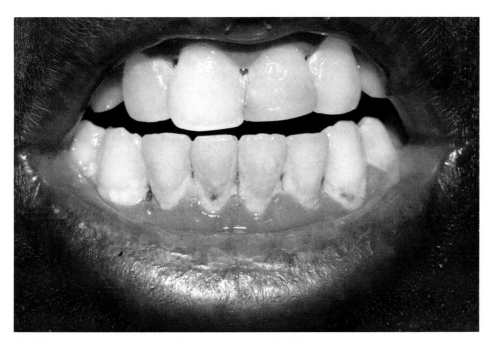

FIGURE 33-8 Acute necrotizing ulcerative gingivitis (ANUG) Very painful gingivitis with necrosis on marginal gingiva, edema, purulence, and halitosis in a 35-year-old female with advanced HIV disease. ANUG resolved with oral clindamycin.

GINGIVAL HYPERPLASIA

- *Findings*: Hypertrophy of both the free and attached gingivae, particularly the interdental papillae (Fig. 33-9).
- *Inflammatory enlargement*: Most common cause of gingival enlargement. Caused by edema and infective cellular infiltration caused by prolonged exposure to bacterial plaque; fibrosis occurs if untreated.
- *Drug-induced fibrous hyperplasia of gingivae*: May cover the teeth and is associated with:
  - Anticonvulsants: Phenytoin, succinimides, and valproic acid.
  - Calcium channel blockers: Nifedipine and verapamil.
  - Cyclosporine.
- *Systemic conditions/disorders:*
  - Pregnancy, puberty, vitamin C deficiency, and glycogen storage disease.
  - Chronic myelomonocytic leukemia (Fig. 33-9).

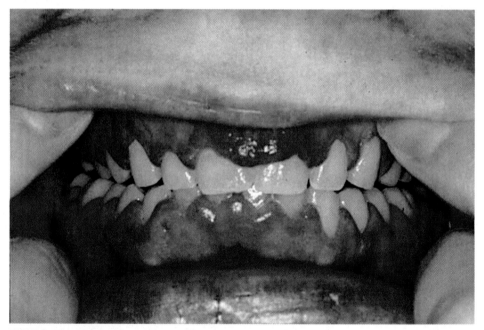

FIGURE 33-9 Gingival hyperplasia: acute monocytic leukemia The gingivae show hyperplasia resulting from infiltration with leukemic monocytes.

APHTHOUS ULCERATION ICD-10: K12.0

- Recurrent painful mucosal lesions.
- Most common cause of oral ulcerations; incidence up to 30% of otherwise healthy persons.
- May be associated with systemic diseases such as HIV/AIDS and Behçet disease.

EPIDEMIOLOGY

ETIOLOGY Idiopathic. Can arise at the site of minor mucosal injury, e.g., bite.
PATHOGENESIS Cell-mediated immune reaction pattern.
AGE AT ONSET Any age; often during second decade, persisting into adulthood, and becoming less frequent with advancing age.

Classification

- Simple: 1 to 3 oral ulcers that recur 1 to 3 times per year.
- Complex: Continuous ulcers and associated with systemic disease or genital ulcers.
- Major aphthous ulcers (AU) may persist for ≥6 weeks, healing with scarring.
- Behçet disease should be considered in patients with persistent oropharyngeal AU, with or without anogenital AU, associated with systemic findings (eye, nervous system). See Section 14.

CLINICAL MANIFESTATION

SYMPTOMS Even though small, AU can be quite painful. In persons with severe AU, weight loss may be associated with persistent pain.

Mucosal Findings

- At times, small, painful red macule or papule before ulceration.
- More commonly, ulcer(s) <1 cm (Figs. 33-10 and 33-11), covered with fibrin (gray-white), with sharp, discrete, and at times edematous borders.
- Herpetiform "or grouped" AU (HAU) and Major AU (MaAU) may heal with white, depressed scars.
- Number of ulcers: Minor AU (MiAU), 1–5; MaAU, 1–10: HAU, up to 100.
- *Distribution*: Oropharyngeal, anogenital, any site in the GI tract. Oral lesions most commonly on the buccal and labial mucosa, less commonly on tongue, sulci, and floor of mouth. MiAU rarely occur on the palate or gums. MaAU often occur on soft palate and pharynx. Also, esophagus, upper and lower GI tract, and anogenital epithelium.

GENERAL FINDINGS With MaAU, occasionally tender cervical lymphadenopathy.
ASSOCIATED DISORDERS Behçet disease, cyclic neutropenia, acute HIV, AIDS (large chronic AU), reactive arthritis; Crohn disease; periodic fever, aphthous stomatitis, pharyngitis, and

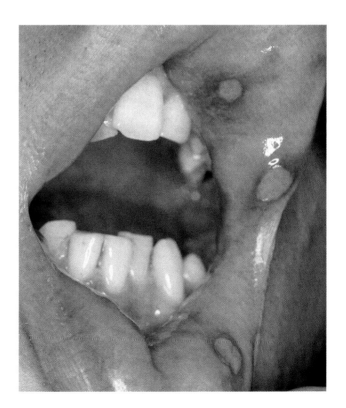

FIGURE 33-10 Aphthous ulcers: minor Multiple, very painful, gray-based ulcers with erythematous halos on the labial mucosa.

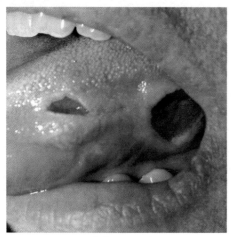

FIGURE 33-11 Aphthous ulcers: major Two large painful deep ulcers on the lateral tongue are seen in a patient with HIV/AIDS. Ulcers resolved with intralesional triamcinolone injection.

adenitis syndrome (PFAPA). The latter occurs in young children with associated high fever occurring periodically every 3 to 5 weeks with AU, pharyngitis, and/or lymphadenitis.

DIFFERENTIAL DIAGNOSIS

Primary herpetic gingivostomatitis, hand-foot-and-mouth disease, herpangina, primary HIV/AIDS infection, Behçet disease, squamous cell carcinoma (SCC), bullous disease, lichen planus, reactive arthritis (Reiter) syndrome, and adverse drug reaction.

LABORATORY

DERMATOPATHOLOGY Nondiagnostic. Rule out specific cause of ulcer, i.e., infection (syphilitic chancre, histoplasmosis, and herpes), inflammatory disorders (lichen planus), or cancers (SCC).

DIAGNOSIS

Usually made on clinical findings, ruling out other causes.

COURSE

Tend to recur during adulthood. Uncommonly, may be almost constant in the oropharynx or anogenitalia, referred to as *complex aphthosis.*

MANAGEMENT

INTRALESIONAL TRIAMCINOLONE 3 to 10 mg/mL in lidocaine very effective for immediate relief of pain and resolution of ulcers. *Amlexanox 5%* can be applied topically four times a day (after meals and before bedtime). *Viscous lidocaine 2%* should only be used for brief, immediate control of pain.

Systemic Therapy

- *Prednisone*: In persons with large, persistent, painful AU interfering with nutrition, a brief course of prednisone is effective (70 mg, tapered by 10 or 5 mg/d).
- **Tetracycline** syrup and **minocycline** 100 mg po BID, reported with variable success.
- *Thalidomide*: Effective in HIV/AIDS, Behçet disease, and large painful AU. Adverse effects: Peripheral sensory neuropathy. Lenalodomide may be used in these cases. Teratogenesis.
- *Tumor necrosis factor- α inhibitor*: Adalimumab and infliximab reported to be effective. Interleukin-1 inhibition shows promise for PFAPA.

LEUKOPLAKIA ICD-10: K13.21

- Leukoplakia is a chronic white plaque/lesion in the oropharynx.
- Premalignant leukoplakia has histologic atypia.
- Leukoplakia is a descriptive clinical term regarding morphology: *squamous cell carcinoma, in situ and invasive, must be ruled out.*
- *Findings*: A white plaque that cannot be wiped off and cannot be diagnosed as any other distinct lesion and may be premalignant or malignant.
- Definitive diagnosis should be made on clinical findings and histology.
- When diagnosis is definitive histologically, "leukoplakia" is no longer appropriate. The differential diagnosis includes SCCIS, invasive SCC, candidiasis, migratory glossitis, radiotherapy and chemotherapy-induced mucositis, lichen planus, and lupus erythematosus.

The differential diagnosis of leukoplakia is shown in Table 33-1.

TABLE 33-1 Differential Diagnosis of Leukoplakia

Lesion/Disorder	Characteristics
Leukoedema (Fig. 33-12)	Grayish-white opalescence of buccal mucosa; variant of normal. Histology: acanthosis.
Frictional keratosis/ lichen simplex chronicus (Fig. 33-13)	Keratosis secondary to friction (e.g., sharp tooth, rough or overextended denture border).
Chronic chewing: lip, tongue, cheek (Fig. 33-14)	Form of frictional keratosis. Surface white, rough. On buccal mucosa, wedge-shaped.
Nicotine stomatitis (Fig. 33-15)	Chemical irritation from smoking pipe, cigar, or cigarette. Occurs on hard palate; obstructs minor salivary glands on palate; ducts become inflamed. Ducts appear raised, erythematous dots on posterior hard palate and soft palate. White appearance resolves with cessation of smoking. Not considered premalignant.
Tobacco chewer's white lesion	Develops where chewing tobacco is held. Mucosa granular or wrinkled. *Location*: mucobuccal fold. Lesion is premalignant. Usually resolves with discontinuation of tobacco.
Hairy tongue (Fig. 33-3)	Elongation of filiform papillae of dorsal tongue; color white, brown, or black. See above.
Aspirin/chemical burn	Occurs following placement of aspirin tablet on mucosal surface. Mucosal surface becomes necrotic; white/painful lesion loosely adherent, easily sloughs off.
Oral hairy leukoplakia (see Fig. 27-66)	See above and HIV disease (Section 27). White corduroy appearance on inferolateral aspect of tongue.
Premalignant leukoplakia	Severity linked to duration and quantity of tobacco and alcohol use. Location: lip, tongue, floor of mouth. Erythroleukoplakia (speckled leukoplakia) has the highest rate of malignant transformation).
HPV: condyloma acuminatum, verruca vulgaris (Fig. 33-16), squamous papilloma	*Findings*: White papules, plaques; small, sessile, papillated, exophytic. Solitary, multiple, mosaic.
Verrucous carcinoma	See below.
Other white lesions	Keratoacanthoma, squamous acanthoma, submucous fibrosis (betel nut chewing), white sponge nevus

FIGURE 33-12 Leukoedema
In this variant of normal, there is bluish and whitish discoloration of mucosa that blanches when the cheek is stretched. (Used with permission from Dr. Nathaniel Treister.)

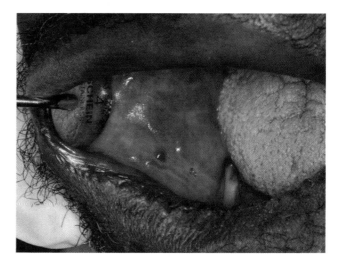

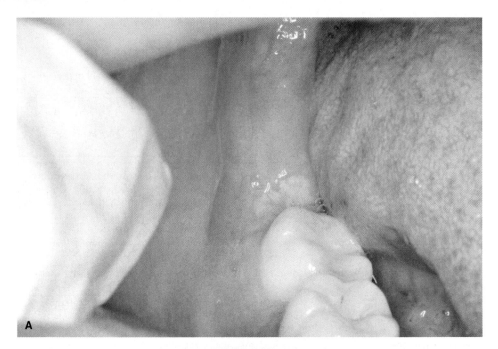

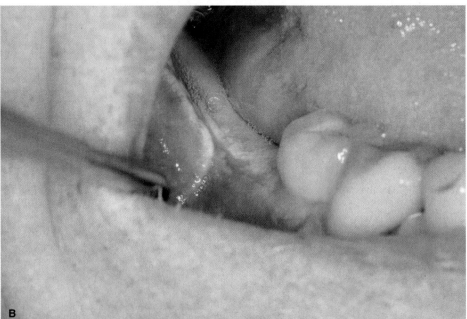

FIGURE 33-13 (A, B) Lichen simplex chronicus Note the white plaque in the retromolar pad (after third molar extractions). These are often seen on edentulous ridge after extractions. (Used with permission from Dr. Sook-Bin Woo.)

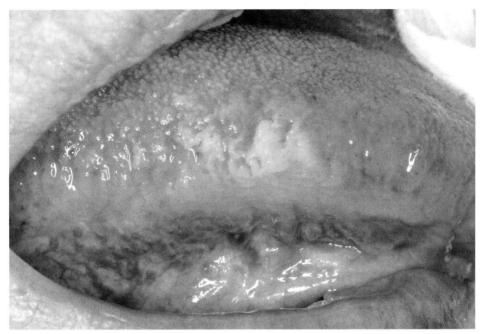

FIGURE 33-14 Chronic chewing A wedge-shaped white papule is noted on the lateral surface of the tongue. (Used with permission from Dr. Sook-Bin Woo.)

FIGURE 33-15 Nicotine stomatitis
Posterior palate shows erythematous pinpoint papules at sites of ducts and white patches where chemical irritation has caused chronic inflammation.

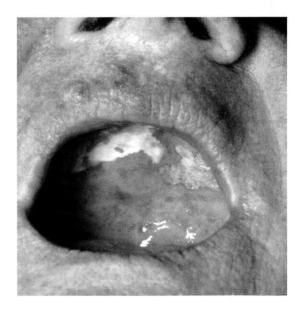

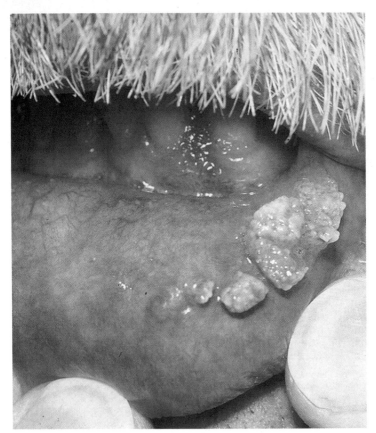

FIGURE 33-16 Condyloma acuminatum: mucosal lip Cluster of white cauliflower-floret-like lesions on the mucosa of the lower lip.

PREMALIGNANT AND MALIGNANT NEOPLASMS ICD-10: C14

DYSPLASIA AND SQUAMOUS CELL CARCINOMA IN SITU (SCCIS)

- *Etiology*: Tobacco-related habits [smoking moist snuff, pan (betel nut)]; human papillomavirus (HPV).
- *Risk factors*: Tobacco use, alcohol use, and oral lichen planus.
- *Findings*: Chronic, ± solitary patch/plaque on oropharyngeal mucosa. ± Reddish velvety appearance with either stippled or patchy regions of leukoplakia (Fig. 33-17). ± Smooth patch with minimal or no leukoplakia.
- *Size*: Usually <2 cm. *Location*: Floor of mouth (men); tongue and buccal surface (women).
- *Course*: Most dysplasias do not progress to invasive SCC; some do.
- Biopsy all lesions that persist for >3 weeks without definitive diagnosis.

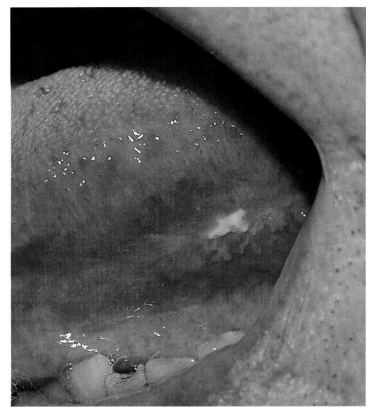

FIGURE 33-17 Squamous cell carcinoma in situ: inferolateral tongue
A 72-year-old male with an asymptomatic lesion on the tongue noticed by his dentist. A 6-mm white plaque (leukoplakia) on the tongue is noted. Biopsy reported SCCIS. The lesion was excised.

ORAL INVASIVE SQUAMOUS CELL CARCINOMA (See also Section 11)

- High associated morbidity and mortality, accounting for about 5% of all neoplasms in men and 2% of those in women.
- *Findings*: Usually appears as a granulating, velvety plaque or nodule with stippled hyperkeratosis ± ulceration (Fig. 33-18) (lips, floor of the mouth, and central and lateral sides of the tongue).
- Biopsy all lesions that persist for >3 weeks without definitive diagnosis.
- *Management*: Aggressive surgical intervention.

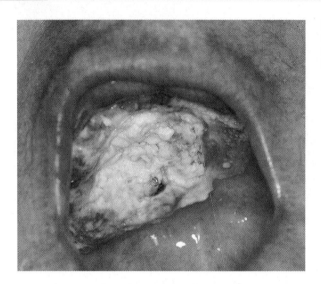

FIGURE 33-18 Invasive squamous cell carcinoma: palate An advanced leukoplakic tumor on the hard palate of a cigarette smoker.

ORAL VERRUCOUS CARCINOMA

- *Etiology*: Oncogenic HPV types 16 and 18.
- *Findings*: Extensive hyperkeratotic white leukoplakia (Fig. 33-19).
- *Course*: Metastasizes late but can be locally destructive. Biopsy all lesions that persist for >3 weeks without definitive diagnosis.
- *Management*: Aggressive surgical intervention.

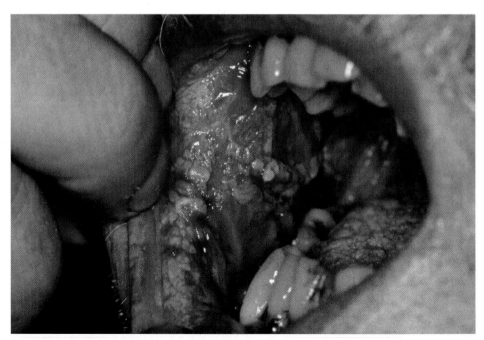

FIGURE 33-19 Verrucous carcinoma: buccal mucosa Extensive thick plaque arising on the buccal mucosa.

OROPHARYNGEAL MELANOMA (See also Section 12)

- *Incidence*: 4% of primary oral malignancies.
- For the most part, lesions are asymptomatic; often advanced when first detected.
- *Findings*: Presents as pigmented lesion (Fig. 33-20), with variegation of color and irregular borders; rarely amelanotic. *In situ* lesions are macular; sites of invasion are usually raised within the *in situ* lesion.
- *Distribution*: 80% arise on pigmented mucosa of the palate and gingiva.
- *Risk factors*: More deeply pigmented individuals (Africans) have higher proportional incidence rates of mucosal melanoma than whites.

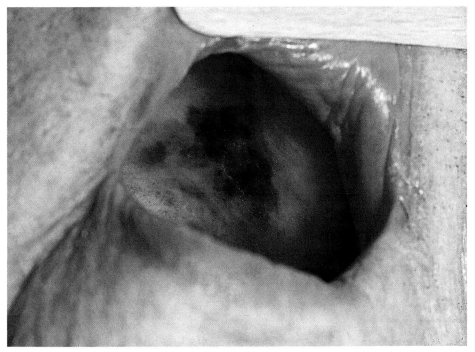

FIGURE 33-20 Melanoma: hard palate A large, highly variegated pigmented lesion in a 63-year-old male. Lesional biopsy of a raised part showed invasive lentigo maligna-like melanoma.

SUBMUCOSAL NODULES

MUCOCELE ICD-10: K11.6

- These arise following rupture of the minor salivary gland.
- *Findings*: Nodule with mucus-filled cavity, with a thick roof (Fig. 33-21). Chronic lesions are firm, inflamed, poorly circumscribed nodules; bluish, translucent; fluctuant.
- *Location*: Develops at sites where minor salivary glands are easily traumatized, mucous membranes of the lip and floor of the mouth.
- *Course*: Chronic, recurrent, and then it presents as a firm, inflamed nodule.
- *Treatment*: Puncuture and withdraw gelatious mucous content. If recurrent, excise.

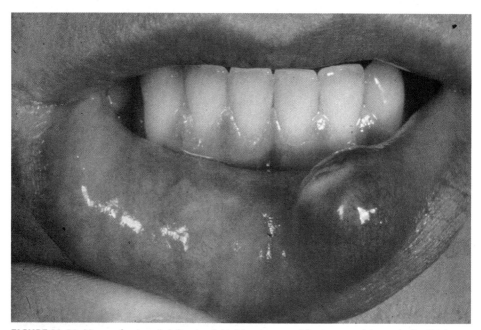

FIGURE 33-21 Mucocele A well-defined, soft bluish submucosal fluctuant nodule on the lip. Thick clear mucus drained when the lesion was incised.

IRRITATION FIBROMA ICD-10: M8810/0

- This is a submucosal nodular scar, occurring at a site of recurrent trauma (Fig. 33-22).
- *Findings*: Sessile or pedunculated, well-demarcated nodule, usually 2 cm in diameter (may be large if neglected). Normal color of the mucous membrane to pink-red; firm to hard.
- *Location*: Buccal mucosa along bite line; tongue, gingiva, and labial mucosa.
- *Synonym*: Bite fibroma.
- *Treatment*: None. If patient is uncomfortable, excise.

FIGURE 33-22 Irritation fibroma: lower lip
A 58-year-old female with a lesion on the lip for
10 years. She frequently bites it when chewing.
There is a rubbery pink nodule at the reflection of
the labial mucosa.

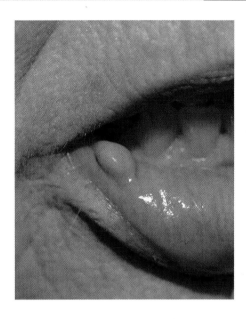

CUTANEOUS ODONTOGENIC (DENTAL) ABSCESS

■ A periapical dental abscess can extend into the overlying soft tissues, tracking and draining on the
face (Fig. 33-23).

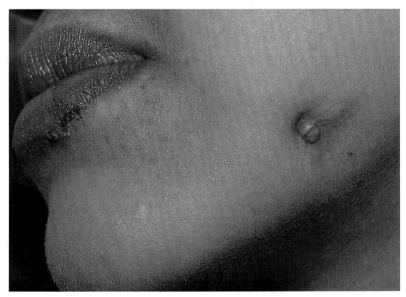

FIGURE 33-23 Cutaneous odontogenic abscess: cheek A 23-year-old healthy
female notes a lesion on the cheek for 6 months. Nodule on the lower left cheek near the
jawline with surrounding erythema and scar-like depression.

CUTANEOUS DISORDERS INVOLVING THE MOUTH

Cutaneous disorders may present in oral mucosa; may be confined to this site for months before cutaneous involvement occurs.

PEMPHIGUS VULGARIS (PV) (See also Section 6) ICD-10: L10.0

- Often presents in oral mucosa; may be confined to this site for months before cutaneous bullae occur. Mucsoal predominant PV shows titers for Desmoglein 3. Mucocutaneous disease more commonly expresses both Desmoglein 1 and 3.
- *Findings*: Blisters are very fragile, rupture easily, and are rarely seen. Sharply marginated erosions of the mouth (buccal mucosa, hard and soft palate, and gingiva) are presenting symptoms. Gingivitis can be a presenting sign. Erosions are extremely painful, interfering with nutrition (**Fig. 33-24**).
- Biopsy, immunofluorescence, or antibody titers against desmogleins 1 or 3 confirm the diagnosis (see "Pemphigus Vulgaris" in Section 6).

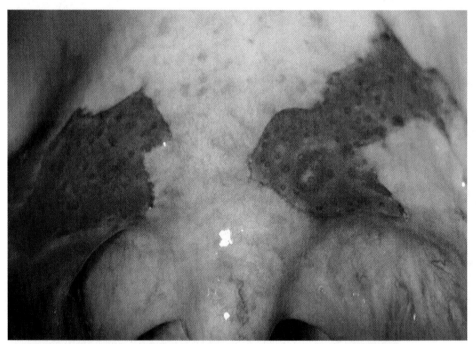

FIGURE 33-24 Pemphigus vulgaris Shallow ulcers and erosions with underlying beefy erythema/dermal tissue are commonly aggravated by trauma from swallowing spicy foods or citrus.

PARANEOPLASTIC PEMPHIGUS (See also Section 19) ICD-10: L10.81

- Painful mucosal erosions, stomatitis; cutaneous blisters, lichenoid papules and erosions; conjunctival erythema can be prominent (see Fig. 33-25). Cutaneous manifestations may be subtle (lichenoid papules), if present at all.
- Confirmed or occult malignancy (though this may precede or lag presentations by 6 months to a year). Can be associated with bronchiolitis obliterans-like pulmonary defects.
- Acantholysis, keratinocyte necrosis, and interface dermatitis. IgG and complement (C3) within the epidermal intercellular spaces and basement membrane seen on immunofluorescence. Circulating antibodies specific for stratified or transitional epithelium can be drawn from blood (ELISA, imuno-precipitation).
- Treatment is generally systemic; topical treatments are symptomatic.

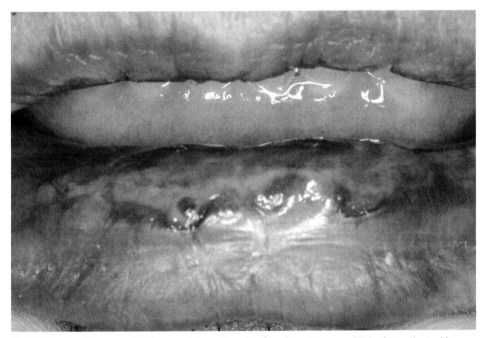

FIGURE 33-25 Paraneoplastic pemphigus Note beefy-red erosive mucositis in this patient with advanced CLL. (Used with permission from Dr. Mark Lerman.)

BULLOUS PEMPHIGOID (See also Section 6) ICD-10: L12.0

- In contrast to pemphigus vulgaris, bullous pemphigoid uncommonly affects the oropharynx.
- *Findings*: Blisters (**Fig. 33-26**), which initially are tense, erupt on the buccal mucosa and the palate, rupture, and leave sharply defined erosions that are practically indistinguishable from those of PV or cicatricial pemphigoid (see **Fig. 33-24**).
- However, erosions less painful and less extensive than in PV.
- Treatment may be topical.
- Diagnosis, see "Bullous Pemphigoid" in Section 6.

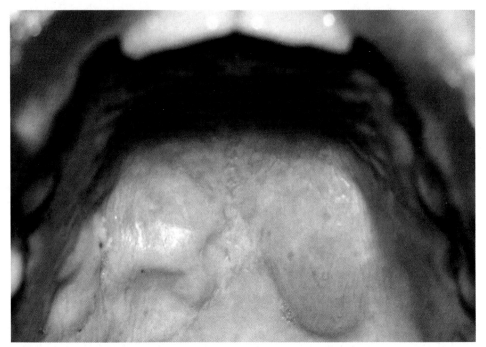

FIGURE 33-26 Bullous pemphigoid In the initial stages, bullae may be seen, which invariably rupture, leaving erosions that are difficult to distinguish from cicatricial pemphigoid or pemphigus vulgaris.

CICATRICIAL PEMPHIGOID (See Section 6) ICD-10: L12.1

- Autoimmune mucosal blistering disease that heals with scarring.
- Clinical manifestations dependent on sites involved. Persistent painful erosions on mucous membranes. Desquamative gingivitis with painful erosions on tongue, buccal, and palatal mucosa (Fig. 33-27). Ocular symblepharon and corneal scarring are feared complications. May be associated with malignancy, particularly if antibodies against epiligrin are noted.
- Sequelae: decreased vision/blindness; hoarseness, upper airway compromise, esophageal stenosis. Eye disease and systemic symptoms necessitate systemic therapy with dapsone, prednisone, cyclophosphamide, intravenuous immunoglobulin, or rituximab.

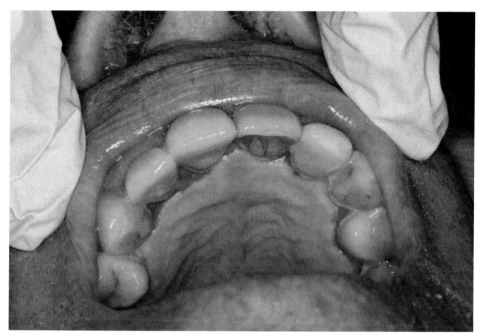

FIGURE 33-27 Cicatricial pemphigoid Gingivitis is seen, which outlines the junction with teeth. Mucosal disease is similar in bullous pemphigoid. (Used with permission from Dr. Sook-Bin Woo.)

SYSTEMIC DISEASES INVOLVING THE MOUTH

BEHÇET DISEASE See the preceding and Section 14.
ADVERSE DRUG REACTIONS See Section 23.

LUPUS ERYTHEMATOSUS (See also Section 14) ICD-10: M32.9

- Mucosal involvement occurs in approximately 25% of those with chronic cutaneous lupus erythematosus.
- *Findings*: Lesions: painless erythematous patches to chronic plaques, sharply marginated, irregularly scalloped white borders, radiating white striae, and telangiectasia. In older lesions: central depression, and painful ulceration.
- *Distribution*: buccal mucosa; palate (Fig. 33-28), alveolar process, tongue. Chronic plaques may also appear on the vermilion border of the lips.
- In acute systemic lupus erythematosus, ulcers arise in purpuric necrotic lesions of the palate (80%), buccal mucosa, or gums.

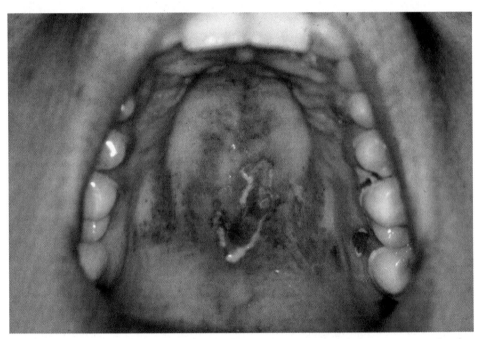

FIGURE 33-28 Lupus erythematosus: hard palate Erythematous eroded plaques were associated with chronic cutaneous LE.

STEVENS-JOHNSON SYNDROME/TOXIC EPIDERMAL NECROLYSIS (See also Section 8) ICD-10: L51.2

- Idiopathic reaction to medications and occasionally viral agents that lead to epidermal necrosis and desquamation. It is essential to discontinue possible culprits as soon as possible. There is a better prognosis with culprit drugs of shorter half-life.
- Classification schemes depend on extent of body surface area involved, but greater than 30% involvement generally agreed to be TEN if mucosal involvement is also noted.
- Most common mucosal location affected is the oropharynx. Mucosal lesions can precede cutaneous involvement by 1 to 3 days. In the mouth, presenting symptoms are burning sensation and decreased oral intake. Erosions are seen in up to 90% of cases. Desquamation can follow soon thereafter (Fig. 33-29).

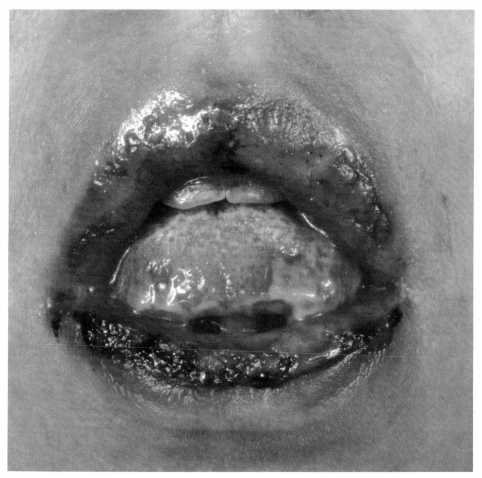

FIGURE 33-29 Toxic epidermal Necrolysis Exuberant desquamation, pyoderma, and hemorrhage accompany oral pain on swallowing, a burning sensation, and, often, dysphonia.

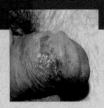

DISORDERS OF THE GENITALIA, PERINEUM, AND ANUS

- Primary neoplasms that arise in anogenital areas are most commonly associated with chronic human papillomavirus (HPV) infection.
- Sexually transmitted as well as other infections also occur commonly.
- Often normal structures, newly observed, give rise to great concerns about sexually transmitted infections such as anogenital warts and molluscum contagiosum.

PEARLY PENILE PAPULES ICD-10: N48.89

- Normal anatomic structures. *Incidence*: Up to 19%.
- *Symptoms*: Asymptomatic; may arouse some anxiety when first noted.
- *Clinical findings*: Skin-colored 1- to 2-mm, discrete, domed papules evenly distributed circumferentially around the corona (Fig. 34-1).
- *Differential diagnosis*: Condylomata acuminatum, molluscum contagiosum.
- *Histology*: Angiofibromas.
- *Management*: Reassurance: Normal anatomic structures. Laser therapy has been reported.

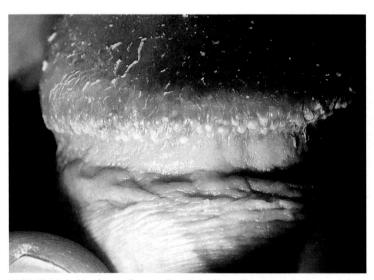

FIGURE 34-1 Pearly penile papules Pink (skin-colored), 1- to 2-mm papules are seen regularly spaced along the corona of the glans penis. These structures, which are part of the normal anatomy of the glans, are commonly mistaken for condylomata or molluscum contagiosum.

SEBACEOUS GLAND PROMINENCE ICD-10: Q89.9

- Normal sebaceous glands. Analogous to sebaceous gland on mucosa of mouth.
- *Locations*: Penis and vulva.
- *Manifestation*: 2-mm dermal papule; cream colored. May be arranged in rows.
- *Synonyms*: Tyson glands, sebaceous hyperplasia, "ectopic" sebaceous glands, and Fordyce condition.

ANGIOKERATOMA (See also Section 9)

- Ectatic thin-walled blood vessels in the superficial dermis with overlying epidermal hyperplasia.
- Increasingly common with aging.
- Multiple purple, smooth, 2- to 5-mm papules. Bleed with trauma. (See Section 9, Fig. 9-26).
- *Location*: Scrotum, glans penis, and penile shaft. Labia and vulva.
- Differentiate from angiokeratomas of Fabry disease (usually pinhead size, found on bathing trunk area and upper thighs), and Kaposi sarcoma.
- *Management*: Reassurance and electrosurgery.

SCLEROSING LYMPHANGITIS OF PENIS ICD-10: N48.29

- *Etiology*: Trauma associated with vigorous sexual activity.
- *Pathogenesis*: Lymphatic stasis may result in thrombosed lymphatic vessels.
- *Clinical findings*: Painless, firm, at times nodular, translucent serpiginous cord appears suddenly, usually parallel to corona; not attached to overlying epidermis (Fig. 34-2).
- *Course*: Resolves spontaneously in weeks to months.
- *Synonyms*: Nonvenereal sclerosing lymphangitis, penile venereal edema, and Mondor phlebitis.

FIGURE 34-2 Sclerosing lymphangitis: penis
A dermal cord on the distal shaft parallel to the corona.

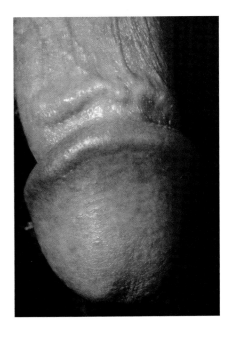

LYMPHEDEMA OF THE GENITALIA ICD-10: I89.0

- Acute idiopathic scrotal edema. Occurs in young boys. Resolves spontaneously in 1 to 4 days. Differentiate from acute scrotum. Also reported in adults with dengue hemorrhagic fever, Henoch-Schönlein purpura.
- Lymphogranuloma venereum (see Section 30). Occurs in chronic undiagnosed infection. Both sexes. Referred to as *esthiomene*: elephantiasis resulting from lymphatic obstruction.
- Chronic recurrent bacterial infection may be causative (**Figs. 34-3A** and **B**).
- Kaposi sarcoma.
- Filarial or lymphatic elephantiasis. Caused by parasitic worms such as *Wuchereria bancroftii, Brugia malayi,* and *B. timori.* Associated with elephantiasis of legs.

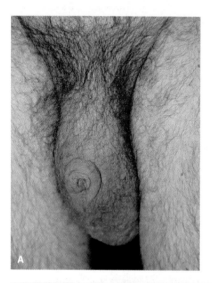

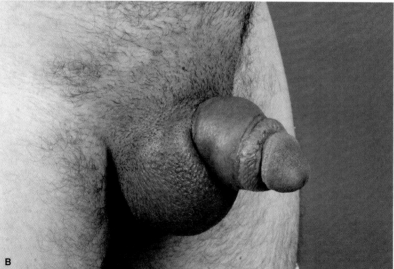

FIGURE 34-3 (A, B) Chronic lymphedema: (A) scrotum A 29-year-old male with history of recurrent scrotal infections that have destroyed lymphatic channels. There is scrotal noncompressible lymphedema and the penis is retracted; **(B) penis** There is erythema and permanent swelling of the penile shaft. Patients often describe a doughy feel to skin.

PLASMA CELL BALANITIS AND VULVITIS

- Asymptomatic red glistening plaque(s) on glans penis (**Fig. 34-4**) or vulva.
- Differentiate from squamous cell carcinoma in situ.
- *Management*: Circumcision is curative in uncircumcised males. Otherwise, topical corticosteroids, calcineurin inhibitors, and imiquimod can be used. Electrosurgery and laser destruction have also been reported.
- *Synonym*: Zoon balanitis.

FIGURE 34-4 Plasma cell balanitis Solitary red glistening plaque in an uncircumcised male.

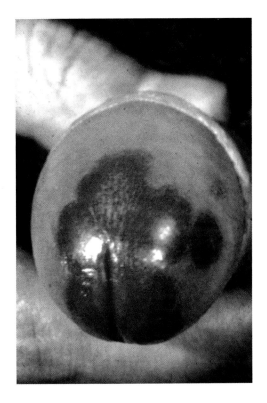

PHIMOSIS, PARAPHIMOSIS, BALANITIS XEROTICA OBLITERANS ICD-10: N48.0

- *Phimosis*: Nonretractable foreskin. *Etiology*: Lichen sclerosus, nonspecific balanoposthitis (posthitis is inflammation of foreskin or prepuce), lichen planus, cicatricial pemphigoid, chronic lymphedema, and Kaposi sarcoma. Precludes examination of glans for precancerous changes (Fig. 34-5).
- *Balanitis xerotica obliterans (BXO)*: End stage of chronic phimosis. Foreskin fibrotic, contracted, fixed over glans and cannot be retracted over glans. Most often end-stage lichen sclerosus, which is commonly referred to as BXO (see Section 14, lichen sclerosus).
- *Paraphimosis*: Foreskin fixed in retraction. *Etiology*: Vigorous sexual activity, acute contact urticaria, acute allergic contact dermatitis, or lichen sclerosus (Fig. 34-6).

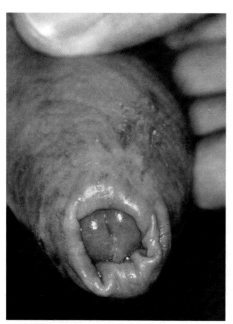

FIGURE 34-5 Phimosis The prepuce or foreskin has been chronically inflamed with scarring and is no longer retractable over the glans penis.

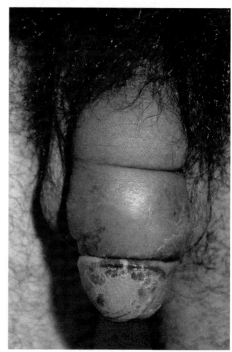

FIGURE 34-6 Paraphimosis The prepuce or foreskin has been retracted proximally over the glans and cannot be replaced to the normal position covering the glans. The shaft is edematous.

MUCOCUTANEOUS DISORDERS

GENITAL (PENILE/VULVAR/ANAL) LENTIGINOSES ICD-10: L98.8

- *Onset:* Adulthood.
- *Clinical findings:* Tan, brown, intense blue-black; usually variegated, 5- to 15-mm macules.
- *Sites:* In clusters on vulva (labia minora, Fig. 34-7), penis (glans, shaft) (Fig. 34-8), and perianal areas.
- *Course:* Persist for years without change in size.
- *Histology:* No significant melanocytic hyperplasia; nevus cells are not present; pigmentation is caused by increased melanin in basal cell layer.
- *Differential diagnosis:* Melanoma in situ, PUVA lentigo, fixed drug reaction, blue nevus, and HPV-induced intraepithelial neoplasia (IN).
- *Diagnosis:* Dermoscopy rules out in situ melanoma; histology confirms diagnosis.
- Extensive lesions that cannot be easily removed should be followed photographically; areas that show significant change should be biopsied.

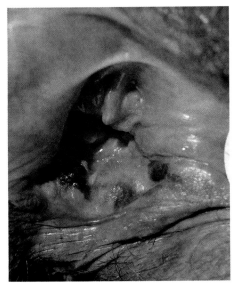

FIGURE 34-7 Genital lentiginoses: vulva
Multiple, variegated dark brown macules, bilaterally on the labia minora. Lentiginous melanoma *in situ* must be ruled out.

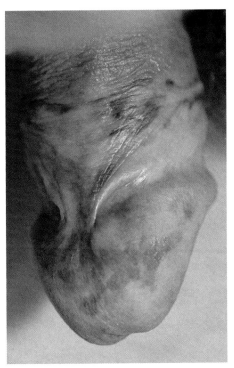

FIGURE 34-8 Genital lentiginoses: penis
Variegated macular pigmentation of the glans and foreskin for over 20 years. Biopsy ruled out melanoma and HVP-infection (SCCIS).

VITILIGO AND LEUKODERMA   (See also Section 13)

- *Etiology*: Loss of melanocytes results in depigmentation.
- *Isomorphic* or *Koebner phenomenon*: Depigmentation at sites of injury: genital herpes, cryosurgery, and imiquimod therapy.
- Wood lamp examination: Differentiates depigmentation from hypopigmentation.
- *Clinical findings*: Sharply demarcated, depigmented, white macules (**Fig. 34-9**); examine skin for other depigmented areas.
- *Differential diagnosis*: Lichen sclerosus, site of genital herpes; iatrogenic after cryo-, electro-, or laser surgery.

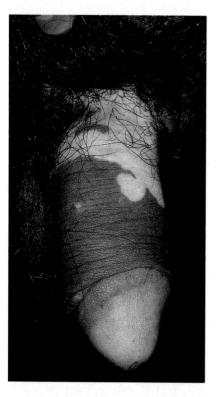

FIGURE 34-9 Vitiligo: penis Multiple depigmented macules have become confluent.

PSORIASIS VULGARIS   (See also Section 3)

- *Incidence*: Most common noninfectious dermatosis occurring on the glans penis and vulva.
- *Onset*: May be initial presentation of psoriasis.
- *Clinical findings*: (1) Erythematous scaling plaques on nonoccluded skin (**Fig. 34-10**); (2) intertriginous psoriasis, well-demarcated erythematous plaques without scale in naturally occluded skin (**Fig. 34-11**).
- *Distribution [intertriginous (inverse) psoriasis]*: Penis, vulva, intergluteal cleft, and inguinal folds.
- *Differential diagnosis*: Lichen planus (LP), fixed drug eruption, condyloma acuminata, HPV-induced IN, squamous cell carcinoma (SCC) *in situ*, invasive SCC, extramammary Paget disease, and migratory necrolytic erythema.

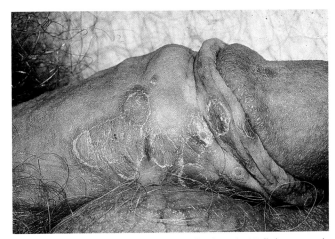

FIGURE 34-10 Psoriasis vulgaris: shaft of penis Well-demarcated scaling plaques on the penile shaft of a 25-year-old male. "Pinking" of the intergluteal cleft and nail findings of psoriasis were also present. The patient presented to a clinic for sexually transmitted disease.

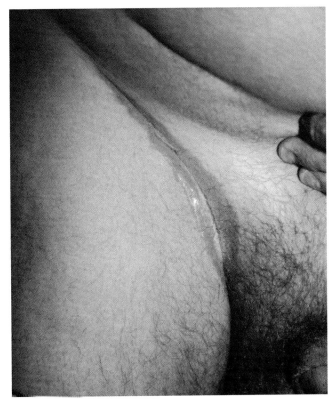

FIGURE 34-11 Psoriasis vulgaris: intertriginous An erythematous plaque, present for decades and unresponsive to topical antifungal agents, is seen in the right inguinal area. Biopsy excluded extramammary Paget disease.

LICHEN PLANUS ICD-10: L43.9 (See also Section 14)

- Commonly associated with LP at other sites: However, may occur as initial or sole manifestation.
- *Symptoms*: Not pruritic; pain in eroded lesions, anxiety about sexually transmitted disease.
- *Clinical findings*: Violaceous flat-topped papules, discrete or confluent. Lacy white surface pattern most commonly on glans. Older lesions may have grayish hue with melanin incontinence. Annular lesions occur on glans and shaft (Fig. 34-12). Bullous and/or erosive LP (Fig. 34-13) on glans, vulva.
- *Distribution*: Glans, penile shaft (Fig. 34-12), and vulva.
- *Course*: Spontaneous remission; erosive LP may persist for decades; SCC complicates rarely.

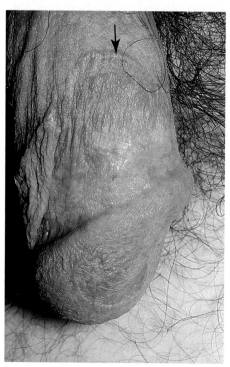

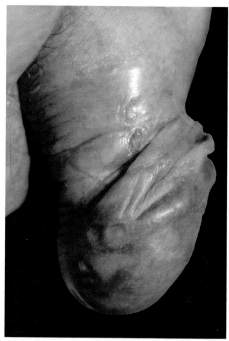

FIGURE 34-12 Lichen planus, annular: penis
Violaceous annular plaques (*arrow*) on the distal shaft and glans of a 26-year-old patient, present for >1 year. White lacelike plaques were also present on the buccal mucosa.

FIGURE 34-13 Lichen planus, erosive: penis
A 36-year-old male with painful erythematous erosions on the glans penis and foreskin for 6 months. Lesions resolved with intralesional triamcinolone injections.

LICHEN NITIDUS ICD-10: L44.1

- 1- to 2-mm papules on shaft of penis (Fig. 34-14).

FIGURE 34-14 Lichen nitidus: penis
Flat-topped papules on the shaft of the penis.

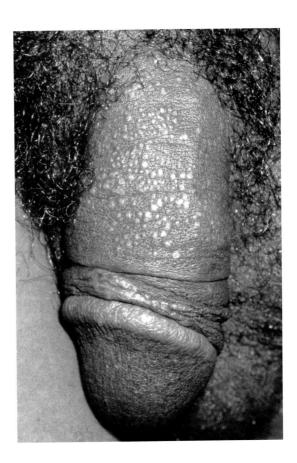

LICHEN SCLEROSUS (See also Section 14)

- *Symptoms*: Pruritus, burning; pain with ulceration.
- *Clinical findings*: Early: erythema ± hypopigmentation. Later: typical ivory- or porcelain-white macules and plaques; white caused by loss of dermal vasculature (Fig. 34-15). Ecchymosis (Figs. 34-15 to 34-17), bullae, and/or erosions may occur in involved sites. May obstruct urethral orifice.
- *Demography*: Ten times move common in female. Causes phimosis (Fig. 34-15) in boys.
- *End stage*: BXO. Effacement of normal architectural features: labia minora and clitoral hood may be absorbed (Fig. 34-16).
- *Course*: Invasive SCC can arise in this site of chronic inflammation.
- *Management*: Clobetasol ointment; monitor for steroid-induced atrophy, pimecrolimus, and tacrolimus.
- *Synonym*: Lichen sclerosus et atrophicus.

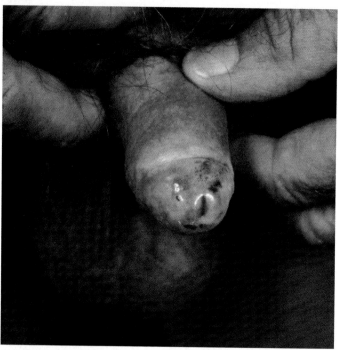

FIGURE 34-15 Lichen sclerosus: penis A male with phimosis (inability to retract foreskin) for 6 months and white sclerotic, adherent plaques on the reflection of the foreskin. Note the shiny gleam on the glans (particularly periurethral), and easy friability of the mucosal surface, and ecchymoses.

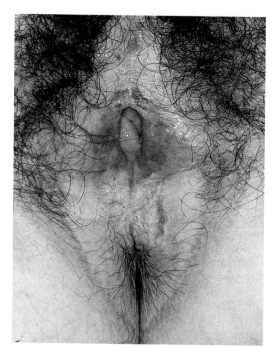

FIGURE 34-16 Lichen sclerosus: vulva and perineum A large white sclerotic plaque extensively involving the anogenital region. The clitoral and labia minora region is completely atrophic (agglutination). Ecchymoses are noted in association with atrophy. Ulcerations can occur and are painful.

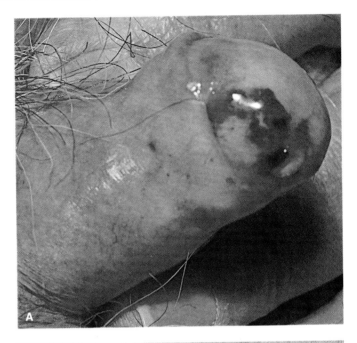

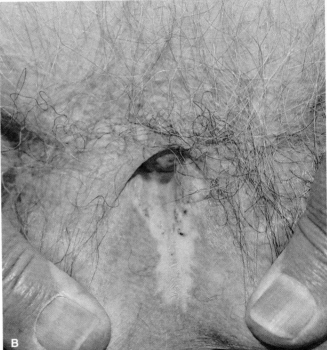

FIGURE 34-17 Lichen sclerosus: penis (A) Whitish plaques on glans with typical ecchymoses; the urethral orifice was constricted. **(B)** Five years later, the penis had become atrophic and submerged within the pubic fat, making urination difficult. A white sclerotic plaque with ecchymoses is seen on the stretched skin of the ventral penile shaft.

MIGRATORY NECROLYTIC ERYTHEMA (See also Section 19)

- Manifestation of glucagonoma syndrome.
- Painful erythematous plaques, glistening surface, and serpiginous border surrounded by scaling (see Fig. 19-10).

GENITAL APHTHOUS ULCERATIONS (See also Sections 14, 30, and 33)

- Idiopathic ulcers on scrotum or vulva. May be associated with oral aphthous ulcerations. May occur as a manifestation of primary HIV/AIDS.
- Occur as part of the syndrome complex of Behçet disease (see also Figs. 14-20 to 14-21).

ECZEMATOUS DERMATITIS

ALLERGIC CONTACT DERMATITIS (See also Section 2)

- On genitalia is often more florid and symptomatic than at other sites.
- *Allergens*: Topically applied agents (medications, lubricants); haptens blotted onto genitals by hands (e.g., poison ivy sap).
- *Symptoms*: Intense pruritus, burning sensation; edema.
- *Clinical findings*: Erythema, microvesicles; edema; exudation of genitals (Fig. 34-18). With phytodermatitis (e.g., poison ivy or oak), lesions are usually present at other sites.
- *Differential diagnosis*: Genital herpes, atopic dermatitis, and irritant dermatitis.

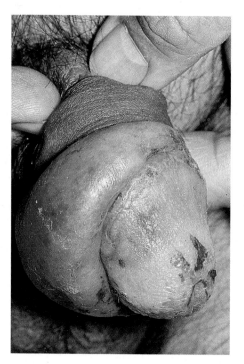

FIGURE 34-18 Allergic contact dermatitis: penis Striking edema of the distal penile shaft associated with severe pruritus in a 21-year-old patient. He had touched poison ivy with his hands, transferring the resin to his penis while urinating. The magenta colored pigment is Castellani paint.

ATOPIC DERMATITIS, LICHEN SIMPLEX CHRONICUS, PRURITUS ANI ICD-10: L29.0

- Atopic dermatitis: Usually associated with more widespread involvement but can be isolated to genitalia.
- Lichen simplex chronicus: Chronic rubbing/scratching results in a single plaque on scrotum (Fig. 34-19), vulva, or anus (Fig. 34-20), persisting for years or decades. In dark skin, hypo- and hyperpigmentation occurs (see Section 2).
- Pruritus ani: Can occur in the absence of any identifiable dermatologic disorder. Chronic pruritus and rubbing often produce some lichenification (Fig. 34-20). *Risk factors*: Atopic diathesis; multifactorial. *Secondary infection: Staphylococcus aureus,* group A and B streptococci, *Candida albicans,* and herpes simplex virus. Can be a sign of lumbosacral radiculopathy. *Management*: Discontinue compulsive rubbing/scratching; maintenance of perianal hygiene. Referral to neurology if radiculopathy is suspected.

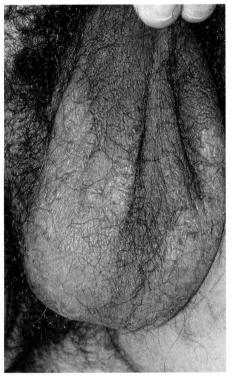

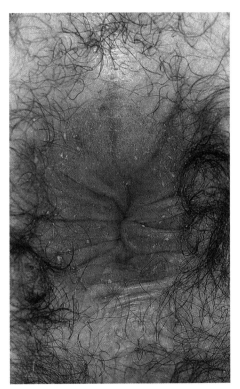

FIGURE 34-19 Lichen simplex chronicus: scrotum Pruritic bilateral erythematous hyper-pigmented plaques present for >20 years.

FIGURE 34-20 Lichen simplex chronicus: pruritus ani The patient had experienced intense anal pruritus for many years. Perianal erythema with mild lichen simplex chronicus and fissure is associated with chronic rubbing of the skin.

FIXED DRUG ERUPTION ICD-10: L27.0-L27.1 (See also Section 23)

- Large blisters occur on the male genitalia commonly; evolve to painful erosion (Fig. 34-21).
- With repeated drug exposure, blisters/erosions recur at the same site.

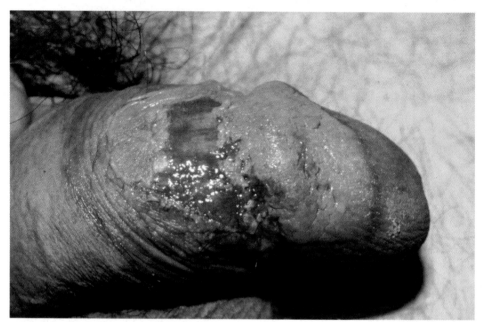

FIGURE 34-21 Fixed drug eruption: trimethoprim-sulfamethoxazole Violaceous bullae that had ruptured, occurring on the dorsum of the penis (glans and shaft), recurring after treatment with trimethoprim–sulfamethoxazole.

PREMALIGNANT AND MALIGNANT LESIONS

SQUAMOUS CELL CARCINOMA (SCC) IN SITU (See also Section 11)

- *Terminology*: Squamous cell carcinoma in situ (SCCIS) is generic; intraepithelial neoplasia (IN) is HPV-induced SCCIS.
- *Etiology*: HPV infection, chronic low-grade balanoposthitis (poor hygiene, LS) in older individuals; chronic dermatoses (ulcerative lichen planus, lichen sclerosus).
- *Clinical findings*: Solitary, well-defined, irregularly bordered, red patch with a glazed-to-velvety surface on the penis (Fig. 34-22) or vulva; associated dermatoses. HPV-associated lesions are usually multifocal, occurring at any sites of the anogenital region (Fig. 34-23).
- *Diagnosis*: Lesional biopsy.
- *Course*: Appearance of a nodule or ulcer suggests progression to invasive SCC (Fig. 34-24). In HPV-associated SCCIS, rate of transformation to invasive SCC is relatively low; rate is higher for vulvar SCCIS: Rate of invasiveness and metastasis higher when associated with poor hygiene/chronic balanoposthitis (see also Section 11).
- *Synonyms*: Erythroplasia of Queyrat; Bowen disease, and bowenoid papulosis.

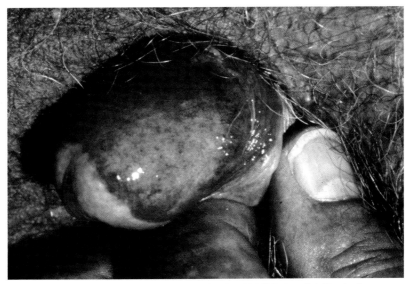

FIGURE 34-22 Squamous cell carcinoma in-situ (SCCis) A well-defined, glistening, irregular red patch. The presence of nodules or ulceration, not seen in this example, would raise suspicion for invasive squamous cell carcinoma.

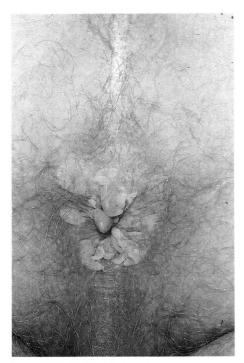

FIGURE 34-23 HPV-induced squamous cell carcinoma in situ: perianal A well-demarcated pink perianal asymptomatic plaque. Anal Pap test showed low-grade squamous intraepithelial lesion (LSIL).

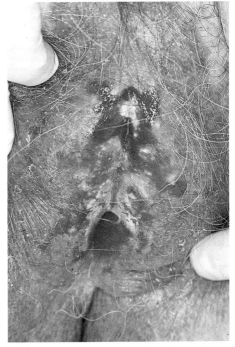

FIGURE 34-24 Squamous cell carcinoma in situ arising in lichen sclerosus: vulva Erythema and erosions with marked atrophy of the labia minora and clitoris in a patient with longstanding genital lichen sclerosus. Lesional biopsy shows associated SCC *in situ* arising in lichen sclerosus.

HPV-INDUCED INTRAEPITHELIAL NEOPLASIA (IN) AND SQUAMOUS CELL CARCINOMA IN SITU (See also Sections 11 and 27)

- *Etiology*: HPV types 16, 18, 31, and 33.
- *Risk factors*: Immunosuppression, occurring in HIV/AIDS disease, iatrogenically induced immunosuppression in solid organ transplantation.
- *Clinical findings*: Erythematous patches and papules (flat-topped) (**Figs. 34-23** and **34-25**); pigmented papules. *Arrangement*: Solitary, clustering, confluence, plaque(s) formation. *Distribution*: Mucosa, anogenital and inguinocrural skin.
- *Course*: Spontaneous resolution; persist for years; multiple new lesions appear; progress to invasive SCC. Progression to invasive SCC highest in cervix, anus. Monitor cervix/anus by periodic Pap testing (cytology) to detect dysplastic changes.

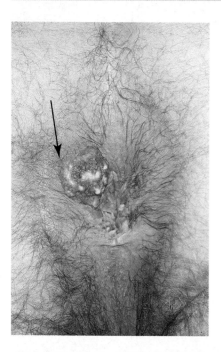

FIGURE 34-25 HPV-induced invasive squamous cell carcinoma: perineum A 34-year-old HIV/AIDS-infected male presented with a perineal tumor (*arrow*) of several months duration.

INVASIVE ANOGENITAL SQUAMOUS CELL CARCINOMA

INVASIVE SCC OF PENIS (See also Section 11)

- *Risk factors*: Lack of circumcision, poor penile hygiene, phimosis (25 to 75%), low socioeconomic status, HPV infection (15 to 80%), UV-radiation exposure, tobacco use.
- *Demography*: More common in developing nations (up to 10% of cancers in men; rare in industrialized nations).
- *Precancerous lesion/disorders*: Phimosis, chronic balanoposthitis, pseudoepitheliomatous keratotic and micaceous balanitis, lichen planus, lichen sclerosus, giant condyloma, and HPV-induced IN.
- *Symptoms*: Precursor lesion, itching/burning under foreskin, ulceration of glans, or prepuce.
- *Clinical findings*: Subtle induration; small excrescence; small papule; warty growth to an obvious extensive carcinoma with sloughing. Necrosis and/or secondary infection in phimotic foreskin. Extends along the penile shaft and involves corpora cavernosa. Rarely, bleeding, urinary fistula, and urinary retention occur.
- *Distribution*: Glans (48%), prepuce (21%), glans and prepuce (9%), prepuce glans and shaft (14%), coronal sulcus (6%), shaft (<2%).
- *Metastasis*: Inguinal lymph node metastases; distant sites rare.

INVASIVE SCC OF VULVA (See also Section 11)

- *Risk factors*: HPV infection, abnormal cervical Pap test, immunosuppression, HIV/AIDS disease, advanced age, increased number of sexual partners, younger age at first episode of intercourse, tobacco use, lichen planus, and lichen sclerosus (Fig. 34-24).
- *Symptoms*: Vulvar pruritus, localized pain, discharge, dysuria, bleeding, and ulceration.
- *Clinical findings*: Bulky whitish or pigmented lesion of thickened or hard skin; verrucoid, polypoid, papular. *Location*: 65% arise on labia majora.

INVASIVE SCC OF CUTANEOUS ANUS (See also Section 11)

- *Etiology*: Oncogenic HPV infection. *Risk factors*: Chronic immunosuppression and HIV/AIDS disease. *Location*: (1) Cutaneous, (2) junction of columnar and squamous epithelium.
- *Precursor lesion*: Anal IN. *Clinical findings*: Papule, nodule, ulcerated nodule (Fig. 34-25).

GENITAL VERRUCOUS CARCINOMA (See also Section 11)

- *Etiology*: HPV infection.
- *Clinical findings*: Large, cauliflower-like, warty tumors.
- *Distribution*: Vulva, penis, and anus.
- *Course*: Slow-growing; rarely metastasize.

MALIGNANT MELANOMA OF THE ANOGENITAL REGION (See also Section 12)

- Incidence: Rare.
- *Precursor lesions*: Preexisting pigmented lesion or *de novo* from epidermal melanocytes.
- *Clinical findings*: Macules or papules with variegation of brown-black color, irregular borders, and often with papular elevation (Fig. 34-26) or ulceration.
- *Distribution*: Males: Glans (67%), prepuce (13%), urethral meatus (10%), penile shaft (7%), and coronal sulcus (3%) (Fig. 34-26); females: labia minora, clitoris (Fig. 34-27).
- *Differential diagnosis*: Genital lentiginosis, old fixed drug eruption, SCC, hemangioma, and Bowenoid papulosis.
- *Histologic types*: Lentiginous melanoma; rarely, desmoplastic melanoma.
- *Prognosis*: Poor because of early metastases via lymphatic vessels; most patients die within 1 to 3 years.

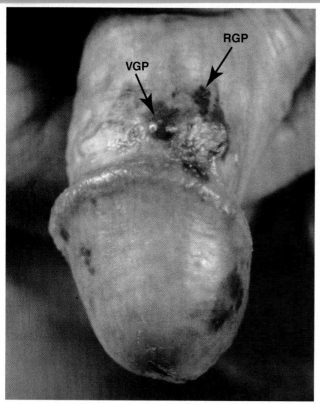

FIGURE 34-26 Melanoma, invasive: penis A violaceous nodule (*arrow*) represents the vertical growth phase (VGP) arising in an area of macular variegated hyperpigmentation (*arrow*) which denotes radial growth phase (RGP) which had been present for 5 years and resembled genital lentiginosis. The most common histologic type of genital melanoma is acrolentiginous melanoma.

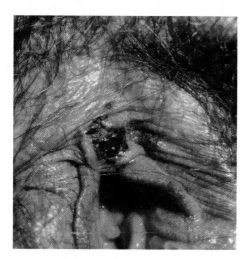

FIGURE 34-27 Melanoma, invasive: vulva A violaceous nodule in a black plaque is seen.

EXTRAMAMMARY PAGET DISEASE (See also Section 19)

- Often undiagnosed for years or decades; treated as intertrigo.
- Well-demarcated plaques in genital area (Fig. 34-28).

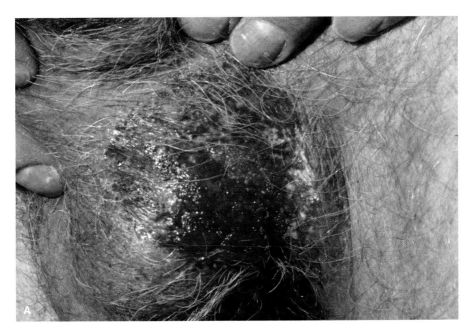

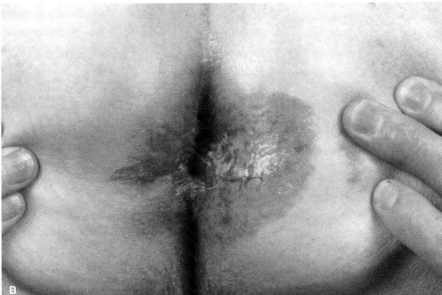

FIGURE 34-28 Extramammary Paget disease: (A) scrotum and inguinocrural, and (B) perianal
Well-demarcated recurrent, bright red plaques for several years. Lesions may be treated via Mohs micrographic surgery but if recurrent, often require treatment with electron beam radiotherapy.

KAPOSI SARCOMA   (See also Section 21)

- Common in advanced untreated HIV/AIDS.
- *Location*: Penis and scrotum.
- *Manifestations*: Violaceous papules, nodules, and plaques; become confluent. Edema of penis and scrotum (Fig. 34-29).

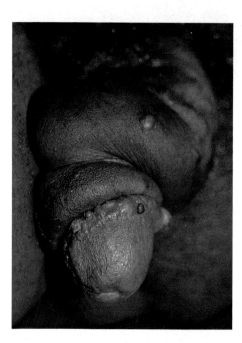

FIGURE 34-29   Kaposi sarcoma: penis   Multiple nodules are seen on the glans and shaft of the penis, present for 8 months in a patient with HIV/AIDS. Massive swelling of the penis was caused by tumor infiltration and lymphatic obstruction, resulting in urinary obstruction. Similar obstruction caused edema of both legs.

ANOGENITAL INFECTIONS   (See also Sections 25, 26 and 30)

- Bacterial infections, see Section 25.
- Mucocutaneous anogenital fungal infections, see Section 26.
- Dermatophytosis and tinea versicolor occur on keratinizing skin only. Rarely occur on the shaft of the penis.
- Candidiasis is common on naturally occluded sites on the penis, vulva, and vagina.
- STI, see Section 30.

GENERALIZED PRURITUS WITHOUT SKIN LESIONS (PRURITUS SINE MATERIA)

- Most skin eruptions and rashes are more or less pruritic, but there are states where there is severe pruritus in the absence of skin lesions, except for scratch marks (Fig. 35-1).
- The diagnostic approach to the patient with generalized pruritus without identifiable skin lesions is a *diagnosis of exclusion*.
- Pruritus is a symptom of skin disease that at the time of examination does not manifest with specific lesions.
- It may be cause by an internal organ disease, metabolic and endocrine conditions, or hematologic disease.
- It may be a manifestation of malignant tumors, psychogenic states, or HIV infection; or it may be related to injected or ingested drugs.
- The various causes of pruritus sine materia are listed in Table 35-1, and an algorithm of how to approach a patient with pruritus sine materia is shown in Table 35-2.
- Skin signs may be clinically inapparent, perhaps confined to only circumscribed areas. This is particularly important with regard to the exclusion of scabies, pediculosis, or conditions such as urticaria factitia.

FIGURE 35-1 Pruritus without diagnostic skin lesions This patient had multiple scratch marks resulting from compulsive scratching because of severe pruritus. There were no other diagnostic lesions. Workup revealed biliary cirrhosis without jaundice.

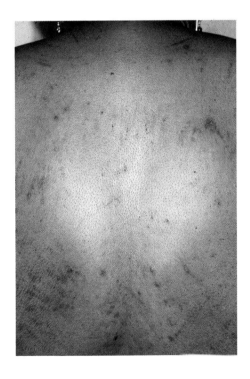

MOST IMPORTANT CAUSES (See Table 35-1**)**

TABLE 35-1 Causes of Pruritus Sine Materia

Metabolic, endocrine conditions
  Hyperthyroidism: probably due to increased blood flow
  Hypothyroidism: probably due to excessive dryness
  Pregnancy related
  Diabetes: pruritus is rarely associated, but can be a symptom of diabetic neuropathy

Malignant neoplasms: can be the presenting feature
  Lymphoma, myeloid and lymphatic leukemia, myelodysplasia
  Multiple myeloma
  Hodgkin disease
  Other cancer (rare)

Drug ingestion
  Subclinical drug sensitivities
  Aspirin, alcohol, dextran, polymyxin B, morphine
  Codeine, scopolamine, D-tubocurarine
  Hydroxyethyl starch

Infestations/Infections
  Scabies[a]
  Pediculosis corporis, capitis, pubis
  Hookworm (ancylostomiasis)
  Onchocerciasis
  Ascariasis
  HIV: can be a primary symptom of infection or a chronic comorbidity

Renal disease
  Renal failure: may develop prurigo nodularis, lichenification, or nummular eczema as a result of scratching

Hematologic disease
  Polycythemia vera: seen in up to 50% of patients upon contact with water
  Paraproteinemia, iron deficiency

Hepatic disease
  Obstructive biliary disease: pruritus starts acrally and then disseminates
  Pregnancy (intrahepatic cholestasis) (see Section 15)

Neurologic disease
■ Peripheral nerve damage: lumbosacral radiculopathy or entrapment neuropathy (anogenital pruritus, meralgia paresthetica)
■ Peripheral nerve damage: lumbosacral radiculopathy [brachioradial pruritus, notalgia paresthetica (Fig. 35-2)]
■ Spinal nerve damage (notalgia paresthetica)

Psychogenic states
  Transitory:
    Periods of emotional stress
  Persistent
    Delusions of parasitosis
    Psychogenic pruritus
    Neurotic excoriations
    Anorexia nervosa

Latent dermatoses and miscellaneous conditions
  Xerosis (dry skin, "winter itch")
  Senile pruritus: very common in people >70 years
  Bullous pemphigoid (without skin lesions)
  Dermatitis herpetiformis (without skin lesions)
  Atopic dermatitis (without skin lesions)
  Factitious urticaria (dermographism)
  Fiber glass exposure
  Aquagenic pruritus: usually in middle aged and elderly; provoked by contact with water of any temperature, lasts up to 1 hour. Different condition from senile pruritus or bath itch from polycythemia. Histamine levels are elevated in blood.

[a]Diagnostic lesions may or may not be present.

MANAGEMENT

1. Identify and treat underlying disease.
2. Treat xerosis (dry skin) with baths and emollients.
3. UVB and narrow-band (311 nm) phototherapy or PUVA (in renal-, biliary-, aquagenic-, and polycythemia vera–related pruritus).
4. Topical agents: Capsaicin, doxepin 5%, camphor/menthol, topical 3% aspirin solution (helps with lichen simplex chronicus (LSC)), pramoxine, and naltrexone cream 1%.
5. Oral agents: Naloxone, naltrexone (25 to 50 mg/d), or ondansetron; antihistamines, tricyclic antidepressants (decrease central itch perception), or thalidomide (especially in HIV), low-dose gabapentin (start at 300 mg/d but may need to titrate up as high 2400 mg/d before deemed ineffective); cholestyramine in cholestatic itch (but ineffective in total biliary obstruction).

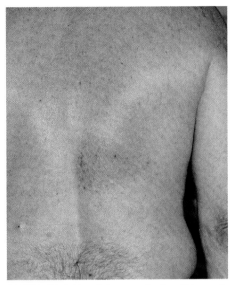

FIGURE 35-2 Notalgia paresthetica This condition in the interscapular region is characterized by intense pruritus without skin lesions. The erythema seen here is caused by rubbing and scratching.

TABLE 35-2 Approach to the Diagnosis of Generalized Pruritus Without Diagnostic Skin Lesions

Initial Visit(s)

1. Detailed history of pruritus:
   - Are there any skin lesions that precede the itching?
   - Is the itching continuous or does it occur in waves?
   - Is the itching related to certain times of the day, does it occur at night, and does it keep the patient awake?
   - Is the itching related to environmental conditions (heat, cold); is it related to emotional stress, physical exertion, sweating, contact with water?
2. Examine carefully for subtle primary skin disorders as a cause of the pruritus; xerosis or asteatosis, scabies, pediculosis (nits?). Discrete papules on elbows, scalp (dermatitis herpetiformis), on scrotum or shaft of penis (scabies).
3. Check for dermographism, rub skin for Darier sign (see "Mastocytosis Syndromes," Section 20).
4. Repeat history related to pruritus. Obtain history of constitutional symptoms, weight loss, fatigue, fever, malaise. History of oral or parenteral medication that can be a cause of generalized pruritus without a rash.
5. General physical examination including *all* the lymph nodes; rectal examination and stool guaiac in adult patients.
6. If dry skin or winter itch is a reasonable possible explanation, give the patient bath oil, followed by an emollient ointment. No soap; the bath is therapeutic, not for cleansing the skin; shower to clean.
7. Follow-up appointment in 2 weeks.

Subsequent Visit(s)

If no relief from symptomatic treatment given on the first visit, proceed as follows:
1. Detailed review of systems.
2. Laboratory tests: complete blood tests including erythrocyte sedimentation rate, fasting blood sugar, renal function tests, liver function tests, hepatitis antigens, thyroid tests, stool and serologic examination for parasites.
3. If the diagnosis has not been established at this point, the patient should be referred for complete workup including pelvic examination and Pap smear.

Source: Adapted with permission from Bernhard JD, ed. *Itch Mechanisms and Management of Pruritus*. New York, NY: McGraw-Hill; 1994, pp. 211–215.

APPENDICES

DIFFERENTIAL DIAGNOSIS OF PIGMENTED LESIONS

Perhaps the most difficult and concerning aspects of the dermatologic physical exam rest on the provider's ability to evaluate pigmented lesions. Such lesions represent a large portion of visits due to patients' concerns regarding rapid growth, change in shape, symptoms such as pruritus, or recent bleeding. The following figures highlight the most reliable features in evaluating pigmented lesions, though overlap does exist between characteristic features. When clinical doubt exists, skin biopsy for histopathologic evaluation or referral to a dermatologist is recommended.

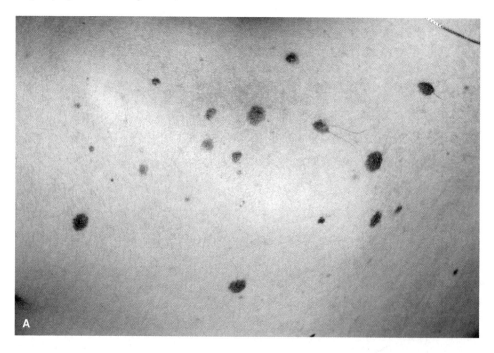

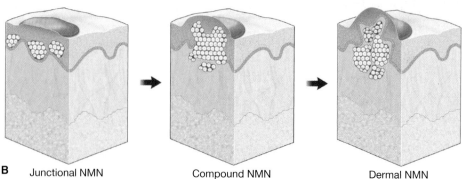

B   Junctional NMN   Compound NMN   Dermal NMN

FIGURE A-1 Common Pigmented Lesions Encountered in Primary Care Medicine.

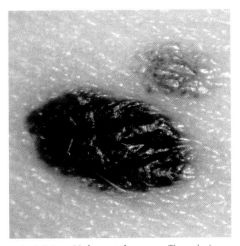

FIGURE A-2 Melanocytic nevus These lesions show even pattern of pigmentation, with regular borders and symmetry. This papule is less than 0.5 cm in diameter.

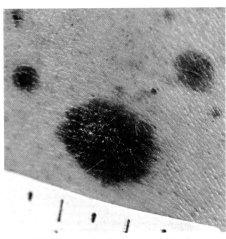

FIGURE A-3 Dysplastic nevus This lesion has both macular and papular components with uneven pigmentation but fairly regular borders and symmetry. There are no areas of "regression" (steel-gray discoloration that is residual from the body's attempt to have the lesion recede).

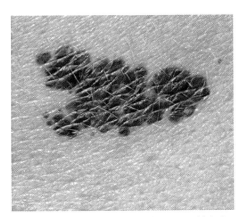

FIGURE A-4 Melanoma This brown and black papule has uneven borders, is asymmetric, and has color variation including red and blue hues. The lesion is larger than 0.6 cm and arose quickly with uneven relief in its surface. Note that there is pigment spread suggesting lateral spread or "radial growth phase."

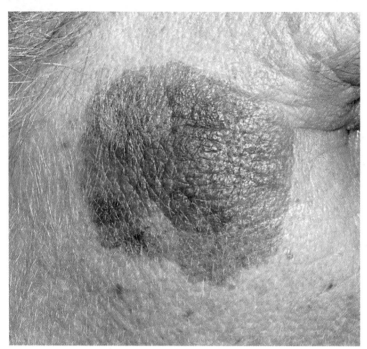

FIGURE A-5 Seborrheic keratosis These lesions usually occur in multiples. A solitary verrucous papule may present diagnostic difficulty and biopsy is often indicated. A verrucous surface with "stuck on" appearance, horn cysts and lack of dermal infiltration, suggests a diagnosis of seborrheic keratosis.

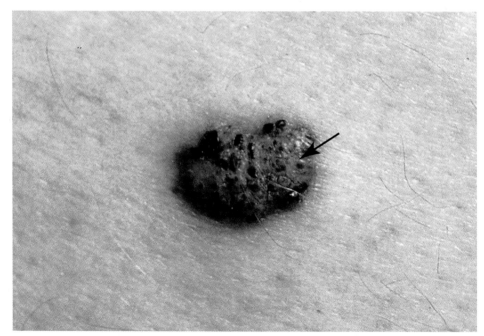

FIGURE A-6 Angiokeratoma This papule has a pebbled surface and is noncompressible (unlike a venous lake). On close examination, thrombosed vascular spaces can be seen (see *arrow*).

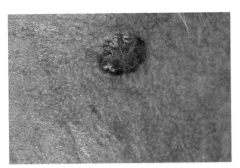

FIGURE A-7 Pigmented basal cell carcinoma
Confusion can arise with a cutaneous melanoma. Translucency in the lesion and a pattern of surrounding telangiectasia are more commonly seen in pigmented basal cell carcinoma.

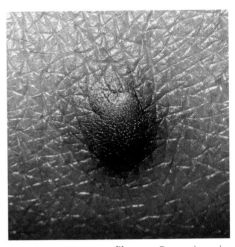

FIGURE A-8 Dermatofibroma Dome-shaped papule with regular and even pigmentation; when pressed from each side, a dimple sign can be elicited.

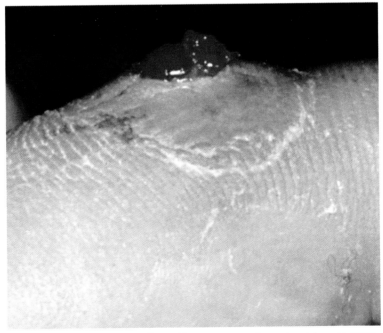

FIGURE A-9 Pyogenic granuloma These acute papules and nodules occur soon after trauma, tend to be beefy-red and in the palms and soles have a collar of thickened stratum corneum at the base.

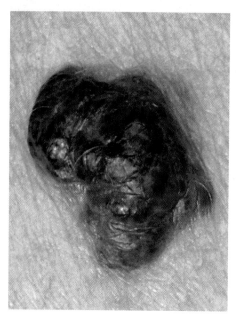

FIGURE A-10 Venous lake This papule has bluish to back coloration, with surface even-nodularity and completely blanches on compression.

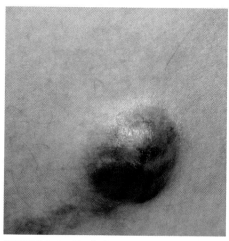

FIGURE A-11 Merkel cell carcinoma This deadly tumor presents on sun-exposed surfaces as a violaceous nodule that does not blanch on compression, often after a very rapid growth phase. This tumor can often grow as cysts, barely noticeable dermal nodules, and venous lake-like lesions. If the diagnosis is suspected, biopsy is paramount.

DRUG USE IN PREGNANCY

The developing fetus can potentially be affected by any medication given to the mother. The disastrous effects of thalidomide and stilbestrol on the exposed offspring led to the development of the U.S. Food and Drug Administration (FDA) categories that are now assigned before a drug is released.

Table B-1 lists safe treatments for dermatologic diseases in pregnancy, and the common dermatologic diseases and drugs used for them. The drugs' pregnancy categories are listed in Table B-2.

TABLE B-1 Safe Treatments for Dermatologic Disorders During Pregnancy

Disease	Medication Name
Acne	Topical clindamycin, erythromycin, benzoyl peroxide
Rosacea	Topical metronidazole, azelaic acid
Psoriasis	Topical glucocorticoids, calcipotriol, broadband UVB
Dermatitis	Topical glucocorticoids, chlorpheniramine or diphenhydramine
Genital human papillomavirus infection	Liquid nitrogen, trichloracetic acid
Herpes simplex virus infection	Acyclovir
Fungal infections	Topical antifungals
Bacterial infections	Penicillins, cephalosporins after first trimester, azithromycin
Urticaria	Chlorpheniramine, diphenhydramine (better to use first over second generation anti-histamines

TABLE B-2 Common Dermatologic Diseases, Drugs used, and Their Pregnancy Categories

Disease	Drug	FDA Pregnancy Category
Acne and rosacea	Topical erythromycin	B
	Topical clindamycin	B
	Topical benzoyl peroxide	C
	Topical tretinoin	C, but not advised
	Topical adapalene	C, but not advised
	Topical tazarotene	X
	Topical metronidazole	B
	Topical azelaic acid	B
	Systemic tetracyclines	D
	Systemic erythromycin	B
	Systemic isotretinoin	X
Psoriasis	Topical glucocorticoids	C
	Topical calcipotriene	C
	UVB phototherapy	Considered safe
	PUVA	Considered potential teratogen
	Systemic methotrexate	X
	Systemic acitretin	X
	Etanercept	B
Dermatitis	Systemic glucocorticoids	C
	Topical tacrolimus	C
	Topical pimecrolimus	C
	Systemic chlorpheniramine	B
	Systemic diphenhydramine	B
Viral infection	Imiquimod	B
	Podophyllin	C, not recommended
	Podophyllotoxin	C, not recommended
	Acyclovir	B
	Famciclovir	B
	Valacyclovir	B
Fungal infection	Topical antifungals	Considered safe
	Systemic terbinafine	B
	Systemic fluconazole	C, not recommended
	Topical fluconazole	C, considered safe
	Systemic itraconazole	C, not recommended
Bacterial infection	Systemic penicillin	B
	Systemic cephalosporin	B; possible association between certain cephalosporins and congenital malformations in first trimester
	Systemic azithzromycin	C
Urticaria	Chlorpheniramine	B
	Diphenhydramine	B
	Hydroxyzine	C; linked to congenital abnormalities (Cleft palate)
	Loratadine	B
	Cetirizine	B
	Levocetirizine	B
	Fexofenadine	C
	Desloratadine	C

FDA Pregnancy Categories for Drugs. A. No fetal risk in controlled studies. **B.** No risk to human fetus despite possible animal risk or no risk in animal studies but human studies lacking. **C.** Human risk cannot be ruled out. Animal studies may or may not show risk. **D.** Evidence of risk to human fetus. **X.** Contraindicated in pregnancy.

DERMATOLOGIC MANIFESTATIONS OF DISEASES INFLICTED BY BIOLOGIC WARFARE/BIOTERRORISM

The use of microbial pathogens as potential or actual weapons of terrorism and warfare dates from antiquity. In 2001, the anthrax attacks via the U.S. postal system resulted in 12 cutaneous and 10 inhalational cases of anthrax with 4 deaths. These caused a tremendous amount of anxiety, had an impact on the U.S. postal system, and led to a functional interruption of the activities of the legislative branch of the U.S. government. The U.S. Centers for Disease Control and Prevention (CDC) has classified potential biologic agents into three categories: A, B, and C (Table C-1). Category A agents are the priority pathogens requiring special attention for public health preparedness. Many of these lead to skin signs and symptoms and are therefore of major concern to dermatologists. The potential bioterrorism diseases with dermatologic manifestations are:

- Anthrax.
- Plague.
- Smallpox.
- Smallpox vaccine (vaccinia).
- Tularemia.
- Viral hemorrhagic fevers.

Full information on plague and the viral hemorrhagic fevers as well as infections with anthrax by inhalation can be obtained at the CDC website: **http://emergency.cdc.gov/agent/agentlist.asp**.

Information on all of these agents and related links can be obtained at the following websites:

- www.bt.cdc.gov/agent/smallpox/diagnosis/pdf/spox-poster-full.pdf.
- http://jama.ama-assn.org/cgi/content/full/287/18/2391.

TABLE C-1 CDC Category A, B, and C Agents

Category A
Anthrax (*Bacillus anthracis*)
Botulism (*Clostridium botulinum toxin*)
Plague (*Yersinia pestis*)
Smallpox (*Variola major*)
Tularemia (*Francisella tularensis*)
Viral hemorrhagic fevers
 Arenaviruses: Lassa, New World (Machupo, Junin, Guanarito, Chapare, Lujo, and Sabia)
 Bunyaviridae: Crimean, Congo, Rift Valley
 Filoviridae: Ebola, Marburg
 Flaviviridae: Yellow fever, Omsk fever, Dengue fever, Kyasanur Forest

Category B
Brucellosis (*Brucella* spp.)
Epsilon toxin of *Clostridium perfringens*
Food safety threats (e.g., *Salmonella* spp., *Escherichia coli* 0157:H7, and *Shigella*)
Glanders (*Burkholderia mallei*)
Melioidosis (*B. pseudomallei*)
Psittacosis (*Chlamydia psittaci*)
Q fever (*Coxiella burnettii*)
Ricin toxin from *Ricinus communis* (castor beans)
Staphylococcal enterotoxin B
Typhus fever (*Rickettsia prowazekii*)
Viral encephalitis [alphaviruses (e.g., Venezuelan, eastern, and western equine encephalitis)]
Water safety threats (e.g., *Vibrio cholerae* and *Cryptosporidium parvum*)

Category C
Emerging infectious disease threats such as Nipah and Hendra, hantavirus, and SARS coronavirus, prions, rabies virus, tuberculosis, influenza

Source: Centers for Disease Control and Prevention and the National Institute of Allergy and Infectious Diseases.

CHEMICAL BIOTERRORISM AND INDUSTRIAL ACCIDENTS

Chemical agents have been used as weapons on a large scale in World War I, in the Iraq-Iran War, by Iraq against Kurdish civilians, and in the Sarin attacks in Japan. Industrial hazardous materials (HAZMATs) produced in chemical plants could also be used as weapons in chemical terrorism.

Table C-2 lists potential agents for such attacks and the symptoms they elicit. Of these, the blistering agent sulfur mustard is one of the most likely agents to be used in a terrorist attack scenario, and it also induces skin lesions (see http://www.cdc.gov/mmwr/preview/mmwrhtml/rr4904a1.htm).

Following exposure and an asymptomatic latent period, erythema, pruritus, burning, and pain may present; initial blistering of the skin will start on the second day after exposure and will progress for up to 2 weeks. Vesicles coalesce, forming large blisters, and wound healing is considerably slower than for a comparable thermal burn. Differential diagnoses are thermal burn or scalding, toxic epidermal necrolysis, and staphylococcal scalded skin syndrome. (See also W R Heymann: Threats of biological and chemical warfare on civilian populations. J Am Acad Dermatol 2004, 51:452.)

TABLE C-2 Recognizing and Diagnosing Health Effects of Chemical Terrorism

Agent	Agent Name	Unique Characteristics	Initial Effects
Nerve	Cyclohexyl sarin (GF) Sarin (GB) Soman (GD) Tabun (GA) VX	Miosis (pinpoint pupils) Copious secretions Muscle twitching/ fasciculations	Miosis (pinpoint pupils) Blurred/dim vision Headache Nausea, vomiting, diarrhea Copious secretions/sweating Muscle twitching/ fasciculations Breathing difficulty Seizures
Asphyxiant/ blood	Arsine Cyanogen chloride Hydrogen cyanide	Possible cherry red skin Possible cyanosis Possible frostbite[a]	Confusion Nausea Patients may gasp for air, similar to asphyxiation but more abrupt onset Seizures prior to death
Choking/ pulmonary damage	Chlorine Hydrogen chloride Nitrogen oxides Phosgene	Chlorine is a greenish yellow gas with pungent odor Phosgene gas smells like newly mown hay or grass Possible frostbite[a]	Eye and skin irritation Airway irritation Dyspnea, cough Sore throat Chest tightness
Blistering/ vesicant	Mustard/Sulfur mustard (HD, H) Mustard gas (H) Nitrogen mustard (HN-1, HN-2, HN-3) Lewisite (L) Phosgene oxime (CX)	Mustard (HD) has an odor like burning garlic or horseradish Lewisite (L) has an odor like penetrating geranium Phosgene oxime (CX) has a pepperish or pungent odor	Severe irritation Redness and blisters of the skin Tearing, conjunctivitis, corneal damages Mild respiratory distress to marked airway damage May cause death Dry mouth and skin
Incapacitating/ behavior- altering	Agent 15/BZ	May appear as mass drug intoxication with erratic behaviors, shared realistic and distinct hallucinations, disrobing and confusion Hyperthermia Mydriasis (dilated pupils)	Initial tachycardia Altered consciousness, delusions, denial of illness, belligerence Hyperthermia Ataxia (lack of coordination) Hallucinations Mydriasis (dilated pupils)

[a]Frostbite may occur from skin contact with liquid arsine, cyanogen chloride, or phosgene.

Source: State of New York, Department of Health. https://www.health.ny.gov/environmental/emergency/chemical_terrorism/poster.htm

INDEX

Page references for figures are indicated by *f* and for tables by *t*.